ESSENTIAL PSYCHIATRY

Essential Psychiatry

Edited by Nicholas D.B. Rose

MB, ChB, FRCPsych
Consultant Psychiatrist
Clinical and Regional Course Tutor
Littlemore Hospital, Oxford
and Honorary Senior Clinical Lecturer in Psychiatry
University Department of Psychiatry
Warneford Hospital, Oxford

SECOND EDITION

OXFORD

BLACKWELL SCIENTIFIC PUBLICATIONS

LONDON EDINBURGH BOSTON

MELBOURNE PARIS BERLIN VIENNA

© 1988, 1994 by
Blackwell Scientific Publications
Editorial Offices:
Osney Mead, Oxford OX2 0EL
25 John Street, London WC1N 2BL
23 Ainslie Place, Edinburgh EH3 6AJ
238 Main Street, Cambridge
    Massachusetts 02142, USA
54 University Street, Carlton
    Victoria 3053, Australia

Other Editorial Offices:
Librairie Arnette SA
1, rue de Lille
75007 Paris
France

Blackwell Wissenschafts-Verlag GmbH
Düsseldorfer Str. 38
D-10707 Berlin
Germany

Blackwell MZV
Feldgasse 13
A-1238 Wien
Austria

First published 1988
Reprinted 1989, 1991
Second edition 1994

Set by Excel Typesetters, Hong Kong
Printed and bound in Great Britain
at the Alden Press Ltd.,
Oxford and Northampton

DISTRIBUTORS

Marston Book Services Ltd
PO Box 87
Oxford OX2 0DT
(*Orders*: Tel: 0865 791155
          Fax: 0865 791927
          Telex: 837515)

USA
Blackwell Scientific Publications, Inc.
238 Main Street
Cambridge, MA 02142
(*Orders*: Tel: 800 759-6102
          617 876-7000)

Canada
Times Mirror Professional Publishing, Ltd
130 Flaska Drive
Markham, Ontario L6G 1B8
(*Orders*: Tel: 800 268-4178
          416 470-6739)

Australia
Blackwell Scientific Publications Pty Ltd
54 University Street
Carlton, Victoria 3053
(*Orders*: Tel: 03 347-5552)

A catalogue record for this title
is available from the British Library

ISBN 0-632-03737-7

Library of Congress
Cataloging in Publication Data

Essential psychiatry/
edited by Nicholas D.B. Rose. – 2nd ed.
        p.   cm.
    Includes bibliographical references
    and index.
    ISBN 0-632-03737-7
    1. Psychiatry.   I. Rose, N. (Nicholas)
    [DNLM: 1. Mental Disorders.
    WM 100 E7856 1994]
    RC454.E78   1994
    616.89 – dc20

Contents

Contributors

S. ABELL MB, BS, FRCPsych, *Consultant Psychiatrist, Oxfordshire Learning Disability NHS Trust, Slade House, Oxford*

J. CATALAN LMS, DPM, MRCPsych, MSc (Oxon), *Senior Lecturer, Charing Cross and Westminster Medical School, Chelsea and Westminster Hospital, London*

P.J. COWEN BSc, MB, BS, MD, MRCPsych, *MRC Clinical Scientist and Honorary Consultant Psychiatrist, University Department of Psychiatry, Warneford Hospital, Oxford and MRC Clinical Pharmacology Unit, Littlemore Hospital, Oxford*

A. CREMONA MRCPsych, *Consultant Psychiatrist, Department of Psychiatry, Wexham Park Hospital, Slough*

N.L.G. EASTMAN MB, BSc, MRCPsych, *Barrister at Law, Head, Academic Section of Forensic Psychiatry, St George's Hospital Medical School, London*

C.G. FAIRBURN MA, MPhil, DM, FRCPsych, *Wellcome Trust Senior Lecturer and Honorary Clinical Reader, University Department of Psychiatry, Warneford Hospital, Oxford*

K.W.M. FULFORD MA (Cantab), DPhil (Oxon), MRCP, MRCPsych, *Research Psychiatrist, University Department of Psychiatry, Warneford Hospital, Oxford*

I.M. GOODYER MB, BS, DCH, MD, MRCPsych, *Professor of Child and Adolescent Psychiatry, Developmental Psychiatry Section, Douglas House, Cambridge*

K. HAWTON DM, FRCPsych, *Consultant Psychiatrist and Clinical Lecturer, University Department of Psychiatry, Warneford Hospital, Oxford*

P.J. HAY MD, FRANCP, *Nuffield Medical Fellow, University Department of Psychiatry, Warneford Hospital, Oxford*

G.A. HIBBERT DM, MRCPsych, *Consultant Psychiatrist and Clinical Lecturer, Warneford Hospital and University Department of Psychiatry, Oxford*

M. HOBBS MA, BChir, MSc, FRCPsych, *Consultant Psychotherapist, and Clinical Lecturer, University Department of Psychiatry, Warneford Hospital, Oxford*

R.A. HOPE MA, PhD, MRCPsych, BMBch, *Leader, Oxford Practice Skills Project and Honorary Consultant Psychiatrist, Warneford Hospital, Oxford*

J.A. MUIR GRAY MD, FRCP (Glas.), FRCP, FFCM, *Director of Health Policy and Public Health, Oxford Regional Health Authority, Oxford*

C. OPPENHEIMER FRCP(UK), FRCPsych, *Consultant Psychiatrist and Regional Tutor, Warneford Hospital, Oxford*

N.D.B. ROSE MBChB, FRCPsych *Consultant Psychiatrist, Clinical and Regional Course Tutor, Littlemore Hospital, Oxford and Honorary Senior Clinical Lecturer in Psychiatry, University Department of Psychiatry, Warneford Hospital, Oxford*

A. STEDEFORD MB, BS, DCH, DObstRCOG, DPM, MRCPsych, *Formerly Consultant in Psychological Medicine, Sir Michael Sobell House, Churchill Hospital, Oxford*

Preface to the Second Edition

Mental health services are in the midst of radical change. This has been caused partly by the controversial shift to more local care provision, and partly as a result of more challenging public and governmental attitudes towards medical services generally and psychiatric services in particular. These changes have resulted in more people needing to be better informed about mental health problems and how they can best be approached. This is particularly so in organizations working with the mentally ill in the community such as social services, voluntary bodies, services for offenders, carer groups and of course general practitioners and community nurses.

Essential Psychiatry is written for readers coming from a range of professional backgrounds. It provides a clear, wide-ranging and practical introduction to psychiatry. Basic principles such as the origin of mental illness, the learning of interview and assessment skills, and an approach to the ethical and moral issues involved are covered in the initial chapters. Later chapters then go on to describe the different forms mental illness takes, illustrated by many case histories. A final group of chapters concentrates on special groups such as offenders, substance abusers, the traumatized, those with sexual problems, and those who pose a risk to themselves or others. There are also separate chapters on psychiatric problems in children, elderly people and people with learning difficulties. Treatment approaches are particularly thoroughly covered and reflect the most up-to-date clinical practices in the use of psychotherapeutic, social and pharmacological approaches.

The first edition of *Essential Psychiatry* quickly became a standard text in many medical schools, as well as being widely used by a range of professional groups including occupational therapists, psychologists, social workers, probation officers, hospital doctors, general practitioners, community and hospital nurses and trainee psychiatrists.

The second edition builds on the successes of the first. It retains the multi-author approach, with contributions from specialists writing to a standard format. Fact sheets at the start of every chapter continue to provide a useful summary to orientate the reader before embarking on a topic, and as an aid to revision. An extensive use of boxes in the layout is used, some containing optional small print material, others highlighting key points.

The range of topics covered has been further widened to include not only areas such as counselling techniques, bereavement, terminal illness, and levels of care from self-care to hospital care; but also areas such as ethics in relation to psychiatry, the effects of abuse and trauma, and eating disorders. Each of these new topics is covered in a number of newly created chapters. Many of the chapters from the first edition have also been extensively revised so that they fully reflect clinical practice in the mid-1990s.

Finally, my thanks are due to all involved in unstintingly burning the midnight oil for *Essential Psychiatry*, not only the authors but all of those who supported them.

Nicholas D.B. Rose
Oxford, March 1994

Preface to the First Edition

A lot of changes are taking place in psychiatry, changes which all too often are not included in introductory text-books: *Essential Psychiatry* is an attempt to rectify this.

The changes are extensive, affecting both patients and those involved in helping them. The organization of clinical services is being revolutionized, with the closure of large hospitals and a shift to more local care. Partly as a result of this, many more people are now becoming actively involved in helping the mentally ill, including those in social service departments, general practice teams and voluntary groups such as MIND. This, of course, means that many more people need to have a familiarity with mental health problems and how they can best be dealt with.

Other areas of change include a new Mental Health Act with greatly improved patients' rights; the contribution psychiatry is making towards areas such as terminal care, psychosexual medicine, and psychological problems seen in general and hospital medical practice; and exciting recent developments both in psychological and physical treatment methods, and in understanding the factors causing mental illness.

This book aims to reflect these changes and communicate them in a clear and authoritative fashion to readers from a range of professional backgrounds. This has been made possible by a multi-author approach with contributions from specialists writing to a clearly defined format.

The range of topics covered is wide, including not only mental disorders but also subjects such as grief, unlawful behaviour, interview and assessment skills, counselling techniques and levels of care from self-care to hospital care. The purpose is to cover the range of topics relevant to someone working in the mental health field, whether they be social worker or general practitioner, medical student or nurse.

Presentation of information has been a high priority. Fact sheets at the beginning of each chapter provide a useful summary to orientate the reader before covering a topic, and as an aid to revision. Other features include frequent case examples and extensive use of boxes – some containing optional small print, others highlighting key points.

Finally, my thanks to all those without whose dogged help this book would still be a day-dream: the authors, their families and their secretaries. Particular thanks go to Michael Gelder, Tony Hope, Basil Shepstone, Pat Greenwood, Carolyn Fordham and Dianne Rose.

Nicholas D.B. Rose
Oxford, July 1988

I
BASIC ISSUES IN
MENTAL ILLNESS

1
Diagnosis, Classification and Phenomenology of Mental Illness

Fact sheet

Principles of diagnosis

Purposes of diagnosis
- Description.
- Aetiology.
- Treatment.
- Prognosis.

Diagnosis in psychiatry
Compared with physical medicine diagnosis in psychiatry is:
- based on symptoms rather than aetiology (cf., neurology);
- dependent on clinical skills rather than laboratory tests;
- divided into two stages, information gathering and formulation (or assessment);
- sometimes concerned with illness as well as particular diseases (e.g. in relation to medico-legal questions).

Psychiatric phenomenology

Psychological symptoms
Mood:
- anxiety;
- affect (happiness—sadness).

Thought:
- stream (slowed/accelerated);
- connection (formal thought disorder/perseveration);
- possession (obsessive—compulsive/schizophrenic);
- content (delusions/overvalued ideas/delusional mood).

Perception:
- hallucinations;
- pseudohallucination;
- illusions.

Cognitive function:
- orientation;
- attention/concentration;
- memory;
- intelligence/IQ (see also p. 134).

Insight.

Physical symptoms
- Autonomic (e.g. in anxiety).
- 'Biological' (e.g. in depression).
- Pain.
- Dissociative ('hysteria').
- Vegetative (appetite, sex, sleep).

Psychological signs
Disturbance of appearance, behaviour and speech may give important clues to the patient's mental state.

Classification of psychiatric disorders

Adult
Diseases:
- organic;
- alcohol/drug related;
- psychotic (other than organic or affective);
- affective;
- anxiety and anxiety related;
- disorders of vegetative functions.

Other disorders:
- personality disorders;
- stress induced.

Child/adolescent
- Mental retardation.
- Specific developmental delays.
- Pervasive.
- Behavioural.
- Emotional.
- Disorders of physiological function.

Diagnosis in practice
The main steps from symptoms to diagnosis are:
Clarification of clinical picture.
Exclusion of:
- organic pathology;
- alcohol/drug related disorders;
- personality disorder;
- stress-induced disorder.

Differential diagnosis of remaining disorders according to symptoms.

Introduction

Most of us come to psychiatry having had experience mainly of physical medicine. The differences between the two subjects are such that the move can involve a degree of culture shock.

This is especially so for diagnosis and classification. In this chapter, therefore, psychiatric diagnosis and classification will be compared and contrasted with their counterparts in physical medicine. First, the principles governing diagnosis and classification in psychiatry will be considered. Then the main psychiatric symptoms and clinical syndromes will be described. Finally, a practical scheme for psychiatric diagnosis will be given. The aim will be to provide an overview. Details will be added in later chapters.

Diagnosis in psychiatry

Why is diagnosis important? Diagnosis in psychiatry serves four main purposes. These are the same as in physical medicine:

1 Descriptive – a diagnostic label is a summary description of a patient's condition, essential for communication, and the key to all other medically relevant information about the patient.

2 Aetiological – diagnoses are sometimes based on, but always imply, information about aetiology (sometimes just that this is unknown).

3 Therapeutic – knowledge of symptoms and of aetiology is the basis for rational decisions about treatment and other aspects of clinical management.

4 Prognostic – symptoms and aetiology, together with the

Fig. 1.1 Different kinds of diagnostic category

The four main purposes of diagnosis in medicine (description, aetiology, treatment, prognosis) are served in different ways by different kinds of diagnostic category.

For example, in physical medicine the diagnosis 'migraine' conveys precise information about a patient's symptoms and their prognosis, but it suggests only a range of possible treatments, and it tells us little if anything about aetiology. With 'diabetes mellitus', on the other hand, the reverse is the case. This diagnosis conveys precise information about aetiology, it suggests certain specific and effective treatments, and it gives an overall idea of prognosis; but, given the wide variety of possible

clinical presentations of this condition, it provides no definite information about the patient's actual symptoms.

In psychiatry, as noted in the text, diagnostic labels are more often defined symptomatically than aetiologically. They are thus more often like 'migraine' than like 'diabetes mellitus' in the kinds of information which they convey. Both types of diagnosis, however, often carry important information about treatment and prognosis. This is illustrated by the following table which shows some of the different implications of four important differential diagnoses of depression*.

Diagnosis	Symptoms	Aetiology	Treatment	Prognosis
Major or psychotic depression (see Chapter 6)	Severe, often relapsing depression with **one or more** of (a) a number of biological symptoms, (b) delusions, hallucinations. Sometimes alternating with periods of mania.	Various theories – see Chapter 2.	Physical treatments (drugs, ECT) likely to be effective and may be life-saving (e.g. with suicide risk). Other treatments important but supplementary.	Good, especially with treatment. Likely to relapse but with (often long) periods of normality. When depressed, beware high suicide risk.
Minor depression (see Chapters 6 and 7)	Usually less severe depression, with **neither** specific biological symptoms **nor** delusions or hallucinations. May be chronic, is often relapsing.	As above.	Behavioural treatments (e.g. cognitive therapy) often helpful together with counselling, support and social intervention. Physical treatments less likely to be helpful.	Generally good; but sometimes condition is chronic and/or relapsing (merging with personality disorder). Risk of attempted rather than actual suicide.
Depressive personality disorder (see Chapter 9)	Depressive symptoms, usually similar to those of neurotic depression; but **continuing largely unchanged** throughout adult life (see Fig. 1.6).	As above.	Treatment unlikely to change the condition. Management thus concentrates on ameliorating the effects of the condition on the patients' life, and on the lives of those around the patient.	Poor. Likely to remain essentially unchanged for rest of patient's life.
Adjustment reaction (see Chapter 12)	May include any of the range of depressive symptoms, but these are **clearly provoked** by loss (e.g. in bereavement) or other psychological trauma.	Experience of loss or other psychological 'trauma' is part of **definition** (see text).	Counselling, support and social intervention indicated; behavioural and physical treatments sometimes helpful.	Good. Even if very severe, likely to resolve; but may recur with further stressors.

*Note that depression, as a symptom, may occur in a number of other conditions beside these; for example in schizophrenia.

---

likely response to treatment, give an estimate of prognosis.

However, diagnosis in psychiatry differs from diagnosis in physical medicine in:

1 the kinds of disease category employed;
2 the clinical skills required;
3 the form of the diagnoses derived ('diagnostic formulation');
4 the importance of the concept of illness.

Disease categories in psychiatry

Disease categories in physical medicine are mostly aetiologically based: 'B_{12} deficiency anaemia', 'aspirational pneumonia', 'mitral stenosis', 'tuberculous meningitis', etc.

In psychiatry, knowledge of aetiology is often too uncertain for such categories to be clinically useful. Mental disorders are therefore classified mainly symptomatically. 'Major depression', 'schizophrenia', 'anorexia nervosa', 'obsessive–compulsive neurosis', and so on, are all defined by particular symptoms or symptom clusters. Aetiology still comes in, for example in the definitions of many organic disorders. Moreover, with future progress in psychology and the brain sciences it is to be expected that symptomatically defined disease categories will increasingly be replaced by aetiological categories: just as in physical medicine aetiological categories have replaced symptomatically defined categories such as 'dropsy' and 'scrofula'. But for the time being this is how it has to be.

In this respect psychiatry is closer to neurology than to other branches of physical medicine. Many neurological disease categories, such as 'migraine' and 'epilepsy', are symptomatically defined. These categories, nonetheless, as in psychiatry, often carry important implications not only for aetiology but also for treatment and prognosis. Careful diagnosis is thus no less important in psychiatry than it is in neurology, or indeed in any other branch of medicine (see Fig. 1.1 for examples, together with the clinical cases described on p. 13).

Clinical skills

Diagnosis in psychiatry, with its mainly symptomatically defined disease categories, is first and foremost a clinical discipline. Laboratory investigations, although sometimes important in excluding physical disease, rarely provide the short cuts to diagnosis so often available in physical medicine. This makes it a difficult clinical discipline. The basic skills required are the same as in physical medicine: **history taking** and examination, the latter in psychiatry involving **examination of the mental state** as well as **physical examination**. Also, the key to success is the same – to know exactly what you are looking for, i.e. the kinds of symptom which may be present, their detailed features, and precisely how they should be elicited.

In psychiatry, however, there are a number of particular barriers to success.

First, the patient may be reluctant to say what is wrong. In physical medicine, patients are usually only too willing to describe their symptoms. But in psychiatry, through fear, embarrassment, guilt, or for many other reasons, they may not be. A depressed patient, for example, with delusions of guilt (see below), may tell you that he feels depressed. But

Fig. 1.2 Differences between diagnosis in psychiatry and in physical medicine

Compared with physical medicine diagnosis in psychiatry is:
1 based on disease categories which are mainly **symptomatically** (rather than aetiologically) defined;
2 dependent largely on the clinical skills of **history taking, mental state examination, and physical examination** (rather than on laboratory and other special tests);
3 clearly divided into two distinct stages, of **information gathering**, and of **formulation** under the headings 'diagnosis', 'aetiology', 'treatment' and 'prognosis';
4 concerned sometimes as much with the **concept of illness** (especially in relation to medico-legal and ethical questions) as with that of disease.

he may hold back what he regards as the real reason for his depression, viz. that he believes he is guilty of some terrible sin, and that he intends to kill himself.

Second, even if the patient is willing to describe his symptoms, these may be so far removed from ordinary experience that he is unable to do so. Imagine, for example, trying to describe thoughts which you think in your own head, and yet which you experience not as your own thoughts but as those of someone else. (This is called 'thought insertion', a symptom of schizophrenia – see later in this chapter and in Chapter 5.)

Third, even though willing and able to describe what is wrong, patients in psychiatry may understand what is wrong quite differently from the way in which it is understood by others. This is especially so with psychotic illnesses (see below). The hallucinating patient, for example, perhaps hearing someone shouting obscenities at him, experiences this not as something wrong with him, but simply as someone shouting obsenties at him . . . and he may react accordingly.

Given these difficulties then, successful diagnosis in psychiatry requires, above all, well-developed interview skills. These are described in Chapter 3. But there is no substitute for clinical experience. You should begin psychiatry by seeing patients.

Diagnostic assessment or formulation

As psychiatry is a clinical discipline, a great deal of information is often required before a diagnosis can be made. This comes not only from the patient but also from friends, relatives and others.

Furthermore, because psychiatric disease categories are mainly symptomatically defined, separate assessments have to be made in each case of the aetiological factors which may be present, and of treatment and prognosis. In physical medicine, the results of a simple laboratory test will often suffice diagnostically: a result such as 'low B_{12}' can tell us everything we need to know about the patient. But in psychiatry diagnosis, aetiology, treatment and prognosis have to be considered separately for each case.

It is thus helpful to think of diagnosis in psychiatry as involving two distinct stages: a stage of **information gathering**, in which data are collected, from the patient and from others, mainly by way of history taking, mental state and physical examination; and then a stage of **formulation or assessment**, in which the information collected is organized and reduced to its relevant essentials under four headings corresponding with the four main purposes of diagnosis: differential (descriptive) diagnosis, aetiology, treatment and prognosis.

Diagnostic assessment is described fully with clinical examples in Chapter 3. It is to the first part of the assessment — the diagnosis proper — that the symptoms and syndromes to be described later in this chapter are mainly relevant.

The concept of mental illness

When a diagnosis is made in physical medicine, it can usually be assumed that if there is anything wrong with the patient at all it will be in the nature of a disease, a wound, a disability, or some other specifically medical kind of disorder. In psychiatry, although this remains largely true, what is wrong can turn out not to be a medical disorder but a problem in the patient's life.

This is sometimes important clinically, especially in relation to medico-legal and ethical decisions such as those involved in compulsory treatment (see Chapter 25). However in practice the first step in psychiatric diagnosis is to decide the more straightforward question — is the patient suffering from any of the particular conditions recognized as psychiatric disorders in the established classifications?

In the remainder of this chapter, therefore, we will be concentrating on these particular conditions, and the symptoms and syndromes in terms of which they are defined. Notes on the concept of mental illness are given in Figs 1.3 and 1.7. An example of a patient requiring compulsory treatment is given in the case studies on p. 13. Selected literature is included in the suggestions for further reading at the end of this chapter, and medico-legal aspects of psychiatry are considered in Chapter 25.

Classification in psychiatry

In all branches of medicine, disease classification develops by a kind of natural selection. As medical knowledge advances, so new and clinically more useful categories gradually replace those which have become less useful.

Medical knowledge in psychiatry has been advancing rapidly in recent years. Psychiatric disease categories are thus correspondingly fluid and this has brought with it a degree of confusion. However, the more widely used classifications are nowadays all broadly similar. They include many of the same overall categories of disorder and they are built up from essentially the same list of basic symptoms and signs. It is mainly in the fine details of particular disease definitions that one classification differs from the next.

In this section, the main psychiatric symptoms and signs will be outlined, together with a summary of the broad categories of disorder common to most modern psychiatric classifications. Details of individual disease categories will be described in later chapters. A practical scheme giving the steps from symptoms to diagnosis in individual cases is described in the final section of this chapter.

Psychiatric phenomenology

Psychiatric phenomenology covers the symptoms and signs of psychiatric disorder. These are of two main kinds, psychological and physical. As to the physical, almost any physical symptom, and many signs, may sometimes be due to psychiatric disorder (just as any psychological symptom may sometimes be due to physical disorder). We will be looking at some of the physical symptoms important in psychiatry in a moment, though, as symptoms, they will already be familiar from physical medicine. Many of the psychological symptoms, on the other hand, will be unfamiliar and it is these we will be concentrating on here.

In what follows you may find it helpful to refer to Fig. 1.4 which gives a checklist of all the main psychiatric symptoms.

Psychological symptoms

As in physical medicine, accurate diagnosis in psychiatry depends on the details of a patient's symptoms. For example, it is not enough to know that a patient is worried by the thought that he is dirty. You have to decide whether the thought in question is, say, an ordinary preoccupation, an obsession, a delusion, or thought insertion. Each of these symptoms has quite different features.

In this section only an outline of the main psychiatric

Fig. 1.3 The concept of mental illness

The diagnostic uncertainties surrounding the concept of mental illness (see text) have led some to claim that the very concept of mental illness is unsound. Those who make this claim do not deny that the conditions conventionally thought of as mental illnesses exist; nor (on the whole) do they deny that these conditions are, like physical illnesses, bad conditions to be in. Their claim is rather that it is a mistake to think of these conditions **as** illnesses at all. Mental illnesses, they say, are not really illnesses, but, variously, learned abnormalities of behaviour (H.J. Eysenck), or responses to being labelled mentally ill by society (T. Scheff), or attempts to adapt to mutually incompatible emotional demands within a family (R.D. Laing), etc.

Many of these 'anti-psychiatry' views reflect important aspects of mental illness: for example, powerful new treatments for the neuroses have been developed from learning theory; some of the clinical features shown by long-stay institutionalized mental patients have been shown to be in part a response to society's expectations of them; and a high level of expressed emotion in a family is now known to be a potent aetiological factor in schizophrenic relapse. Where these views fail, however, is in attempting to reject the concept of mental illness **as a whole** simply by exaggerating one or other aspect of it. The anti-psychiatry movement has been important in raising awareness of the clinically important ethical and conceptual aspects of psychiatry. The most obvious way of defining illness, in terms of disturbed functioning, works only up to a point with mental illness, and this remains an area of active research interest.

This research is important, if only because of the growing importance of ethical and medico-legal problems in practice (see text). However, that mental illness is difficult to define is not, in itself, grounds for doubting the validity of the concept. Even if a concept has not been adequately defined it may still be put to good use — try defining 'time' for example.

References for further reading on the concept of illness are included at the end of this chapter.

symptoms will be given. You will find more detailed accounts in later chapters, though, as has already been emphasized, there is no substitute for first-hand clinical experience.

The psychological symptoms of psychiatric disorder can be divided up for descriptive purposes into disorders of mood, thought, perception, and cognitive function. Insight is not a distinct symptom but a feature of other symptoms and is dealt with separately.

Mood

Mood is the prevailing feeling state. Disorders of mood include extreme, or otherwise maladaptive, states of (a) anxiety, and (b) affect (sadness/happiness).

'Anxiety'

Morbid states of anxiety are commonly relatively persisting and generalized. This is sometimes called **free floating anxiety**. Anxiety which is directed or focused is called **phobic anxiety**. A phobia is an unreasonable or unfounded fear of an object or situation usually leading to avoidance behaviour. Phobias are of three main kinds: phobias of specific objects or situations, e.g. fear of thunder, spiders, etc.; social phobias, in which anxiety is experienced in social situations, such as speaking or eating in public; and agoraphobia. Agoraphobic symptoms are diverse but are related mainly to two situations, leaving one's home or other familiar surroundings (sometimes called the 'housebound housewife syndrome'), and being in crowded places. **Panic attacks** are what their name implies, brief but usually very intense attacks of anxiety. They are associated with other symptoms, especially autonomic symptoms of anxiety.

'Affect'

The term 'affect' is used in psychiatric phenomenology to refer to the sadness/happiness aspect of mood. Depression of mood is a more common symptom than elation. Together with anxiety, depression is probably the most common psychiatric symptom (anxiety and depression commonly occur together). When depression is relatively mild it is like ordinary sadness, except that it is inappropriate to the patient's circumstances. More serious states of depression on the other hand ('**major depression**' – see below) differ qualitatively from normal. Often the seriously depressed pa-

---

Fig. 1.4 Psychiatric symptom check-list (not exhaustive)

Psychological symptoms

Mood: morbid states of:
anxiety
• generalized (free floating)
• phobic: specific object, social phobic, agoraphobic
• panic attacks;
affect = sadness/happiness
• depression
• elation (hypomania)
• mixed
• diminished.

Thought: disorders of:
1 stream
  • slowed
  • accelerated, pressure of thought; flight of ideas;
2 connection
  • thought block
  • knight's move
  • positive formal thought disorder (asyndetic thinking, interpenetration of themes, overinclusiveness)
  • negative formal thought disorder ('concrete' thinking)
  • 'word salad' (severe formal thought disorder+neologisms and metonyms)
  • perseveration;
3 possession
  • obsessive–compulsive symptoms
  • thought insertion **/withdrawal**/broadcasting** (schizophrenia);
4 content
  • delusions**; differentiated by content (paranoid/self-referential; persecutory; grandiose; hypochondriacal; nihilistic; of guilt; of poverty) and origin (primary and secondary)
  • partial delusions*
  • morbid fears
  • overvalued ideas;

Perception
1 Hallucinations**, differentiated by mode (auditory, visual, olfactory, gustatory, tactile) and form (simple, complex).
2 Pseudohallucinations*.
3 Illusions/distortions.

Cognitive function: disturbances of:
1 orientation (for time, place, person);
2 attention/concentration;
3 memory
  • recent
  • remote;
4 IQ (verbal, performance).

Insight: for any symptom, lack of:
1 awareness that something is wrong and/or;
2 recognition that what is wrong is a symptom of mental illness.

Physical symptoms
Any physical symptom may be due to a psychiatric disorder. Important examples include:
1 autonomic symptoms of anxiety (palpitation, tremor, globus, etc.);
2 biological symptoms of depression;
3 pain (e.g. in 'masked' depression);
4 disorders of primary sense and voluntary motor systems (in hysteria);
5 disturbances of vegetative functions
  • appetite (loss, anorexia, bulimia); sexual (drive, orgasmic); sleep (increased, decreased).

Psychological signs
Disturbances of appearance, behaviour and speech. Important but mainly as pointing to psychological symptoms; e.g. 1 expressed affect (facial, postural, speech), 2 self-neglect (e.g. in dementia).

* = partial insight   ** = psychotic symptoms

tient does not complain of depressed mood as such though they usually appear extremely sad, unsmiling and inert. Depression of this kind is associated with motor and psychological slowing (**psychomotor retardation**), though sometimes with the opposite, **agitation**. There may be associated **biological symptoms** (fixed diurnal variation of mood, together with loss of appetite and weight, and early morning waking) and delusions (see below). A state of pathologically elevated mood is called **hypomania**. This is the counterpart of major rather than of minor depression in that the patient generally does not complain of their altered mood state as such. Also, there are associated biological and other symptoms, and often delusions and hallucinations (all as described later). **Mixed affective states** are sometimes seen, in which features of both depressed and elated mood co-exist. These are quite different from states of diminished affect in which the patient's capacity to feel happy or sad is reduced, e.g. **flattened** affect in schizophrenia, '**belle indifference**' in hysteria.

Thought

Disturbances of thinking are usually divided into disorders of (a) stream, (b) connection, (c) possession, and (d) content.

'Stream'

The stream of thought—how fast one thought follows another—may be **slowed** (as with psychomotor retardation in depression) or **accelerated**. Acceleration of the stream of thought occurs typically in hypomania and may take the form of **pressure of thought** (thoughts rushing out one after another) and/or **flight of ideas** (rapid changes of topic which are nonetheless still connected up, e.g., through meaning, rhyme, pun, or metaphor).

'Connection'

A variety of disorders of the connections between thoughts are seen in normals, in schizophrenia, in hypomania and in organic disorders. **Thought block** is a simple stopping of the line of thought. It can be a normal phemonenon in states of anxiety, fatigue and stress. As a psychiatric symptom, however, it often occurs in an extreme form in schizophrenia when it may be associated with others symptoms of **schizophrenic thought disorder**; e.g. **knight's move** in thought, a shift from one topic to another without any logical connection. A more general loosening of the associations between thoughts occurring in schizophrenia is called **asyndetic thinking**. This may be combined with **interpenetration of themes** (two or more topics woven more or less haphazardly into the patient's speech) and with **overinclusiveness** (a tendency to excessive generalization beyond the normal boundaries of a given topic). The overall picture of schizophrenic disconnected thinking is sometimes called '**positive formal thought disorder**'. The corresponding '**negative formal thought disorder**' is the rather different phenomenon of so-called 'concrete thinking', viz. an acquired inability to think in abstract terms (demonstrated by over literal proverb interpretation). In addition to formal thought disorder, schizophrenic patients sometimes produce **neologisms** (invented new words) and **metonyms** (approximately correct, idiosyncratic uses of real words and phrases). The net effect of schizophrenic thought disorder is to leave the listener baffled. In extreme form, the patient's speech may become wholly unintelligible (called '**word salad**' or **verbigeration**). Neologisms and metonyms also occur in hypomania and, combined with flight of ideas, this may give a picture not unlike formal thought disorder. Note, however, that flight of ideas differs from schizophrenic thought disorder in that there is always a residual logical connection between the thoughts expressed (as described above). Phenomena similar to those seen in schizophrenic thought disorder may occur in organic states, though usually associated with disturbance of cognitive function (e.g. clouding of consciousness, memory impairment, etc.—see below and Chapter 11). In addition, organically impaired patients may show other disturbances of the connections between thoughts such as **perseveration**—an inability to switch topics, manifesting as a senseless repetition of the last part of what is said...is said...is said; i.e. like a gramophone getting stuck. Perseveration may be shown in behaviour as well as in speech.

'Possession'

Disorders of possession of thought are of two main kinds, obsessive–compulsive and schizophrenic (thought insertion, withdrawal and broadcasting). An **obsessional thought** is stereotyped in form and comes back repeatedly into the patient's mind. The patient regards the thought as foolish and unpleasant and tries to resist it but is unable to do so. More generally, an obsession is any mental content with these features; e.g. ruminations, doubts, images, impulses, series of numbers, repeated words and phrases, and so on. **Compulsive acts** are the motor counterpart of obsessions. Common examples include compulsive handwashing, tidying, touching and cleaning. Obsessional thoughts, although resisted by the patient, remain their own thoughts, i.e. thoughts which they are thinking. With **thought insertion**, on the other hand, the patient actually experiences the thoughts in their head as those of some other person or agency, as thoughts put there by somebody else. **Thought withdrawal** is the experience of one's thoughts being taken out of one's head. **Thought broadcasting** is an extension of thought withdrawal, in which the patient experiences their thoughts travelling out of their head and being available for other people to inspect. Obsessional thoughts differ only quantitatively from normal experiences, e.g. the experience of getting a tune stuck in one's mind. Obsessional thoughts are 'out of control' but otherwise remain one's own thoughts. Thought insertion, withdrawal and broadcasting on the other hand, differ qualitatively from normal (see also p. 59).

'Content'

Delusions are abnormal beliefs. They are the most important of the abnormalities of thought content. **Delusions** take various forms but are usually defined as (a) false beliefs, which, (b) are not susceptible to the ordinary processes of reasoning and appeal to evidence, and which, (c) are culturally atypical, i.e. out of step with the beliefs conventionally held among people of the same cultural and ethnic background as the patient. To be a delusion, a belief must be held with complete conviction. Delusions are divided up mainly according to their subject, i.e. what they are about. The most important kinds are: **paranoid**, reflecting a distorted relationship between the patient and the world about them, e.g. persecutory, self-referential, and grandiose delusions; **hypochondriacal; nihilistic** (beliefs involving the idea that the patient is already dead, that their body is rotting away, etc.); delusions of **guilt**; delusions of **poverty**. Delusions are also divided up according to their origin. Most delusions are **secondary**, that is delusions which are secondary to some other morbid phenomenon, e.g. delusions of guilt or of impoverishment in depression. Some delusions are **primary**, springing into the patient's mind apparently without morbid antecedents. A **delusional perception** is a primary delusion sparked by some quite normal percept. Primary delusions are nearly always symptoms of schizophrenia – see Chapter 5. **Delusions of control** are also usually schizophrenic symptoms. Although called delusions, they are not so much beliefs as experiences of the will being taken over by some other agency: movements, volitions, even feelings are experienced as being out of one's own control and manipulated by someone or something else (these are sometimes called 'made phenomena', e.g. made acts, made volitions, made affect). **Partial delusions** are like delusions except that they are not held with complete conviction. They are ideas with which the patient is much preoccupied while yet not quite believing that they are true. **Delusional mood** is a state of perplexity in which the patient senses that something important is going to happen but they are not sure what. With delusional mood, the patient often experiences brief delusion-like ideas which fluctuate in content over short periods of time. Besides delusions, patients may show other abnormalities of the content of thinking, e.g. **morbid fears** in anxiety states, such as a fear of collapsing or of 'losing control' in public, **overvalued ideas** – beliefs of a highly idiosyncratic nature with which the patient is much preoccupied. Overvalued ideas are like delusions in being firmly held, but are understandable given the patient's particular circumstances and background.

Perception

The most important abnormalities of perception in psychiatry are hallucinations. **True hallucinations** are perceptions occurring in the absence of a stimulus which the patient takes to be real, e.g. the example above of a patient hearing voices shouting obscenities at him. Hallucinations come in many forms. Besides auditory, as in this case, they may be visual, olfactory (smell), gustatory (taste), tactile (touch), or somatic (bodily or visceral sensations). Then again, they may be well or ill defined in content – simple or complex hallucinations respectively. Voices speaking clearly would be complex hallucinations; simple auditory hallucinations would include mutterings, scrapings, slitherings. Similarly, complex visual hallucinations include well-formed images of people, animals, etc., while simple visual hallucinations may take the form of geometric shapes, or brief flashes, or patches of colour. **Pseudohallucinations** are similar to true hallucinations except that they lack the full qualities of true perceptions; for example, an auditory hallucination heard in one's head rather than in outside space; or voices coming from the outside world but which the patient regards as possibly not being real. **Illusions** differ from hallucinations in being deceptions of the senses, e.g. a

stick which looks bent when it is partly immersed in water. Unless very frequent or bizarre, illusions are not generally of pathological significance. Certain **distortions of perception** may be pathological, however, e.g. micropsia (things looking too small) and hyperacusis (things sounding too loud). **Déjà vu** and **jamais vu** experiences, things seeming excessively familiar or excessively unfamiliar respectively, are sometimes significant, e.g. in temporal lobe epilepsy. **Derealization** is the experience of things appearing unreal, like a stage set, or as though made of cardboard. **Depersonalization** is a similar experience of one's self or one's body feeling unreal. These are often anxiety-related symptoms but may occur in other psychiatric conditions.

Cognitive function

Disturbances of cognitive function include: (a) disorientation (time, place and person), (b) defects of attention and concentration, (c) impaired memory (recent and remote), (d) reduced general intelligence or IQ (for both verbal and non-verbal tasks). All these symptoms are described fully in Chapter 11. A mild global impairment of cognitive functions is called **clouding of consciousness**. This is the first slip away from full consciousness towards coma. **Delirium** is clouding of consciousness with a high output of verbal and non-verbal behaviour. **Stupor** is a state of consciousness in which the patient is inert and mute but appears nonetheless to be conscious of his surroundings (e.g. with severe psychomotor retardation in depression). **Dementia** as a descriptive term means an acquired impairment of cognitive function of a long-term nature, usually progressive, and with marked impairment of memory function. The term is also used of a group of specific diseases.

Insight

Insight is not a symptom as such. It is the degree of understanding that a patient has of their symptoms. Understanding is a complex matter involving, among other things, **awareness** that there is something wrong, and **recognition** of the nature of what is wrong as illness. Insight in the former sense may be lacking with any symptom, psychological or physical. However, insight in the second sense is typically lacking in respect of certain particular psychological symptoms, specifically with delusions, hallucinations and certain kinds of thought disorder (marked with ** in Fig. 1.4, * indicating partial insight). With these symptoms the patient is well aware that something is wrong, but fails to recognize that what is wrong is that he or she is mentally ill. Such symptoms are called psychotic symptoms. Conditions in which symptoms of this kind typically occur are called psychotic conditions. Assessment of insight is important diagnostically, and to medico-legal issues involving compulsory treatment and legal competence (see Chapter 25).

Physical symptoms

Among the physical symptoms of particular importance in psychiatry are the following.

Autonomic symptoms

A variety of autonomic symptoms are associated with anxiety, including palpitation, tremor, sweating, blurring of vision, loose stool and frequency of micturition. Sometimes these may be the presenting symptoms of an anxiety disorder. Certain specific symptoms are recognized, e.g. 'globus hystericus' (psychogenic difficulty swallowing).

Biological symptoms of depression
As noted earlier, with major depression there may be marked biological symptoms such as reduced appetite and extreme weight loss. Depressed patients may sometimes complain of these or of other physical symptoms rather than of lowered mood. This is called 'masked depression'.

Pain
Pain is an important presenting symptom in psychiatry as well as in physical medicine. Besides hypochondriacal conditions, it is common in both anxiety disorders and depression. In anxiety disorders, chest pain, colicky abdominal pain, and headache is common. Headache and facial pains are common in depression.

Dissociative symptoms
These are symptoms usually either of the primary sense and voluntary motor systems or of memory, which turn out to be due to psychological rather than to physical factors. None of these symptoms is common but examples include paralysis, blindness and memory loss. Symptoms of this kind are traditionally called 'hysterical'. The term 'dissociative' is sometimes restricted to disorders of memory (memory loss and fugue states), the term 'conversion' then being used for the remainder. This distinction is derived from a psychoanalytic theory of the origin of these symptoms.

Vegetative symptoms
These include disorders of appetite, of sexual drive, and of sleep. Specific distrubances of appetite include reduction and loss of appetite, anorexia (a persistent active refusal to eat) and bulimia (binge eating). The sexual symptoms included under this heading are those involving drive and performance; drive may be reduced (impotence in men, frigidity in women); difficulties of performance are called 'orgasmic' difficulties, e.g. premature and delayed ejaculation in men, vaginismus in women. Disorders of sleep include insomnia, hypersomnia (excessive sleeping), disorders of sleep rhythm, and a variety of specific disorders such as sleep walking and night terrors (attacks in which the patient wakes screaming and apparently terrified but with little or no recall the next morning).

Psychological signs
Signs of disorder are as important in psychiatry as they are in physical medicine. Specifically psychiatric signs are limited to disturbances in the patient's appearance, behaviour and speech. These are described fully in Chapter 3, under the assessment of the mental state. Observations of the patient are as important diagnostically as simply listening to what they say. Changes in their appearance, behaviour and speech may all provide vital clues to underlying psychological symptoms. Important examples include (1) expressed affect (e.g. in depression – unsmiling and immobile face, minimal eye contact, slumped and inert posture, monot-

onous speech, slowed movements), (2) dress (e.g. flamboyant in hypomania, bizarre in schizophrenia, neglected in dementia).

Categories of psychiatric disorder

The two most widely used classifications of psychiatric disorders are of the International Classification of Diseases (the 'ICD'), published by the World Health Organization, and the American Psychiatric Association's Diagnostic Statistical Manual (the 'DSM'). Both classifications have been developed in a series of editions over a number of years, the current versions being ICD-10 and DSM-III. A fourth edition of the DSM is due out shortly.

As already described, although these classifications differ in detail they include much the same broad categories of disorder. These are summarized in Fig. 1.5. An initial division is made between disorders in adults and disorders in children and adolescents. Adult disorders are further subdivided into disease categories proper (defined partly in terms of symptoms partly in terms of aetiology, as described above), personality disorders and stress-induced disorders.

Adult disease categories
There are six main categories of psychiatric disease in adults.

Organic
Organic disorders are usually defined partly in terms of organic symptoms (i.e. certain specific symptoms which suggest the presence of underlying organic pathology) and partly in terms of organic aetiological factors. The most important organic symptoms are disturbances in cognitive function, especially clouding of consciousness and impaired memory as described above. However there are other organic symptoms, for example, 'organic hallucinations' 'are formed (of people, etc.), often show size distortion (Lilliputian characters are characteristic), coloured (rather than black and white) and moving: and they are usually worse in the evenings (i.e. when it is getting dark).

Organic states are mental states showing one or more organic symptoms. Organic mental states are non-specific: they point to gross pathology of some kind (space-occupying, cardiovascular, infections, etc.) affecting the brain, but tell us very little about the nature or precise location of the pathology. They are affected by the rate at which the pathology develops, however. Hence they are subdivided broadly into **acute** and **chronic organic states**. An example of the former would be a toxic confusional state in which there is clouding of consciousness with disorientation especially for time, progressing to semi-coma and unconsciousness. Dementia is the most familiar example of a chronic organic state. Here the earliest change is usually a disturbance of memory, especially for recent events. But as with acute organic states, as the condition progresses impairment of all cognitive functions, usually with organic hallucinations and other organic symptoms is the rule – see also Chapter 11.

Fig. 1.5 Main categories of psychiatric disorder

Adult disease categories (symptoms and aetiology)
Organic
• Acute (confusional states).
• Chronic (dementias—primary, secondary).
• Special syndromes (e.g. frontal lobe syndrome).

Alcohol/drug related
• Addiction states.
• Complications of use/abuse.
• Withdrawal syndromes.

Psychotic disorders other than organic and affective
• Schizophrenia (simple, hebephrenic, paranoid, catatonic).
• Persistent delusional disorder.
• Brief psychotic episode.

Affective disorders
(happiness/sadness)
• Depression—major ('psychotic'/biological').
• Minor ('neurotic').
• Hypomania.
• Bipolar.
• Schizoaffective.

Anxiety and related disorders
• Anxiety disorder (generalized, phobic, panic).
• Obsessive–compulsive.
• Dissociative (hysteria).
• Somatoform (e.g. psychogenic pain, hypochondriasis).

Disorders of vegetative function
• Eating (anorexia nervosa, bulimia).
• Sexual function (orgasmic, drive).
• Sleeping (insomnia, hypersomnia, sleep terrors, etc.).

Other categories of adult disorder
• *Personality disorder:* very long-term maladaptive personality traits.
• *Stress-induced disorders:* psychiatric disorder as a reaction to extreme stress; 'psychological trauma'.

Child/adolescent disorders
• *Mental retardation:* mild, moderate, severe, profound.
• *Specific developmental delays:* e.g. speech, reading, spelling, arithmetic.
• *'Pervasive disorders':* autism; disintegrative psychosis; schizoid disorder of childhood.
• *Behavioural disorders:* hyperkinetic syndrome; conduct disorder, socialized and unsocialized.
• *Emotional disorders:* e.g. separation anxiety, school phobia.
• *Disorders of physiological functions:* e.g. enuresis, encopresis.

The term 'secondary dementia' means a dementia caused by some other medical condition (e.g. myxoedema), with the implication that the condition can be arrested or reversed with treatment. Most dementias are 'primary'. A number of **specific organic syndromes** are recognized, e.g. frontal lobe syndrome (a syndrome of disinhibition, see Chapter 11), and various kinds of memory disorder such as Korsakoff's psychosis (short-term memory loss with confabulation). Finally, any other mental disorder clearly due to brain disease, damage or dysfunction, or to other physical disease, is sometimes included as an organic disorder, e.g. '**organic depressive state**'.

Alcohol/drug-related disorders
These are generally divided up partly according to the substance involved (alcohol, opioids, cocaine, hallucinogens, etc.), partly by clinical syndrome. The clinical syndromes are of three main kinds, **addiction states**, direct **complications of use/abuse**, and **withdrawal syndromes**.

Psychotic disorders other than affective and organic
As we saw earlier a psychotic disorder may be thought of as one in which hallucinations and/or delusions and/or certain types of thought disorder typically occur. In ICD-9 these disorders were classed together as a separate category distinct from all non-psychotic disorders (sometimes called 'functional' disorders). In ICD-10 and in DSM-III, they are included partly in the categories of organic and affective disorders, partly in a residual category for psychotic disorders of other kinds. These latter disorders include **schizophrenia** (defined by certain specific kinds of delusion, hallucination and thought disorder; and subdivided, according to the predominant symptomatology, into simple, hebephrenic, paranoid and catatonic forms), **delusional disorders** (disorders in which delusions predominate, without specific symptoms of organic, schizophrenic or affective psychoses), and **brief psychotic episodes** (any psychotic disorder of acute onset, limited duration, and without serious sequelae).

Affective disorders
The most common affective disorders are depressive. Depressive disorders are subdivided into major and minor according partly to the depth of depression, partly to the presence or absence of associated symptoms. **Major depression** is associated with biological symptoms as described earlier. It is in major depression also that psychotic symptoms (mainly delusions, sometimes hallucinations) occur. Major depression is sometimes called 'psychotic depression'. **Minor depression** is often associated with anxiety symptoms. It is sometimes called 'neurotic depression', **Hypomania** (together with its more severe form mania) is the elevated mood counterpart of major depression. It is a psychotic disorder, commonly associated with hallucinations and delusions. There are often biological symptoms (e.g. reduced sleep, increased sexual appetite) and specific forms of thought disorder (e.g. pressure of speech and flight of ideas). **Bipolar affective disorder** is a condition in which episodes of major depression and of hypomania alternate. In **schizoaffective disorder** specific schizophrenic symptoms occur in association with marked mood change, either depressive or hypomanic (see Chapter 6).

Anxiety and related disorders
The disorders in this category are sometimes referred to as 'neurotic disorders'. These disorders cluster together — mixed forms are common, and different forms may occur at different times in the same patient. They are defined by their predominant symptomatology, as described above in the section on phenomenology. The main categories are **anxiety disorders** (generalized, phobic and panic), **obsessive–compulsive disorders**, **dissociative (hysterical) states**, and **somatoform disorders**. The latter is really a residual category

Clinical examples (depression)

Depression is a very common psychiatric symptom occurring not only in major and minor depressive illnesses but also in many other conditions. The following cases illustrate some of the differential diagnoses of this symptom.

Case 1: minor (neurotic) depression

Mrs A.B., a 28-year-old housewife, presented with complaints of *low mood, loss of interest* in her hobbies (reading and badminton), and *difficulty in coping* with her home and family. She said that she felt *tired* much of the time and *worried* a good deal, mainly about the family finances. She had become *irritable* with her children. She had been suffering these symptoms *increasingly over the preceding 9 months* but was usually a cheerful and optimistic person. Her youngest child was just under 12 months, and she had two other children under 5. Her husband had been made redundant 2 weeks before she went to see her doctor. Since that time she had been *tearful* and had had *occasional suicidal ideas*. She had had *difficulty getting off to sleep* but had been waking later than usual. Her weight had been unchanged. She was a little pale but her general physical health was good.

Comment. This patient showed the symptoms of *minor depression.* There was *no evidence of organic disorder.* There was a clear change from her normal personality. Although stress factors were important her symptoms were more than merely a response to these. She responded well to *counselling and social support*, working jointly with her husband.

Case 2: major depression

Mr D., a 48-year-old bank manager, was brought to his general practitioner by his wife. He had become increasingly *low in mood over the preceding 3–4 weeks* and in the last few days had *stayed off work*, sitting at home, largely mute and immobile. His doctor could get little from him but his wife said that he had been *sleeping badly, waking early and wandering round the house*. He had *stopped eating* and she thought that he had *lost weight*. She had found that his mood lifted *a little in the evenings*, but was otherwise unresponsive to her efforts to cheer him up, or to any other distraction. He had told her the previous evening that *he believed he was dying of cancer and that there was 'no hope' for him.* In fact, he had *not been eating*. His wife *was afraid that he was planning to kill himself*. He had had *previous illnesses* similar to the present on two occasions, aged 30 and 38. On the last of these he had made a serious *suicide attempt*. Mr D. refused treatment but was eventually admitted to hospital as an involuntary patient under *Section 2 of the Mental Health Act,* 1983.

Comment. In this case, both biological symptoms and a delusion were present. The Section 2 order was justified, given the high risk of suicide (see Chapter 19). It is important to be aware that *depression is sometimes symptomatic of serious underlying physical disease.* However, in this case, careful investigation showed no organic pathology and Mr D. made a full recovery on antidepressant medication.

Case 3: early dementia

Mrs C.W., a 66-year-old *recently widowed* woman, went to see her general practitioner complaining of *headaches*. Physical examination showed no definite abnormalities but the GP felt that she was rather *depressed*. He found she was waking early and had *lost some weight*, and he started her on an *antidepressant*. Three weeks later she returned for a follow-up appointment with her daughter. On this occasion, she seemed *perplexed and tearful*. Her daughter said that she had been *frightened by repeatedly thinking that she had seen rats in her kitchen* in the evenings. Her daughter had been with her on one occasion and there were definitely no rats there. The daughter was able to tell the general practitioner that *her mother's memory had seemed to be deteriorating* for some months though she had put this down to the upset of her bereavement. Cognitive function testing confirmed the loss of short-term memory.

Comment. It is not unusual for *dementia to present with depressive symptoms.* A failure to respond to antidepressants in an elderly patient, especially with the appearance of *organic symptoms* (this woman's hallucination of seeing rats occurring in conditions of low illumination was a typical organic hallucination), should all *raise the possibility of dementia.* In this case *withdrawal of the antidepressants improved her mental state temporarily. Social support and sheltered accommodation* were organized.

Case 4: grief reaction

Mrs K.L., a 46-year-old woman whose *husband had died six months previously*, saw her general practitioner complaining of *low mood and a feeling of hopelessness* about the future. She was *sleeping badly*, having *difficulty getting off to sleep, waking frequently and often early. Her appetite was poor*, though she had not lost weight. She had *difficulty concentrating.* She felt *unable to face going out* with her friends who had been encouraging her to join various social activities. She said that she continued to *think about her husband* a great deal and commonly *heard his voice speaking to her*, especially as she was falling asleep. She knew that he was not really there, although the voice seemed very real and she thought that 'there might be something in spiritualism'. It seemed that she had *initially shown little reaction to her husband's death* but that it had 'hit her' just two months previously.

Comment. Here the patient's *depression is clearly related to* bereavement. Her symptoms, including *pseudohallucinatory* experiences of hearing her husband's voice, are all typical of bereavement. In addition, the time course of the symptoms were consistent with this diagnosis, i.e. a delay followed by a severe reaction. Treatment consisted of what is called *'grief work',* i.e. counselling directed towards helping the patient come to terms with the death of their loved one (see Chapter 22).

Antidepressant medication is not usually indicated despite the presence of a number of biological symptoms.

Case 5: depressive personality disorder

Mr R.B., a 38-year-old unmarried man was referred to psychiatric out-patients *18 months after the death of his mother*, with whom he had lived all his life. He was complaining of *low mood, tiredness and difficulty sleeping.* Initially, it was thought that he was suffering a protracted grief reaction. However, on direct questioning, it turned out that he had never really been close to his mother. Indeed, as he had had to spend most of his spare time looking after her, her death had really been something of a relief to him. His sister, who had come with him, said that she felt the real problem was that although he resented looking after his mother, this had given him a focus for his life. She said that *he had always been inclined to take a bleak view of things and that she did not regard his present symptoms as significantly different from usual.*

Comment. The history here suggested that the patient's *depressive symptoms represented a very long-term personality trait.* Prior to the death of his mother, the patient had rationalized his gloomy feelings as being due to having to look after her. Treatment was only partially effective. A combination of *cognitive therapy and task-oriented counselling* (see Chapter 18) helped him to reshape his attitudes but he remained generally gloomy and lacking any real interest or enthusiasm for life.

Case 6: masked depression

Mrs C., a 58-year-old barrister, was referred to psychiatric out-patients from the local neurology department. She had been referred there with *persistent headaches for which no organic cause had been found.* However, her husband had told the neurologist that he thought she had got very *depressed* of late and they had persuaded her to agree to a psychiatric opinion. The patient herself *denied feeling depressed* but said she had been *sleeping badly, waking earlier than usual.* Also she had *lost some weight.* She admitted to a *previous depressive illness* as a young woman. On reflection, she recalled that she had *suffered from headaches during the course of that illness.* She agreed to a trial period on antidepressants. During follow-up, her headaches improved and she became more talkative and animated. She eventually admitted to marital difficulties and she and her husband benefited from a short period of joint counselling.

Comment. Although this lady was not complaining of low mood as such, her husband considered her *mood to be depressed compared with normal.* In addition, there were *biological symptoms* consistent with depression, and a *history of a previous similar episode.* The antidepressants helped to lift her mood and to relieve her headaches. As she gained confidence in the psychiatric services, she was able to admit to background marital difficulties which had been an important aetiological factor in her depression.

for conditions presenting with physical symptoms of psychogenic origin not catered for elsewhere in the classification, e.g. psychogenic pain, hypochondriasis.

Disorders of vegetative functions
These disorders are defined by the presence of specific vegetative symptoms as described above under Phenomenology. The most important categories are disorders of **eating** (e.g. anorexia nervosa and bulimia), of **sexual function** (disorders of drive and of performance), and disorders of **sleep** (insomnia, hypersomnia, sleep terrors, etc.).

Other categories of adult disorder
Two main groups of condition are included here, personality disorders (together with certain long-term behavioural disorders) and stress-induced disorders.

Personality disorder
Personality disorder can be thought of as a maladaptive exaggeration of a personality trait. Symptomatically, a personality disorder may appear very similar to one or other of the diseases described above. However, where a disease represents a **change** from what is normal for the patient concerned, a personality disorder is normally established by late adolescence and continues more or less **unchanged** into old age. Thus, in order to decide whether someone is suffering from a personality disorder or a disease proper, you have to establish the longitudinal pattern of their symptoms. This is illustrated in Fig. 1.6.

Stress-induced disorders
Stress-induced disorders are analogous to physical trauma. Stress is of course an important aetiological factor for both physical and psychological disease. However, where a psychiatric condition is very clearly and manifestly a reaction to major stress, the diagnosis is of a stress-induced disorder, e.g. grief reaction, battle fatigue. The symptoms of stress-induced disorders are very varied. Anxiety and depression are common, as are somatic complaints. But hallucinations, confusion, mania, and many other symptoms also occur.

Both personality and stress-induced disorders are divided into subtypes according to the main symptoms.

Disorders of childhood and adolescence
Many of the disorders of childhood and adolescence are different from those occurring in adults, and they are conventionally classified separately. The main groups of disorder are listed in Fig. 1.5. **Mental retardation** and **specific developmental delays** are separated out as distinct categories. The so-called '**pervasive disorders**' correspond approximately with adult psychotic disorders, the **emotional disorders** of **childhood** with adult anxiety related (or neurotic) disorders. The remaining groups of disorder include **behavioural disorders** (e.g. conduct disorder), and disorders of **physiological functions** (e.g. enuresis and encopresis). The multiaxial classification system used for childhood disorders is described on p. 186.

From symptoms to diagnosis

Diagnosis in adult psychiatry can be thought of as involving three main stages (Fig. 1.8): (a) clarification of symptoms, (b) exclusion of organic, drug/alcohol-related, personality and stress-induced disorders, and (c) differential diagnosis of remaining disorders according to symptomatology.

1 Clarification of symptoms. This is the basis of diagnosis in psychiatry as it is in physical medicine.

2 Exclusion of (a) organic disorder, (b) drug/alcohol-related problems, (c) personality disorder, and (d) stress-induced disorders. Excluding organic and drug and alcohol-related disorders depends partly on identifying any organic symptoms which may be present, partly on history, physical examination and appropriate laboratory tests. This is described further in Chapters 10 and 11. Excluding personality disorder depends on establishing the long-term pattern of a patient's symptoms (see above and Fig. 1.6). Excluding stress-induced disorders involves establishing whether the patient's condition is mainly a direct reaction to some major stress factor. The latter two kinds of category should be used only very sparingly and when they are quite definitely present.

Fig. 1.6 Definition of personality disorder

In this diagram, the four longitudinal axes represent the lifetimes of four people, from late adolescence through to old age (this being the period over which personality is normally stable). The four horizontal axes represent, for purposes of this example, mood swings – up for happy, down for sad. This axis could represent any other personality trait.

1 Normal This shows the regular, moderate mood swings of a normal individual subject to the normal exigencies of an average life.

2 Depressive personality disorder Here the subject's mood swings are mainly depressive.

3 Illness superimposed on a normal personality The subject suffers a depressive illness, followed by a manic illness. Note that his symptoms during his first illness are the same as those which subject number 2 suffers most of the time. But for this subject, they represent a *change* from the norm.

4 Illness superimposed on an abnormal personality Again, the essential difference between illness and personality disorder is a change from the norm for the patient in question, either quantitative (i.e. the first and second blips on the trace) or qualitative (the third, square-shaped blip). Here the personality disorder is cyclothymic, i.e. with excessive mood swings both up and down.

Fig. 1.7 When is a symptom not a symptom?

The principle of defining diseases symptomatically may seem simple enough. However, symptoms are incorporated into the definitions of particular disorders in a number of different ways and this can lead to complications.

These complications, in psychiatry as in physical medicine, are apparent at three main levels. In descending order of importance (from the point of view of practical diagnosis) these are: (a) in distinguishing one disease from another, (b) in distinguishing diseases from disorders of other kinds, especially from disabilities and wounds, and (c) in distinguishing disorders generally from normality.

Distinguishing one disease from another

Symptomatically defined disease categories are marked out one from another partly by particular symptoms and partly by particular symptom patterns.

Particular symptoms. Thought insertion (p. 59), is an example of a symptom which, in the absence of evidence of organic disease, is pathognomonic of schizophrenia. Such a symptom is thus said to be a 'discriminating' symptom for schizophrenia: if thought insertion (and/or one or more of a number of other similar symptoms, see Chapter 5) is present, then the diagnosis is schizophrenia.

Symptom pattern. Most psychiatric symptoms, such as anxiety and depression, are not discriminating symptoms. They occur in more than one disease. Most psychiatric disease categories are thus defined in terms of characteristic patterns of symptoms, or 'syndromes'.

The basis on which these patterns are identified varies widely. Most are hybrids of:

1 *Simple association*; e.g. manic-depressive depression is defined by depression in association with one or more of certain biological and/or psychotic symptoms (see Fig. 1.1 and Chapter 6).
2 *Relative severity*; e.g. depression is common in anxiety neuroses and vice versa, the two kinds of neurosis thus being distinguished by whichever symptom is the more severe (Chapter 7).
3 *Course*; e.g. depression may be complicated by the appearance of obsessional symptoms and vice versa, the distinction between depressive and obsessional illnesses thus depending (in part) on which symptoms appear first (Chapters 6 and 7).
4 *Importance*; i.e. some symptoms 'trumping' others, creating simple hierarchies; e.g. anxiety is trumped by a first rank symptom of schizophrenia – if both are present, however severe the anxiety, the diagnosis is schizophrenia. The rules here are *ad hoc*, but in general organic symptoms trump psychotic. which in turn trump all other symptoms.

Note, however, that the symptomatic disease categories employed in psychiatry are not all mutually exclusive; a patient may have dementia, for example, as well as depression. Also, the categories may overlap, some patients showing a combination of symptoms from more than one disease category.

Distinguishing diseases from other disorders

In physical medicine diseases are distinguished on the one hand from chronic disabilities and on the other from trauma (wounds and injuries). In psychiatry the disorders most closely corresponding with these are respectively:

1 *Personality disorders*. The symptoms of a personality disorder may be the same as those of a psychiatric disease. They differ in being generally life-long rather than of limited duration. The patient with a personality disorder usually has the symptoms with which he presents; the patient who is ill does not (see text, Fig. 1.6 and Chapter 9).
2 *Disorders induced by stress*. Acute reactions to stress (e.g. battle fatigue) and adjustment reactions (e.g. grief reaction). As with personality disorders, the symptoms of these conditions may be identical with those of a psychiatric disease; the patient may be anxious, depressed, manic, confused, hallucinating, amnesic, etc. In this case, however, the difference is that the symptoms are clearly a response to extraordinary stress. Stress is of course a common aetiological factor for all kinds of psychiatric (and physical) illness, and these categories of disorder should be used only in cases in which, by analogy with physical trauma, the symptoms are very **clearly** a response to quite **extraordinary** stress (see text and Chapter 20).

The diagnostic distinctions between psychiatric disease proper, personality disorder and stress-induced disorder, may have important implications for prognosis and treatment (see Fig. 1.1 and clinical examples, p. 13).

Distinguishing disorders from normality

Many phenomena which are sometimes recognizable as psychiatric symptoms (whether of disease, of personality disorder, or of mental 'trauma') may also form part of normal experience, e.g. depression, anxiety, obsessions. Psychiatric symptoms are in this respect no different from many physical symptoms – not all pains, episodes of nausea or of dizziness are symptoms of physical illness. Just what marks out a symptom **as** a symptom is a large question which overlaps with the question of how illness itself, physical or mental, should be defined (see Fig. 1.3). It has something to do with (a) duration and severity, (b) the presence of associated symptoms and signs, and (c) appropriateness, i.e. whether the symptom is one which is appropriate to the circumstances in which it occurs – nausea with something nauseating, or anxiety with something anxiety provoking, are not normally symptoms of illness. In practice, however, diagnosis in psychiatry (as in physical medicine), is mostly concerned not with the general question of whether a particular symptom is morbid or healthy but with whether a pattern of symptoms corresponds with one or more recognized disorders.

Fig. 1.8 From symptoms to diagnosis

Diagnosis in psychiatry involves three main steps.
1 **Clarify the symptoms**—from history, mental state and physical examination.

2 **Check**
  • Whether due to physical disorder (if so, = organic disorder).
  • Whether due to alcohol/drug abuse.
  • Whether symptoms represent a change for that patient (if not, probably = personality disorder).
  • Whether clearly a reaction to exceptional stress (if so = stress induced disorder).

3 **Decide differential diagnosis of remaining conditions according to:**
  • specific symptoms and symptom clusters (syndromes);
  • most prominent symptoms;
  • time course (e.g. which symptoms come first);
  • hierarchy (organic > psychotic > others);
  • other *ad hoc* rules.
    (See also Fig. 1.7).

Note. (a) Most psychiatric diagnoses are made at stage 3. (b) Patients presenting psychiatrically, especially in general practice, do not always have anything medically wrong with them. Sometimes they just have problems in their life with which they need help.

3 Differential diagnosis of remaining disorders. This covers all the symptomatically defined categories, i.e. *3rd category on,* in Fig. 1.5. Anxiety and related disorders, together with minor depression, are the most common, followed by disorders of appetite and sexual function. Psychotic disorders are the least common. Finally, it should not be forgotten that many patients presenting psychiatrically, especially in general practice, do not have anything wrong with them as such. They have life problems and difficulties with which they need help.

The ways in which disease and other categories of disorder are built up from symptoms and symptom patterns are described further in Fig. 1.7. Practical aspects of diagnosis are described fully in Chapter 3.

QUESTIONS

1 How do the disease categories employed in psychiatry differ from those employed in physical medicine?
2 In connection with what particular kinds of clinical problem is the concept of mental illness important?
3 Which of the following are **least**, and which **most**, variable from one psychiatric disease classification to the next — main categories of disorder, individual diseases, particular symptoms?
4 What are the key defining features of (a) hallucinations, and (b) delusions?
5 Name some physical symptoms important in psychiatry.
6 What is the essential difference between personality disorder and other kinds of psychiatric disorder?
7 What are the main steps from symptoms to diagnosis in psychiatry?

FURTHER READING

Psychiatric symptoms
Leff J.P. & Issacs A.D. (1981) *Psychiatric Examination in Clinical Practice.* 2nd Edition. Blackwell Scientific Publications, Oxford. [Clear descriptions of all the important psychiatric symptoms together with clinical examples.]

Psychiatric disease classification
The two main classifications are:
The ICD-10 Classification of Mental and Behavioural Disorders: Clinical Descriptions and Diagnostic Guidelines (1992). World Health Organization, Geneva.
The Diagnostic and Statistical Manual, 3rd Edition – Revised, (1987). American Psychiatric Association.
Gelder M., Gath D. & Mayou R. (1989) *Oxford Textbook of Psychiatry.* Oxford University Press, Oxford. [Some of the issues and difficulties raised by disease classification in psychiatry are examined in Chapter 3.]
Kendell R.E. (1975) *The Role of Diagnosis in Psychiatry.* Blackwell Scientific Publications, Oxford. [Technical and research aspects.]

The concept of mental illness
Clare A. (1979) The disease concept in psychiatry. In: Hill P., Murray R. & Thorley A. (eds) *Essentials of Postgraduate Psychiatry.* Academic Press, Grune & Stratton, New York. [A review of different views on the concept of mental illness.]
Caplan A.L., Engelhardt H.J. & McCartney J.J. (eds) (1981) *Concepts of Health and Disease.* Addison-Wesley Publishing Co., Reading, Massachussetts. [A useful collection of papers for further readings.]
Lewis A.J. (1955) *Health as a Social Concept, Br. J. Sociol.,* **4**, 109–24. [A classical paper on the functional account of mental illness.]
Fulford K.W.M. (1989) *Moral Theory and Medical Practice.* Cambridge University Press, Cambridge. [Recent research extending this account to specific symptoms.]

2
Causes of Mental Illness

Fact sheet

Introduction

Human behaviour can be explained either in **objective** terms (e.g. events in early childhood or biochemical events in the brain) or in **subjective** terms (e.g. a person's motives, desires or feelings). This chapter is concerned mainly with objective explanations.

What is the cause of a particular mental illness?

In asking this question two points must be remembered:

1 that **there is no single answer** to this question;

2 that the demonstration that a **particular physical** (or social) **event is a cause** of a particular mental illness **does not imply that treatment should** necessarily **be physical** (or social).

A particular cause may be important for one purpose, but not for another, for example, the genetic component to the cause of a particular illness may be important for genetic counselling but not for treatment.

Establishing causal links

In general this is a two-stage process. First, it must be shown that the supposed cause is **associated** with the supposed effect; and second, non-causal explanations for this association must be ruled out. In order to rule out non-causal explanations a study must be **well designed**. Several aspects of study design are discussed in this chapter.

This chapter considers in particular four main categories of cause.

Genetic theories of mental illness

There are three main types of study.

1 Family studies: the rate of the illness is compared between the relatives of those with the illness and those without.

2 Twin studies: the rate of the illness is measured in a group of people who have a twin who is affected with illness. The rate is compared between those who are monozygous twins (MZ) and those who are dizygous twins (DZ).

3 Adoption studies: the purpose of adoption studies is to try and separate genetic from environmental factors. One study design is to see whether amongst adopted children those who have a biological parent affected with the illness have an increased chance of being affected compared with adopted children whose biological parents were not affected. Despite the problems in interpreting these studies **genetic factors appear to play an important role in the aetiology of: schizophrenia; major affective disorder; alcohol abuse; and in some cases of Alzheimer's disease**.

Biochemical theories

There are three main kinds of study:

1 the **comparison of biochemical measures** in tissues under investigation and from normal controls;

2 establishing **the biochemical effects of treatments** for the illness in question;

3 establishing **the biochemical effects of drugs which can precipitate the illness** or mimic the symptoms of the illness.

Biochemical theories which have been particularly important in stimulating research are: **the dopamine hypothesis of schizophrenia; the monoamine theory of depression; and the cholinergic theory of Alzheimer's disease**.

Social theories

To what extent do psychiatric disorders result from living in a particular environment? Both schizophrenic and depressive illnesses appear to be more common amongst those of low social class. In the case of schizophrenia this is probably because the schizophrenic illness causes a drift towards lower social class (**the drift hypothesis**). In the case of depressive illness the lower social class appears to cause the increased prevalence in the illness. But through what mechanism? The evidence supports the view that those of lower social class have more adverse experiences and it is those experiences which lead to the depression. Two types of adverse experience are distinguished:

1 life-events (such as changes in job, housing or important personal relationships) which can precipitate the depressive illness in those already vulnerable to depression;

2 vulnerability or predisposing factors (such as the absence of a close confiding relationship) which make someone vulnerable to depression when they experience a life-event.

Psychological theories

Four areas in particular are discussed.

1 Learning theory. Operant conditioning in particular has influenced aetiological theories of psychiatric problems. For example, a child's **behaviour problems** may be fruitfully looked at from the point of view of what system of rewards and punishments may have led to the problems.

2 Cognitive theory. This has led to an interest in the importance of beliefs and patterns of thinking in causing and maintaining psychiatric illness. **Depressive illness** and **anxiety neurosis** in particular have been looked at in this way.

3 Psychoanalytic theory. This stresses the importance of unconscious motives and desires in the cause of psychological problems. As such, psychoanalytic explanations tend to be subjective. However, psychoanalytic theory sees early childhood experience as important in the development of unconscious desires, and has led to research into such experience and subsequent psychological problems.

4 Personality theory. The connection between personality and the major 'psychotic' illnesses is weak, but certain types of personality can be seen as **predisposing factors in the aetiology of neuroses**.

Conclusion

Many factors interact in causing mental illness, and for most illnesses none is predominant. The psychiatrist must be alert to the various categories of cause, and must be able to consider the relevance of each to the problem in hand.

Introduction

This chapter is about how the causes of mental illnesses can be investigated, and its purpose is to encourage a critical approach to evidence. The chapter is organized around four main areas: **genetics**; **biochemistry**; **social science**; and **psychology**. The discussion of these four areas is preceded by an introduction to the concept of causation and by a consideration of the difficulties in establishing causal links.

Two models of explanation for human behaviour

We make use of two rather different ways of explaining human behaviour and feelings:
- objective;
- subjective.

Consider the action of a car thief. I might explain what he does objectively by pointing to his deprived childhood, or even the biochemistry of his brain. On the other hand, I might explain his action subjectively in terms of his own motives, desires or feelings, for example that he stole the car to buy a package holiday to Greece.

This chapter is mainly about objective explanations. However, I do not wish to imply that subjective explanations should be avoided in psychiatry, nor that they are inferior. When the psychiatrist ceases to think about the desires, motives and experiences of patients, then he or she will cease either to understand or to help them.

Psychoanalytic theory encompasses both subjective and objective explanations. One of its major contributions is to have extended the realm of subjective explanation by including **unconscious** motives, desires and feelings. In addition it has laid stress on the importance of the early development of interpersonal relationships. This has paved the way for a fruitful empirical approach in which the attachment between mother and child is studied in relation to subsequent development.

Causation

There are several points to make about causation with respect to mental illness. The first is that the question 'what is the cause of X?' has no single or basic answer. Thus the answer to the question of what is the cause of an event will depend on the reason we have for asking the question (Fig. 2.1). For example, any one of the following may be the reason why we want to know what causes depressive illness:
- to give genetic counselling;
- to develop a new drug for treatment;
- to design a new housing estate;
- to develop a psychological treatment;
- to advise an individual about employment;
- to counsel a family in crisis.

Depending on our interests, we will choose one or other

aspect to study. These various different causes of a single event may relate to each other in various different ways (Fig. 2.2).

The second point is that the demonstration that a particular physical (or social) event is a cause of mental illness does not imply that treatment should necessarily be physical (or social). For example, we may show that depressive illness is caused by a particular physical state of the brain. However, this does not mean that we cannot treat the condition successfully through psychotherapy. Conversely, from the demonstration that losing a job can be a cause of depressive illness, it does not follow that treatment with tablets will be ineffective. This point is taken up in the **conclusion** to this chapter.

Fig. 2.1 Some causes of a forest fire

Any one of the following could be a cause of the same forest fire. There is no single fundamental answer to the question: what is the cause of X? The relevant answers depend on our reasons for asking the question.
1 The lack of rain over the previous months.
2 The match which was dropped.
3 The carelessness of the person who dropped the match.
4 The pile of leaves where the match was dropped.
5 The oxygen content of the air.
6 The narrowness of the fire-break paths in the forest.
7 The inaccessibility of the forest to fire-engines.

Fig. 2.2 Three ways in which two causes of X, A and B, may relate to each other

1 A → B → X
For example, unemployment may lead to marital problems which lead to depression.

2 A ⎫
        + ⎬ → X
       B ⎭

For example, an anxiety neurosis may occur in someone who has an anxious personality and who has just started a new job.

3 A → X ← B
For example, depressive illness can result from bereavement; or it may be secondary to Cushing's disease.

Fig. 2.3 Causes of behaviour and attitudes to patients

What would your attitude be, to a patient who had been dangerously violent, for each of the explanations of the behaviour given below: (a) if the person were in a court of law and you were judging the verdict and the sentence; and (b) if the person were an out-patient of yours?
1 A brain tumour.
2 Schizophrenia.
3 A depressive illness.
4 Pre-menstrual tension.
5 Drunkenness.
6 Violent personality.
7 Hypoglycaemia.
8 Having been brought up in a violent family.

Causes of illness and attitudes to patients

Our view of the causes of mental illnesses and our understanding of why a particular patient behaves in a particular way affect our attitude to that patient (Fig. 2.3). The central reason for this is the close relationship between cause and responsibility.

The difficulty in establishing causal links

The first clue that there is a causal link is usually the discovery of an association between an event and the mental illness. However, **correlation is not causation**. If we observe a correlation between the wearing of a raincoat and the wearing of boots, it does not follow that one is the cause of the other; the rain may be the cause of both.

The problem is: **how can we avoid the trap of seeing a causal link where none exists?** Good research design is concerned, first, with maximizing the chances of discovering

---

Fig. 2.5 The data from a hypothetical study to look at the relationship between the loss of a job and depressive illness

a, b, c, and d represent the number of people in each category from a total sample size of $n = a + b + c + d$

	Job lost	No job lost
Depressive illness	a	b
No depressive illness	c	d

---

whether an association does exist or does not exist; and second, if an association does exist, it is concerned with ruling out non-causal explanations. Good research design is formalized common sense. We will now consider each component in turn.

Evidence for association

Suppose that we are interested in the question of whether the loss of a job is associated with an increase in the rate (Fig. 2.4) of depressive illness. Imagine that we have some data which can be expressed in the form of Fig. 2.5.

In psychiatry the association between two factors is rarely complete; not all those who lose a job become depressed, nor have all the depressed lost a job. This is, no doubt, because there are many paths to depression, and many ways of avoiding it. However, we may find that losing a job and depression tend to go together. Thus if a multiplied by d is greater than c multiplied by b in Fig. 2.5, we have *prima facie* evidence that there is an association between depression and losing a job. But, such a finding could occur by chance. Probability theory (usually called 'statistics' in this context) can give some quantification to this possibility. It is usually possible to answer the following question: supposing that there were no association between losing a job and be-

---

Fig. 2.4 Rates of disease

The fundamental measures used in most large studies of the causes of disease are rates of disease within a population. Of particular importance are **prevalence** and **incidence**.

The **prevalence** of a disease is the number of cases with the disease, at any time during the study period, divided by the population at risk (midway during the study period). The length of the study period should be specified.

The **incidence** of a disease is the number of **new** cases of the disease within the study period, divided by the population at risk (at the start of the study). The length of the study period should be specified.

The usual time period is a year, giving **annual prevalence**, and **annual incidence**. The **point prevalence** is the prevalence at a given point in time.

Annual prevalence = point prevalence + annual incidence (where the point prevalence is for the first day of the year in question).

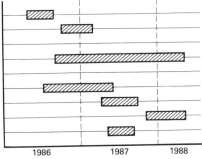

The diagram above represents a population of nine individuals over a two-year period. The hatched area indicates the time over which an individual suffers the disease (seven of the people have the disease at some time). What is the **annual prevalence** and **annual incidence**, for the year 1987, and what is the **point prevalence** on January 1st 1987 and 1988?

(Answers: annual prevalence 1987 = 6/9; annual incidence 1987 = 3/9; point prevalence 1987 = 3/9; point prevalence 1988 = 2/9.)

Fig. 2.6 Some ways of accounting for an association between A and B

1 A causes B.
   A → B
2 B causes A.
   B → A
3 The method of sampling the population has tended to select those individuals with both A and B (or those with neither A nor B) more frequently than by chance (i.e. the sample does not truly reflect the population).
4 A does not cause B, but it alters the time when B occurs (in particular it causes B to happen earlier than it would have done in the absence of A).
5 A is an early sign of B.

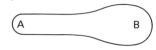

6 P (another factor) causes both A and B.

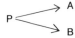

---

coming depressed, then what is the probability of obtaining a particular result? On the basis of this probability we must decide whether or not to believe in an association. If we conclude wrongly that there is an association we make what is called a 'type 1' error. If we conclude falsely that there is no association we have made a 'type 2' error.

Evidence for a causal connection

There are many ways of accounting for an association between two factors: A and B. Figure 2.6 gives a number of these ways. **Good research design is about eliminating as many non-causal explanations as possible.** Let us consider the work of Brown and Harris. They were interested in the social causes of depression and assessed whether major events in a person's life ('life-events') (e.g. losing a job, illness, job promotion) could cause depression. They did a retrospective study (Fig. 2.7) and compared the number of life-events in the previous year in a group of depressed women, with the number of such events in a group of non-depressed women. **They found that there had been more life-events amongst depressed women than amongst non-depressed women.**

Could this be an artefact of sampling (point 3, Fig. 2.6)? Could it be, for example, that the occurrence of life-events affected the chance of depressed women being entered into the sample? This is unlikely because they studied women chosen at random from the household register.

Could life-events have caused depression to occur earlier than it would otherwise have done, but not have affected the chance of depression happening (point 4)? This is difficult to rule out although by making a number of assumptions it is possible to get an answer to this question. The results suggest that life-events can cause a depressive illness to occur which would otherwise not have occurred; but that with schizophrenia, life-events simply bring forward the time when the symptoms occur.

Could life-events have been an early sign of the depressive illness (point 5)? This is certainly possible for some of the life events. If a person is dismissed from a job this might be for behaviour which is due to the, as yet undetected, depressive illness. However, for other life-events such an explanation for the association looks most unlikely, as is the case if the loss of the job is due to the factory closing down.

Could another factor have caused both the depression and the losing of a job (point 6)? For example excess alcohol intake may increase the chances of losing a job and of depression, without the job loss and the depression being causally related. To assess this possibility the samples would have to be matched (Fig. 2.7) for the number of people who drank excess alcohol.

Having discussed briefly some points about evidence for causes in general, I will now consider four specific areas in turn: genetics, biochemistry, social science and psychology.

Fig. 2.7 Study designs

Suppose we are investigating the question of whether A causes B (e.g. does unemployment cause depression?).

Case control (retrospective) study

The study group consists of subjects with condition B (depression). The control group consists of subjects without condition B. The previous occurrence of A in subjects within the study group is compared with that in subjects within the control group. Such a study will give information on the question of what proportion of those with B (depression) were exposed to A (unemployment).

Cohort (prospective) study

The study group consists of those subjects exposed to factor A (unemployment). The control group consists of subjects not exposed to factor A. The incidence of B (depression) is compared between the two groups. Such a study will give information on what proportion of those with A (unemployment) go on to develop B (depression). **A cohort study generates incidence data; whereas a case control study does not.**

NB. A cohort study may be carried out 'retrospectively', for example, a group of people unemployed a year ago could be compared with a group of employed people with respect to the incidence of depression over the last year.

Matching

This is the most powerful way of dealing with explanation 6 (see Fig. 2.6). If both study and control groups are matched for P (i.e. factor P occurs with the same frequency in both groups), then any association found between A and B is unlikely to be due to the influence of P.

In general, those factors should be matched which are associated with both A and B, independently of any causal connection between A and B. For example, the age of subjects may affect both the chance of unemployment and the chance of depression independently of any direct association between unemployment and depression. Study and control groups should be **matched** for age.

In a cohort study in which the experimenter has control of whether a subject receives A (e.g. in a treatment trial), a powerful way of matching is for subjects to be allocated **randomly** to either study group or control group. With such an allocation method it is unlikely for there to be any systematic difference between the two groups for any factor other than A.

Over-matching

It would be wrong to conclude that the study and control groups should be matched for everything possible. Suppose that unemployment causes low income and low income causes depression. If we were to match the two groups for low income then we would not pick up the genuine causal link between unemployment and depression. In general, those factors should not be matched which may intervene in the causal chain linking A and B.

Masking

In assessing B both the subject and the experimenter may be influenced by a knowledge of whether this particular subject has been exposed to A. Thus, if the study aims to assess the effect of a new antidepressant, the judgement as to whether a particular subject's depression has improved may be influenced by knowing whether that subject received the active drug or placebo. If the subject does not know which he is taking, but the experimenter does know, the study is said to be **single blind**. In a treatment trial, the better design is for neither subject nor experimenter to know. The trial is said to be **double blind**. **In a good treatment trial, the blind lead the blind.**

Genetic theories of causation

Introduction

The shape of a stone on the beach is a result of the action of the sea and the wind on the constituents of the stone. It might seem odd to ask: how much of the shape is due to the sea and how much is due to the calcium carbonate? The matter of the stone is sculpted by the environment.

There appears a strong tendency for doctors to ask: how much is this disease due to genetic factors and how much is it due to environmental factors? But our physical and mental life is a result of the action of the environment on our genetic constitution. When we say that Huntington's disease is genetic, we mean that given one genetic constitution (the possession of the Huntington gene) we have not found any environment which prevents the disease short of one which kills the person, and, given another genetic constitution (the absence of the gene), we have not found any environment in which the disease manifests itself.

None of the major mental illnesses is determined so forcibly by the genetic constitution as is Huntington's disease. In the cases of **schizophrenia, major affective disorder** (depression and manic-depressive disorder), **alcohol abuse**, and at least some cases of **Alzheimer's disease**, there is good evidence that genetic factors play a significant aetiological role.

However, the conclusions which we can draw from such evidence are limited. It does not necessarily tell us whether we can treat or prevent the disease better by manipulating the social, psychological or biological environment. The conclusion that a genetic component to aetiology favours 'biological' treatments and an environmental component to aetiology favours 'psychological' treatments is unsound.

Study designs

There are three main types of study which provide evidence for the importance of genetic factors in the aetiology of mental illness:
- family studies;
- twin studies;
- adoption studies.

Family studies

For a general description see Fig. 2.8. **The central problem with such studies is that family members share both environmental and genetic factors.** For example, family studies show that alcoholism occurs in the children of alcoholics at a much higher rate than in the general population. This could be because genetic factors are important in its aetiology. However, members of the same family will tend to share a large number of environmental factors, and it may be these factors which are of importance. Nevertheless, family studies have been useful in providing the initial evidence for the importance of genetic factors. A different approach to family studies is to look at the pattern of inheritance of the disease in question within large families, over several generations. Occasionally, as in the example of Huntington's disease, this pattern of inheritance strongly suggests that the presence of the disease is principally determined by a single gene.

Fig. 2.8 Types of study used to examine the genetic bases of mental illnesses

Family studies

The prevalence (or incidence) of the illness is compared between the relatives of probands* and the relatives of non-affected controls. The general population is often used for controls, in which case it is important to match, at least for sex and age.

Twin studies

Probands are those with the disease who have a twin. For each twin pair it is determined whether the twins are monozygotic (MZ) or dizygotic (DZ). The prevalence of the disease in the MZ twins is compared with the prevalence in the DZ twins. This gives the MZ:DZ prevalence ratio.

Adoption studies

Two different types of design are shown below. In the first type the prevalence of the disease is compared between an adopted group who are the biological children of affected parents, and a control adopted group whose biological parents are not affected.

In the second type of design the subject group consists of adopted people affected with the disease, and the control group of adopted people not affected. The prevalence of the disease is compared between the biological parents of the affected group and the biological parents of the non-affected group. Interesting comparisons can also be made between biological and adoptive relatives of the two groups.

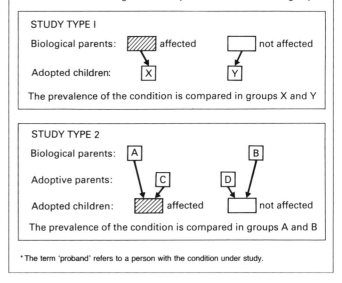

* The term 'proband' refers to a person with the condition under study.

Several family pedigrees suggesting single gene inheritance have also been identified for Alzheimer's disease of presenile onset. Once such families have been identified it becomes possible to carry out **linkage studies**. The purpose of linkage studies is to find out where the gene which determines the disease is located. The method involves finding a 'marker' for which the gene location is known and which segregates with the disease, i.e. the marker is present in those individuals within the family who have the disease and absent in those who do not have the disease. The gene is likely to be on the same chromosome, and close to, the marker. This method has been used, for example, to show that the Huntington gene is on chromosome 4, and that in some families Alzheimer's disease is likely to be caused by a gene located on chromosome 21. In both cases, this initial localization has allowed the gene itself to be identified, and thereby to discover the mutations in the gene which cause the disease.

Twin studies

If the MZ:DZ ratio (see Fig. 2.8) is significantly greater than unity, this is evidence for the importance of genetic factors since MZ twins share more genes than DZ twins. **The main problem in interpreting twin studies is that MZ twins may share more environmental factors than DZ twins**. This could, for example, be because by looking identical they tend to evoke similar responses from others. They may also tend to choose very similar environments. Twin studies are more powerful than family studies in the investigation of genetic factors, but the results remain open to various interpretations.

Adoption studies

Adoption studies (see Fig. 2.8) **provide the most powerful design in attempting to understand the interaction between genes and the environment.** They provide the opportunity of comparing people with similar genetic constitutions who are brought up in different environments, and of comparing those with different genetic constitutions who are brought up in similar environments. It is as though one were to take stones of varying composition and see what shapes they developed in different places. However, **the fundamental difficulty in interpreting the results from adoption studies is to determine whether two environments are similar or different**. The answer is, of course, that any two environments are similar in some ways and different in other ways. Returning to the analogy of the stone, if we were to find that stones of one chemical constitution tend to be of one shape, whether in Bognor or Barbados, we might conclude that the shape is strongly determined by the composition. But, perhaps, all the environments we have explored are very similar in the factors which are important in the sculpting of the stone. We may have explored places as different as Barbados and Bognor, but we may have only been where the land emerges from the sea. Children brought up in different families may share important environmental features. Conversely, there may be important differences in the environments of children brought up in the same family. Adoption studies can be used to test the relative importance of genes and **specified** environmental factors, but it does not make sense to contrast genes with the environment *in toto*.

Monogenic and polygenic theories

If genetic composition plays a significant role, then the question arises: is it one gene which is important, or many? This turns out, in general, to be a very difficult question to answer. Classic Mendelian modes of single gene inheritance are rare. If, in a large family, only affected parents have affected children, and if the disease appears in about 50% of those in each generation, we have good evidence for a single dominant gene. But if we don't get this pattern, a single dominant gene might still be important. With reduced penetrance, and variable expressivity, a very wide range of patterns can be accommodated. The data concerning most major psychiatric illness, including schizophrenia, affective disorder and Alzheimer's disease, are compatible, in general, with both monogenic and polygenic theories of inheritance.

Conclusion

The question of whether genetic factors are important in the aetiology of mental illness turns out to be a surprisingly difficult one to answer. Genetic factors probably play a significant aetiological role in schizophrenia, major affective disorder, alcohol abuse and in some cases of Alzheimer's disease. However, the conclusions we can draw from these facts with regard to the treatment of patients are limited.

Biochemical theories of causation

Behind every mental phenomenon there is a physical event within the brain. But what are the relationships hidden by the word 'behind'? We are imprisoned within our concepts. Centuries from now we will be seen to have been using a quaint picture of mind and brain.

The only questions we can ask, at present, about the connection between the brain and mental illness are cast in the form of what biochemical measures correlate with mental illnesses. For the most part, the biochemical measures made use of are either the concentration of neurotransmitters and their metabolites, or the number of receptors. There are, of course, many other features about the brain which are relevant to its functioning (the specific connections made by neurons; the shape and positioning of the dendritic branches), but these are difficult to study and they do not readily suggest drug treatments.

Figure 2.9 lists the most common study designs which are used to investigate the relationship between mental illness and brain biochemistry.

Fig. 2.9 Types of study used to examine the biochemical bases of mental illnesses

1 The comparison of biochemical measures in tissues from those with the illness, and from those without the illness. The tissues can be taken:
- post-mortem (usually the brain);
- ante-mortem (CSF, blood, urine, brain biopsy).

2 Establishing the biochemical effects of treatments for the illness (for example, studying the mode of action of phenothiazines as a way of shedding light on schizophrenia, or of antidepressants to understand the biochemistry of depression).

3 Establishing the biochemical effects of precipitants of the condition [for example, reserpine (which reduces monoamine stores) can cause depression, and amphetamine can lead to schizophrenic symptoms].

NB. Biochemical studies may be aimed at looking for **trait** or **state** markers. Thus, if a measure is altered in someone who has had depressive illnesses compared with controls, and this alteration remains whether or not that person is currently depressed, this measure is a **trait** marker. If, however, a measure is found to be abnormal only when someone is currently depressed, it is a marker of the **state** of depression.

Problems in the interpretation of biochemical studies

There are many problems in interpreting the results from such studies as evidence that the biochemical changes are a cause of the illness.

Problem 1

The biochemical changes may *result* from some aspect of the illness. For example, some of the biochemical changes found in people with depressive illness (for example, altered results from the dexamethasone suppression test) may be due to the altered patterns of eating or exercise which are found in depression.

Problem 2

The biochemical changes may be a result of treatment. This problem has confounded post-mortem studies of schizophrenia since most subjects will have been taking major tranquillizers.

Problem 3

In post-mortem studies, the biochemical measure will be affected by extraneous factors, for example, by both the precise mode of death and by how the brain is treated after death.

Problem 4

In post-mortem studies the diagnosis of the mental illness may be uncertain. Post-mortem studies have been carried out on people who have committed suicide in an attempt to study the biochemical basis of depression. But it is uncertain how many such people had a depressive illness.

Problem 5

Many of the tissues examined (e.g. blood, CSF and urine) **are an indirect way of looking at the brain.** For example the breakdown products of neurotransmitters are often measured. There are two problems with this. Firstly, there may be sources of the product other than from the brain. In one study urinary dopamine was found to relate to the intelligence of monkeys as measured by a learning task. However, it was discovered that the dopamine came from the bananas which were given as reward. Secondly, there may be quite different changes in the brain which could be expressed by the same change in the concentration of substance in the periphery. For example, an **increase** in brain noradrenaline may lead to an increase in the peripheral concentration of its breakdown product MHPG. However, an increase in the metabolism of noradrenaline with consequent increase in peripheral MHPG may result in a decrease of brain noradrenaline. Thus, raised levels of peripheral MHPG might be associated either with raised or lowered levels of brain noradrenaline.

An interesting use of blood cells is as a 'model' of the brain. Thus, on platelets, there are α_2-adrenergic receptors which have many properties in common with α_2-adrenergic receptors in the brain. *In-vivo* experiments can be undertaken in which these receptor numbers and properties are studied in various mental illnesses, in the hope that the brain receptors behave similarly. There is, for example, some evidence that the number of these receptors decreases in the days following childbirth, and that this decrease is greater in women who experience a markedly depressed mood.

Conclusion

There are a number of biochemical theories of mental illnesses, although none is certain. Their main value is in suggesting what properties therapeutic drugs might be expected to have. Amongst the more important biochemical theories of mental illness are:

1 **the dopamine hypothesis of schizophrenia;**
2 **the monoamine theory of depression;**
3 **the cholinergic theory of Alzheimer's disease.**

According to the first, schizophrenia is due to **elevated** levels of dopamine, at least in some areas of the brain. The second theory claims that depressive illness results from **reduced** levels of the monoamines, noradrenaline and 5-hydroxytryptamine. According to the third theory the clinical features of Alzheimer's disease are due mainly to the loss of neurones containing acetyl choline.

Social theories of causation

To what extent do psychiatric disorders result from living in a particular social environment? This question is raised, although not answered, by the observations that a particular psychiatric disorder is found more commonly in one social group, or in one society, than in another. Depression is found more commonly amongst working class than middle class women. Schizophrenia is found more commonly in inner city areas. Such observations are essentially of correlations. What are the causal links?

Consider first the observation of Faris and Dunham. Schizophrenia was found to have a higher prevalence amongst those living in the central districts of Chicago. It is known that in this inner city area there are proportionately

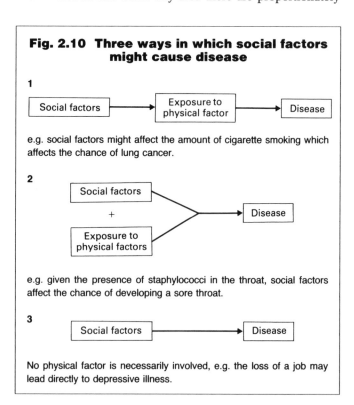

Fig. 2.10 Three ways in which social factors might cause disease

1

e.g. social factors might affect the amount of cigarette smoking which affects the chance of lung cancer.

2

e.g. given the presence of staphylococci in the throat, social factors affect the chance of developing a sore throat.

3

No physical factor is necessarily involved, e.g. the loss of a job may lead directly to depressive illness.

more people of lower social class. **Is lower social class therefore necessarily associated with schizophrenia?** The answer is **no**. This is because those with schizophrenia within the inner city may not be the same people as those of lower social class. To discover whether or not schizophrenia is associated with low social class, the social class distribution of people with schizophrenia has to be examined and compared with a suitable control group. In fact, an association has been found between schizophrenia and low social class. There can be several explanations for such association (see Fig. 2.6). Two alternative theories in particular have been proposed. The first is that the low social class is a factor in causing the schizophrenia (the **generation hypothesis**). The second is that having schizophrenia has led to a drift towards lower social class (the **drift hypothesis**). This second explanation is supported by the subsequent observation that the social class of those with schizophrenia is lower than that of their fathers.

In the case of depression, however, the explanation for the higher rate in women of lower social class cannot be accounted for by the 'drift' hypothesis. In this case the depression appears to be caused by the low social class. But through what mechanism? Social factors might cause disease by a number of different means (Fig. 2.10).

Brown and Harris, in this study of depression in women in Camberwell, London, took as their starting point the fact that the rate of depression was greater in those women of lower social class. They were interested in the question of why this is the case. They took a simple model in order to design their study (Fig. 2.11). This model is no different from that generally used in psychiatry to think about aetiological factors, viz. that there are **predisposing** and **precipitating** factors, which in this context were called **vulnerability factors** and **provoking agents**. They carried out a case control study (Fig. 2.7) and took detailed histories which were designed to do two things. Firstly, to find out about major events occurring in the months prior to the onset of depression. Such events, for example, changes in job, housing and personal relationships, have come to be known as **life-events**, and have been studied a great deal in connection with psychiatric problems. This is because an important theme in psychiatric aetiology is the idea that mental illness is often precipitated by stress which itself is caused by important changes in life.

The second part of the history was to find out about possible vulnerability factors. This covers many of the aspects covered in taking a 'personal history' from a psychiatric patient.

The results of this study showed that the increased rate of depression amongst women of lower social class could be accounted for by an increase in vulnerability factors and provoking agents. Four **vulnerability factors** in particular were identified:

1 the absence of a close, intimate and confiding relationship;
2 the loss of mother before the age of 11 years;
3 having three or more children under 14 living at home;
4 the lack of employment outside the home.

The first of these was found to be the single most important factor and this has been confirmed in subsequent studies. The provoking agents which were important were found to be severe agents which had long-term consequences, for example giving up an enjoyable job to look after an invalid parent.

Another theme in looking at social causes of mental illness has been the role of communication. There is a long history of interest in the possibility that poor communication between family members can contribute to schizophrenia. This idea has proved difficult to research, and there is no good evidence that it is an important **causal** factor. However, there is evidence that if the family tends to make critical comments about the patient then the relapse rate is significantly higher (Chapter 5). In other words aspects of family communication are important in the **outcome** of schizophrenia rather than in its cause.

Family communication and relationships have been studied extensively with regard to child and adolescent problems, and **family therapy**, in which change is brought about in the way family members interact with each other, is now a major form of treatment.

Psychological theories of causation

It is impossible in this chapter to do more than to sketch some of the concepts which psychiatry has taken from psychology. Four areas will be mentioned:
- learning theory;
- cognitive theory;
- psychoanalytic theory;
- personality theory.

These are all areas which have had a profound effect on psychiatric treatment, although the aetiological theories on which the treatment methods are based are less well grounded than the treatments themselves.

In genetic, biochemical and to a large extent in social theories the explanations of mental illnesses are in objective terms. Some approaches to experimental psychology explicitly keep within the bounds of objective explanations, and avoid concepts such as **motives**, **desires**, and **feelings**. The most important of these from the point of view of its

---

Fig. 2.11 A simplified model of the causes of depressive illness used by Brown and Harris

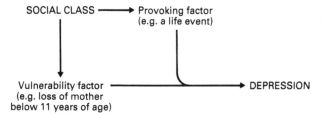

A simplified picture of Brown and Harris' model of the social causes of depression. Depression is seen as the result of a provoking agent acting on a vulnerable person. The association between low social class and depression can be accounted for by the effect of low social class on the frequency of vulnerability factors and provoking agents.

impact on psychiatry is **behaviourism**, with learning theory at its core. At its most extreme this perspective sees the mind as a **black box**, and the rules which govern learning are specified in terms of what objectively describable conditions must obtain in order for learning to take place. But a black box model invites the question of what is inside the box. What is not clear is whether the inner workings of the box can be adequately understood without the use of **subjective** concepts.

Learning theory

Classical conditioning
During the process of learning by **classical conditioning** (first explored by Pavlov) an **unconditioned stimulus** (e.g. the sight of food) and a **conditioned stimulus** (e.g. the sound of a bell) occur simultaneously (or nearly so). Each such occurrence is called a **trial**. The unconditioned stimulus causes some (unconditioned) response (e.g. salivation, in response to the sight of food). Given sufficient trials the animal will salivate in response to the sound of the bell (conditioned stimulus), in the absence of the sight of food (unconditioned stimulus).

This learnt response can be unlearnt (extinguished) if the conditioned stimulus is repeated many times in the absence of the unconditioned stimulus. Thus, if the animal keeps hearing the bell without seeing food, it will, in due course, cease to salivate on hearing the bell.

This principle of extinction has led to the development of 'behaviour therapy'. Consider for example a man who has a phobia for spiders. In behaviour therapy he would be gradually exposed to spiders in increasingly stressful situations (starting for example with small spiders 12 feet away and progressing to large spiders crawling over him). At each stage of treatment he would be helped to relax and to dissipate the feeling of anxiety. Thus by exposing him to spiders under circumstances where little anxiety is felt, the association of spiders with anxiety is gradually extinguished.

The fact that behaviour therapy can be effective treatment does not prove the phobia to have originated by means of classical conditioning. How many people fear spiders because of an accidental association between seeing a spider and an independently anxiety provoking event? Very few, if any. A much more convincing example of classical conditioning encountered in medical practice is sometimes seen in patients who are receiving regular injections of chemotherapy. These drugs when injected often cause nausea. After several injections, patients may come to experience nausea simply on meeting the doctor whom they have come to associate with giving the injections.

Operant conditioning
Operant conditioning plays a much greater part in the aetiology of psychiatric problems than does classical conditioning. This is the form of learning exemplified in the training of animals where rewards are given whenever the animal does (approximately) what you want it to do. It can be very fruitful in the practice of psychiatry to consider what might be the rewards to the patient of behaving in the way which has been identified as the problem. A child whose

---

Fig. 2.12 Examples of classical and operant conditioning in the treatment of psychiatric disorders

Classical conditioning
'Bed and buzzer' treatment for nocturnal enuresis
In this treatment, if the child starts to wet the bed, a buzzer rings. It is unclear why this treatment is effective but classical conditioning may play a part. Thus the buzzer (unconditioned stimulus) wakes the child (unconditioned response). The sensations just prior to wetting the bed (e.g. of urine starting to pass down the urethra) are the conditioned stimulus and lead to the child waking before wetting the bed. This allows conscious delay of urination.

Graded exposure in the treatment of phobias
As is explained in the text, the concept of classical conditioning led to the development of graded exposure as a treatment for phobias. The association of relaxation with the feared situation may be part of the mechanism by which this treatment works. However, the situation is complex and cognitive processes undoubtedly also play a major part.

Operant conditioning
Star charts used for nocturnal enuresis
The reward (a star) is given whenever the child is dry at night and this leads to more and more dry nights.

'Token economy' in the management of people with chronic schizophrenia
On wards which specialize in the treatment of people with chronic schizophrenia, a 'token economy' may be adopted. Essentially patients can 'earn' tokens by behaving in ways considered desirable.

The management of behavioural problems in mental handicap
In people with severe mental handicap it may be difficult to manage disruptive behaviour by talking and listening. In such cases, rewarding the absence of the behaviour will often significantly decrease the frequency of the troublesome behaviour.

---

tantrums are causing endless problems may be being inadvertently rewarded for this behaviour because it is the only time the parents pick the child up and give him or her their attention.

Operant conditioning has also been seen as the mechanism underlying the cause of depressive illness. The idea originates from the rather unpleasant observations that when animals have been given electric shocks from which they cannot escape, they subsequently fail to learn tasks as effectively as before, and they behave in a depressed manner. This has led to a view of depression as 'learned helplessness'. That is, if earlier experience has taught that whatever the person does they cannot escape from unpleasant experiences, they continue to believe this even when it is inappropriate to do so.

Figure 2.12 gives some more examples of the use of classical and operant conditioning in psychiatric treatments.

Cognitive theory
There is increasing interest in the role of beliefs and patterns of thinking in the cause and maintenance of psychiatric disorders. Particular attention has been paid to depressive illness, although other conditions, for example anxiety neurosis, are being analysed in similar fashion. The putative role of beliefs in the cause of depressive illness is shown in

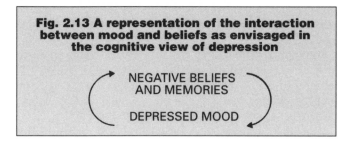

Fig. 2.13. The central idea is that low mood leads to a number of changes in the pattern of thinking. One change is that faulty generalizations of the kind: 'I did badly in that exam therefore I'm useless and stupid' become more persuasive. Another is that unpleasant events in the past are remembered selectively in preference to good (bad exam results are remembered but not good exam results). These changes in thinking lead to lower mood which causes still gloomier thoughts and so a vicious cycle is set up. Cognitive therapy is aimed at confronting patients with the irrationality of their thoughts and seeking to change the pattern of thinking and so to reverse the vicious cycle.

Psychoanalytic theory

In contrast with learning theory, and with the thrust of experimental psychology, psychoanalytic theory not only works explicitly with the concepts of motivation desires, etc., but sees these as being much more pervasive than does 'common sense psychology'. Mental illness is seen as resulting often from conflicts between different unconscious motives and desires. For example the conflict between sexual urges and what is socially acceptable leads to anxiety. According to Freudian theory it is the attempts to reduce this anxiety which lead to neurotic behaviour.

Psychoanalytic theory, however, also has important implications for objective explanations of behaviour. For example, it stresses the importance of the early experiences of children in psychological development, and in particular the attachment of the infant to its mother. This has led to animal experiments, mainly with monkeys. These experiments have shown that abnormal attachment between infant and mother can have a profound and detrimental effect on the former's later social and mothering abilities. It has also led to observational studies in humans. On the basis of these studies, it has been found that some babies appear less secure in their attachment to their mothers. In such cases, the mothers have been found to be less responsive to their babies' needs. The nature of the early attachment of a child to its parents is probably of great importance to the development of the child's self-esteem. A person who experienced parental love as being conditional on his/her achievements is likely to be vulnerable to depression when self-esteem is threatened. The response of a person to bereavement is probably similarly affected by that person's early parental attachment. A secure attachment helps to engender an inner self-esteem which supports the person through the loneliness of the loss.

Personality

What is the connection between personality and mental illness? The history of psychiatry is rich with suggestions that a particular kind of person is prone to develop a particular kind of illness. The term **schizoid** was coined to describe a person who is detached, cold and self-sufficient, because it was believed that such personality characteristics predispose to schizophrenia. The belief in a close connection between personality and illness can lead to the unfortunate consequence that mental illness is seen as an aspect of personality. It is a short step to see mental illness as a weakness and as something shameful.

The evidence suggests that the connection between personality and the major 'psychotic' illnesses is weak. For the **neuroses**, the connection is somewhat stronger. Certain types of personality can be seen as **predisposing** factors in the aetiology of neuroses – in particular high levels of 'neuroticism'. Such people have obsessional traits and are prone to becoming anxious.

The study of the determinants of personality is one of the most difficult areas in psychological research. Within the first few weeks of life, babies can differ one from another in characteristics such as mood and attention span, and these characteristics persist at least into childhood. This observation suggests either that genetic factors or that very early childhood experiences are important in the shaping of personality. The importance of childhood experiences is stressed in psychoanalytic theory. Freudian theory has put emphasis on the importance of the interaction of specific events with the developmental stage of the child. Social learning theory emphasizes the effect of rewards and punishments that a child gets when he or she behaves in various ways.

Conclusion

I have discussed four categories of cause of mental illness and have given an account of the kinds of evidence which may support each category. How do we put all this together?

There is an unfortunate tendency amongst psychiatrists for one or other category of cause to be considered supreme. Thus there are 'biological psychiatrists' who view biochemical and genetic theories of cause as more fundamental and important than other categories and similarly for 'social psychiatrists' and psychologically minded psychiatrists. One of the reasons behind such narrowmindedness is a mistaken view that it is not possible for there to be different kinds of cause for the same event and that, therefore, one kind of cause has to be the **major** cause. Figure 2.2 shows that there are several ways in which different causes for the same event can interrelate.

These different categories of cause are relevant even if one's philosophical view of the mind is at one extreme. To illustrate this I will take as an example a thorough going 'organic' view of depressive illness. On this view depressive illness results if and only if the brain is in a particular state or states. For the sake of exposition I will call this state (or these states) D.

A **biochemical approach** to causation will be aimed at describing the biochemical aspects of state D. **Genetic factors**, clearly, may determine the composition of the brain and may affect the chance of its being in state D. Thus, it is quite clear that both biochemical and genetic theories of causation make sense within this organic account of depression. This is also true of **psychological and social theories**. If one takes the view that mental phenomena depend ultimately on the physical state of the brain, then one must accept that the physical state of the brain is altered by our social and psychological experience. So, for example, if a person's mother dies when that person is still a child, the brain will be affected by this. Experiences involving loss may well alter the brain so as to make it more likely that it will be in state *D*. To describe these changes which take place in the brain in biochemical terms may or may not be more helpful for a particular purpose than to describe the situation in terms of the type of loss experienced by the person. No *a priori* decision can be made as to which approach is more useful. Furthermore when it comes to treatment there can be no *a priori* reason for rejecting physical or psychological methods. Even were we to have a complete physical description of brain state *D*, the best way of changing that state to normal may be through psychological or social means rather than through physical means.

Philosophically there is no reason to prefer one category of causal explanation or treatment. **In clinical practice much is to be gained both in theoretical understanding and in helping patients by thinking about all categories of causal explanation**.

QUESTIONS

1 It has been suggested that unemployment may be a cause of depressive illness. How might you set up a study to investigate this possibility, and what will be the problems in interpreting your results?

2 The prevalence of Alzheimer's disease for those aged 80 years is about 15%. What further information would you require to calculate the annual incidence of the disease? Why do you think that the incidence of the disease is not known?

3 The pharmaceutical company for which you work is putting a large research effort into developing a new drug for the treatment of morbid jealousy. You are asked to advise on the biochemical properties you would be looking for in such a drug. What kinds of research study might help you to give good advice?

4 Sitting in your local pub you overhear an argument about what causes alcohol abuse. One person's view is that it is determined mainly by your genes, whereas the other person is of the opinion that it is the price of alcohol that matters most. What studies might help to resolve the conflict?

Later that evening in a drunken brawl between two customers who are habitual heavy drinkers, the bartender gets seriously hurt. The two customers are eventually found guilty of grievous bodily harm. Could the results of the studies affect your view as to what sentence the court should impose?

5 A patient of yours becomes excessively anxious when travelling on a train. How might the origins of this anxiety be accounted for from the viewpoints of **classical conditioning**, **operant conditioning** and **cognitive theory**?

FURTHER READING

Atkinson R.L., Atkinson R.C., Smith E.E. & Bem D.J. (1993) *Introduction to Psychology*, 11th Edition. Harcourt Brace Jovanovich, Fort Worth. [An excellent and attractively produced book.]

Brown, George W. & Harris, Tirril (1978) *Social Origins of Depression – a Study of Psychiatric Disorder in Women*. Tavistock Publications, London. [Contains the results of a classic study by the authors, and surveys the strengths and weaknesses of applying the social sciences to a study of the aetiology of mental illness.]

Dinan T. (ed.) (1990) *The Principles and Practice of Biological Psychiatry*, Volume 1. CNS Publishers, London. [A general survey which covers the biological basis of psychiatry in more depth than standard textbooks.]

Hart H.L.A. & Honoré T. (1985) *Causation in the Law*, 2nd Edition Oxford University Press, Oxford. [Chapter 1 contains an excellent account of the philosophical problems which surround the concept of *cause*.]

McGuffin P. & Murray R. (eds) (1991) *The New Genetics of Mental Illness*. Butterworth Heinemann, Oxford. [An up-to-date textbook of molecular genetics in relation to psychiatric disorders.]

Tsuang T.S. & Vandermey R. (1980) *Genes and the Mind*. Oxford University Press, Oxford. [A clear, readable and fairly detailed survey of the genetics of mental illness.]

3
Assessment of the Patient

Fact sheet

Aims of psychiatric assessment:
- establish **diagnosis** and **differential diagnosis**;
- identify **causal factors**;
- identify **risks** associated with the illness;
- make a **therapeutic plan**;
- start the **therapeutic process**.

Psychiatric assessment methods
Information from four sources is usually needed:

1 The psychiatric history
The history from the patient and others should aim to do the following.
- Identify the symptoms of illness, their development over time, and the effect on the person's life.
- Detect and understand the significance of factors which caused the illness. These may be: longstanding **predisposing factors** such as family history of illness, or personality; **precipitating factors** such as recent stressful events; or **maintaining factors** such as marital problems.
- Identify factors which influence the management, and outcome of the illness.

The psychiatric history is therefore a structured means of establishing important information. This is recorded under the following headings:
- circumstances of interview;
- account of present problems;
- family history;
- personal history;
- menstrual, marital and sexual history;
- medical, surgical and psychiatric history;
- present life circumstances;
- normal personality.

2 Mental state examination
The main aim is to establish the evidence for mental illness, showing itself during the interview.

Information about a patient's mental state is obtained by making systematic observations and by direct questioning in the following areas of functioning:
- behaviour and appearance;
- mood;
- speech;
- thinking;
- perceptions;
- cognitive abilities (orientation, concentration, memory, intelligence);
- insight.

3 Physical examination
The aim is to exclude:
- physical causes of psychiatric symptoms;
- co-existent physical disorder;
- physical consequences of psychiatric disorder.

4 Further laboratory or special physical investigations; and further psychological, social or occupational assessments
The aim is to assist in correct diagnosis and in planning appropriate management.
- Important laboratory investigations to consider include: Hb, ESR, Fbc, blood glucose, thyroid function tests, liver function tests, serology for syphilis and tests for HIV.
- Important special investigations to consider include: skull and chest X-ray, lumbar puncture, electroencephalogram, electrocardiogram, and brain scan.
- Psychological assessment may identify specific areas of cognitive or behavioural dysfunction.
- Occupational assessment may provide information on impairments of working or living skills.
- Social assessment may provide more information on environmental causative factors, and on impairments of general functioning.

Skills and attitudes needed for psychiatric assessment

1 Interview skills
- Establishing a therapeutic relationship.
- Managing the interview.
- Obtaining information.

2 Diagnostic and management planning skills
- Making a diagnosis.
- Formulating an assessment summary.
- Making a problem orientated care plan.

3 Attitudes towards the patient
- Empathy.
- Self-evaluation.
- Scientific inquiry.
- Ethical considerations.

Circumstances of psychiatric assessment

1 Circumstances leading to the assessment
- Degree of urgency involved.
- Level of anxiety of patient and relatives.
- Expectations of patient, relatives, and referer.

2 Circumstances in which assessment is done
- Home, clinic, GP surgery, etc.
- Appropriate people to be included during the assessment.

3 Consequences of the assessment
- Clear communications.
- Impact on patient and relatives.
- Danger of subsequent diagnostic bias.

Special groups
Children, elderly patients, the dangerous, and people with learning difficulties require modifications of the basic assessment model.

Introduction

Psychiatric illness is highly invasive. It strikes at the heart of how we experience the world. Confidence and sense of identity may be undermined, and grasp of reality distorted or severed.

Assessing psychiatric illness is a necessary first step in providing specialist help. Yet this assessment brings with it special challenges. Perhaps the most formidable is the task of assessing someone else's internal world. You can't slap a stethoscope on the brain; you have to gain the patient's confidence to enable them to disclose their innermost thoughts and experiences. In this way you can painstakingly build up a picture of the patient's internal world.

This relies above all else on a facilitating quality of trust building up between the patient and interviewer. Thus, psychiatric assessment is a deeply interpersonal affair, easily sabotaged by insensitivity on the part of the interviewer. It also comprises a curious mix of science and art in that it combines the rigours of scientific method with the skill of relating in a special therapeutic way to other people. This, of course, is so in medicine generally, but it is especially important in psychiatry where the interviewer is much more likely to be entering the private world of the patient.

Purpose of assessment

A psychiatric assessment is the means by which a diagnosis of mental illness is established and an appropriate therapeutic plan of action made.

The assessment encompasses a wide area of enquiry covering psychological, social and illness factors both in the present and the past. This is necessary partly because the diagnosis of psychiatric illness requires a meticulous assembly of evidence from across a wide range of symptoms and areas of functioning; and partly because the causation of psychiatric illness often involves a complex interaction of long-term vulnerability factors and more recent precipitating and maintaining stressors which have to be understood if an effective management plan is to be found.

Thus a psychiatric assessment must do more than just focus on the conspicuous features of illness. It must actively delve behind the scenes, building up a three-dimensional picture of the psychological and social context in which the illness arises.

There are five key tasks to achieve in any psychiatric assessment. These are as follows:

Diagnosis

This depends on the build-up of information from a number of sources, and involves looking for patterns of symptoms or clinical features which provide evidence of illness. A range of diagnoses is initially considered giving a differential diagnosis which by further enquiry or investigation can usually be narrowed down to a favoured diagnosis. Differentiating between illness and normality can sometimes be problematic in psychiatry: for example in assessing whether a person's psychological and physical symptoms following the death of a loved one are normal given the circumstances, or whether they go beyond normality into the realm of illness.

Causative factors

An understanding of why a particular individual should develop an illness at a particular time is central to appreciating causality. Causative factors can be usefully grouped into vulnerability factors, for example a family or personal history of illness; precipitating factors, for example loss of a job or relationship; and maintaining factors, for example ongoing family tensions or social isolation. Since relevant causative factors may not be volunteered or even appreciated by the patient, careful history taking is important. This needs to take into account not just the nature of past and current events, but also the special significance these events have for the individual. The same event can have a totally different impact on differing people, depending on the meaning attached. For example a diagnosis of angina can be shrugged off by some, yet experienced as life shattering by others who see it as evidence of declining health and loss of former physical prowess.

The importance of a good understanding of causation lies in the way this will influence the therapeutic plan. For example focusing on persisting causative factors such as job or relationship stresses may play an important part not only in helping to resolve a current illness, but in reducing the risk of a subsequent relapse.

Risks associated with the illness

Some psychiatric illnesses are associated with high-risk consequences such as suicidal behaviour or impulses to harm others. Other less spectacular risks include progressive self-neglect or reduced ability to take proper safety precautions at work or while driving. Often these potentially harmful even fatal consequences of illness are not immediately obvious, and need to be the focus of careful enquiry. Evaluating these risks is an important part of every psychiatric assessment.

Therapeutic plan

Once a diagnosis is made, and the relevant causal and risk factors taken into account, a therapeutic plan can be discussed with the patient and action agreed. It is useful for such plans to be problem orientated and subject to regular review. A therapeutic plan may also include an account of the likely outcome or prognosis for the patient.

Starting the therapeutic process

A psychiatric assessment can be therapeutic of itself by providing an opportunity to unburden difficulties and feelings to someone who listens; by enabling greater insight and understanding of influential problems; by bringing rationale to a previous sense of chaos and lost control; by giving hope of relief or recovery; and finally by the creation of an all important trusting relationship with the interviewer, without which help may neither be accepted nor complied with.

These five tasks seem straightforward enough, but of course problems inevitably arise. Patients may not be cooperative, or they may lack insight and believe they do not have a problem. On the whole however, those assessed are likely to

Fig. 3.1 Taking a psychiatric history

Checklist	Checklist (continued)

Circumstances of the interview
- Date and place of interview
- Source of referral
- Reason for referral
- Informant including their name, relationship to patient, and an impression of their reliability

Account of present problems

Main problems volunteered by patient?
- Nature of problem
- Date of onset
- Duration
- Severity

Include psychiatric and physical symptoms together with social, relationship or work difficulties

Associated problems?
- Include problems not necessarily volunteered by the patient
- These may include disturbances of concentration, appetite, weight, etc.

Understanding of onset of problems?
Was onset related to any particular factor or event? If so, describe in detail nature of event and relationship to onset of problems

Understanding the development of the problems?
- How did the problems develop?
- When were they at their worst?
- Have there been any changes in the development of the problem?
- If so, was this related to any particular factors or events?
- Are there factors which increase or decrease the severity of the problems?

Effects of the problem?
Effects on the following activities
- Work
- Domestic tasks
- Leisure activities, interests
- Social activities
- Family and other relationships
- Sexual activities

Treatment so far?
- Nature and effects of psychological or physical treatment given
- Dose and duration of any psychotrophic medication given, together with an assessment of compliance

Patient's understanding of the problems?
Attitude to and understanding of problems

Patients resources and strengths?
- Identify strengths in patient and existing helping resources such as family and friends as shown during the development of the problems

Family history

Parents
- Ages, or age at death
- Cause of death
- Health
- Occupation
- Personality

Siblings
- Ages
- Marital status
- Health
- Occupation
- Personality

Family history
Mental illness, personality disorder, epilepsy, alcoholism, or important medical conditions. Where family members have similar problems, describe in as much detail as possible, including nature of treatment and outcome

Family relationships
The influence these have had on patient from childhood to the present time

Family events
- Important family events in patient's early years
- Physical and/or sexual abuse

Personal history

Early development
Details of
- Pregnancy
- Birth
- Habit training problems (e.g. incontinence)
- Developmental milestones (e.g. talking)

Childhood
- Health
- Early neurotic traits (e.g. stammer, fears, school refusal)

School
- Age when attended
- Number and type of schools
- Academic and non-academic progress
- Relationships with peers and teachers

Higher education/occupations
- Higher education progress
- List of jobs, duration of jobs
- Reason for job changes
- Current employment situation
- Current job satisfaction
- Current financial situation

Menstrual history
- Age of menarche
- Menstrual pattern
- Premenstrual tension
- Pain
- Date of last period
- Menopause (if appropriate)

Sexual history
- Heterosexual and homosexual experience
- Contraception
- Current sexual practice and attitudes
- History of any sexual problems
- History of sexually transmitted diseases

Marital history
- Length of courtship
- Age and circumstances when married
- Age, occupation, health and personality of spouse
- Details of live births, stillbirths and abortions
- Children's ages, names, health, personality
- Quality of marital relationship

Continued

Fig. 3.1 (Continued)

Checklist (continued)

Past medical and surgical history	• Past medical disorders and review of recent physical health • Include accidents, allergic reactions and drug intolerances • Include current or recent medication for physical disorder
Past psychiatric history	Episodes where treatment received • Date • Nature and duration of symptoms • Effects on work, social and relationship functioning • Nature of treatment, and response • Hospital and doctor concerned • Include GP, and specialist treated episodes Episodes where no medical help sought • Specify date, nature and duration of symptoms, and effects on functioning
Present life situation	• Housing • Composition of household • Social contacts and supports • Finances
Personality (NB. Informant other than patient needed)	*Lifelong personality traits* Useful checklist comprises • Worry prone/anxiety prone • Depressive prone • Self-depreciative/lack self-confidence • Overdependency on others • Immature, need for attention • Impulsive, irritable • Overmeticulous, perfectionist • Introspective, emotionally cool • Suspicious, jealously prone • Antisocial, lack of feeling for others *Lifelong coping resources* Usual capacity to cope with life's stresses in the past *Social, work, and relationship adjustments* • Ability to make and keep friendships • Ability to maintain close relationships • Hobbies and interests *Beliefs and attitudes* • Religious and moral • Attitude to own health *Habits* • Food and tobacco • Alcohol and drugs *History of offending* • include alcohol/drug-related offences • outcomes, e.g. probation order, prison, etc.
Information check	• Is the information you have reliable? • Are there any omissions? • Do you need to contact further informants? • What must you be particularly sure to concentrate on in mental state examination?

work hard with the interviewer in the process of clarifying and understanding their problems.

Who should be familiar with psychiatric assessment techniques?

All health professionals should have a basic knowledge of the techniques used to identify and assess patients who may have mental illness.

This is because over 95% of patients with mental illness are managed by general practice teams, and never see a psychiatrist. Similarly, patients in hospital because of physical disorder, but who also have mental illness, are usually not seen by a psychiatrist.

Hence, a wide range of health workers, particularly doctors and nurses both in hospital and the community, should be familiar with basic mental health assessment techniques. This will keep them alert to the possibility of mental illness, will help them best manage the illness, and will help in making appropriate decisions concerning referral for more specialist assessment or help.

How does psychiatric assessment differ from medical assessment?

There are three main ways in which psychiatric assessments differ.

• *Assessment may be more time consuming.* This is because psychiatric diagnosis rarely depends on any single clinical or laboratory test. Instead it relies on a painstaking build-up of precisely defined features, a diagnosis only being made when certain combinations of features are found (see Chapter 1).

• *Other informants are particularly invaluable.* This is because many features of psychiatric illness may be distorted, or even omitted, in the patient's inevitably subjective account. For example, the relevance of recent stressful events, the contribution of long-standing personality characteristics, or a slowly progressive decline in functioning not noticed by the patient.

• *Patients are likely to feel particularly vulnerable.* There are two main reasons for this. First, the patient may feel a failure having to seek help at all. This is because for many people there is still a degree of stigma attached to psychiatric illness. Admitting to emotional problems may therefore be hard, especially it seems for men. On the whole our society values competitiveness and individual achievement, and emotional or psychiatric vulnerability is often experienced as failure. The act of seeking help may therefore be accompanied by feelings of shame and self-consciousness, which are rarely encountered in other branches of medicine.

Second, the patient is likely to be disclosing their innermost painful thoughts and feelings, perhaps putting them into words for the first time. However, it is crucial that they are able to do this in order for the interviewer to carry out the assessment. Thus reliance on the enabling therapeutic realtionship is especially important in psychiatry. Indeed a brusque or indifferent clinical manner is likely to be particularly damaging, since it may result in important diagnostic information being withheld, as well as making the patient less likely to engage in treatment.

Fig. 3.2 The mental state examination
(For a more detailed description of individual symptoms see Chapter 1)

Behaviour and appearance

Important observations may be made as the patient walks in the door.

Social manner
- Disinhibition, e.g. in mania.
- Physical tension together with signs of anxiety, such as sweating, blushing or rapid and shallow breathing.
- Withdrawal, poor eye contact, e.g. in depression.

Dress
Self-neglect, flamboyancy.

Movement
- Reduced, e.g. in parkinsonism, severe depression, some schizophrenic patients.
- Increased, e.g. in agitation, restlessness or overactivity.
- Abnormal movements, e.g. fine tremor of hands, facial movements of drug induced oral dyskinesia.

Psychodynamic
E.g. a patient appearing very regressed or immature in behaviour; a patient denying the obvious importance of critical aspects of their problem; an overcritical distressed or angry relative.

Mood

- Mood is assessed by combining observations of behaviour and appearance, particularly facial expression and posture, with what the patient tells you about how he's feeling, e.g. depression, anxiety, anger, emotional and physical tension, elation.
- Some moods rely on your observations rather than what the patient tells you, e.g., perplexity, suspiciousness, irritability, incongruity or blunting of affect, emotional lability.
- Some moods have associated features to look out for, e.g. depression and suicidal thoughts; suspiciousness and persecutory ideas; incongruity of affect and schizophrenia; emotional lability and dementia.

Speech

Quantity of speech
- Rapid speech, e.g. in elated or very anxious patients. Can result in incoherence.
- Slow speech, e.g. in depressed, suspicious or uncooperative patients.
- Muteness, e.g. in severe depression, schizophrenia or certain organic states.

Quality of speech
- Speech difficulties, e.g. dysarthria, dysphasia or stammer.
- Flatness or excitability of speech.
- Creation of new idiosyncratic words as in neologisms.

Thinking

Altered stream of thoughts
- Altered speed of thinking, e.g. accelerated or retarded thinking. This can be inferred from the patient's speech, or asked about directly.
- Discontinuity of thinking, e.g. perseveration of thoughts, or thought blocking.

Altered connection between thoughts
The thoughts themselves may be normal, but there is a lack of coherence in the way they are linked together, making the person's train of thought hard to follow, e.g. 'knight's move' thinking (positive formal thought disorder) or concrete thinking (negative formal thought disorder tested by proverb interpretation: p. 9).

Altered control or possession of thoughts
- Loss of control of thoughts, e.g. obsessional thoughts (which recur against the patient's will).
- Loss of possession of thoughts, e.g. thought insertion and withdrawal, thought broadcasting (thoughts are no longer the patient's own: these experiences are known as passivity phenomena).

Abnormal content of thinking
1 Abnormal thoughts and worries.
- Morbid beliefs or fears, as in ideas of guilt and suicide in depression, or fears of collapse in anxiety.
- Overvalued ideas (distinguish from delusional beliefs).
- Ideas of self-reference, where chance observations may be misinterpreted as having some special persecutory or depressive meaning particular to the patient.
2 Delusional beliefs.
- False unshakeable beliefs out of keeping with a person's educational and cultural background are called delusions. They arise from internal morbid processes.
- People may be unforthcoming about their delusional beliefs, e.g. if they are of a persecutory nature. Following up hints of underlying beliefs, such as suspiciousness, is important.
- Record what the patient tells you about the beliefs, writing this down verbatim where possible. Challenge beliefs to test their incorrigibility. If the patient expresses doubt, then the belief is not delusional at that time.
- Distinguish between primary and the more common secondary delusional beliefs.
- Delusional beliefs may be of persecution, jealousy, grandiosity, hypochondriasis, guilt, poverty or nihilism.
- Beware! Certain delusional beliefs may be associated with at-risk behaviour, e.g. morbid (delusional) jealousy of a spouse's fidelity is associated with a risk of assault.

Continued

Fig. 3.2 *(Continued)*

Perception

Sensory distortions and illusions
- A sensory distortion results in a change in the perceived intensity or quality of the stimulus. e.g. in depression voices may seem very distant; in drug induced states there may be heightened perception.
- An illusion is a misperception of a real stimulus, e.g. a depressed man thinks that the shadow of a lampost on his curtains is the gallows.

Hallucinations
1 Hallucinations are perceptions without any external stimulus. They can be of hearing (the most common, usually voices), vision (second most common, often associated with organic states), and smell, taste or touch (all less common).
2 Abnormal perceptions are commonly not volunteered by the patient, and should be carefully inquired about. Clues that the patient may be hallucinating include:
- episodes of apparent distraction, when he may be listening to voices;
- apparent unpredictable outbursts, responding to voices, arguing back;
- a history of regularly talking or muttering to himself.
3 Distinguish between true and pseudohallucinations.

Other abnormal perceptions
e.g. Déjà vu, jamais vu.

Cognitions

Cognitive impairments may indicate organic aetiology. (More detailed assessment details pp. 131–135.)

Orientation
- Orientation in time. Usually indicates an altered level of conciousness caused by an organic state, although it may occur in chronic dementia and acute (non-organic) psychotic states where contact with reality is severely disturbed. Test by asking time of day, day of week, date and year.
- Orientation in place and person: disturbance usually indicates altered level of consciousness. Test by asking where patient thinks he is, how he got there, who you are, etc.
- Disorientation is usually worse at night due to lack of sensory cues.

Recent memory
1 The ability to register information. Test by asking the patient to immediately repeat name and address you give.
2 The ability to recall recent information. Test by:
- ask patient for details of recent events that can be checked, e.g. what did they have for their last meal;
- give 'name and address'. Check that patient has registered the information. Ask them to repeat the name and address after 5 minutes.

Remote memory
1 The ability to recall information learnt before the onset of any memory difficulties, and after a considerable time has elapsed. Test by:
- asking about general knowledge, e.g. key dates (the Second World War) or people (a Prime Minister);
- asking about the patient's knowledge in an area familiar to him (date of marriage, number of flowers known if a gardener).
2 Take into account the patient's age and normal intelligence. Watch for gaps of knowledge, confabulation or perseveration which may indicate organic impairment.

Concentration
1 Apparent poor concentration may be due to a number of causes:
- distraction by intrusive thoughts or abnormal perceptions;
- impaired reasoning, as in formal thought disorder;
- impaired concentration ability, as in severe depression or delirium.
2 Concentration problems may present with poor ability to cope with complex questions, with a tendency to stray off the point, to get lost or to give up easily. Tests of concentration are:
- serial sevens ($100 - 7 = 93$, $93 - 7 = 86$, etc.);
- months of the year backwards;
- ask patient to immediately repeat a sequence of digits you give, firstly forwards (normal digit span 6–7) then backwards (normal span 5).

General intelligence level
- Previous levels can be assessed from education and work history.
- Present level by history, simple tasks, and clinical impression.

Insight

Patient's attitude and beliefs
- Towards the illness.
- Towards the consequences of and limitations imposed by the illness.
- Towards any help offered.

Fig. 3.3 Mental state examination: checklist of sample questions

Introductory questions.

I would like to get an idea of the problems that have been troubling you recently. What have been the main difficulties?...Can you say more about that?...Is there anything else that has been troubling you?...Could you give me an example?

Mood	How have you been feeling in yourself recently?...Have you felt anxious or frightened?...or irritable?...How have you felt in your spirits?...How did it affect you?...
Speech	(In slow speech or muteness) I recognize you find it hard to put things into words: you can indicate your answer by a movement of your head.
Thinking	Do you ever experience your thoughts stopping, quite unexpectedly so that there are none left in your mind even when your thoughts were flowing freely before? (thought block).
	Do you spend a lot of time on tidyness or cleanliness or constantly double checking things?...get worried about contamination with germs?...get terrible thoughts coming into your mind despite trying to stop them?...What happens when you try to stop? (obsessional thoughts and rituals).
	Are thoughts (*not* voices) ever put into your head which are not your own? (thought insertion)....Or do you ever seem to hear your own thoughts spoken aloud in your head so that others could actually hear what you were thinking?...Give me an example...How do you explain this? (thought broadcasting).
	How do you see the future?...Have you felt life wasn't worth living?...felt like ending it all?...How might you do it?...How close have you got to doing that?...What has prevented you so far? (suicidal thoughts and plans).
	Have you ever felt people were against you in any way?...wish to hurt or harm you?...How do you explain this?...Do you have any doubts at all about what you have told me? (persecutory beliefs).
	Have you ever felt under the control of a force or power other than yourself?...like a robot with no will of its own?...Does this force take over your movements?...Can you resist? (delusions of control; passivity feelings).
Perceptions	Is there anything unusual about the way things sound, or look or smell or taste? (perceptual distortion).
	Do you ever hear noises or voices that others may not hear?...What do the voices say?...Do they talk to you or about you?...Do you hear them when you are alone?...Do you hear voices inside your head (pseudohallucinations) or through your ears (true hallucinations)?
	Do you ever see things that others couldn't see?...with your eyes or in your mind?...when you are fully awake?
Cognitions	Have you had any lapses of memory recently?...times when you've completely forgotten what happened?...had to start making lists?
	Do your thoughts tend to be muddled or slow?...Can you make up your mind about simple things fairly easily? (subjective assessment of inefficient thinking).
	What has your concentration been like recently?...Could you read an article, watch a television programme right through?...Do your thoughts tend to wander so you don't take in things?
Insight	Do you think there is anything the matter with you?...What?...Do you feel you need any form of help?

Learning to carry out psychiatric assessments

In any assessment a lot is going on at a number of levels all at the same time: gathering information, analysis, hypothesis, therapy even, and more. The assessment process will therefore be broken down into its component parts, each described in turn.

In order to carry out a psychiatric assessment you need three things: (a) a knowledge of the psychiatric illnesses; (b) a knowledge of assessment methods including structured history taking and mental state examination; and (c) the necessary interview and diagnostic skills and attitudes to use these methods sensitively and to good effect.

The psychiatric assessment methods together with the skills and attitudes needed to apply them will now be covered in turn.

Psychiatric assessment methods

Psychiatric assessment involves taking a detailed history, examining the patient's mental and physical state, and arranging for further investigations where appropriate.

The psychiatric history

History taking is central to any psychiatric assessment for two reasons: firstly, it generates information essential to the process of making a psychiatric diagnosis and management plan; secondly, it is a vehicle for getting to know the patient and, of course, for the patient to know you. This is important not only in enabling the patient to share their innermost thoughts and feelings, but also in enlisting their cooperation in any help or advice you may recommend.

Structure of the psychiatric history

Information from the patient's history is collected systematically under a number of sub-headings similar to those used in general medicine. These are listed in Fig. 3.1 together with explanatory notes about the importance of each sub-heading. The sub-headings also act as a useful checklist, to ensure that important areas of enquiry are not left out by mistake.

Order in which information is obtained

Although you should guide the patient to unfold information in the order given in Fig. 3.1 flexibility is needed since the patient may need to relate information in their own way. You should certainly not stick rigidly to the interview structure at all costs; this would be insensitive and might jeopardize your relationship with the patient.

However, information should always be recorded in a clear, organized and chronological fashion, since records are an important means of communicating with other professionals.

Quality of information obtained

It is important that information obtained during history taking is as accurate and comprehensive as possible. Unreliable or omitted information may influence diagnostic and management decisions. Thus where possible, relatives or close friends should be interviewed. In addition, contacting other professionals involved, obtaining past medical records or even (with the patient's permission) obtaining information about functioning at work may all help in the building up of a thorough assessment.

The mental state examination

The purpose of the mental state examination is to detect abnormal features in a patient's behaviour and state of mind at the time of the assessment. If abnormal features are found this information contributes to the diagnostic process.

The examination consists of systematic observations of the patient during the interview, together with specific inquiries into various aspects of their thinking, feelings, perceptions and cognitive functioning.

These specific areas of inquiry are usually done after the history taking, since by this time the patient is more familiar with the interviewer.

Where the patient has impairments which make interviewing difficult, such as memory, orientation, or concentration problems, these should be assessed first since the impairments will influence the way you carry out the assessment.

Although the mental state examination is mainly designed to detect abnormal symptoms, such as false beliefs or the hearing of voices, observations of psychodynamic abnormalities should also be made. For example, a denial of feeling concerning a recent bereavement; or a tendency to deflect all responsibility for self onto others. Such observations may reflect lifelong personality traits, or they may be a temporary result of stress or psychiatric illness.

Observations of psychodynamics are also important when interviewing a family, or couples. The way the family or couple interact during the interview may give important clues to both the contributing causes of the problem (as in the case of the overcritical relatives of a patient relapsing with schizophrenia) and to the type of help you should offer.

Structure of the mental state examination

Observations are grouped into seven broad categories, and these are summarized in Fig. 3.2 together with explanatory notes.

As with history taking, it is not always possible to elicit features in the order outlined in Fig. 3.2. However, they should always be recorded in this way.

Three additional points are worth stressing.

1 Establish individual features of symptoms with as much accuracy as possible. This is because they may be of critical diagnostic importance. In practice, this means asking the patient to describe the feature of symptom **in detail**. Avoid putting words into the patient's mouth and where possible carefully record the patient's own words. To establish whether all the characteristics of a specific symptom are present, be prepared to ask further supplementary questions. Familiarity with the characteristics of symptoms is important, and refer to a glossary when in doubt. Time spent in clearly establishing the presence and character of individual symptoms is rarely wasted. This is particularly true of the more unusual symptoms such as obsessional thoughts or ideas of reference.

2 Follow-up earlier clues or warning signs. For example, if there is a family history of suicide, be sure to establish whether the patient has had thoughts of suicide. Or if a relative has complained that the patient has become increasingly forgetful, be sure to carefully test for cognitive impairment.

3 Because the mental state examination **focuses on the 'here and now'** it may alter over short periods of time. Indeed, consecutive examinations are an important part of evaluating progress. You should be careful therefore to distinguish between recent and current features.

The physical examination

A physical examination should be done where indicated, and this is particularly important in the following circumstances.

1 Where physical symptoms such as weight loss, or pain are present.

2 Where the psychiatric state is atypical, for example first time depression in a late middle-aged woman with no obvious precipitants.

3 Where the patient has a history of potentially relevant physical disorder, for example a history of endocrine disorder, or treatment of carcinoma.

4 Where the nature of the psychological features suggests an underlying physical cause, as for example in the case of progressive memory impairment, amnesia, or florid visual hallucinations.

Further assessment methods

In order to complete a psychiatric assessment, further investigations may be needed as indicated:

Laboratory or special physical investigations

The most relevant laboratory investigations are ESR, haemogloblin and full blood count, liver function tests, thyroid function tests, serology for syphilis and screening for illicit drugs. The most relevant special investigations are X-rays, EEGs, brain scans and ECGs. Testing for HIV antibodies or infection may also be indicated on occasions (see p. 146).

Non-medical assessment: by a social worker, psychologist or occupational therapist

A **social worker** may gain valuable social background information, usually by visiting the patient's home. If social factors such as isolation, debt or housing problems have influenced the development or continuation of the illness, social worker intervention can then be considered for the management plan.

A **clinical psychologist** can provide detailed assessments of a patient's cognitive functioning, for example if cognitive impairments are suspected which may indicate focal or generalized cerebral pathology. In addition, clinical psychologists assess suitability for an increasing range of cognitive behavioural therapies and coping techniques; for example exposure therapy for agoraphobia, social skills training for those with chronic social skills problems, and anxiety and stress management training for those with anxiety or stress-related problems.

An **occupational therapist** is able to assess a patient's occupational, self-care and general living skills, either during a home visit or during hospital attendance. This form of assessment is particularly useful for those with chronic mental health problems, and those recovering from an acute illness.

Extended behavioural or mental state assessment

This can be done either during day attendance, or alternatively during a brief hospital admission. It would be used if more information about the patient's symptoms, level of functioning and potential risk factors is needed than could be obtained during an interview; or alternatively if a series of special investigations need to be completed quickly.

The assessment of risk of suicide or dangerousness is covered in further detail in Chapters 19 and 24.

Skills and attitudes needed for psychiatric assessment

The methods just described give you a system of obtaining information. But they only tell you **what** to do. **How** to obtain the information, and **what to do with it** depends

---

Fig. 3.4 Establishing a good relationship with the patient

Be genuine	A friendly, open and non-judgemental manner will help gain the patient's trust and confidence.
Communicate clearly	Avoid jargon. Use plain English. Use words the patient has used (e.g. feeling *low*).
Be empathic	• Show concern. For example, don't constantly ask questions, but make occasional empathic remarks such as 'That must have been a very difficult time for you'. The patient will then feel he is being taken seriously. • Avoid burying your head in notes. Look at your patient. Employ 'active listening'.
Deal with your patient's emotions appropriately	• Intense emotions may be stirred up during an interview, for example, weeping. It is usually best to acknowledge the emotion in a supportive way, and then to facilitate it. Associated thoughts and triggers should be gently inquired about. As a result, both you and your patient may reach a clearer and deeper understanding of the problem. • Physical contact: sometimes a touch on the elbow or shoulder from the interviewer may help the patient through a time when they feel especially vulnerable in the interview. • Be cautious, however, about facilitating emotions of anger or irritability, particularly in patients with personality disorders or psychotic illnesses.
Monitor your own feelings about the patient	*Affection* It is usual and therapeutic to feel affection for the patient. However, avoid overinvolvement, which the patient may feel as burdensome, and which may interfere with your ability to take objective decisions. If you begin to feel overinvolved with a patient, for example by identifying very strongly with them, then do discuss these feelings with a supervisor. *Frustration, irritation or dislike* • These feelings are less common, but inevitably occur. Monitor whether you are acting out such feelings, for example by giving the patient less time. Do not share these feelings with the patient, but do discuss them with a supervisor. Unchecked, these feelings may be harmful to the patient. • Other feelings include fear or uncomfortableness (e.g. with severely paranoid patients), the feeling of being manipulated (e.g. with a personality disordered patient), or a feeling of being very worried (e.g. with a suicidal depressed patient). Being aware of these feelings is important, since they may influence decisions you take about the patient. • Some feelings towards a patient may be triggered from the interviewer's own past experience. For example, if the interviewer grew up feeling intimidated by an authoritarian parent he may continue to feel intimidated in the presence of similar older figures later in life, making certain groups of patients difficult to interview. This 'transference' of feelings may not be obvious to the interviewer. Discussion with a supervisor may help detect and understand these responses (see also p. 227).

Fig. 3.5 Managing the interview as a whole

Before seeing the patient

Prepare yourself
- Read any available information carefully.
- Get the patient's name right.
- Dress appropriately.
- Be a good time-keeper.

Prepare the setting
- Use a quiet room.
- Place interviewer's and interviewee's chairs at right angles to each other.
- If desk is used, it is often best to place the patient beside this rather than on the other side of it.
- Avoid placing yourself in front of a bright window.

Other informants
If patient is accompanied: always see patient first.

The beginning of the interview

Introductions and explanations
- Introduce yourself fully. If you are a student, explain this.
- Explain the purpose and duration of the interview.
- Explain about note taking and confidentiality.
- Explain how the interview time will be used, i.e. an opportunity for patient to describe problems; your need to ask questions about their background; and finally the fact that you will then discuss your understanding of the problems with them, together with any advice concerning treatment.

Anticipate concerns
Many patients may be concerned or reluctant to see someone about psychological problems. Where appropriate, invite the patient to discuss these concerns.

Invite the patient to describe the problem
The patient should have ample opportunity to do this, in their own words.

The interview proper

Control
Maintain control of the interview to ensure that all areas of inquiry can be covered in the time available.

Flexibility
Be flexible in the order in which information is obtained. All areas of history taking and mental state examination must be covered, but not necessarily in a rigid order.

Facilitation
- Help the patient tell you what you need to know not only by direct questioning, but by giving reinforcing comments or gestures when you are told something important.
- Periodically summarize to the patient your understanding of what you've been told. This reassures the patient that you are listening, helps keep the interview focused and double checks information gained.

The end of the interview

Summarize to the patient
Appropriately summarize your assessment and opinion in a clear way to the patient.

Check patient's understanding
Ensure that your patient understands the main points you have explained.

Decision making
Include the patient as much as possible in any decision making. Where appropriate, also include relatives.

Clear plan of action
Summarize the final plan of action agreed upon, and again check that all involved are clear on the main points. Also, check that you have your patient's consent for any further actions such as contacting relatives.

---

firstly on interview and diagnostic skills, and secondly on the attitude of mind with which you approach your patient and his problems.

Each of these areas will now be dealt with. You should remember, however, that skills and attitudes cannot be learnt from books. You need on-the-job experience, with appropriate training, supervision and discussion. What follows is given as a checklist to augment that practical experience, drawing together the main elements of the skills and attitudes involved.

Interview skills
All health workers who see patients need good interview skills, and this is particularly important for those who see

Fig. 3.6 Obtaining information

Care in observation	In addition to systematic observations described under history taking and mental state examination, **watch for clues:** as when a person shows increased emotion when talking about a particular situation. This may lead you to an important area of inquiry. **Watch for omissions or inconsistencies:** sometimes information that is withheld from the history may be just as important as what is reported, e.g. the existence of an extramarital affair.
Care in questioning	The phrasing of questions tends to alter during an assessment interview. Initially, questions are 'open-ended', whilst later they become much more specific and are then termed 'closed questions'. **Open-ended questions:** these are non-specific questions designed to allow the patients to express problems in their own way and ensure a wide trawl for information, e.g. 'Tell me, what brought you here today?' or 'You say you are feeling low, could you tell me about that?'. **Closed questions:** focus on eliciting specific items of information, e.g. 'How has your sleep been recently' . . . At what time do you wake?' . . . 'How long has that been for?' . . . Note that there are degrees of openness and closedness in questions. **Avoid asking questions which imply the answer or questions that can be answered with a simple yes or no:** this is because patients often have a tendency to say what they believe the interviewer wishes to hear. Consequently the answers will be of doubtful validity, e.g. avoid asking 'Do you feel worse in your spirits when you wake up in the morning?'. Instead ask 'Is there any time when you feel worse in your spirits?'
Quality of information	**Don't make assumptions about information:** inquire into each feature on its own merits. For example, just because a person is depressed, it doesn't mean that he is failing to cope in various areas of his life. These other features should be inquired about separately. **Confirm information with the patient:** repeat your understanding of key events, problems or symptoms back to the patient to check their correctness. **Confirm information with other informants:** this should be done where possible, and with the patient's consent.

patients with mental health problems. In relation to psychiatric assessment, these skills are needed to do the following:

- build up a good relationship with the patient;
- manage the assessment interview as a whole;
- obtain information important to the diagnostic process.

Each of these areas is described in further detail in Figs 3.4–3.6.

To learn interviewing skills, first you must understand what they consist of (Figs 3.4–3.6); then as early as possible sit in on assessments done by experienced interviewers. This will give you the opportunity to observe their technique. Then, you should start to interview patients yourself, obtaining regular feedback from a supervisor. This feedback can be either by discussion about the assessment; by jointly looking at a videotaped recording of your interview; by rehearsing an interview using role play; or by inviting your supervisor to sit with you during an assessment. Ideally a combination of these methods should be used, videotaped recordings being a particularly potent form of learning interview skills.

Diagnostic and management planning skills

Diagnostic skills are needed to convert a mass of information about a patient into a reasoned diagnosis and appropriate plan of action.

The skills are not easy to define, but include the following three main elements.

1 Sifting and categorizing of information. The aim is to pick out patterns of clinical features suggestive of particular diagnoses, or aetiologies.

2 Making judgements about the relative importance of information. The aim is to evaluate the significance of information. For example, judgements need to be made about

the relative importance of causative factors in the patient's illness; about the seriousness of risk factors; and about the relevance of certain symptoms.

3 Decision making. Decisions are usually the main outcome of an assessment, and will include choices in diagnoses and management.

In practice, the diagnostic process takes place in parallel with information gathering, and both start the moment you see the patient.

These two activities are closely interrelated, each constantly influencing the other. For example, your focus of questioning will be influenced by the diagnoses you are considering; in turn, new information may cause you to think of alternative diagnoses, or causative factors.

Making a diagnosis

An early task in the assessment interview is to consider a provisional differential diagnosis. Initially, this should be overinclusive. As the interview proceeds, more information is sifted and arguments for and against particular diagnoses and causative factors emerge more clearly. However, constant revision may be needed in the light of new information. It is also important not to make a firm diagnosis too early, since this may bias the way you collect and interpret subsequent information. Always try to keep an open mind until you are satisfied you have assembled all the data you need.

Making a care plan

Towards the end of the interview when a much clearer idea of the diagnosis and relevant aetiological factors has been developed, a care plan together with an assessment of the prognosis can be considered.

A care plan should have two main features. Firstly, it

should be problem orientated. Secondly, it should distinguish between immediate plans and longer term plans.

A problem orientated plan summarizes the problems relevant to the patient's mental health and lists actions to address these problems. The problems themselves may be psychological (e.g. depression, suicidal impulses), social (e.g. isolation, lack of day activity) and physical (e.g. untreated hypotension, early dementia).

When patients are admitted to hospital, the Department of Health requires that they have a care plan on discharge. The plan is drawn up with the full participation of the patient and circulated to key people involved including relatives or carers where the patient is in agreement. Care plans are particularly important if patients have severe illness with a number of ongoing psychiatric needs (p. 67).

Distinguishing between immediate and longer term plans is important. After an assessment, some actions may need to be taken immediately. For example, admitting a suicidal patient to hospital. Other actions will be less urgent. For example, reducing social isolation by gradually building up day activities at a centre.

The prognosis of a patient's illness can never be predicted with certainty. Helpful indicators include outcome after previous illnesses, speed of onset of illness, the resolvability of any relevant stress factors, the extent to which the illness fully resolves after an acute episode, and the coping resources and personality of the individual concerned. The likely long-term outcome of the illness is a frequent and understandable concern for patients and relatives, and information and counselling in this area is often needed.

Fig. 3.7 Assessment summary

Introduction	Outline the presenting problem.	Mrs A. is a 25-year-old housewife with a 3-year history of increasing difficulty in getting out of the house.
Differential diagnosis	• Consider each possible diagnosis in turn in order of their probability. • Concisely assemble evidence for and against each diagnosis. • Include only evidence which discriminates between different diagnoses. • Don't forget to include organic states if there is sufficient evidence.	**Agoraphobia**: on leaving the house, Mrs A. experiences episodes of panic characterized by physical symptoms of palpitations and breathlessness, and thoughts of fearfulness. As a result, she avoids leaving the house. She experiences no anxiety when at home. **Depression**: Mrs A. has been weepy, sad, and lost interest in household activities in recent months. However, she has not experienced biological symptoms of depression such as early morning wakening, and she has had no thoughts of suicide. **Thyrotoxicosis**: Mrs A. has a fine tremor and a preference for the cold. However, her weight has been steady and on examination she has a normal heart rate and rhythm, a normal thyroid gland, and no evidence of exophthalmos, lid retraction or lid lag.
Aetiology	Summarize the aetiological factors relevant in the patient's illness. Distinguish between predisposing, precipitating, and maintaining factors.	Mrs A.'s mother and sister have been treated for agoraphobia (predisposing factor). Mr A. threatened to leave Mrs A. 6 months ago resulting in a general worsening of the chronic problem (precipitating and maintaining factor).
Conclusions about diagnosis and aetiology	A concluding statement giving the most likely diagnosis, and linking this with the main aetiological factors concerned. In addition, highlight outstanding problems or further investigations needed.	Mrs A. has agoraphobia with secondary mild depression of more recent onset. There is a family predisposition to this disorder. However, the recent worsening of symptoms seems to be related to marital problems which are still outstanding. Thyroid function tests need to be done in order to exclude the unlikely possibility of thyrotoxicosis.
Treatment/care plan	Summarize problems and main features of appropriate plan, taking into account illness severity, risk factors, available helping resources, and the influence of aetiological factors.	• Agoraphobia: *in vivo* exposure treatment combined with anxiety management initially at the patient's home. • Marital problem: joint counselling. • Depression: addition of antidepressant if initial response to treatment is poor.
Prognosis	Consider both outcome of the current illness (short-term outcome) and the possibility of further illnesses in the future (long-term outcome) giving your reasons.	Short term: high motivation and good previous personality adjustment argue for a good outcome; however, if resolution of marital problems proves impossible, response may be less good. Long term: family predisposing factors indicate that Mrs A. may develop further illnesses, particularly at times when she encounters stressful circumstances.

Assessment summary

The assessment process just described can be summarized in the form of an assessment summary. An example, together with a commentary is given in Fig. 3.7.

Your attitudes towards the patient

The attitudes you adopt towards your patient and your assessment task are important, and influence the effectiveness and quality of your work. Three attitudes are particularly important.

1 You should be **empathic and accepting** in your relationship with the patient. The importance of this has already been underlined in the section on interview technique.

2 You should develop an attitude of **constant self-evaluation**, and be prepared to look at your own behaviour and feelings in relation to patients or situations. For example, if the patient arouses strong feelings in you, whether of anger, anxiety, or overprotectiveness, it is important to understand these feelings, and the way they may influence your behaviour and decision making.

3 You should maintain an attitude of **vigorous scientific inquiry**. Always be prepared to ask the question 'why?', and to continue to evaluate and re-evaluate your opinions and decisions, particularly concerning diagnosis and management.

Ethics

Ethics mainly concern the rights and wrongs of the actions and motives of a person, in this case the health worker. Ethical considerations thus form an integral part of our attitudes and behaviour towards patients. Their importance is shown in two particular areas.

1 **The relative power health carers have over their patients**: this arises from a number of sources including the formidable tradition of special healing knowledge; the disparity between patient and professional in level of personal disclosure and of information held; and the inherent vulnerability associated with having an illness and seeking help. The health professional is thus in a position of considerable relative power over the patient, and must be careful not to abuse this, by for example imposing his own values. This would be the case if a doctor with well-defined ideas on sexuality, relationships or religion, sought to influence the patient according to those views.

In addition, doctors, nurses and social workers have the even more tangible powers entrusted by society, in that they can take away a person's rights and deprive them of liberty (see Chapter 25).

2 **The health carer is trusted by the patient**: most patients tend to place their trust in health professionals. This is partly because the doctor or nurse represents a tradition of expertise and good conduct, and partly because patients have a need to develop trust in order to be helped. The individual health professional builds on this trust, by his personal conduct.

The patient's trust manifests itself in a number of ways, but is most obvious in a preparedness to reveal confidential information or vulnerable feelings, and a preparedness to accept that advice is given in good faith, and in their best interests.

Thus, this trust carries with it considerable responsibilities for the professional. Three common areas of ethical concern, all related to issues of trust, and relative power, are summarized in Fig. 3.8. For a more detailed review of ethical considerations, see Chapter 4.

Circumstances of psychiatric assessment

Any assessment must take into account the context in which it occurs. This can be conveniently divided into the circumstances leading up to the assessment, the circumstances

---

Fig. 3.8 Ethical considerations

Confidentiality	• As a health care worker you will be entrusted with confidential information. To maintain confidentiality, explain that anything the patient tells you will be in confidence.
	• Explain the purpose of note keeping.
	• Obtain the patient's permission before talking to others, including relatives, friends and other health staff.
	• Breaches of confidentiality may endanger the therapeutic relationship, and hinder work with the patient.
	• Sometimes a patient's right to confidentiality conflicts with society's rights, for example when a serious crime is admitted to (see Chapter 25).
Rights of the patient	Important because of the relative power of the health care professional. Specific rights are incorporated in the 'Patients' Charter', and in the Access to Medical Records Act implemented from 1991. Important general rights include:
	• the right to privacy;
	• the right to be helped in the least restrictive setting;
	• the right to participate as much as possible in decision making;
	• the right to be kept fully informed of what is happening and why. This is particularly important in relation to informed consent to treatment such as medication or ECT.
Intimacy with the patient	• Concern and regard for a patient should be differentiated from overinvolvement, and intimate or sexual feelings. Such overinvolvement may interfere with objectivity, and may be experienced as burdensome by some patients. For this reason it is rarely appropriate to share intimate feelings or personal worries.
	• However, you are more likely to help patients if you like them, and your behaviour should certainly communicate this liking and concern.

in which the assessment is done, and the consequences of the assessment. These will be dealt with in turn. Considering all of these areas is important if an assessment is to fulfil its purpose and have an effective outcome.

Circumstances leading to the assessment

Two factors are important. Firstly, **you must have an understanding of how the patient came to see you**. Did he for example come of his own accord, or was he persuaded by well-meaning friends or relatives? If he was reluctant to come, you may have to pay special attention towards motivating him to take part in any treatment you offer.

Was he seen as a matter of urgency, or was the consultation more of a routine matter? Clearly emergency assessments are usually a response to rapidly deteriorating or at-risk behaviour, and you will need to respond appropriately.

Secondly, you must understand **what expectations others have of the assessment**. For example, relatives may be at the end of their tether and be fully expecting you to arrange hospital admission. Alternatively, a doctor referring someone to a specialist may only wish for an opinion, and want to continue management himself. All of these expectations may or may not be reasonable, but this is not the point. Unless they are enquired about, misunderstanding may occur which could adversely affect the management of the patient.

Circumstances in which the assessment is done

Where should the assessment be done?

Assessments are usually done in the patient's home or in some form of medical setting such as a health centre or hospital. Occasionally they may be done in prisons or police stations.

Assessing the patient at home has a number of advantages.
1 They are seen in their normal surroundings. Their behaviour is therefore not distorted by an unfamilar setting. This is particularly useful in assessing people with psychotic illnesses, as well as those with certain neurotic illnesses such as agoraphobia or obsessional illnesses.
2 Careful observation of the home can give important clues about the patient's level of functioning; for example an uncharacteristically neglected home, or a lack of food supplies in the kitchen.
3 Relatives or friends may be more readily available during a home visit.

Thus for certain patients, a home visit may be the best way of carrying out an initial assessment. Where an assessment is done in a medical setting, limitations imposed by the setting should always be recognized.

Who should be included in the assessment?

Combined assessments are very often helpful, and may assist subsequent management. For example, a GP and a community nurse, a GP and a psychiatric specialist, or a psychiatric specialist and a social worker may jointly see and assess a patient. In particular, where the patient has a history of violence, or is extremely disturbed, he should generally not be seen alone, particularly on a home assessment.

Consequences of the assessment

Clear communications

The outcome of assessment usually involves making decisions about diagnoses and future plans. Always communicate this information clearly to the patient, and to others who are involved.

Where you need to communicate with other people quickly, do this by telephone or personal contact, but don't forget to back this up with letters where appropriate. Finally, make a clear written record of your assessment, remembering that the patient has a right to read these records under the Access to Medical Records Act of 1991.

Impact on the patient

An assessment interview may have a considerable impact on the patient. Although most patients feel reassured at the end of the interview, sometimes the result may be an exacerbation of painful feelings, or even an escalation of difficult behaviour. If this is the case, you may need to make special arrangements. For example, making sure someone remains with the patient, or arranging for further early contact.

Beware subsequent diagnostic bias

Do not let the initial assessment bias your subsequent understanding of the patient. Always be prepared to challenge and reassess your opinions and plans.

Common problems in psychiatric assessment

The patient refuses to be seen

Check whether there are any circumstances in which the patient would agree to be seen, for example at home or with a friend or relative. From the available information, establish whether there appear to be any at-risk factors as a result of possible mental illness, since if there are you may need to consider using the Mental Health Act (1983) in order to assess the patient (see Chapter 25).

The patient is unforthcoming

This may be due to a number of reasons; for example anxiety, depressed mood or persecutory beliefs. The history from other informants will be critically important, as will gaining the patient's trust. You may also need to allow more time to complete the assessment, as well as concentrating on key areas of information you need to know; for example an assessment of suicidal thoughts.

The patient 'takes over' the interview

This is commonly due to overtalkativeness, which may itself be a result of anxiety concerning the interview. Thus, acknowledging how anxious the patient is about the interview may be helpful. A clear statement at the beginning of the interview concerning how much time is available and approximately how it will be used also helps. Where the patient is frequently distracted by detail, and you wish to move on to other areas of inquiry, avoid 'cutting across' the patient. This may be interpreted as disinterest or irritation, and may actually worsen the problem. Instead, acknowledge the importance of what the patient is saying, then firmly remind him that there are other important areas you must now cover.

The overdemanding patient
This may be due to a variety of causes including disinhibition (as in mania or alcohol intoxication), an immature personality under stress, or the anxiety of a worried relative. Remember, a demanding patient is often an insecure and frightened one, and it is important not to be cold or rejecting in the face of unrealistic demands. Reassurance, clear information, and the setting of firm (and caring) limits may all help depending on the reasons for the demands.

Tearfulness
It usually helps to acknowledge the tears and explain that is part of the reason they have come to see you. The trigger that sets off the tears may be an important clue in understanding the patient's problems. Successfully coping with a tearful patient will also help your therapeutic relationship with that patient.

Hostility or suspiciousness
This may be due to the patient's personality or it may indicate underlying persecutory beliefs. The first task is to build up a relationship with the patient, to gain his trust. Avoid too many questions initially, concentrating more on facilitative comments. If the patient is highly irritable, or has a history of violent behaviour, take necessary precautions. For example do not do a home visit alone.

The patient is restless, irritable or over-active
You may have to accept that brief interviews only may be possible. Thus, concentrate on important areas of inquiry relevant to the decisions you have to take. Arrange further brief interviews if appropriate.

Patient and interviewer see the problem quite differently
For example, the patient sees his problem as one of acutely furred-up arteries, whilst the doctor sees it as depression, of which the worry about arteries is but one symptom. The doctor should take the worry seriously, acknowledging the distress it causes, but at the same time actively treat the underlying depression.

Diagnosis and management plan remains unclear after assessment
Consider further sources of information, for example contacting relatives or other professionals. Also consider further assessment, for example by seeing the patient again or by asking for a second opinion.

If the patient refuses any help offered
Check that the patient understands the nature of the help offered. Review whether alternative forms of help would be acceptable. However, in the end the patient has the right not to accept help unless you believe he is at risk of harming himself or others as a result of mental illness.

Hidden psychiatric illness
Psychiatric illness may go unrecognized, and remain hidden from health carers. Over a third of significant psychiatric disorders among attenders at GP clinics go unrecognized.

The more severe the disorder, the more likely it will be detected. However, those with certain severe disorders such as schizophrenia and depression may not seek help and can remain undetected for that reason. Alcohol and drug abuse, eating disorders and early dementia also commonly go undetected.

A high index of suspicion for the presence of psychiatric disorder, combined with the knowledge about the presentation of psychiatric disorders, assists detection, especially in high-risk groups such as young mothers with babies, the elderly, the bereaved, and those with chronic physical disorders.

QUESTIONS

1 Outline the skills required in order to do a psychiatric assessment, and state why they are important.
2 An interviewer needs to be very directive in order to make the best use of the assessment time: discuss the advantages and disadvantages of this approach.
3 The patient's wife discloses that she is having a secret affair. You believe that these marital difficulties are contributing to your patient's depression. Discuss the ethical issues involved.
4 Justify inquiring into the patient's life and circumstances prior to the onset of psychiatric symptoms.
5 Discuss the relationship between the diagnostic process and obtaining information from the patient.
6 Your patient becomes at first angry, then tearful during the assessment interview. Discuss how you would handle this situation.
7 Discuss how the circumstances leading up to an assessment may influence both the assessment itself, and its outcome.

FURTHER READING

Cooper J.E. (1983) Diagnoses and diagnostic practice. In: Shepherd M. & Zuagwill O.L. (eds): *Handbook of Psychiatry*, Volume 1, pp. 199–209. Cambridge University Press, Cambridge. [Gives a more detailed discussion of the diagnostic process.]

Leff J.P. & Isaacs A.D. (1990) *Psychiatric Examination in Clinical Practice*. Blackwell Scientific Publications, Oxford. [A concise paperback introduction.]

Pendleton D. & Hasler J. (1983) *Doctor–Patient Communication*. Academic Press. [An introduction to consultation technique, intended for general practitioners but of relevance to other disciplines.]

Sims A. (1988) *Symptoms in the Mind*. Baillière Tindall, Edinburgh. [A stimulating and sympathetic introduction to psychiatric symptoms.]

4
Ethics and Psychiatry

Fact sheet

Ethics is central to medical practice in general and psychiatric practice in particular. Apprenticeship is an excellent method of training for many of the scientific and technical aspects of psychiatry, but doing what is ethically right is not like learning a technique. There must be the opportunity during the training of every psychiatrist to reflect on the ethical aspects of practice.

Treating patients against their will

One of the most ethically difficult and frequently encountered situations met with in the practice of psychiatry is the question of when is it right to treat someone against their will. In most situations where this question arises there is a clash between two major ethical principles. The **principle of respect for the patient's autonomy** requires us in general to allow patients to choose whether to accept the treatment offered or not. The **principle of beneficence** states that that action should be taken which has the best consequences. A theoretically simple solution to this clash is to say that if the patient is **competent** then he should not be treated against his will, but if he is not competent then that treatment should be given which is in his best interests. The problem with this solution is that competence is not an all-or-none phenomenon, but is graded.

A structured approach to psychiatric ethics

Ethical issues arise frequently in the practice of psychiatry and not simply around the issue of treating patients against their will. It is suggested that there are four components necessary for a thoughtful approach to the ethical dimensions of practical medicine.

1 Attitude: an attitude that it is important to practice to high ethical standards.

2 Awareness of when an issue is an ethical issue.

3 Analysis: the ability to analyse the ethical aspects of the situation.

4 Action: taking the right action in the light of the analysis. It is further suggested that in carrying out the analysis it can be helpful to consider different **perspectives**, different **principles** and different **paradigms**.

Communication skills

Good communication with patients, their relatives, and with other members of the health care team is a vital component of ethically good practice.

Introduction

In common with medicine and surgery, training in psychiatry is primarily an apprenticeship: we learn on the job under the guidance of senior and experienced practitioners. For many purposes such apprenticeship is excellent; but doing what is ethically right is not like learning a technique. We must be careful not simply to copy the practice we observe; it is also important to think about the practice and to decide what we believe to be right or wrong. There must be the opportunity during the training of every psychiatrist to reflect on the ethical aspects of practice. Such opportunities should begin when future doctors first encounter psychiatric practice as medical students.

An ethical problem which arises with particular prominence in psychiatric practice is the treating of people against their will. Because this situation is so important and common I will devote the first part of this chapter to a consideration of some of the ethical issues raised. However, this is by no means the only important ethical problem. Indeed there is hardly a psychiatric consultation which does not raise ethical questions. In the second part of this chapter I will suggest a simple system for organizing a structured approach to the ethical aspects of psychiatric practice.

Treating patients against their will

It is a part of everyday clinical medical practice to meet patients who refuse the treatment offered. Normally such refusal does not pose any difficult ethical problems, both because the patient is normally competent to decide on treatment, and because the consequences of not accepting treatment are rarely dreadful. There are however occasions when a patient's refusal of treatment does pose problems, and such occasions are encountered more often in the practice of psychiatry than in other branches of medicine. The Mental Health Act in the UK, and similar legislation in other countries, gives powers to psychiatrists to bring patients into hospital, and to institute treatment, against their will. The law allows considerable room for manoeuvre. The question is raised therefore in psychiatric practice as to when is it right to enforce treatment.

If treatment is enforced then we may trespass upon the right of patients to determine their own lives; if treatment is not enforced we may be abdicating our responsibility to help patients to a healthy life.

Two principles

There are two principles which are of major importance in trying to answer the question of when it is right to enforce treatment. The first is **the principle of respect for the patient's autonomy** – that each person has the right to choose for him or herself whether to accept treatment or not; the second is **the principle of beneficence** which, in the present context, states that that action should be taken which has the best consequences. The problem when a patient refuses beneficial treatment is that these two principles are in apparent conflict.

Competence

The usual solution to this dilemma is to make use of the concept of **competence**. Thus, if the person is competent and refusing treatment, treatment should not be enforced. If the person is not competent, then the refusal is not given weight and that treatment should be given which is in the best interests of the patient.

The Mental Health Act does not use the concept of competence directly. Instead it employs the terms mental disorder and mental illness (see Chapter 25). The main defence for treating someone against their will because of mental disorder must, presumably, be on the grounds that the mental disorder affects competence to refuse. The fact that mental disorder and incompetence are not synonymous raises interesting questions concerning the moral basis of the Act.

If competence is to be the decisive factor in deciding when it is right to enforce treatment then this concept needs to be looked at carefully. How is the question of whether someone is competent or incompetent to be decided?

Figure 4.1 describes four vignettes and asks you to decide how competent each person is to refuse treatment. What do you think and what reasons do you have for your particular decision? There are a number of points to be made about competence.

Competence is particular to the decision and is not global

The question of whether a person is, or is not, competent is incomplete. One can only talk of competence *for a particular task* (Buchanan & Brock, 1989). This point is recognized by English law in the context of 'testamentary capacity', i.e. whether a person is competent to make a valid will. The criteria for testamentary capacity include the following.

1 Whether the testator knows the nature and extent of his property, although not in detail.

2 Whether he knows the names of close relatives and can assess their claims to his property.

3 Whether he is free from an abnormal state of mind that might distort feelings or judgements relevant to making a will.

4 Whether he knows what a will is, and what its consequences are.

The key point is that these criteria are not to do with the *global* question (is this person competent or incompetent?) but with the *specific* question (is this person competent *to make a valid will*?). The same is true of competence to refuse beneficial treatment. An assessment of competence must be made with respect to the knowledge and capacities which are crucial in deciding whether to accept or refuse the treatment offered.

Competence is a graded concept

The decision method outlined above treated competence as a binary concept: a person is either competent or incompetent, and the right action follows directly from which of these is true. However, even when we consider competence with regard to a particular decision, it is highly debatable whether competence is a binary concept. Consider the fol-

Fig. 4.1 How competent are these patients?

Using a scale from 0–100, rate the following people for competence to choose their own treatment: 0 = competence of an unconscious patient; 100 = competence of a normal healthy adult.

Assume that there are no features which could compromise their competence other than those mentioned. If you need more information to come to a decision clarify in your own mind what this information is, and why.

Case 1

A depressed 40-year-old housewife who is eating and drinking sufficiently, believes that she is worthless and undeserving of medical care. On testing her intellectual abilities she is found to be slow but otherwise normal in her thinking. ECT is recommended. How competent is she to consent to, or refuse treatment?

Case 2

A 64-year-old publican is brought in to casualty having vomited blood. He is found to be bleeding from his stomach, and also to be suffering from Korsakoff's psychosis (an intellectual defect, resulting from excessive alcohol intake, in which memory of recent events is severely impaired but other intellectual functioning is unaffected). He is advised to have an operation to stop the bleeding, and the reasons for this advice are clearly explained to him. However, he is unable to give an account of these reasons immediately after you have given them. How competent is he to decide whether or not to accept this treatment?

Case 3

A 60-year-old woman believes that she is playing a key role in the defence of Britain by observing every aeroplane that passes over her house. She believes her observations are 'taken' from her mind and displayed at the headquarters of British intelligence. She is diagnosed as suffering from schizophrenia and medication is offered. How competent is she to consent to or refuse treatment?

Case 4

A 22-year-old unmarried woman suffering from anorexia nervosa, is severely underweight as a result of prolonged voluntary restriction of diet together with laxative abuse. She wishes to lose more weight because she thinks she is still heavier than she should be. She is strongly advised to have treatment but refuses. How competent is she to do this?

lowing argument. There must be an IQ so low that someone with that IQ is not competent to make a choice about whether or not to receive a particular treatment. Or, alternatively, there must be a level of consciousness (for example, delirium) at which someone is not competent. Conversely, there must be an IQ or level of consciousness at which someone is fully competent. Both IQ and level of consciousness are graded features so that there is a range within which competence lies somewhere between full competence and full incompetence. To deny this would require justification of the view that there is a level of IQ or of consciousness at which the slightest increase renders someone fully competent whereas the slightest decrease renders them fully incompetent.

Did you, in deciding on the level of competence of the people described in Fig. 4.1 tend to rate competence in a binary fashion (rating each person either as less than 10 or greater than 90), or in a graded fashion?

The capacities needed for competence to accept or refuse treatment

In deciding a person's competence, to accept or refuse treatment, a variety of capacities are relevant. What features seemed relevant to you when considering the cases in Fig. 4.1? The ability of a person to understand, in broad terms, the nature of their illness and the prognosis with and without treatment would seem central. This requires a degree of **intellectual** ability.

Competence requires, too, some capacity for reasoning making use of the relevant information. How much memory is needed for such reasoning to be valid (see Case 2, Fig. 4.1), and in what way do **hallucinations** and **delusions** affect competence?

How did you rate the competence of the person with anorexia nervosa? If her competence is low, what is your justification? If her competence is high would you treat her against her will if she were at substantial risk of dying? How would this situation compare with a Jehovah's witness who refused life-saving blood transfusion?

Balancing competence and consequences

The solution outlined above to the conflict between the principles of autonomy and beneficence is to apply them in a 'hierarchical' fashion; that is, to ask first whether the patient is competent. If the answer is *yes*, then treatment should not be given, whatever the consequences for the patient. If the answer is *no* then beneficial treatment should be given. The problem with this solution is that it enforces a binary decision on what, I have argued, is the continuous concept of competence. The result is that above the threshold of competence total weight is given to the patient's decision, ignoring altogether the consequences. Below the threshold of competence no weight at all is given to the patient's view.

An alternative to this 'hierarchical' method of application of these principles is to trade them off against each other. Thus, the worse the consequences of not treating, compared with treating, the more competent the person would need to be with respect to the treatment decision in order for his refusal to be accepted. Conversely, if the consequences of not treating are not so serious, then the patient's decision is more likely to be followed, even if his competence is less (Eastman & Hope, 1988).

A structured approach to psychiatric ethics

Ethical problems arise throughout psychiatric practice. Figure 4.2 gives three examples of situations, identified by a group of junior psychiatrists from their recent clinical practice, which raised ethical issues. The three case examples considered below were supplied by the same group of psychiatrists. You may be able to add examples from your own recent experience. There are, I believe, four components necessary for a thoughtful approach to the ethical dimensions of practical medicine: attitude; awareness; analysis; and action (Hope, 1993).

Attitude

The scientific training which is a necessary foundation of medical education can lead to the ignoring of the non-scientific aspects of medicine. It is vital for the practice of good medicine to realize the importance of a thoughtful approach both to the scientific and to the ethical aspects of medical practice.

Awareness

No matter how important a doctor thinks the ethical aspects of practice are, this attitude will be useless unless she is also aware of when there is an ethical issue. These ethical aspects of medical practice can be hidden from doctors because a particular way of acting becomes so much of a routine that it is accepted unquestioningly. Consider the following case.

In choosing treatment for a 16-year-old patient with behavioural problems it was decided that family therapy would be the best approach. In pursuing such treatment it became necessary to explore problems within the family and not simply the problems of the patient who was referred for treatment. Some family members complained that the therapists had no right to probe into their lives in this way.

Had the family not complained, it is unlikely that the ethical issues raised in changing the focus for treatment would have been noticed because such changes of focus are routine in family therapy. In order to try and increase awareness of ethical issues it is important to make time to consider what issues arise. Medical students can be particularly helpful here because they bring a fresh outlook unsullied by experience of routine practice.

Analysis

Once you are aware of the ethical issues, you are in a position to analyse them. There is no single method of analysis; and it is usually best to apply more than one approach. Three approaches which provide complementary methods of analysis are: *perspectives*, *principles* and *paradigms*.

Perspectives

In order to make sure that you consider the range of relevant factors it is helpful to think about the issues from the differing perspectives of the various people concerned. Consider the following case.

A 23-year-old patient with a severe depressive illness was admitted as a voluntary patient for treatment. The patient frequently rang her parents and sister using either the ward phone, or the pay phone which was in the corridor outside the ward. The family found her frequent phone calls, in which she sought constant reassurance, very wearing and asked the ward staff to stop the patient from phoning so frequently. The staff were uncertain how they should respond.

In this example the perspectives of the patient, her family and the ward staff are all relevant in ensuring that the range of ethical issues is properly considered before a decision is reached as to what to do. From the patient's perspective, she

is a voluntary patient and her normal rights should not be restricted. However, the reassurance which she receives each time from her relatives does not appear to give her relief for very long. It is unclear how much these phone calls are helping her. The family's perspective is provided by their complaint to the ward staff about the frequent phone calls. However, assuming that they care about the patient, they may also be distressed to know how the patient is likely to feel if unable to call them. It would be important to understand why exactly the family finds the phone calls so wearing. Perhaps it is the feeling that they are powerless to help when the patient phones them, rather than the amount of time they spend on the phone, which is distressing. If the patient does appear to benefit, even if only for a short time, it would be important for ward staff to let the relatives know.

Principles

Four principles have been identified as central to medical ethics and have proved their worth in thinking about clinical situations (Gillon, 1985; Beauchamp & Childress, 1989). These principles are:
1 the principle of respect for the patient's autonomy;
2 the principle of beneficence;
3 the principle of non-maleficence;
4 the principle of justice.

The first two have already been discussed. The third principle states that in general we should not harm other people. In much of medical practice, if we are to have a chance of benefitting a patient, we have to accept some risk of doing harm. For many purposes principles 2 and 3 can be combined into the single concept of maximizing benefit and minimizing harm. The main reason for keeping them separate is that they have different scopes. Our duty not to harm may encompass all of human kind, but we do not owe a duty to benefit everyone.

Justice is a complex concept related to fairness and entitlement. Two broad kinds of justice can be distinguished. *Distributive justice* is concerned, in the medical setting, with questions like how resources should be distributed. *Retributive justice* is concerned with how those who break the law should be punished. This latter question arises, although often somewhat covertly, when psychiatrists are asked to report on a patient who has broken the law. The Court looks to the psychiatrist for some guidance on the extent to which the mental state, and background factors, might reduce the responsibility of the patient for the crime and thus affect what is a just punishment.

Paradigms

A third way of helping to analyse an ethical problem is to compare the problematic situation with other related settings which are not so puzzling. Through identifying the similarities and differences it is often possible to clarify the puzzling situation. Consider the following case example.

A 35-year-old man had a car crash as a result of driving uncharacteristically fast and carelessly. It became apparent that he was suffering from a manic illness. He was admitted to hospital and treated. Because of the accident his driving license was taken away.

After treatment of the acute episode of mania he returned to normal. He remained well on no medication for almost 3 years at which point he again became unwell. Treatment was started straight away and he required only a couple of days in hospital. When he had returned to normal it was recommended that he take lithium, as standard prophylactic treatment, to decrease the chance of further relapse. He was not willing to do this. He remained well, however, and 18 months later asked his doctor to support an application for the return of his driving license. The doctor was uncertain whether it was right for him to support this application.

In this situation there is a conflict between the man's wish to resume driving, and the possible danger to the public should he become ill and drive dangerously before treatment is started. It may not be immediately obvious what the doctor should do. There is, however, a comparable situation which can give some guidance. The question of epilepsy and driving is one which has received considerable attention and for which there are clear legal guidelines. In the UK the law states that a person may not drive unless free from fits for two years. This gives some guidance on what society is willing to risk. Society does not take the view that a person should not be allowed to drive if there is *any* risk of an illness leading to dangerous driving. Neither does society demand that the person who has had fits should be on prophylactic medication, as long as there have not been any fits for two years.

A consideration of epilepsy is helpful but it is important to think about the similarities and differences between epilepsy and mania. Important issues are: the degree of warning which the patient and others have of the onset of the illnesses; the degree to which the patient is likely to take heed of the warning; and the likelihood of further illness given that there have been no relapses for two years.

Action

The purpose of taking ethics seriously is to ensure that psychiatric practice is of high ethical standard. In practice it is impossible to separate the ethical aspects of medicine from good communication skills, and this is the reason why the concept of **practice skills**, involving the integration of ethics, communication skills and the law, has been advanced (Hope & Fulford, 1993). For example, when faced with the question of whether to enforce admission, it is not simply a question of deciding what is ethically right, and then either leaving the patient at home, or bustling him into an ambulance. The communication between the doctor and the patient is a critical aspect of good practice, and, indeed, what the patient wants may depend on such communication. It is vital also that different members of staff communicate closely with each other and this is particularly true in situations of ethical complexity, as is illustrated in example 1 of Fig. 4.2.

Conclusion

Good psychiatric practice requires a thoughtful approach to the ethical aspects. These aspects are not a side issue but are a central part of everyday practice. I have suggested that

Fig. 4.2 Three examples of ethical problems identified by a group of psychiatrists from their recent clinical practice

1 A 30-year-old man had suffered all his life from severe learning difficulties. A year ago his mother had died and because he was unable to care for himself he had become resident in a hostel. His behaviour caused problems in the hostel and it was thought that he was suffering from depression, probably as part of the grief following his mother's death. He was admitted as a voluntary patient to a psychiatric ward for assessment and treatment. On the ward he would go into the bathroom and drink large quantities of water. When it was pointed out to him that he was becoming dangerously overhydrated and could die from doing this, he indicated that he was quite happy to die and continued to drink excessively. The only way he could be stopped from doing this was to keep him within a restricted area of the ward, using force when necessary. Staff were divided as to whether this was justified.

2 A mildly manic inpatient went home from the ward for a trial week-end. On returning from the week-end away it became apparent that she had taken a taxi home, and had had sexual intercourse with the taxi driver in lieu of payment of the fare. The HIV status of the patient was not known as she had never given consent for testing, but there was concern that she was at some risk of being HIV positive. Some members of staff thought that the taxi driver, whom they could identify, should be told of the risk of HIV infection.

3 An 80-year-old woman was suffering from a moderate degree of dementia. She was living alone. There was concern that she was not feeding herself adequately and she was certainly losing weight. However, she adamantly refused to leave her home although a suitable residential placement had been found. It was thought that if she could be taken to the residential home she would probably settle into it well and forget about her own home. The question arose as to whether she should be taken against her will to the residential home.

there are four components to good ethical practice: **attitude**; **awareness**; **analysis**; and **action**. The analysis of the ethical issues does not give an answer in the manner of a proof in geometry, but it is a vital component in coming to a well-considered judgement.

ACKNOWLEDGEMENTS

My thanks are due to Sidney Bloch, Bill Fulford, Nigel Eastman and many trainee psychiatrists on the Oxford Rotational Scheme, for useful discussions of ethical issues in psychiatry.

REFERENCES

Beauchamp T.L. & Childress J.F. (1989) *Principles of Biomedical Ethics.* 3rd Edition. Oxford University Press, New York.

Buchanan A.E. & Brock D.W. (1989) *Deciding for Others: the Ethics of Surrogate Decision Making.* Cambridge University Press, Cambridge.

Eastman N. & Hope R.A. (1988) The ethics of enforced medical treatment: the balance model. *J. Appl. Philos.* **5**, 49–59.

Gillon R. (1985) *Philosophical Medical Ethics.* John Wiley & Sons, Chichester.

Hope T. (1993) Medical ethics. In: C. Bunch *et al.* (eds) *The Oxford Principles of Medicine.* Oxford University Press, Oxford, in press.

Hope T. & Fulford K.W.M. (1993) Medical education: patients, principles and practice skills. In: R. Gillon (ed.) *Principles of Health Care Ethics*, pp. 697–709. John Wiley & Sons Ltd.

FURTHER READING

Anzia D.J. & LaPuma J. (1991) An annotated bibliography of psychiatric medical ethics. *Acad. Psych.* **15**, 1–17. [A useful annotation of over 100 articles in psychiatric ethics.]

Bloch S. & Chodoff P. (eds) (1991) *Psychiatric Ethics.* 2nd Edition. Oxford University Press, Oxford. [A useful collection of 24 papers covering a wide range of ethical and political issues raised by the practice of psychiatry.]

Bloch S. & Hope R.A. (1988) Ethical issues in psychiatry. *Curr. Opin. Psych.* **1**, 630–7. [Reviews a number of recent articles which address a range of issues in psychiatric ethics.]

Committee on Medical Education (1990) *A Casebook in Psychiatric Ethics.* Brunner Mazel, New York.

Fulford K.W.M. (1989) *Moral Theory and Medical Practice.* Cambridge University Press, Cambridge. [The author argues that the concepts of illness and disease are necessarily value-laden. The evaluative nature of delusions is discussed in particular detail.]

Fulford K.W.M. & Hope T. (1993) Psychiatric Ethics. In: R. Gillon (ed.) *Principles of Health Care Ethics*, pp. 681–95. John Wiley & Sons Ltd. [The strengths and weaknesses of the application of the four principles to psychiatric ethics are discussed.]

Holmes J. & Lindley R. (1991) *The Values of Psychotherapy.* Oxford University Press, Oxford. [A clear and detailed account of ethical issues raised by psychotherapy. The authors also argue forcefully for psychotherapy to be a profession in its own right.]

Hope R.A. (1990) Ethical philosophy as applied to psychiatry. *Curr. Opin. Psych.* **3**, 673–6. [Reviews a number of recent articles which address a range of issues in psychiatric ethics.]

Hope T. (1991) General and applied psychiatric ethics. *Curr. Opin. Psych.* **4**, 778–81.

Lidz C.W., Meisel A., Zerubavel E., Carter M., Sestak R.M. & Roth L.H. (1984) *Informed Consent: a Study of Decision Making in Psychiatry.* The Guilford Press, New York. [The results of an empirical study in how psychiatric patients came to a decision. The results suggest that psychiatrists are not good at enabling patients to come to their own informed decisions.]

II
THE COMMON SYNDROMES

5
Schizophrenia

Fact sheet

Definition

Schizophrenia is a mental disorder defined in terms of abnormal clinical features of behaviour, affect, thinking and perceptions.

Schizophrenia takes a wide variety of forms, and almost certainly represents a group of disorders which share some characteristics, but are as yet only poorly defined.

Clinical presentation

Very variable.

- *Acute form*: florid or 'positive' symptoms such as bizarre beliefs and hallucinations.
- *Chronic form*: deficit or 'negative' symptoms such as underactivity, low motivation and flattening of emotional responsiveness.
- *Behavioural presentations of schizophrenia include*: social withdrawal, disturbed or agitated behaviour, downward drifting lifestyle, minor offences, self-harm and substance abuse.

Diagnosis

Based on observations of the clinical features of the disorder.

- *Discriminating features*: first rank symptoms (Schneider); blunting and incongruity of affect; formal thought disorder.
- *Associated features*: 'negative symptoms'; secondary delusions.

The presence of discriminating features in the absence of organic disorder or major affective disorder is highly suggestive of schizophrenia.

Classify into acute and chronic forms of the illness, with a description of main clinical features.

Distribution

- *Worldwide distribution*, differing little between countries.
- *Incidence of new cases*: 10–20 cases per 100 000 population per year.
- *Prevalence*: all cases at particular point in time: 2–9 per 1000.
- *Lifelong risk of developing schizophrenia*: approximately 0.5–1% during years of highest risk 15–45 years.
- *Number of new cases seen/year by average GP*: less than one every two years.
- *Hospital bed occupancy*: half of patients in psychiatric hospitals for 6 months–3 years have a diagnosis of schizophrenia.

Factors associated with schizophrenia

- Increased risk of suicide.
- Onset during early adulthood – peak age 25–35 years.
- Increased risk of alcoholism.
- No increased risk of gross intellectual deterioration.
- Normal life-expectancy.
- *Males and females* affected about equally.
- Onset later in women.
- *Social classes* affected equally.
- *Tendency to drift* to urban areas.
- *Social isolation*: two-thirds of those with schizophrenia in developed countries live away from family or friends, usually alone. (In developing countries most live with their family.)
- *Depression*: up to a half of patients have depressive symptoms at some time during the 6 months following acute schizophrenia.

Aetiological factors

- Largely unknown. Probably an interaction between environmental factors and individual's inherited vulnerability.
- Inherited factor: lifetime expectancy of schizophrenia in first-degree relatives raised over tenfold (to 8–16%) of general population.
- Environmental factors: stress may precipitate or maintain schizophrenia.
- Minimal brain damage may predispose to schizophrenia.
- Mechanism of schizophrenia: unknown.

Assessment

Of particular importance is: (a) information from informants other than patient; (b) exclusion of risk factors; (c) obtaining cooperation of patient who lacks insight.

Main differential diagnosis

Organic conditions (including alcohol/drug withdrawal). Severe mania and depression.

Management

Acute illness

- Nursing care, usually in hospital.
- Sedation, e.g. chlorpromazine.
- Family work – support and information.
- Compulsory admission if appropriate.

Chronic or intermittently relapsing illness

Reduce relapse risk by: (a) prophylactic medication with supervision; (b) family counselling where patient lives with relatives; (c) appropriate use of therapeutic and care facilities.

Care plan focusing on: (a) personal functioning, e.g. individual counselling, support; (b) social functioning, e.g. social skills groups, day centres; (c) occupation, e.g. sheltered workshops; (d) accommodation, e.g. hostels, group homes; (e) relatives' needs, e.g. problem-orientated counselling.

Aim of care plan: to minimize disabling effects of illness and institutional care. Emphasis on early return to supported living in the community.

Prognosis

Varied outcome.

- A quarter recover completely.
- One-tenth become severely disabled.
- The remainder: occasional acute relapses, may develop mild to moderate chronic impairment.

Syndromes sharing some of the features of schizophrenia

- Paranoid states.
- Schizoaffective disorders.

What is schizophrenia?

Schizophrenia is the name given to a psychiatric syndrome which can be both severe in its effects, and diverse in its course and outcome. Clinically, the syndrome can be divided into an acute and chronic form.

Acute schizophrenia is characterized by florid symptoms such as delusional ideas or auditory hallucinations. Contact with reality may be lost, and disturbed and even dangerous behaviour may be a feature. The patient's mental and social functioning is usually greatly impaired, and hospital admission is often needed.

Chronic schizophrenia, by contrast, is characterized by lack of motivation, social withdrawal and affective flattening. Florid symptoms are uncommon, but do occur. Chronic impairment of work, or social or mental functioning may result in severe lifelong disablement.

The range of the severity and diversity of schizophrenia is thus vast. It may present as a once-in-a-life time brief acute illness, or it may result in lifelong dependency, its chronic course periodically interrupted by acute relapses.

Since we know little about the underlying aetiology of schizophrenia, any definition must be based on descriptions of the clinical features of the illness, much as TB was defined before the discovery of the tubercle bacillus. Such descriptions confirm that schizophrenia not only occurs worldwide, but also has almost certainly existed for very many centuries.

Given the extraordinarily diverse nature of schizophrenia, psychiatrists have spent over a century attempting to define clinical sub-groups of the disorder. The most enduring subdivision has been by Kraepelin (see Fig. 5.1) who described four sub-groups of schizophrenia: simple, hebephrenic, catatonic and paranoid. However, the validity of these subgroups is doubtful on three counts: (a) they have proved indistinguishable genetically; (b) the same patient may present with different clinical sub-groups of schizophrenia during his lifetime; and (c) in clinical practice, the subgroups are often not clearly distinguishable. The usefulness of these sub-groups is therefore limited, although they do appear in the two most popular international classification systems covering mental illness: the *International Classification of Diseases*, and the *Diagnostic and Statistical Manual* (see Chapter 1).

In general therefore, schizophrenia is best described as acute or chronic. A group of syndromes sharing some of the clinical features of schizophrenia is described at the end of this chapter.

How is schizophrenia diagnosed?

The clinical features of schizophrenia are divided into two groups: discriminating features and associated features.

Fig. 5.1 Historical perspective on schizophrenia

19th century. County asylums were built for the care of the severely mentally ill, taking over from a variety of informal care arrangements, including workhouses.

1890s. Emil Kraepelin (1855–1926) distinguished between dementia praecox (schizophrenia) and manic depressive psychosis, correlating symptomatology with prognosis. Kraepelin noted that patients with dementia praecox had their symptoms of hallucinations, delusions and reduced attention to the outside world **in a state of clear consciousness** and with unimpaired perception and memory. He described four clinical sub-groups: dementia simplex, hebephrenia, catatonia and paranoid.

Simple: characterized by insidious fading of personality beginning during adolescence or early adulthood. The main feature is of progressive disinterest in social and emotional relationships with reduced work ability leading to resultant isolation and general impoverishment. Florid symptoms such as hallucinations or delusions are usually absent.

Hebephrenic: usually starts before the age of 25. Associated with florid symptoms including hallucinations and delusions. Unpredictable or irresponsible behaviour common, as are affective symptoms and thought disorder.

Catatonic: usually starts before the age of 25. Psychomotor disturbances of overactivity or stupor predominate. More rarely stereotyped movements are a feature.

Paranoid: later age of onset. Frequently has an insidious onset. Persecutory delusions predominate. Patient's behaviour and general functioning can be minimally affected, which may lead to late presentation to a doctor.

1900s. Eugen Bleuler (1857–1939) introduced the term schizophrenia. Bleuler felt the term dementia praecox inappropriate first because he recognized that intellectual deterioration did not occur, and second because the syndrome could occur at any age, not just in the young.

1950s. Kurt Schneider (1887–1967) described first rank symptoms of schizophrenia. Schneider felt these symptoms were of empirical importance in diagnosis.

Introduction of effective drugs, particularly chlorpromazine, for the treatment of schizophrenia.

Mental Health Act (1959) resulted in non-compulsory stay in psychiatric hospitals becoming more widespread, and combined with drug efficacy and changing public attitudes this resulted in patients with schizophrenia beginning to move from hospital back into the community.

1970s. A white paper entitled 'Better services for the mentally ill' (DHSS, 1975) recommended movement from institutional care to community-based care.

1980s and 1990s. Mental Health Act (1983) further protects the rights of particularly the severely mentally ill.

The closure of large institutions (county hospitals) commences during the 1980s on the assumption that care will be provided for the severely mentally ill on a more local basis. The Community Care Act implemented from 1993 makes local authorities (social services departments) responsible for ensuring that the social care needs of the severely mentally ill are provided for. We have yet to see how effective this arrangement will be.

Discriminating features

Discriminating features are so called because they are highly specific, distinguishing one syndrome from another. The most discriminating clinical features of schizophrenia are first rank symptoms and these are listed in Fig. 5.2, with examples included in Fig. 5.3. If first rank symptoms are found, then, in the absence of an underlying organic pathology, a firm diagnosis of schizophrenia is made. First rank symptoms have the advantage of having an all-or-nothing quality to them. They are either present or they are absent. This has led to their popularity as criteria for diagnosing schizophrenia, since reliability between psychiatrists is likely to be greater. About 80% of patients diagnosed by UK psychiatrists as having schizophrenia will have one or more first rank symptoms at some stage in their illness. A diagnosis of schizophrenia can be made in the absence of first rank symptoms, although with lesser degree of certainty.

Discriminating features other than first rank symptoms

These are listed in Fig. 5.2. These features lack the all-or-nothing quality of first rank symptoms, and in their mild form it may be difficult to decide whether they are present or not. Formal thought disorder would be one example, where the feature may be anywhere on a continuum from vague eccentricity of thought to complete incoherence.

Associated features

Associated features of schizophrenia are those which commonly occur in the syndrome, but are not specific to it. The most frequently occurring are listed in Fig. 5.2, with examples included in Fig. 5.3. In arguing for a diagnosis of schizophrenia, relatively little weight is put on these features.

Fig. 5.2 Features of schizophrenia

Discriminating features
First rank (Schneider)
Delusional perception.
Thought insertion, withdrawal and broadcasting.
Voices discussing subject's thoughts or behaviour.
Voices repeating or anticipating subject's thoughts.
Passivity experiences.

Non-first rank
Formal thought disorder.
Chronic negative symptoms (not associated with depression):
● marked apathy;
● paucity of speech;
● blunting or incongruity of emotional responses;
● resultant social withdrawal.
Catatonic behaviour (uncommon and less discriminating):
● excitement, stupor, mutism, and negativism;
● posturing or waxy flexibility.

Associated features
Persecutory delusions.
Ideas of reference.
Suspiciousness.
Lack of insight.
Stereotypies or mannerisms (uncommon).

In addition, schizophrenia is often associated with symptoms lower in the diagnostic hierarchy, such as depression, anxiety, irritability or worrying. These features play no part in the diagnosis of schizophrenia.

Making the diagnosis

The usual requirement for a diagnosis of schizophrenia is at least one first rank symptom, or two non-first rank discriminating symptoms, to have been clearly present for most of the time during a period of a month or more. The ICD-10 classification states that if duration of symptoms is less than a month (whether treated or not), the diagnosis should be of an acute schizophrenic-like psychotic disorder and should only be reclassified as schizophrenia if the symtoms persist for a longer period. The DSM-III classification system is a little more restrictive needing a duration of symptoms or dysfuntion of at least 6 months.

ICD-10 and DSM-III classifications both subdivide schizophrenia into paranoid, hebephrenic, catatonic and simple types. However, as mentioned previously, this is of limited value.

How does schizophrenia present?

The commonest features shown by patients with acute schizophrenia are listed in Fig. 5.4. Remarkably, these features are common in all countries where careful observations have been made of acutely ill schizophrenia patients. This includes America, Russia, UK, Nigeria, India and Taiwan.

Schizophrenia may initially present acutely, or less commonly insidiously. In either case, the patient will rarely seek medical help directly. Even where symptoms cause great distress, as in the case of persecutory beliefs or voices, patients are reluctant to see themselves as ill, and believe they do not need medical help.

Presentation to the doctor is therefore often late, and this results in schizophrenia being a common reason for both emergency psychiatric admission and for the use of compulsory powers of admission under the Mental Health Act.

Presentation, broadly speaking, occurs in one of three ways. Firstly, concerned people, often relatives or friends but sometimes a social worker or hostel warden, may observe **bizarre symptoms** or a **behaviour change**, and instigate a medical referral. Secondly, **consequences of the illness** may result in a medical referral, for example unlawful behaviour, alcohol abuse, attempted suicide or social deprivation. Thirdly, and more rarely, the **patient may seek medical help with specific symptoms associated with the illness**. These symptoms may include: unrealistic concerns about a supposed physical deformity; unreasonable or bizarre complaints about family members, neighbours, employers, or even other doctors; or neurotic symptoms such as depression or anxiety associated with the underlying schizophrenic illness.

In the **acute** form of schizophrenia, florid symptoms will usually develop over a period of weeks or months. The most

Fig. 5.3 Clinical features of schizophrenia (see also Chapter 1)

Delusional perception: a primary delusional belief (and therefore arising inexplicably) triggered by a normal percept. The belief usually has some special significance for the subject. Primary delusions are rare, and should be distinguished from the more common secondary delusional beliefs (see p. 10).
Example: 'I saw the light turn green, and I suddenly knew that I had to lead the world from sin.'

Thought insertion: experience of alien thoughts put into one's mind.
Example: 'I'm driving along, thinking of the weather, but then the thoughts of God come into my mind forcing my own thoughts out.'

Thought withdrawal: experience of thoughts being taken out of one's mind as if by some external force.
Example: 'I'm thinking about my work, and suddenly my thoughts are sucked out of my mind, leaving it completely empty for a time.'

Thought broadcast: experience of one's thoughts being known to others.
Example: 'As I think, people around me, even down the street, know precisely what I am thinking. It's because I am telepathic.' (Associated secondary delusion.)

Voices discussing subject's current thoughts or behaviour, some as a running commentary.
Example: 'I hear the voice from across the park. It is always there, and it has just said: He's going to the cupboard, now he is behaving like a fool and getting out too many plates, now he's having nasty thoughts about being asked questions.'

Voices discussing or arguing about subject in the third person.
Example: 'When I'm alone, I hear these four voices; I hear them clearly through my ears. They say things like: "He shouldn't be allowed to go free, he should be locked up". "No he shouldn't" argues another, "he should be given more rope to hang himself with".'

Voices repeating subject's own thoughts aloud, or anticipating subject's thoughts.
Example: A woman complained that every time she had a thought of doing something, a second or so later a voice from outside of herself quietly repeated the thought. The thoughts 'I'll go to the shop today', or 'I'll just make the beds', were repeated in this way.

Passivity experiences: the subject experiences 'made' emotions, specific bodily movements, or specific sensations being caused by an external agency or being under some external control which cannot be resisted.
Example: A man experiences the movements involved in cleaning his teeth as being made and controlled by an alien force by means of magnetism. (Associated secondary delusion.)

Formal thought disorder: subject has an impairment of connection between thoughts sometimes distinguished into positive and negative formal thought disorder (see p. 9). May result in incoherent or irrelevant speech. Distinguish from flight of ideas characteristic of mania where connection between thoughts is retained.
Example: 'My house needs a lot doing to it, but he is not the man I thought him to be because the train always waits for people like me, people who live in glass houses like me'.

Negative symptoms: main features are persistently reduced social activity, speech and energy unexplained by mood change or neuroleptic medication.

Blunting of affect: subject has reduced emotional responses.
Example: Persistently expressionless face and voice.

Incongruity of affect: subject expresses emotions inappropriately.
Example: Outbursts of giggling when discussing sad issues.

Catatonic behaviour: characterized by bizarre posturing and extreme motor under- or over-activity.

Persecutory delusions: delusions where the content of the false belief is persecutory. Persecutory delusions are usually secondary delusions.
Example: 'You see, I *know* they want to kill me, the voices talk about it. And the people I met this morning are in on the conspiracy.'

Ideas of reference: subject feels extremely self-conscious, believing others take particular notice of him. Ideas may become delusional, where the subject believes events have a special significance referring just to him.
Example: A cup placed in a certain way is taken to mean that subject is homosexual. A TV programme about the Pope is believed to include material put in specifically for the subject's benefit.

Suspiciousness: suspiciousness of mood despite there being no justification for this. Often associated with unforthcomingness concerning symptoms.

Lack of insight: subject does not accept he is ill, or if he does will explain it in delusional terms.

Stereotypies: repetitive movements. For example rocking or grimacing. Stereotypies may also be found in organic cerebral conditions (see p. 135).

Mannerisms: odd stylized movements or postures often suggesting a special meaning or purpose. For example, the subject wrings his hands before sitting.

---

common associated behaviour changes are firstly increasing social withdrawal, and secondly restless unpredictable and sometimes bizarre behaviour. Unlawful or dangerous behaviour can also occur (see Chapter 24).

The patient's behaviour may be directly influenced by specific underlying psychotic experiences. For example the patient may converse with himself (responding to auditory hallucinations), shout at passers-by (responding to persecutory ideas of reference or auditory hallucinations) or send abusive communications (in response to persecutory beliefs).

Generally, the patient's day-to-day functioning will be impaired. This results from the compelling and persistent quality of the florid psychotic experiences, and the commonly associated features of poor concentration, poor volition, difficulty with thought processes and subjective distress.

Where schizophrenia has an **insidious onset**, it may develop over some years. There may be a progressive development of negative symptoms (see Fig. 5.2) such as loss of volition and poverty of speech content, resulting in an increasing loss of skills, social withdrawal, and downward social drift. Alternatively, social withdrawal may be the

Fig. 5.4 Common symptoms in acute schizophrenia
(source: WHO, 1973)

Symptom	Frequency of occurrence (%)
Lack of insight	87
Auditory hallucinations	74
Ideas of reference	70
Suspiciousness	66
Flatness of affect	66
Voices speaking to the patient	65
Delusional mood	64
Delusions of persecution	64
Thought alienation	52
Thoughts spoken aloud	50

result of an encapsulated system of persecutory delusional ideas, as is sometimes the case in schizophrenia occurring later in life.

Where schizophrenia becomes a recurrent illness, there is a tendency for the same features of the illness to recur. In addition, where schizophrenia affects more than one member of a family, there is a tendency for the features to be broadly similar. However, this is by no means always the case.

In order to highlight the main features of the various presentations of schizophrenia, a series of case studies is given on p. 61. In each case, clinical details are accompanied by a commentary on special features of note.

Aetiology of schizophrenia

An understanding of the aetiological factors contributing to an illness is important, since it may help in the management of that illness, and in the prevention of recurrences.

However, care should be taken to distinguish aetiological factors which may provoke or predispose to illness from factors which result from illness. The latter are thought to explain the high incidence of schizophrenia among those with low socio-economic status, among those in urban as opposed to rural areas, among the socially isolated and among certain migrant groups.

Aetiological factors can be divided into those that predispose to, those that precipitate, and those that maintain an illness. Commonly, aetiological factors from all three of these areas frequently co-exist in the same patient.

Predisposing factors
Only one convincing predisposing factor has been found to be associated with a person's risk of developing schizophrenia for the first time, and that is genetic inheritance. Neither personality factors, such as schizoid personality traits, nor the type of family environment an individual grows up in have convincingly been associated with an increased risk of the disorder. There is evidence that pre- and perinatal brain injury caused by infection or anoxia may in some people slightly increase the risk of developing schizophrenia later on in adulthood. However, this apparent causal association is largely speculative at present.

Once an individual has had schizophrenia, that person is predisposed to a recurrence of the illness. This knowledge may be of particular value in detecting and helping those most at risk of developing the illness at stressful times such as after surgery or in the puerperium.

Genetic inheritance
To distinguish the effects of genetic inheritance from those of family environment, follow-up studies have been done on children separated from their schizophrenic parents soon after birth, and brought up in non-schizophrenic families. These individuals still retain the increased risk of developing schizophrenia of between 8–16%. It seems therefore that genetic factors do influence the risk of developing schizophrenia, and that if environmental factors have a part to play it is in those patients already genetically at risk. It is unclear, however, what the genetic mode of inheritance is. Figure 5.5 gives a summary of the lifetime expectancy of developing schizophrenia in relatives of schizophrenics.

Precipitating factors
Stressful life-events may precipitate schizophrenia in those already predisposed to the condition. The nature of the stress seems to be non-specific, and includes events which in other people might provoke affective disorders. Two-thirds of patients with acute schizophrenia have experienced a stressful event independent of the illness in the previous 3 weeks. Amongst the stressful events which may provoke acute illness are pregnancy (leading to puerperal psychosis), physical illness, surgery, major loss or change, and family conflict.

Maintaining factors
Social or family circumstances may maintain an illness by maintaining stress, or by depriving a patient of opportunities for help. Overcritical families, isolated digs, unemployment and financial problems are some examples.

Further information on causative factors and schizophrenia can be found on pp. 22–27.

Mechanism of schizophrenia
This is not known. One theory is that schizophrenia results from an imbalance of the central neurotransmitter dopamine in the brain. This could be caused by a variety of influences. The theory is supported by the observation that dopamine receptors are blocked by drugs which control schizophrenia symptoms. However, there is as yet no evidence that this is the central underlying malfunction in schizophrenia.

Although some schizophrenics have enlarged cerebral ventricles, some have abnormal EEGs, and some have abnormal sensory neurological signs, no consistent neurological abnormalities have been found. The significance of these physical findings has been attributed to brain damage early in life which as previously described may predispose to the disease in some people.

Fig. 5.5 Lifetime expectancy of developing schizophrenia in relatives of schizophrenics

1st degree relatives	Siblings Children Non-identical twin	8–16%
	Identical twin Children of two schizophrenic parents	over 40%
2nd degree relatives	Grandfather, nephews nieces, first cousins	2–4%

Influence of aetiological factors on management

Treatment and prevention

Identifying factors which provoke or maintain an illness is important for both effective treatment and future prevention. For example, if family stress precipitates an acute schizophrenic illness, treatment and future prevention measures should aim to reduce this source of stress. Where there is a complete absence of apparent aetiological factors, this should be recognized as atypical, and the possibility of a hidden organic causation be considered.

Prevention during at-risk times

People with a known vulnerability for developing schizophrenia may need to be carefully monitored during at-risk times, when prophylactic medication should be considered. For example, the woman who has had an acute schizophrenic illness after her first baby will need to be carefully observed after her second.

Genetic counselling

Patients and relatives will commonly want to know the risks of other family members developing the disorder. Counselling should be based on an accurate diagnosis and a thorough family history. The figures given in Fig. 5.5 represent average expectations based on a number of studies, and can only be put forward as a rough guideline in the individual's case. It should be noted that the lifetime risk for second degree relatives is not so very different from that of the general population. Also, very acute or paranoid illnesses probably carry a lower risk than chronic or other forms of the disorder.

Genetic counselling is usually done by a psychiatrist, and must be done with considerable tact and sensitivity. In particular, feelings of guilt among relatives should be anticipated, and these feelings can often be helped by explaining that neither early family environment nor parental upbringing are thought to cause the illness.

Assessment

Assessment of acute schizophrenia

Acute schizophrenia poses two particular assessment problems: first, it is often associated with a total lack of insight

on the part of the sufferer leading to a reluctance to seek help and a frequent lack of subsequent cooperation; second, it can be associated with alarming and sometimes life-threatening consequences including gross self-neglect, suicide, assault and self-mutilation. Assessment skills are rarely better tested.

In relation to the five main tasks of psychiatric assessment (p. 31) the following are of especial importance when seeing someone who may have acute schizophrenia.

Diagnosis

Much time may need to be spent talking with the patient in order to build up a detailed picture of their state of mind, focusing in particular on the psychotic experiences they are having which may determine their behaviour. This process is crucial for diagnostic and risk assessment purposes. It may however be fraught with difficulty if the patient is unforthcoming, terrified, hostile or otherwise unable to co-operate. Information from past records and from those who know the patient is likely to be of great importance.

Causal factors

Again information from relatives and friends can be invaluable, since the acutely ill sufferer may be unable to give a coherent history of relevant factors. A common reason for a relapse of the illness is failure to comply with prophylatic medication, perhaps at a time when stresses are occurring. Drug- or alcohol-related states must be excluded.

Risks

A small but important proportion of people who have acute schizophrenia may endanger their own or other people's health and safety as a result of their illness. This can either be as a direct result of psychotic experiences, for example where voices tell the patient to set fire to himself; or as part of a general disorganized response to distressing symptoms as in the patient who is irritable and frightened, then becomes quickly aroused to aggressiveness when over-stimulated.

Therapeutic plan

Since people with acute schizophrenia commonly believe there is nothing wrong with them, they often present late, reluctantly, and in crisis. This combined with the rapid onset of at least some forms of the illness means that emergency assessment is frequently needed. Any therapeutic plan drawn up in these circumstances has to address immediate needs, the most important being the following.

1 *The need to reduce risk*, for example by admission to the relative safety of a hospital. Sometimes if the risks are unacceptably high, yet the sufferer rejects all help, compulsory admission under the Mental Health Act may be needed.

2 *The need for intensive support, reassurance and care*, to help settle acute symptoms. This can be provided by relatives with the help of psychiatric staff working in the community, or more commonly by a period of hospital care.

3 *The need for medication* to help settle acute distress and disturbance, and to begin treatment of the underlying illness.

4 *The needs of relatives and other carers* to be kept informed and supported.

Case 1: the sudden religious inspiration		Case 2: the man who went on a walkabout		Case 3: the paranoid bridge player	
Mrs R. was a deeply religious 39-year-old accountant. She was admitted to a psychiatric hospital following a week of increasing religious preoccupation associated with agitation. This appeared to follow an accumulation of stresses at work.	*Acute onset. Stress related. Good previous personality adjustment.*	Mr W. was a man in his early 30s who was detained by the police after wandering in traffic and threatening passers-by. Six months previously he had moved to the area, remaining socially isolated, living in local bed and breakfast accommodation and without a job.	*At least two-thirds of patients developing acute schizophrenic illnesses live alone.*	Mrs B. was a 67-year-old widow who had lived on her own for many years. A year ago she moved into a new flat. Within a few months, she became convinced that neighbours were spying on her. She believed they had bugged the lights with listening devices, and kept a 24hr vigil outside her windows. At times she could clearly hear their voices talking about her, and planning her death. As a result she frequently became afraid and would then phone the police at all hours.	*Organic state more common in the elderly: beware.*
On examination, she described a vivid internal struggle between good and evil in which she was constantly tested by God. Through her ears, she heard the voices of God and the Devil arguing about her, but she denied passivity experiences.	*Probable first rank symptom (Schneider): external voices discussing subject in third person.*	At the police station, he was abusive and accusatory. He said he threatened passers-by because of the conspiratorial way they had looked at him. He believed there was a political conspiracy to kill him.	*Risk of danger to others as a result of mental illness. Section 2 allows period of observation in psychiatric hospital for 28 days.*		*First rank symptom (Schneider): voices discussing patient in third person. Fearfulness common in acute schizophrenia.*
18 hours after admission the patient suddenly enucleated her right eye with her fingers. She had interpreted the bible passage 'if your right eye offendeth, pluck it out' as having a special reference to herself.	*No evidence of acute organic confusional state.*	He was admitted to a psychiatric ward as an involuntary patient under Section 2 of the Mental Health Act (1983). He agreed to take neuroleptic medication and over a period of 8 weeks his florid symptoms disappeared. He was left with poor motivation, flat affect and concentration difficulties.	*Poor motivation, etc.: probably residual negative symptoms of schizophrenia. However depression (common after acute schizophrenia) and drug-induced akinesia would need to be excluded.*	Mrs B. remained active in many of her interests, continued to have excellent powers of memory and concentration and maintaining a regular game of bridge with two trusted friends. At no stage was she depressed. Eventually however Mrs B. abandoned bridge as she became increasingly reluctant to leave the house, for fear of her life.	*Symptoms relatively encapsulated, allowing patient to continue functioning in many areas of her life (common in schizophrenia occurring for the first time late in life). Lack of cognitive impairment or depressed mood are important negative findings, since they make an organic state or major depression less likely causes of the patient's symptoms. Physical examination and screening laboratory tests should be done however*
	Risk of self-harm or harm to others must always be considered in acute schizophrenia: *1 as a result of acting on delusional ideas, acting on instructions of auditory hallucinations or in association with passivity experiences;* *2 as a result of the patient's frightened, agitated and unpredictable state.*	Mr W. had a long history of similar acute symptoms treated in a number of psychiatric hospitals.	*Chronic schizophrenia when associated with social disablement and persistence of negative symptoms may*	Mrs B. had never previously been psychiatrically ill, although she had always had	

Case history	Comment
Details of a past illness in Ireland 17 years previously, which was unknown to the husband, revealed that in a similar illness the patient had attempted to set fire to herself with petrol, while ruminating on a passage from the bible. Mrs R. was treated with neuroleptic medication, and she returned to her normal self within 6 weeks. She had permanently lost the sight in one eye, however. Three years later she remained symptom free, was continuing to take depot injections, and continued to successfully further her career.	*Predictors of high risk: a good predictor of high risk behaviour is past high risk behaviour.* *Prompt response to treatment.*
Previous attempts at rehabilitation and aftercare had been initially successful, but the patient usually 'went on walkabout', leaving the area. His medication would then stop, and he would eventually relapse. He had no family, had been unemployed for many years and periodically abused alcohol and slept rough. With Mr W.'s participation, a discharge care plan was made and he moved to a supervised hostel, from where he attended occupational therapy workshops. He was seen regularly by a community psychiatric nurse, who supervised his prophylactic depot medication, given to prevent the recurrence of florid symptoms. After 6 months, Mr W.. decided to leave the area, and follow-up proved impossible.	*Despite good prognostic features (acute onset, good previous personality, lack of negative symptoms) the consequences of a further illness are potentially very serious. Aftercare was therefore long term, and included prophylactic medication, careful supervision, and counselling to encourage the patient and relatives to seek help early in the event of signs of illness relapse.* *result in progressive social decline, a drift towards urban centres, and associated alcohol abuse.* *Rehabilitation plan included accommodation provision, day activity, supervision and counselling.* *Mobile lifestyle, low motivation and/or ambivalence concerning help may limit what the patient will accept.*
a rather quiet, suspicious predisposition. In recent years she had become midly deaf but refused to see anyone about it. Mrs B. was treated with neuroleptic medication on a day patient basis. A community psychiatric nurse also visited her at home. Slowly, over 3 months, her persecutory ideas left her, and she became active in local clubs and a community day centre. Two years later, she remained on a low dose of neuroleptic medication, since a trial off all medication 6 months before had resulted in a return of her persecutory ideas. Her bridge playing remained highly competitive.	*because patient is in at-risk age group for an underlying organic disorder. Deafness and blindness predispose to paranoid illnesses in the elderly.* *Patients with persecutory ideas are often reluctant to take medication or to seek help. Day attendance and community nurse follow-up assisted with this problem.* *Long-term medication indicated.* *Unimpaired cognitive abilities at follow-up confirm that chronic dementia unlikely.*

Therapeutic process

Part of assessment involves trying to engage the acutely ill person in the treatment you may be recommending. Developing a sympathetic relationship will help, since you may be expecting someone who is suspicious and frightened to trust the advice of a stranger on such fundamental matters as moving from the familiarity and privacy of home into the unknown hectic and very public world of hospital; or the taking of medication which may have very unpleasant side effects.

These five tasks of assessment are carried out using the method of history taking, examination, diagnosis and care planning described in Chapter 3. Figure 5.6 highlights features to look for when using these methods to assess a person who may have acute schizophrenia, and includes a clinical example.

Assessment of post-acute and chronic schizophrenia

Assessment of those recovering from acute schizophrenia or who have chronic schizophrenia needs to include the following.

Fig. 5.6 Assessment of someone who may have schizophrenia

History taking

	Special features to look for	Clinical example
Circumstances of assessment	• **Often done as emergency.** • **Information often hard to establish:** patient may be unwilling to be seen and family may feel under great stress. Obtaining information from relatives, other involved professionals, and where appropriate home assessment is of particular value.	John aged 19 punches his mother. The district nurse involved with the family then alerts the GP, observing that John had become overly suspicious and withdrawn recently. The GP gets little out of John and requests a psychiatric opinion. The psychiatrist suggests a joint home visit, when John and parents were seen separately.
History of symptoms	• **Inaccessible clinical features:** patient may be unforthcoming about important diagnostic symptoms. Therefore, question patient and relatives thoroughly, observe for behavioural clues of underlying psychotic experiences. • **Atypical features:** look for atypical features, such as disorientation, memory disturbance or visual hallucinations, since these may suggest an alternative diagnosis. • **High-risk features:** look for high-risk features such as thoughts of self-mutilation, or assaults on others. • **Aetiological factors:** look for precipitating or maintaining causative factors, particularly those related to stress.	John was well until 6 months ago. He then became increasingly withdrawn, abandoning his job and spending most of the time in his bedroom. He is irritable when confronted by increasingly critical and exasperated parents. Recently, he told his mother that alien forces controlled some of his movements, and that he was in the centre of a battle between good and evil. On two occasions recently he has assaulted his mother, accusing her of controlling his thoughts. A possible recent source of stress was his difficulty coping with an increasingly busy job.
Family history	**Aetiological factors:** look for predisposing inherited aetiological factors.	Father killed himself during an acute schizophrenic illness when John was aged 2.
Personal history	**Chronic adjustment difficulties:** even before the first florid illness, schizophrenia can be associated with progressive social isolation or increasing underachievement in jobs.	Prior to 6 months ago, John presented as a moderately well-adjusted individual, with an appropriate steady job.
Past medical history	• **Physical illness which can resemble schizophrenia:** including vitamin B_{12} deficiency, myxoedema, epilepsy, substance abuse, porphyria. • **Allergies or drug reactions:** e.g. hypersensitivity to chlorpromazine.	No previous medical history of note.
Past psychiatric history	**Establish details of past mental illnesses:** psychiatric illness tends to run true to form in subsequent relapses — check characteristics, risk factors, duration and response to treatment in relation to all previous psychiatric illness.	No previous psychiatric history.
Personality	• **Features associated with schizophrenia:** include progressive personality change unexplained by mood and characterized by loss of sociability and motivation. • **Alcohol, drug or solvent abuse:** patients with schizophrenia may drift into these abuses. Alternatively substance abuse may present with features similar to schizophrenia.	Always a bit of a loner. No substance abuse admitted to.

Continued

Fig. 5.6 (*Continued*)

Mental and physical state examination

	Special features to look for	Clinical example
Behaviour	*Behavioural clues to underlying psychotic experiences:* e.g. distraction by hallucinations: caution resulting from persecutory beliefs.	*Unkempt. Avoided eye contact. Restless.*
Talk/speech	*Incoherence or poverty of speech:* neologisms.	*Normal.*
Mood	*Blunting or incongruity of affect:* fear, suspiciousness, anger, irritability, depression.	*Irritable. Frightened.*
Thoughts	• *Abnormal connection between thoughts:* e.g. formal thought disorder (discriminating feature). • *Abnormal possession:* thought insertion and withdrawal. Thought broadcasting (first rank symptoms). • *Abnormal content:* distinguish between primary (first rank symptom) and secondary delusions. Establish the risk of a patient acting on a delusional belief.	*John had the delusional belief that his mother was an imposter substituted to spy on him. This belief appeared to be secondary to his experience of hearing constant persecutory voices (secondary delusion). John sometimes felt so frightened of his experiences that he had considered suicide as the only way out (possible suicide risk). He did not, however, have symptoms of depression.*
Perceptions	• *Auditory hallucinations:* distinguish between voices in the second person and third person (first rank symptom) and true and pseudohallucinations. Establish the risk of a patient acting on instructions from voices. • *Special forms of auditory hallucinations:* voices repeating subject's thoughts out loud or anticipating subject's thoughts. Voices commenting on subject's thoughts or behaviour (first rank symptoms). • *Visual hallucinations:* if present, exclude organic cause. • *Other hallucinations:* e.g. tactile or olfactory hallucinations. • *Passivity experiences:* (first rank symptoms) often associated with secondary delusions.	*John described continually hearing through his ears the voices of two unknown men arguing with each other over whether he should harm his mother. (Voices discussing subject in third person: first rank symptom. In addition, there is a possible risk of John assaulting his mother in response to his morbid symptoms.) John also described experiencing some of his movements as being 'made' by intrusive alien forces over which he had no control. For example he experienced his hand being moved in a threatening gesture towards his mother. (Passivity experience with increased risk of assault.)*
Cognition	*Exclude* altered level of consciousness and memory or intellectual impairment, since these features would indicate an underlying gross organic aetiology.	*No abnormality found.*
Physical examination	*To exclude gross organic aetiology.*	*No abnormality found.*

Outcome

	Diagnostic assessment: common differential diagnoses to always consider are mania, depression, and organic states including alcohol- and drug-related states.	*First rank symptoms in the absence of organic or affective disorder confirmed a diagnosis of schizophrenia. The family's history of schizophrenia predisposed him to the condition; possible precipitating and maintaining stress factors were recent work problems and the family's increasing intolerance of John's behaviour.*
	Management plan: to include immediate measures taking into account risk factors, together with plans for long-term rehabilitation and preventative measures.	*John reluctantly agreed to hospital admission where because of the suicide risk he was put under careful nursing observation, and commenced on a trial of neuroleptic medication. Long-term plans would include a review of accommodation and employment needs; the provision of ongoing psychological help to patient and family; and ensuring effective arrangements for giving prophylactic medication combined with careful monitoring for recurrence of at-risk symptoms.*

Diagnosis

Depression is common in those diagnosed as having schizophrenia, particularly after an acute phase of the illness. Alcohol and drug misuse may also occur. The degree of control exerted by medication over schizophrenic symptoms also needs to be regularly reassessed.

Causal factors

Ongoing causal factors should be identified since they increase the risk of an acute relapse of illness. Likely factors include housing problems, family tensions, lack of support and poor compliance with medication.

Risks

Suicide is a lifelong risk for those with schizophrenia, usually but not always occurring during depressive illness. Young people gaining insight following an acute schizophrenic illness and who have been high achievers in the past may be at particular risk. Schizophrenic symptoms may persist despite treatment in some patients and can be associated with an ongoing risk of unpredictable behaviour, for example by acting on delusional ideas or instructions given by voices. Finally those with so-called negative features of schizophrenia may be particularly at risk of gross self-neglect.

Therapeutic plan

Once the acute phase of the illness is over, the longer term care needs of the patient and their family have to be assessed. The aim is to help the individual return to as normal and independent a life as possible, and to lessen the risk of the acute phase of illness returning. Likely needs are as follows.
1 *Medical supervision*: e.g. monitoring progress of illness; reviewing medication and side effects.
2 *Personal and social functioning*: e.g. needs arising from lost confidence, poor social skills, problem behaviours and social isolation.
3 *Daytime activity/occupation*: e.g. need for structured daytime activity.
4 *Accommodation*: e.g. need for sheltered accommodation.
5 *Family/carers*: e.g. need to help family and patient live together or separate.
Assessment of these needs may be done by different members of a multidisciplinary team including occupational therapists, community nurses, social workers, psychologists and psychiatrists. Assessment after acute illness is usually done whilst the patient is still in hospital, often involving visits to day activity centres or accommodation on a trial basis. The final outcome of the assessment for the patient and relatives or carers should be a *care plan* which meets their illness related needs as far as is practical, and which can be reviewed on a regular basis.

Continuing the therapeutic process

People with schizophrenia often have long-term needs requiring long-term help. Good ongoing relationships between professionals and the patient and relatives are therefore vital. Since the assessment process leading to a care plan usually involves much discussion between all involved, this is often a time when these relationships can be firmly established.

Management of schizophrenia

Management can be broadly divided into the management of the acute illness, and the management of the chronic or post-acute phase of the illness.

Management of acute schizophrenia

The management of acute schizophrenia aims to effectively treat the illness as safely and rapidly as possible, taking due account of any risk factors present as well as the needs of concerned relatives. The acute illness is usually treated by a combination of intensive care and support, together with medication.

Intensive care and support

This is usually provided by nurses following an admission to hospital. Admission is usually indicated because the florid symptoms of the acute illness are frequently associated with behavioural disturbances. High levels of nursing care and supervision are then needed in order to look after the patient. Occasionally it may be possible to manage a less disturbed patient at home, providing the family is supportive and community psychiatric nurses are readily available.

Wherever the patient is looked after, it is essential for the professional carers to develop a supportive relationship with the patient. This will help make the alarming psychotic experiences less frightening and will also increase the likelihood of cooperation with treatment.

Where the acute illness is associated with high-risk features, such as assaults or self-harm, and the patient refuses to come into hospital, compulsory admission under the Mental Health Act 1983 (see Chapter 25) should be arranged. Irrespective of whether the Mental Health Act is used, patients who have high-risk features should be carefully nursed with appropriate levels of observation and care (see pp. 252 and 304).

Medication

Medication has an important part to play in the treatment of acute schizophrenia where two particular needs exist: firstly, to settle acute agitation and fear rapidly, together with the often associated unpredictable and disturbed behaviour; secondly, to begin treatment that over a period of weeks is likely to resolve the underlying acute symptoms of illness.

Where disturbed behaviour or distress is not a prominent feature medication can be withheld for a time, since a small but significant proportion of patients will settle spontaneously within a week of coming into hospital.

Chlorpromazine is the medication of choice in the acute phase of the illness. In sufficient dose, its sedative action on agitated or disturbed behaviour is effective within hours although its influence on symptoms such as delusions or voices usually takes at least 3 weeks, having its full effect only after about 6–12 weeks. Most patients will respond to daily doses of up to 800 mg of chlorpromazine. Where acute agitation or behaviour disturbance is not a feature, Sulperide or Risperidone may be used since they are less likely to cause side effects. Up to 5% of patients with acute schizophrenia will, however, fail to respond to adequate doses of medication, and may then have persistent florid symptoms together with the chronic disability that this entails. Details of the neuroleptic group of drugs commonly given to people with schizophrenia, including dosages and side effects, are given on p. 213.

Support and information to relatives

This is an important aspect of managing acute schizophrenia, particularly if this is a first illness and if the patient lives with relatives. Misconceptions about severe psychotic illnesses are commonplace, and may need to be corrected. Information should be provided at a level relatives can cope with, and a series of meetings is usually needed. A firm diagnosis of schizophrenia should only be made if there is sufficient evidence for this, and statements about outcome should be given with caution, since the long-term outcome of the illness is so difficult to predict.

Management of post-acute and chronic schizophrenia

The management of patients who are recovering from acute schizophrenia, or who have chronic schizophrenia, has two main aims: firstly, to return the patient to their best possible level of functioning; and secondly, to prevent recurrences of the acute illness.

At least a half of patients having an episode of acute schizophrenia will be left with some degree of disability. This usually takes the form of residual symptoms and personal or social re-adjustment problems. These in turn may lead to social disadvantages, particularly with accommodation, occupation and social isolation. The aim of ongoing care after the acute phase has settled will differ greatly between individuals. In some, return to work or previous activities may be realistic. In others, long-term sheltered activities and residence, perhaps over many years, may be more appropriate, the main goals being to arrest any further deterioration of functioning, and reduce the possibility of relapse.

Aftercare in the community

Most people with schizophrenia live in the community, coming into hospital only during acute relapses of illness. Only a tiny minority, less than 5%, need long-term hospital care usually because of very severe disablement and dependency, or chronic dangerousness. This is the reverse of the trend in the first half of this century when care was provided in large centralized asylums with all the inherent dangers of institutionalization, segregation and stigma. Now, with the closure of most of the old county asylums, care is increasingly provided away from hospitals and closer to where people live allowing them to carry on a more normal lifestyle with greater privacy and more control over their surroundings.

The mental health care needs of someone with chronic or post-acute schizophrenia are usually assessed while they are still in hospital, and are summarized in a care plan (Fig. 5.7). The patient, and where appropriate relatives and carers, should fully participate in the creation of the care plan. Frequently this is done during one or more case conferences involving all concerned. Since 1992, all patients in the UK

Fig. 5.7 Care plan

A 23-year-old man recovering from a first episode of schizophrenia and about to leave hospital who normally lives with parents and is at present unable to cope with open employment.

Need	Action	Responsibility
Ongoing support and problem orientated counselling	Weekly sessions with community nurse	CPN Z. Smith
Ongoing depot medication to reduce relapse risk	GP to prescribe; community nurse to give injection	GP Dr Ra CPN Z. Smith
Periodic medication review	Medical follow-up bimonthly	Dr Jones
Family support, counselling and education	Family sessions. Initially monthly. Information given about relative support groups, e.g. NSF	Dr Jones and CPN Z. Smith
Day activity	Attend day centre twice a week and community OT unit twice a week	OT P. Smith
In longer term, maybe need for sheltered accommodation away from home	Social worker to investigate options	SW S. Reed

Date of last review: ......
Keyworker: CPN. Z. Smith

---

discharged from psychiatric hospital are required by the government to have a care plan. In addition, the Community Care Act which came into force in 1993 has given Social Service departments responsibility for assessing and where possible meeting the social care needs of those with mental illness.

A keyworker, usually a community nurse or social worker, ensures that the care plan is put into effect and periodically reviewed. This person also acts as a link between the various professionals involved. These may come from a number of different agencies including Social Services, general practice, probation, housing, voluntary bodies, and of course various parts of the Health Service.

A care plan is likely to involve the patient in using some combination of the following resources.

Medical supervision

Periodic medical contact is important not only to review medication and its side effects, but also to monitor the underlying illness and associated risks. Since many patients require long-term contact with Mental Health Services, doctors who can see a patient regularly over a long period can best provide the follow-up needed.

Personal and social functioning

Help with four problem areas may reduce the disabling effect of the illness: the patient's loss of confidence; loss of social skills; social isolation; and the presence of recurrent problem behaviours.

Regaining confidence takes time, and can be helped through a supportive relationship with a member of the aftercare team, as well as by the experience of achieving some successes however small. Support groups and evening clubs also help (see p. 231 on supportive psychotherapy).

Training in new behaviours, such as social skills may assist a person's confidence and ability to be independent.

Problem behaviours, for example behavioural outbursts, inactivity or poor self-care, may be lessened by using behavioural therapy approaches. These would encourage appropriate behaviours, whilst ignoring inappropriate ones (see p. 26 and pp. 229, 230).

Daytime activity

Structured activity at a level the patient can cope with is likely to provide companionship, reduce boredom and give a sense of purpose to the week. It may also relieve relatives. A variety of day activities are needed to suit differing needs. These range from the more informal and supportive community mental health day centres to the structured occupational therapy units, sheltered workshops and gardening groups which may prepare people for a return to open employment.

Sheltered accommodation

Those leaving hospital after an acute episode of illness may not be able to live independently, needing varying amounts of support linked to their accommodation. These accommodation needs are likely to be met by choice from a range of differing types of 'sheltered' accommodation, including friendly landlady schemes; hostels with 24 hr live-in staff; bed sits or single person flats with day carers or wardens on hand; and group homes where three or four residents live in an ordinary house with regular visits by a member of a community mental health team.

Fig. 5.8 Living with a person who has schizophrenia

Relatives living with people who have schizophrenia report the following behaviours as most common, the features of social withdrawal and socially embarrassing behaviour being particularly hard to deal with (after Creer & Wing 1975).

Percentage of relatives reporting the problem	Problem behaviours
74	Social withdrawal
56	Underactivity
54	Lack of conversation
50	Few leisure interests
48	Slowness
41	Overactivity
34	Odd ideas
34	Depression
34	Odd behaviour
30	Neglect of appearance
25	Odd postures and movements
23	Threats or violence

Helping the family

At least a fifth of patients with schizophrenia live with close relatives in Western countries. Living with someone who has symptoms of schizophrenia can be stressful, and relatives report that problems associated with social withdrawal or socially embarrassing behaviour are both common and difficult to deal with. A list of problem behaviours reported by relatives is given in Fig. 5.8.

Supportive family therapy and problem-orientated family therapy are likely to be particularly valuable (see p. 237 including Case 11).

Help should recognize the important role of the caring relative, provide adequate information and support, and assist the family to find ways of reducing or coping with difficult behaviours as well as making sure that local aftercare resources are being used to the full. In addition, organizations such as the National Schizophrenia Fellowship provide information and support, giving families an opportunity to meet others who share the same problems (see also p. 201 for further discussion of types of care involved).

Patient and carer involvement

Imposing a care plan on someone is doomed to failure. The patient and if appropriate the family should actively participate in care planning. This is likely to involve looking at various choices. For example, should a patient stay with his family or live in sheltered housing? If in sheltered housing, then what types are there and what are the advantages and disadvantages of each? As a general rule the more the patient has contributed to the care plan and exercised choice within it, the more likely he is to adhere to it rather than rebel against it. Beware the tendency of professionals to take over, thinking they know best but in the process disempowering and institutionalizing the very people they are seeking to help towards greater independence.

Finally, any care plan may be limited by two realities. Firstly, not all mental health needs can be met. There is for example a widespread shortage of sheltered housing and support staff in the community. Secondly, not everyone wants to cooperate with aftercare (Case 2, p. 62). In a society that values individual freedom and self-determination this choice must be respected, even if you believe it puts the person's mental health at risk.

Prevention of relapse

Two measures are of proven value in reducing the risk of relapse in vulnerable individuals: prophylactic medication, and stress reduction.

Prophylactic medication

In the year after the acute illness, the relapse risk for those on no medication is at least 2–3 times that for matched patients continued on medication. Prophylaxis, either by using oral neuroleptics or depot preparations, is therefore advised in most patients who have had acute illnesses particularly if these show a recurrent pattern, are associated with severe disruption of the patient's life, or are associated with high-risk features.

Regularly taken, prophylactic medication can be expected to reduce the relapse rate to below 10% during the year after an acute illness. Compliance with medication is however a crucial factor, and this can be assisted by regular aftercare supervision, for example by a psychiatric community nurse, or general practitioner, and also by using depot injections.

Details of prophylactic neuroleptic medications in use are given in pp. 213–215.

Stress reduction
Over two-thirds of acute schizophrenic illnesses occur within 3 weeks of stressful circumstances not brought on by the effects of the illness itself. Thus, the timing of relapses is often related to stress, and this is at least as important a factor as the cessation of prophylactic medication.

Although many stressful events are unavoidable, two particular sources of stress commonly causing relapse can be reduced: stress arising from living with relatives, and stress arising from a rehabilitation programme.

Family stress: this is most evident in so called 'high expressed emotion families' where typically key relatives are highly critical of the patient yet also spend a lot of time with them. Patients from such families have a higher risk of relapse than those living in other circumstances, even if they are taking prophylactic medication. Family counselling may help such relatives cope more constructively with the problems of living with a person suffering from schizophrenia, and in addition, face-to-face contact with relatives can be reduced by for example, encouraging the patient to attend a day centre. However, where difficulties persist the patient may be best living away from their relatives.

Care programme stress: over-energetic aftercare or premature return to work and previous responsibilities may precipitate a relapse. This reinforces the importance of creating an appropriate initial care plan, and the need to continually review its progress and goals.

Fig. 5.9 The expected range of outcomes over a period of at least 5 years

Good outcome 50%
No problems (25–35%)
- No ongoing symptoms.
- Normal social integration.
- Able to work.
- Long-term medication not required.

Minor problems (15–25%)
- Relapse is likely.
- Risk of some social or work impairment.
- Independent living possible.

Intermediate outcome 25%
- Episodic course with relapses of acute illness.
- Significant social and work disablement likely.
- Limited ability for independent living.

Poor outcome 25%
- May have persistent negative symptoms.
- May have persistent florid symptoms (5–10%).
- Moderate to severe social and work disablement.

Fig. 5.10

Good prognostic factors	Poor prognostic factors
• Sudden onset.	• Insidious onset.
• Florid rather than negative symptoms.	• Prominent negative symptoms.
• Presence of depression.	• Flattening of mood.
• Well-adjusted previous personality.	• Social isolation.

In addition to reducing stress at source, patients can be taught strategies which help them cope with unavoidable stressful events. Again, the psychiatric community nurse is often in the best position to do this.

The course and prognosis of schizophrenia

The follow-up studies of patients who present with acute schizophrenia indicate a varied long-term outcome. Figure 5.9 outlines the expected range of outcomes over at least a 5-year period.

Given the particular patient, however, can we tell in advance which outcome group they will fall into? To do so would obviously be of value in both counselling relatives and in developing a therapeutic plan for the patient. In general, information from three areas can help in predicting the future course of the illness: clinical presentation, social factors, and factors known from the patient's personal history. These factors, together with the outcome they are associated with, are listed in Fig. 5.10. It must always be remembered, however, that they are only informed guesses based on the results of a range of follow-up studies, and in the case of an individual patient they may be misleading. Prediction should thus be made with considerable caution.

Related syndromes

Persistent delusional disorders
These comprise a variety of disorders where long-standing delusions are the only or most conspicuous feature, and there is an absence of an organic or schizophrenic mood disorder. The relationship of these disorders to schizophrenia is uncertain. The delusions may be persecutory hypochondriacal or grandiose, and may for example be concerned with litigation, jealousy or bodily appearance. Features such as auditory hallucinations are absent. Three examples are given.

Morbid jealousy
The central feature is a delusional belief that the partner has been unfaithful. This may lead to persistent questioning of the spouse, together with exhaustive checks and searches for evidence of the supposed infidelity. Morbid jealousy is

commoner in men, and may lead to violence and even murder (see also p. 302).

Paranoid state
The patient may have a highly encapsulated belief of being the victim of a conspiracy. Alternatively the patient may believe that others think he smells, or is homosexual.

Monosymptomatic hypochondriacal psychosis
The patient may have the delusional belief that his bodily functioning is diseased or abnormal, or that his body is misshapen. Persistent attempts to obtain treatment or cosmetic surgery may result. People with persistent delusional disorders can be very reluctant to accept appropriate help. They may repeatedly visit physicians, lawyers, the police or cosmetic surgeons, but are unlikely to want to see a psychiatrist.

Diagnosis involves the exclusion of underlying primary disorders such as depression or organic states, and the appraisal of any risk factors such as danger to the spouse in the case of morbid jealousy. Treatment with neuroleptics may be helpful if the patient is willing to accept this.

Acute and transient disorders
These comprise disorders with acute (within 2 weeks) or abrupt (within 48 hours) onset, are often stress related, and appear to be particularly common in developing countries. Symptoms of schizophrenia such as hallucinations may be present, but are short lived (less than a month) and rapidly changeable. Outcome is generally good.

Schizoaffective disorder
An episodic disorder in which both affective (manic or depressive) and schizophrenic symptoms are prominent within the same episode of illness, usually simultaneously but at least within a few days of each other. The relationship to typical mood and schizophrenic disorders is uncertain. The prognosis is significantly better than for schizophrenia.

QUESTIONS

1 What criteria would you use in order to establish a diagnosis of schizophrenia? What syndromes may clinically resemble schizophrenia?

2 Discuss the importance of the family in the assessment and longer term management of a person who has acute schizophrenia.

3 A man with a history of schizophrenia is in a police cell after assaulting a neighbour. What would you try to establish in your psychiatric assessment of this man?

4 A patient's acute schizophrenic illness is resolving. How would you assess the need for aftercare, and what should be the main features of an appropriate care programme?

5 Discuss critically the factors which might influence the course and prognosis of schizophrenia.

6 Outline the factors which may put an individual at risk of developing schizophrenia.

FURTHER READING

Gelder M., Gath D. & Mayou R. (1989) Schizophrenia. In: *Oxford Textbook of Psychiatry*. Oxford University Press, Oxford. [A good comprehensive review.]

Sims, A. (1988) *Symptoms in the Mind*. Ballière, Tindall, London. [A stimulating and engaging introduction to symptoms found in schizophrenia.]

Wing J. & Wing L.C. (eds) (1983) *Handbook of Psychiatry, Volume 3, Part 1, Schizophrenia and Paranoid Psychoses*, pp. 3–95. Cambridge University Press, Cambridge. [A more detailed multi-author review of important clinical, aetiological and management topics.]

USEFUL ADDRESSES

National Schizophrenia Fellowship, 28 Castle Street, Kingston Upon Thames KT1 1SS (tel: 081-547-3937).
MIND, 22 Harley Street, London W1N 2ED (tel: 071-637-0741).

6
Affective Disorders

Fact Sheet

Definition
Clinical disorders of mood, including a wide range of conditions, from depression to elation, and characterized by abnormalities of speech and thought, bodily functions and behaviour.

Classification
By reference to their clinical picture, they can be classified into manic disorders, depressive disorders and dysthymic disorders (depressive neurosis). By reference to their course, they are classified into bipolar disorders and unipolar disorders.

Presentation
Manic episodes are characterized by:
- elated or irritable mood;
- pressure of speech, flight of ideas, grandiosity and mood congruent delusions;
- insomnia without tiredness, increased appetite and libido;
- illusions and mis-interpretations;
- hyperactivity, overspending, tendency to unlawful acts.

Depressive episodes can present with:
- sadness, worthlessness, anxiety;
- poverty of thought, pessimistic thoughts, suicidal ideas, impaired concentration, mood congruent delusions;
- early morning waking, lack of appetite, reduced libido;
- perceptual abnormalities;
- self-neglect, avoidance of social interaction, impaired performance, suicidal ideation.

Dysthymic disorders share many of the symptoms of a depressive episode, but they are less severe, variable in response to external events and associated with other neurotic symptoms.

Bipolar disorders are those with recurrent episodes of mania and depression. Recurrent manic episodes without depressive phases are rare and patients with such disorders are in practical terms regarded as suffering form bipolar conditions. **Unipolar** disorders are characterized by recurrent depressive episodes.

Distribution
1 Bipolar disorders:
- prevalence: under 1% (men and women combined);
- incidence: 9–15 per 100 000 per year for men and 8–30 per 100 000 per year for women;
- lifetime expectancy: about 1% for men and women.
Onset usually before 30 years of age.

2 Unipolar depression:
- prevalence: about 3% for men and 9% for women;
- incidence: 80–200 per 100 000 per year for men and 250–600 per 100 000 per year for women;
- lifetime expectancy: 10% for men, 20% for women.
Peak age for women 35–45 and for men after the age of 55.

3 Dysthymic disorders:
- prevalence and incidence unclear because of different diagnostic practices;
- lifetime prevalence of about 5%.

Aetiological factors
Causes and mechanisms are not fully understood. Predisposing factors include genetic characteristics, early social factors, personality traits and attitudes, current social difficulties and biological factors. Precipitant factors include adverse life events and biological factors. Maintaining factors include personality, social difficulties and biological factors.

Assessment
Careful evaluation is needed to establish the nature and extent of the disorder, aetiological factors and need for further treatment. Attention needs to be paid to suicide risk and risk to others, and to the need for admission to hospital.

Differential diagnosis
This will include normal reactions to stress, schizophrenia, organic syndromes and personality disorders.

Management
Short-term management includes:
- psychological treatments from simple information and support to specialized techniques;
- physical methods, such as neuroleptics, antidepressants and ECT;
- social measures.

Long-term treatment will include psychological treatments, physical methods like lithium and antidepressants and social measures.

Prognosis
Short term: the large majority of patients recover from an episode in less than 1 year. Long-term relapse is common and a proportion of patients experience chronic disorders. About 15% commit suicide. A significant minority experience social impairment.

What are the affective disorders?

The affective disorders, or disorders of mood, include a wide range of abnormalities, from mild states to severe and even life-threatening conditions. Mild forms are relatively common and usually self-limiting, but the more severe forms, while less common are very important and need to be recognized. This is so, first, because of the associated risks, such as suicide, and second because of the existence of very effective treatments for these conditions.

Disorders of mood can present to the clinician with a large range of symptoms and different clinical pictures, but in all such disorders, the predominant abnormality is one of mood or affect. Other symptoms commonly found in addition to mood abnormalities are disorders of thinking or perception, and changes in biological functions, such as sleep, appetite, interest in sex, or levels of energy.

The affective disorders are usually divided into:
1 minor affective disorders, consisting of conditions of mild symptomatology and of generally good short-term outcome;
2 major affective disorders which, as their name suggests, are characterized by severe symptoms. These major disorders include depressive disorders, when the predominant mood is low, and manic disorders, when the mood is elevated. Only severe disorders will be considered here, whilst the minor affective disorders will be discussed elsewhere (see Chapter 12, p. 143).

In contrast with other psychiatric conditions, such as schizophrenia, the symptoms that characterize the affective disorders can be found to a certain degree in healthy or normal individuals, or in people who are faced with stressful situations, but who would not otherwise be regarded as psychiatrically disturbed. For example, most people have experienced feelings of sadness, insomnia, or elation. The distinction between normal and pathological mood is crucial, and one that can usually be made without difficulty when dealing with the major affective disorders. Thus, an abnormal mood will be characterized by its persistence and lack of response to changing situations; its degree of severity and association with other typical symptoms, and its being out of proportion to the circumstances.

In the case of the minor affective disorders, it may be harder to differentiate between a normal and a pathological mood. As a rule, the difference will be one of degree, rather than one concerning the quality or nature of the reported symptoms. The individual's own subjective perception of the symptoms, and social expectations as to what degree of distress is considered abnormal, will also contribute to determine whether the person seeks help from doctors or others.

Classification and terminology

The general classification of psychiatric disorders has been dealt with in Chapter 1 (p. 12) but some issues of relevance to the affective disorders need to be considered here in some detail.

A wide variety of terms are commonly used to refer to the affective disorders, and these can lead to a good deal of confusion. For example, depression is sometimes referred to as 'reactive' or 'endogenous', depending on the presence or absence of clear precipitants; the terms 'psychotic' and 'neurotic', also in relation to depression, are sometimes used to classify the condition by referring to some of the symptoms of the disorder. Unfortunately, it is sometimes assumed that 'reactive' and 'neurotic', or even mild depression, are synonymous; this can often be wrong as for example in the case of a severe depressive disorder ('psychotic' depression) following a bereavement ('reactive' depression).

Some terms used commonly in relation to the affective disorders are listed here.
- Bipolar disorder: depressive, manic, or mixed episodes have occurred in the past.
- Unipolar disorder: only depressive episodes have occurred, either once only, or in a recurrent pattern.
- Manic depressive disorder: this is synonymous with bipolar affective disorder.
- Endogenous depression: depressive disorder without known external precipitants.
- Reactive depression: depressive disorder with obvious external precipitants.
- Psychotic depression: depression with 'psychotic' symptoms, such as delusions or hallucinations.
- Neurotic depression: depression with 'neurotic' features, such as anxiety, phobias, or obsessional symptoms.
- Dysthymic disorder: this term is synonymous with neurotic depression.
- Melancholia: depressive disorder with marked loss of pleasure in usual activities, severely low mood, and somatic symptoms such as early waking, loss of weight, etc.
- Involutional melancholia: depressive illness occurring late in life.
- Hypomania: manic disorder of mild or moderate degree.

Figure 6.1 shows a working classification of the affective disorders.

In practice, it is useful to try first to describe the clinical syndrome in terms of whether it is a depressive or a manic disorder, or one where both depressive and manic symptoms co-exist, and to establish the severity of the syndrome by noting the nature and extent of its symptoms.

After the clinical picture has been clarified, it is useful to comment on the history of the disorder, and in particular, on whether the current disorder is a one-off episode or whether

---

Fig. 6.1 Classification of affective disorders

1 *Major affective disorders*
By reference to the clinical syndrome:
- manic episode;
- major depressive episode;
- dysthymic disorder (depressive neurosis).

By reference to the course over time:
- bipolar disorder;
- unipolar disorder.

2 *Minor affective disorders*
- With predominant depressive symptoms.
- With predominant anxiety.

previous depressive or manic, or both, types of episodes are known to have occurred (Fig. 6.2).

Finally, it is important to establish whether the current episode appears to be related to obvious environmental factors, and to list them, or to state whether such precipitants are largely absent.

How can they be recognized?

The diagnosis of affective disorder is essentially a clinical procedure, and is is therefore based on the careful assessment both of the person's symptoms at the time of the interview (mental state examination), and of the history (recent and distant), as provided by the individual or close relatives. Although research is being carried out in search of tests or biological markers of affective disorder, this work remains experimental, and does not, as yet, have direct clinical application.

The psychiatric assessment of patients and history taking have been considered in Chapter 3, and it should only be necessary to mention here the need to observe the patient's appearance and general behaviour, to listen to the patient's spontaneous utterances, and to ask specific questions to clarify particular aspects of the patient's symptoms or history.

In affective disorders, most areas of psychological func-

tioning can become impaired, but the key abnormalities of interest to the clinician are likely to be concerned with:
- mood;
- thinking, both its content and form;
- bodily or somatic functions;
- perceptions;
- behaviour.

Manic episode

The main characteristic of a manic episode is mood elevation, but a wide range of other abnormalities can also appear, Manic episodes are circumscribed, with return to normality between bouts of ill-health. The clinical features of a manic episode are described below, and are summarized in Fig. 6.3 (see also atypical features of mania in the elderly, p. 162).

Abnormalities of mood

The patient presents with elated and expansive mood, with a marked subjective feeling of well-being. The patient's mood is often out of keeping with the circumstances, and tends to remain elevated for long periods of time. There can also be some lability of mood, with brief periods of sadness.

Some manic patients show irritability and a tendency to become angry, rather than a clear elevation of mood. Here too, the abnormal mood is persistent and unrelated to environmental events, although the patient may become sensitive to criticism or to efforts to exert some control over his or her behaviour, and in response may behave in an aggressive way towards others.

Abnormalities of speech and thought
Manic patients are usually over-talkative and speak rapidly, showing a characteristic pressure of speech. The patient may speak in an unnecessarily loud voice, without regard to social conventions, or burst into song. The patient may show flight of ideas, with rapid changes in thought content, and a tendency to distractibility in response to environmental stimuli.

The patient's thoughts are consistent with the elevated mood, and are characterized by increased self-esteem, and the belief in the possession of special abilities and powers. Sometimes, these ideas can reach delusional intensity, when they would be known as grandiose delusions. Manic patients can also suffer other types of delusions, such as of persecution or of jealousy, and they are usually consistent with elevated mood (also known as mood congruent delusions).

Abnormalities of bodily functions
Sleep is very often disturbed, and this can be one of the earliest signs of an impending manic episode. The patient may be reluctant to retire to bed at the habitual time, and remain awake and active. After a brief period of sleep the patient may wake up full of energy and ideas once more, with little sign of exhaustion.

Appetite is usually increased, and food is consumed in an indiscriminate way. In the untreated, hyperactive patient, weight can actually decrease, in spite of the increased food intake.

Sexual interest and activity usually become heightened, and together with elated mood and grandiose ideas can lead the patient to become sexually disinhibited, and to commit unlawful acts.

Perceptual abnormalities
Illusions and misinterpretations consistent with a euphoric mood are common. In severe forms, the patient may suffer hallucinations, auditory or visual, and of content related to the euphoric mood.

Abnormal behaviour
The patient is usually hyperactive, often in a purposeful way, but likely to fail to accomplish tasks, and in general remains easily distractible. Not infrequently, the patient may set off on a journey, or make unrealistic travel plans. Business ventures may be started, and large sums of money spent sometimes before the patient's relatives have come to realize. Aggressive and disinhibited sexual behaviour may occur, and the patient may break the law as a result.

The patient may show an excessively familiar attitude to strangers, and behave in an over-friendly and socially inappropriate fashion.

Major depressive episode
The principal characteristic of a depressive episode is the presence of low mood, although other symptoms may also be present. As in the case of manic disorders, the disturbance

---

Fig. 6.4 Main features of a major depressive episode

1 Abnormalities of mood
- Sadness.
- Tearfulness.
- Anxiety.
- Worthlessness, hopelessness, self-blame.
- Loss of feeling.

2 Abnormalities of speech and thought
- Slow speech, poverty of thought.
- Agitated speech.
- Pessimistic thought content.
- Suicidal ideas.
- Impaired attention and concentration.
- Mood congruent delusions.
- Other delusions.

3 Abnormalities of bodily functions
- Early waking, restless sleep.
- Lack of energy.
- Psychomotor retardation or agitation.
- Loss of appetite.
- Loss of weight.
- Reduced sexual interest and activity.
- Constipation, menstrual problems.

4 Perceptual abnormalities
- Illusions.
- Misinterpretations.
- Hallucinations.

5 Abnormal behaviour
- Avoidance of social interaction.
- Impaired work performance.
- Self-neglect.
- Neglect of responsibilities.
- Actions in preparation of suicide.

---

is circumscribed and episodic in nature, and the patient usually returns to a normal state between episodes of ill health. The clinical features of a major depressive episode are described here, and they are summarized in Fig. 6.4 (see also typical features of depression in the elderly, p. 162).

Abnormalities of mood
The predominant mood is one of sadness, which the patient may describe as one of depression, feeling low or down, or in similar terms. The low mood is persistent, without sudden changes, although there may be some variation in the degree of mood disturbance during the day: for example, in severe forms, the patient's mood is characteristically worse in the morning, showing some improvement as the day goes by, and being at its best in the evening.

Depressive feelings may range in intensity from a mild dysphoric state, to one of deep and all-pervasive sadness and unhappiness. Low mood is often accompanied by tearfulness, although in severe forms the patient may complain of inability to cry. Feelings of subjective anxiety and distress, as well as anxious foreboding, are not uncommon. Patients often complain of lack of enjoyment in their usual activities,

Case 1: manic episode	Case 2: major depressive episode	Case 3: dysthymic disorder (depressive neurosis)
Gradual onset over several weeks. Good previous adjustment.	*Recent onset. Precipitants present.*	*Suicide attempt associated with alcohol. Domestic problems as precipitant.*
Richard was a 26-year-old self-employed carpenter who was admitted to a psychiatric hospital under *Section 4 of the Mental Health Act.* During the previous 6 weeks he had become increasingly *hyperactive and irritable* and had been getting involved in *arguments with strangers.* His admission was precipitated by a row at a public house, when the police had to be called, and Richard was taken to the police station, where he was seen by the police surgeon who was concerned about his mental state. There had been *no obvious stresses or problems associated with the change in his behaviour.*	Elizabeth was a 62-year-old retired school teacher, who was admitted to a psychiatric hospital voluntarily. *For the previous 5 weeks or so she* had become socially *withdrawn, gradually* dropping her social commitments and had begun to *lose interest in her* appearance or her house. Her husband had become concerned about her, and in the week prior to admission had given up his part-time job as a caretaker to look after her, but by now he was finding it increasingly difficult to do so. There had been some *minor disagreements with one of the children, and a close friend had died 2 months previously.*	Christine was a 32-year-old married woman with four children who was admitted to the general hospital following an overdose of *sleeping tablets and alcohol.* Her act was precipitated by a *row with her husband and one of the younger children who had been unusually demanding.* Her overdose had been of *low suicidal intent,* and she denied any *wish to die. However, she* had felt desperate and when she was seen by the psychiatrist in hospital, she remained unhappy and despondent about her problems.
Elated mood with marked irritability. Grandiose ideas.	*Marked retardation, but some agitation present, self-blame, sadness, impaired concentration.*	*Chronic difficulties.*
On examination, he looked unkempt and was angry and verbally abusive to everyone around him. He spoke in a *loud voice and behaved in a threatening manner* but was not actually violent. The content of his speech was mostly about his concern about nuclear power, and the risk of nuclear leaks. He claimed to be a nuclear expert, and to have the power to control nuclear energy and release it at will. He was *very sensitive to events around him, and*	On examination, she looked *sad and uncommunicative, with very little spontaneous movement, and with a rather fixed posture. Her hands moved restlessly,* straightening her skirt or picking at her cardigan. She *spoke in a very monotonous voice* and usually hesitated for a few seconds before answering questions. She felt she should not be wasting the doctor's time, and that she should be at	Her problems had begun about 2 years previously, when her 13-year-old son by a previous marriage had got into trouble with the police. The situation had continued to deteriorate since then and for the last 6 months the boy had been taken into care because of the family's difficulty coping with him. During the last year, Christine had felt *unhappy and tearful, with better periods in between.* She had felt guilty about not being able to cope with her son, but at the same time felt *unable to look after her*
		Fluctuating symptoms of depression, but no marked somatic features.

could easily be distracted from his discussion of nuclear topics. At times he would smile broadly and wink, but his *cheerful mood tended to be short-lived*. He was *fully orientated* but he would not cooperate with memory tests. He denied hearing voices or having any difficulty with his thinking. Richard had a *history of three* previous admissions to hospital, the first one at the age of 19 and the other two at intervals of about 18 months. The first and third admissions had been as a result of manic episodes, while the second one followed an episode of depression. Following his third admission he had been put on *lithium*, but he had only taken it for 6 months after discharge.

Previous history of marked mood swings.

Following admission, Richard was treated with *chlorpromazine*. He absconded several times, and his *Section 4 was converted to a Section 2*. By the end of his third week in hospital, his mood and behaviour began to improve, but he did not return to normal for another 5 weeks, in which time he had become an informal patient. After his second week of in-patient

Compulsory admission required.

Difficulty accepting the illness is common in young patients.

home trying to finish her housework and looking after her husband.

At the same time she admitted she felt very tired, and *unable to plan what to do next*. She *felt she was letting her husband down* and at that point cried silently. She was orientated, but had *difficulty with tasks involving mental arithmetic*. Her husband confirmed that she had been *waking up early* in the morning, and that he had become worried when he found her standing in her nightdress looking out of the window on the last two mornings. She had had a lot of *difficulty getting dressed and he had to take responsibility for getting her ready in the mornings*, and preparing her food. She had *hardly eaten and she had lost weight*.

Loss of appetite and weight.

She had had *two previous episodes similar to the present one*, one following the birth of her first daughter who was now 40 and the second time shortly after her menopause. On the first occasion she was admitted to hospital where she had ECT and stayed for 2 months. On the second occasion she was treated by her GP with antidepressants.

Past history of depressive episodes.

husband and the other children properly. She had been occasionally tearful, especially recently when her husband had begun to resent her involvement with the boy.

There had been no change in *appetite, or weight, but she had tended to have difficulty getting off to sleep*, and had had occasional periods when *she had tended to wake up early in the mornings*. Over the last 6 weeks or so she had begun to *drink wine at home*, especially at weekends when it was expected that Stewart would be coming home. Her *relationship with her husband had deteriorated and she had lost interest in sex*.

Alcohol abuse.

She had also *begun to worry about heart disease*, and on one occasion had become very *worried about the possibility of having breast cancer*.

Hypochondriacal concerns.

Her husband was seen after she had been admitted to the general hospital and he admitted *he had become irritable lately and perhaps had been less supportive*. A joint discussion followed and they agreed to discuss fully the implications of Stewart's return home, and

Planning how to tackle problems.

Continued on p. 78

Case 1 (Continued)

care *lithium was added to his regime and by the time he was discharged to outpatient care he had begun to accept the need for continuous lithium therapy,* although he was still finding it difficult to accept that he had a bipolar affective disorder, and that he would need long-term medication. Five years later he continues well and has accepted the need to receive lithium. He has now married, and his wife has taken an interest in helping him come to terms with his condition. He continues to be followed up as an out-patient.

Good outcome and good response to lithium.

Case 2 (Continued)

Following admission, Elizabeth was treated with *amitriptyline* in increasing doses but after 3 weeks there had been only limited improvement and she was beginning to feel distressed and anxious because of her failure to return home. After discussion with her and her husband *a course of ECT was given and her mood and general behaviour improved rapidly,* so that by the end of nine treatments she was discharged home. Three years later she continued to do well.

She was *continued on antidepressant medication for a year,* after which the medication had been gradually reduced without difficulties.

She had returned to her usual full social life and involvement in local activities having made a full recovery.

Antidepressants and ECT were needed.

Antidepressants were useful as prophylatic.

Case 3 (Continued)

whether it would be in fact better to have the boy fostered.

They agreed to discuss the matter with the boy's social worker. Christine also agreed to stop drinking alcohol, whilst she was looking at other ways of dealing with her problems.

Over the next 4 months, Christine and her husband were seen together on five occasions. After several discussions with the GP and Social Services, Stewart was placed with foster parents which were acceptable to him and to Christine. Relations with the boy and his mother had improved and her mood was now returning to normal.

Her relationship with her husband had also improved and the sexual relationship had now resumed.

Counselling and social intervention were successful in improving her symptoms and domestic problems.

and in some cases, patients may experience a subjectively distressing lack of feeling for their children or other loved ones.

Patients may experience feelings of hopelessness, self-blame and self-reproach, and worthlessness. Complaints of subjective lack of energy are common.

These depressive symptoms show limited reactivity to external events. In mild cases, the patient's mood may improve to a certain extent for brief periods in response to circumstances, but in severe forms, all reactivity may be lost.

Abnormalities of speech and thought

The depressed patient's talk is usually slow and monotonous, with a tendency to brief utterances, and showing a limited range of expression. There may be a marked poverty of thought content, and little spontaneous speech.

On the other hand, depressed patients who also have symptoms of agitation, may be very talkative, but the content of their speech is restricted to a limited range of distressing topics concerned with illness, death or impending disaster. In extreme cases, the patient may shout or call for help in a persistent and distressing way.

Thought content, as described above, is consistent with low mood, and centred on pessimistic and distressing ideas. Patients regard themselves in a negative way, showing decreased self-esteem and abilities, and viewing their past achievements as worthless, and the future as hopeless and doomed.

Suicidal ideas are common in depressive disorders. They may range from fleeting suicidal thoughts or ill-formed ideas about wishing to be dead, which the patient can dismiss easily, to carefully thought out suicidal plans, including details of the procedure to be used. Suicidal thoughts can be very distressing to some patients, who may fear they are losing control, or that they are going mad, while others may respond to such ideas with a fatalistic sense of inevitability. Suicidal thoughts are sometimes at their most intense in the early hours of the morning, accompanying the diurnal variation in depressed mood (see also p. 246).

Patients may complain of difficulty thinking, with subjective feelings of impaired concentration, reduced ability to carry out mental tasks, or difficulty making decisions. For example, patients may describe problems when trying to read the newspaper or watch TV.

Depressed patients' beliefs about ill-health, financial ruin, guilt, punishment, etc., may reach delusional intensity, and this is characteristic of severe depression. As described above, this type of depressive syndrome is sometimes called 'psychotic depression'. The content of the delusional ideas is usually consistent with the depressed mood (or mood congruent).

Abnormalities of bodily functions

Sleep is usually impaired, and in severe depression it is characterized by persistent early waking, generally several hours before the patient's usual time, followed by inability to go back to sleep. Patients can also experience difficulty getting off to sleep, or restless, disturbed sleep, often interrupted by distressing dreams or nightmares. Whatever the pattern of sleep disturbance, patients often complain of exhaustion on getting up, and of a feeling of dread at the prospect of having to face the day. In some cases, hypersomnia is seen, although this is not common in severe depressive disorders.

Complaints of subjective tiredness and lack of energy are accompanied by slowness and hesitation in the way routine activities, such as getting up, dressing, etc., are carried out. In severe forms, the term 'retarded depression' is used to refer to patients with marked psychomotor retardation. In other cases, a picture of purposeless activity and restlessness is seen, so that the patient paces up and down, or starts tasks which are soon abandoned. This syndrome is described clinically as 'agitated depression'.

Appetite is usually decreased, and patients often describe loss of interest in and lack of enjoyment of food. The result is loss of weight, which in some patients can be very marked. Some depressed patients increase their food consumption, and also their weight, and this is sometimes the result of comfort eating, aimed at providing relief from depression.

Sexual interest and activity are reduced, and psychosexual dysfunctions, such as erectile impotence and impaired interest, can sometimes be an early sign of depression (see Chapter 23, p. 290).

Other bodily manifestations of depression include constipation, difficulties with micturition, and menstrual problems, such as irregular periods and amenorrhoea.

Perceptual abnormalities

Illusions and mis-interpretations consistent with the predominant depressed mood are often present, and can be very distressing to the patient. In severe disorders, hallucinations and pseudohallucinations of a depressive content can occur.

Abnormal behaviour

As described above, psychomotor retardation or agitation may be present. In addition, a patient's loss of interest in things may lead to avoidance of social situations, impaired work performance and loss of job, neglect of family responsibilities, failure to maintain usual standards of hygiene, and self-neglect. Patients with serious suicidal ideas may take steps towards self-harm, for example, purchasing firearms, making a will, or making financial arrangements in anticipation of death.

Dysthymic disorder or depressive neurosis

In contrast with manic or depressive episodes, dysthymic disorders are characterized by their chronicity, so that they can be present for many months. Depressive symptoms are less severe than in major depressive disorders, and their range is limited. Thus, delusions, hallucinations, and severe bodily abnormalities are absent. In addition, symptoms respond significantly to external events, and low mood can improve as a result of favourable circumstances.

The main symptoms of dysthymic disorders are described below.

Abnormalities of mood

Sadness of mild to moderate degree and lack of interest in usual activities are common, but they are not persistent, and the patient is able to respond to favourable external events.

Irritability, anxiety, obsessional symptoms, phobias and hypochondriacal preoccupations are often present. Feelings of lack of confidence, of difficulties in social interactions are common.

Abnormalities of speech and thought

Delusions do not occur. The patient may be worried about the future, jobs, health, etc., and the content of the patient's speech may reflect these concerns, but it is possible to divert the patient from these preoccupations. Suicidal ideas may be present, but they are usually transient, and ill-formed.

Abnormalities of bodily functions

Sleep is usually disturbed, with difficulty getting off to sleep, or late awakening, rather than early waking, which is characteristic of severe depression. Patients often complain of restless sleep. Tiredness and subjective lack of energy may be present. There may be appetite changes, usually of a mild nature, including over-eating, as well as anorexia. Comfort eating is not uncommon. Sexual interest and satisfaction are usually reduced, although some degree of sexual responsivity can be present.

Perceptual abnormalities

Hallucinations do not occur. Illusions and other minor abnormalities may be present.

Abnormal behaviour

A mild degree of impairment of social interactions may be present, including difficulties with work, family, and leisure. Irritability and anger may contribute to the problems. Suicide attempts of low suicidal intent and minimal preparation can occur. Shoplifting is occasionally associated with depression (see Chapter 24, p. 306).

What are the causes of the affective disorders?

The problems involved in clarifying what is meant by 'cause' in relation to psychiatric disorders have been discussed in Chapter 2 (p. 20) and, in particular, the difficulty in establishing the relative contribution of a variety of likely aetiological factors, and the reader should turn to that chapter for a general review of this topic. Here, the causes of the affective disorders will be discussed, with emphasis on the examination of factors associated with them, and the mechanisms involved. Figure 6.5 summarizes the main aetiological factors.

Factors associated with the affective disorders: predisposing factors

Genetic factors

There is strong evidence for a genetic contribution to the major depressive and manic disorders. Thus, patients are likely to have relatives with a history of affective disorder; twin studies show very high concordance rates for MZ twins and somewhat lower rates for DZ twins; and adoption

---

Fig. 6.5 Aetiology of affective disorders

1 Predisposing factors
- Genetic factors: genetic sub-groups related to clinical syndromes and epidemiological features.
- Early social factors: loss of parent; disturbed family relations.
- Personality traits and attitudes: obsessionality; learned helplessness; 'negative cognitive set'; 'low self-esteem'.
- Current social factors: lack of confiding relationship.
- Biological factors: neurotransmitter vulnerability.

2 Precipitating factors
- Life-events: threat, loss.
- Physical disorders.

3 Maintaining factors
- Personality traits and attitudes: 'negative cognitive set', etc.
- Current social factors: chronic and persistent difficulties.
- Biological factors: neurotransmitter abnormality.

---

studies indicate that the incidence of affective disorder in the biological parents of adoptees with affective disorders is much greater than in their adoptive parents.

There is also evidence for genetic differences between bipolar disorders (those with a history of manic and depressive episodes, or of manic episodes alone) and unipolar (depressive) affective disorders: patients with a bipolar illness are likely to have relatives with the same form of disorder, whilst those with unipolar disorders have relatives both with unipolar and bipolar conditions. Genetic sub-groups have been identified in both bipolar and unipolar disorders, which take into account the patient's sex and the age of onset of the condition.

Genetic evidence is less clear in the case of dysthymic disorders, although it has been suggested that a range of problems including depression, alcoholism and personality disorders are likely to be present in relatives of such patients.

The mechanisms of genetic transmission are not known, and hypotheses such as the single major locus (SML) model and the multifactorial (MF) model are currently under consideration.

Early social factors

It is generally agreed that early environmental experiences are important in relation to the subsequent development of affective disorders, but it is notoriously difficult to be sure as to the degree and specificity of its contribution, and research in this area is a minefield of methodological problems. Even when studying events as objective as the loss of a parent in childhood, for example, the evidence remains contradictory. The same applies to other experiences, such as the presence of uncaring or rejecting parents.

Personality traits and attitudes

It has been suggested that some personality traits predispose to affective disorders: for example, people with obsessional, perfectionistic personalities and ambitious or competitive traits may be prone to depression. Similarly, there are theories which suggest that individuals who have learnt throughout their lives that their efforts usually result in failure ('learned helplessness') may be likely to give up when faced with fresh difficulties, or that those who become depressed may have a tendency to develop a 'negative cognitive set' in the presence of stress, or that they have chronically low self-esteem. Apart from begging the question as to how these traits and attitudes develop, the evidence to support these explanatory models is very limited.

Current social factors
The presence of chronic social difficulties is associated with an increased risk of depression and, in particular, the lack of social supports increases the person's vulnerability. There is a good deal of evidence for the role of confiding intimate relationships as protective against depressive disorders.

Biological factors
Although there is still no evidence for the existence of predisposing biological features apart from the general influence of genetic factors, it could be argued that individuals likely to become depressed may be different in terms of the action and metabolism of the neurotransmitters involved in the regulation of mood.

Factors associated with affective disorders: precipitating factors
Stressful events are often associated with the onset of affective disorders, and it has been estimated that depressed patients experience three times as many life-events in the preceding 6 months as normal controls. In general, threatening events or those involving losses, such as death or separation, are of particular relevance. A variety of physical disorders, such as glandular fever or cancer, can be associated with affective disorders, although the mechanisms involved are unclear. In some cases, the abnormal mood can be secondary to a physical disorder, and this may raise important diagnostic and treatment issues. For a discussion of the organic psychiatric disorders, see Chapter 11.

Factors associated with affective disorders: maintaining factors
Many of the factors that predispose to or precipitate affective disorders can have persistent effects, and so contribute to the perpetuation of the abnormal mood. For example, the loss of a partner by death may lead to social isolation, financial difficulties, and lack of a confiding relationship or longstanding low self-esteem may also be associated with a 'negative cognitive set' which may cause the loss of a job, etc.

It could be argued that in predisposed individuals, the interaction of a variety of biological, psychological and social factors can lead to a pathological state characterized by abnormalities at many levels, psychological as well as biological, with the neurotransmitter abnormalities acting as the common pathway. The precise biological abnormalities are not known, although there are many theories that attempt to explain the biochemistry of the affective disorders. The biogenic amines theories are concerned with the role of dopamine, noradrenaline and serotonin (5-HT), whilst other theories involve the possible role of endocrine abnormalities, in particular, cortisol or electrolyte disturbances involving sodium and potassium.

How should the affective disorders be managed?

In discussing the management of affective disorder, attention will be given first to its assessment, and then to the description of the main lines of treatment.

Assessment of affective disorder
This could be best understood as the process of obtaining answers to a series of questions (Fig. 6.6).
1 Is the person suffering from a primary disorder of mood? The differential diagnosis will include:
  - normal reaction to adverse circumstances;
  - schizophrenic disorder;
  - organic syndrome, including dementing illness;
  - personality disorder.
2 What is the nature (mania, severe depression, dysthymic disorder) and extent (range of symptoms, degree of reactivity, severity) of the disorder?
3 Is there a past history of affective disorder?
4 What are the likely causes? In other words, are there any obvious aetiological factors?
5 Is there a risk of suicide or of acts of deliberate self-harm? The reader is here directed to Chapter 19, for a detailed discussion of this question.
6 Is further help indicated or necessary, and, if so, what kind of help and who should provide it – the general practitioner, the psychiatrist?
7 Is the person willing to receive help? If not, is the person able to make this choice or is his or her judgement impaired

Fig. 6.6 Assessment of affective disorder
1 Is there a primary mood disorder?
2 What is the nature and extent of the disorder?
3 Is there a past history of affective disorder?
4 What are the likely causes?
5 Is there a risk of suicide or deliberate self-harm?
6 What kind of treatment is needed?
7 Is the person willing to receive help?

Fig. 6.7 Management of affective disorder

Short term

Psychological	Physical	Social
Explanation and advice	Neuroleptics	Family support
Specialized therapies:	Antidepressants	Social intervention
• cognitive therapy	ECT	
• psychodynamic therapy		
• bereavement counselling		

Long term

Psychological	Physical	Social
Counselling	Lithium salts	Family support
Specialized therapies	Antidepressants	Rehabilitation
		Social intervention

by the disorder? Should admission to hospital against the patient's wishes be considered? The uses of the Mental Health Act (1983) are discussed in Chapter 25.

Answers to these questions can usually be obtained by means of careful interview of patient and relatives, although at times it can be difficult to be certain about some aspects of the assessment, for example the degree of suicidal risk, or the need for compulsory hospitalization.

Management of affective disorder

Management can be considered in terms of immediate, or short-term management, and long-term management (Fig. 6.7). In both instances, a range of psychological, physical and social measures could be used.

Short-term management

The first decision that has to be made is whether to treat the patient in hospital or at home. Admission to hospital will be indicated when the disorder is of severe degree, and when there is a significant risk of suicide or of harm to others. The nature of the patient's domestic circumstances will also influence the decision whether to admit: absence of home supports may require the admission of a person with a mild degree of depression, while other patients with much more severe conditions may be managed at home if there are capable partners or children.

Psychological measures

In all cases, efforts should be made to provide the patient with an explanation about the nature of the disorder, its causes, and the treatment and likely prognosis. In some severely ill patients, it may be necessary to delay detailed discussion until the patient is in a position to grasp what is happening. More specific psychotherapeutic interventions may be of value, depending on the nature of the problems. For example, bereavement counselling (see Chapter 22, p. 273), cognitive behavioural therapy for depression, crisis counselling or psychodynamic psychotherapy (see Chapter 18, pp. 229–235) could be used. Full use of these specialized therapies may be more appropriate as part of the long-term management.

Physical methods

Medication and other physical methods of treatment have an important place in the treatment of severe affective disorders, both short and long term. Physical treatments and their use are discussed in Chapter 17, and they will only be mentioned briefly here.

Manic episodes: neuroleptics are the main drugs used in the acute treatment of manic disorders, in particular phenothiazines, such as chlorpromazine, and butyrophenones, such as haloperidol. Lithium salts have anti-manic properties as well, and they are sometimes added to neuroleptics in the treatment of resistant manic disorders.

Depressive episodes: antidepressants, including both tricyclic and monoamine oxidase inhibitors, and the newer antidepressants, such as the SSRI, are the treatment of choice in most cases of depression. However, in very severe depressive disorders, and where urgent treatment is needed because of serious suicide risk or risk of self neglect, ECT is indicated. Other treatments, such as lithium, can be considered in cases of resistant depression.

Social management

The patient's relatives are likely to require some help to understand the nature of the disorder, and they may need support while the patient is receiving treatment. In some cases, family and social difficulties may contribute to the disorder, and so it may be necessary to take steps to advise the patient and relatives, or to provide specific help.

Long-term management

Long-term management will be concerned with the prevention of relapses, and the reduction in the adverse consequences of the disorder.

Psychological measures

As described above, specialized forms of psychotherapy may be required to help the patient understand the nature of the problems, their causes, and to find effective ways of solving them. Patients with recurrent affective disorders often find it difficult to cope with the knowledge that they have a chronic condition which can be very disruptive to their personal and professional lives, and such patients and their relatives may need a good deal of support over the years. In some cases, patients learn to recognize the kind of situations likely to precipitate relapses, and so take steps to avoid them, or they may develop ways of initiating treatment at the first sign of ill-health. Cognitive behavioural techniques may help the person identify persistent patterns of thinking which contribute to depressive mood, and to develop ways of successfully altering them. For some people, the experience of major affective illness may lead to the re-examination of earlier experiences during childhood or adolescence, which have played a part in the development of later problems. Psychotherapeutic approaches that explore and help resolve early traumas may be indicated.

Physical methods

Medication has an important place in the prevention of recurrent affective disorders. Lithium salts are the treatment of choice in bipolar disorders, and antidepressants appear to be of value in the case of unipolar disorders. Antidepressant medication should be continued for at least 6 months, with close monitoring when medication is tailed-off, in case of relapse. Lithium therapy may be continued indefinitely while monitoring regularly thyroid and renal function.

Social measures

As described above, family and social difficulties may act as long-term aetiological factors, and attention should be paid to this possibility, and the necessary measures used.

What is the course and outcome of the affective disorders?

Short-term outcome refers to the course of an episode, and in particular to its duration and chances of recovery. Long-term outcome refers to the likelihood of relapse and of the development of a chronic disorder.

Short-term outcome

It is not always easy to determine the duration of an episode of mania or depression, and using the time of referral to the psychiatric services or admission to hospital as the starting point will naturally tend to underestimate its duration, especially if the disorder had a gradual onset. In general, an episode of major affective disorder lasts between 3 months and 1 year, with an average of about 6 months. Manic episodes tend to be of more rapid onset and recovery than depressive episodes, and they also tend to be of shorter duration.

Factors associated with a prolonged episode of affective disorder include gradual onset, the presence of delusions, and development late in life.

Most patients recover from their first episode of illness, and in some reports this applies to over 90% of patients.

Long-term outcome

Most patients with affective disorders will experience minor exacerbations over time. A significant proportion will suffer major relapses, which may include the need for hospitalization. It has been estimated that over a 10-year period, more than 50% of patients will have a severe relapse, and almost 80% will relapse at some stage during the rest of their lives.

Some patients may experience persistent difficulties. These can be the result of chronic symptoms, or a consequence of the social impairment caused by repeated episodes of illness. Research has shown that between 20 and 50% of bipolar patients show deterioration in their employment capabilities. A smaller proportion, between 5 and 10%, may need persistent in-patient treatment.

The risk of suicide in patients with affective disorders, especially depression, is significant. As many as 15% of bipolar patients die by suicide, and similar proportions have been reported for patients with dysthymic disorders (depressive neurosis). There is a good deal of evidence to suggest that a very high proportion of individuals who take their lives were suffering from severe depression at the time (see Chapter 19, p. 246).

It has been suggested that patients with chronic depressive disorders have an increased risk of developing physical illnesses, especially cardiovascular disorders. Apart from the interesting theoretical issues that it raises, this suggestion also highlights the need to assess depressed patients fully, and not assume that all their complaints are necessarily secondary to their mental state.

QUESTIONS

1 How would you differentiate between a normal reaction to an adverse event and a depressive episode?
2 What aspects of a patient's mental state and history would make you decide that admission to hospital was indicated?
3 How would you estimate the short-term risk of suicide in a patient suffering from a major depressive episode?
4 How would you manage a young patient with a clear history of bipolar disorder who refuses to take lithium?
5 In what circumstances would you think of using a compulsory treatment order under the powers of the Mental Health Act 1983?

FURTHER READING

Gelder M., Gath D. & Mayou R. (1989) *Oxford Textbook of Psychiatry*. 2nd Edition. Oxford University Press, Oxford.

Kaplan H.I. & Sadock B.J. (1985) *Modern Synopsis of the Comprehensive Textbook of Psychiatry/IV*. 4th Edition. Williams & Wilkins, Baltimore and London.

Wing J.K. & Wing L. (eds) (1982) *Handbook of Psychiatry 3: Psychosis of Uncertain Aetiology*. Cambridge University Press, Cambridge.

All of these references give more detailed reviews of the affective disorders.

7
The Neuroses

Fact sheet

Definition
Neuroses are exaggerated and disabling forms of the normal reactions to stressful events.

Classification
The main syndromes to be considered here are:
1 Undifferentiated neuroses.
2 Anxiety states.
3 Phobic states: (a) agoraphobia; (b) social phobia; (c) simple phobia.
4 Obsessive–compulsive disorders.
5 Hysteria.
Depersonalization syndrome and **hypochondriasis** are dealt with only briefly. **Neurasthenia**, which is no longer regarded as a syndrome distinct from depression or anxiety, is not described. **Neurotic depression** is described in Chapter 6 along with other types and degrees of depression.

Presentation

Usual age of onset
● Anxiety states, agoraphobia, social phobia and obsessive compulsive disorders most commonly present between the ages of 17 and 35.
● Simple phobias develop in childhood.
● Hysteria may present at any age, usually before 35.

Clinical presentation
● Neurotic symptoms frequently mimic physical illness.
● Psychiatric referral only follows careful physical examination and investigation.
● Psychiatric out-patients with neuroses commonly present several years after the onset of their disorder.
● Syndromes represent clusters of neurotic symptoms with major overlaps between diagnostic categories.

Differential diagnosis
1 Depression.
2 Physical illness.
3 Alcohol or drug abuse.
4 Personality disorder.

Aetiology
A combination of predisposing factors (inherited vulnerability/predisposing early experience) and stressful experiences. There is a concordance for neurosis of 40% in MZ twins and 15% in DZ twins.

Distribution
Neuroses comprise 67% of psychiatric cases in general practice.

Lifetime prevalence
● Undifferentiated neuroses: 20/1000–140/1000.
● Anxiety states: 17/1000 men, 38/1000 women.
● Phobias: 6/1000 (in adults, agoraphobia is the most common).
● Hysteria: 3–6/1000 for women, less common in men.
● Obsessive–compulsive disorders are very uncommon.

Sex distribution
Most neuroses are twice as common in women, but social phobia appears to be equally distributed.

Associated factors
● Depression may cause neurotic symptoms or may develop as a consequence of a neurosis.
● There is an increased incidence of suicide in the neuroses.
● Excessive alcohol consumption may be a cause of neurotic symptoms or may develop as a consequence of a neurosis.

Assessment
● Identify the pattern of neurotic symptoms present.
● Exclude depression, substance abuse and physical illness.
● Assess family attitudes and support.

Management
Patients are usually managed either by the GP or as an out-patient.
● *Psychological*: first choice is cognitive behavioural therapy.
● *Physical*: minor tranquillizers (effective for a brief course, but addictive); antidepressants.
● *Social*: family needs education, guidance and support.
● *General*: measures to restore self-esteem.

Outcome

For neuroses in general

Patients identified by:	Approximate recovery rate:
community survey	50% in 3 months
general practice	50% in 1 year
psychiatric out-patients	50% in 4 years

i.e. recovery rate falls abruptly with increased severity and duration

For specific syndromes
● Anxiety states: if more than a few months' duration, generally a poor outcome with treatment. If short duration, outcome of treatment often good.
● Phobias: simple phobias, good outcome with treatment.
● Agoraphobia/social phobia, generally a good response to cognitive behavioural treatment.
● Obsessive–compulsive disorders: spontaneous fluctations in severity are common. Treatment outcome poor.
● Hysteria: treatment outcome is generally poor.

Indicators of good outcome
● No family history of neurotic disorder.
● Robust personality (previously coped well with stress).
● Clear precipitating stress.
● Brief illness before referral.
● Mild illness.
● Presence of avoidance or overt rituals.
● Stable/supportive family or others.
● Absence of other disorder (e.g. alcohol abuse).

What are neuroses?

Definition

Neuroses are mental disorders without any demonstrable organic basis, in which the patient does not lose touch with external reality or experience psychotic symptoms.

Individual symptoms such as anxiety, transient obsessional thoughts and physical symptoms without organic pathology are all experienced by many normal people in response to the demands of everyday life. In the neuroses these become more intense and are out of proportion to the severity of the stressful circumstances. Like other psychiatric disorders the neuroses are syndromes and therefore consist, not of an individual symptom, but of a recognizable combination of neurotic symptoms. In the more severe cases particular symptoms predominate leading to the diagnosis of a specific syndrome. In the milder (and most common) cases, no specific syndrome is identifiable (Fig. 7.1). These milder states are sometimes called 'undifferentiated neuroses' or 'minor emotional reactions'. Undifferentiated neuroses are very common in general practice but are not often referred to in psychiatric out-patients.

Individual neurotic symptoms, such as anxiety or obsessional thoughts, frequently occur in other psychiatric disorders, particularly depression. In these cases the diagnosis would be of depression (or other major psychiatric disorder),

Fig. 7.1 Frequency of symptoms in undifferentiated neuroses

Anxiety and worry	93%
Despondency and sadness	81%
Fatigue	81%
Somatic symptoms (of anxiety)	59%
Sleep disturbance	57%
Irritability	43%
Obsessions and compulsions	22%

What are the causes of neuroses?

In most patients the onset of their neurosis is a consequence of the combination of stressful experiences and a vulnerable personality (see also Chapter 2).

Stress

Stressful living and working conditions play a part in causing neuroses. Stressful events which could not be the result of the neurosis itself occur more commonly than expected in the 3 months before the onset of neuroses. Stressful events which pose a threat to the individual (rather than those which represent a loss) are particularly associated with the onset of neuroses (rather than depression).

Personality

Whether or not stressful events lead to the onset of a neurosis may depend on inherited aspects of the individual's personality, early experiences in life or on social factors such as those implicated in causing vulnerability to depression (Chapter 6, p. 80). The more vulnerable the individual is, as a result of such aspects of their personality or experience, the less stress will be needed to precipitate a neurosis. This means that in extreme stress, normally robust people may develop neuroses. In contrast, those who are particularly vulnerable will develop neuroses in the context of everyday stress.

The contribution of inherited predisposition

An inherited component of vulnerability to neuroses has been demonstrated by studies of adult twins. This approach has shown a concordance for neurosis of 40% for MZ twins and 15% for DZ twins.

The contribution of early experience

The capacity to withstand stress or a predisposition to neurosis may also arise from aspects of upbringing. Psychoanalytic, learning and cognitive psychology theories have all attempted to explain how particular experiences might be important. However, in spite of their intellectual appeal these have not led to any significant factual knowledge about how early experience contributes to vulnerability to neuroses.

The significance of childhood emotional disorders

Although emotional disorders are common in childhood, only a minority persist into adult life. The majority of emotional disorders in childhood appear to be reactions to current circumstances. Most neurotic children grow up to be normal and most neurotic adults did not present with neuroses in childhood.

Personality disorder and neuroses

Patients who develop neuroses may have vulnerable personalities but not satisfy the criteria for a personality disorder. Personality disorders are characterized by persistent disorders of behaviour since early adulthood, whereas many patients with neuroses have many years of normal behaviour.

Assessment of neuroses

It is essential that any primary cause, such as physical illness, depression, alcohol dependence, dementia or schizophrenia, is not overlooked. It is particularly important to reconsider these if no evidence emerges of a vulnerable personality or of sufficient precipitating stress. An alternative diagnosis must also be considered if there is no improvement with adequate treatment.

Treatment of neuroses

Specific aspects of treatment of particular neurotic syndromes is considered with the description of each syndrome. A number of general points about the treatment of this population should be borne in mind. Spontaneous remission is common (see below) but those who do not improve spontaneously within the first few weeks are likely to remain disabled if they do not receive treatment. The great majority of patients with neuroses can be treated by their general practitioners or as out-patients. Detailed assessment, followed by explanation, information about the nature and origin of symptoms, and encouragement is always useful and in mild cases of recent onset may be sufficient to bring about recovery. Patients should be encouraged to feel responsible for carrying out treatment procedures themselves and for actively attempting to solve their problems in life.

The therapist does not 'do' the treatment to a passive patient but has responsibility to motivate, inform, advise and encourage the patient to act on their own behalf. In addition to specific treatment measures, efforts should always be made to help patients to rebuild their self-confidence and self-esteem. This may involve encouragement to take up work or social pursuits.

Anxiety management training

Training in anxiety management lies at the centre of the treatment of anxiety states, phobias and obsessive–compulsive disorders because it is only when patients feel that they can manage anxiety independently that they will be willing to confront factors promoting their disorder, such as external stresses, avoidance, frightening thoughts or a compulsion to carry out rituals. It is not helpful in patients not experiencing anxiety such as those in remission or those with dissociative disorders (Fig. 7.2).

Fig. 7.2 Anxiety management training

The rationale for anxiety management training
Anxiety cannot be abolished but it can be controlled and the ability to control it can be learned. Anxiety is maintained by three factors.

Psychological factors
Upsetting thoughts, worries or fears, in particular a fear of symptoms so that the patient anticipates having an attack of anxiety symptoms. Fearful anticipation brings on the anxiety attack itself.

$$\text{fear} \longrightarrow \text{bodily feeling}$$
$$\nwarrow \qquad \swarrow$$
$$\text{fearful mis-interpretation}$$

Aspects of behaviour, typically avoidance as a maintaining factor because:
- relief obtained by avoidance is temporary;
- in the long run it makes facing things harder;
- avoidance tends to spread to other things;
- the patient knows that the situations avoided are not really dangerous and this is demoralizing.

Loss of confidence, with the result that:
- easy things become hard;
- patients tend to withdraw from rewarding activities;
- their anxiety becomes the centre of their attention.

General components of anxiety management
- Defining the problems in detail.
- Record keeping and symptom monitoring (diaries).
- Reviewing and setting new 'homework' during treatment sessions.
- Reviewing progress and identifying helpful strategies.
- Preparing for the future, in particular, predicting and being prepared for setbacks.

Specific components of anxiety management
- Learn to control symptoms by:

relaxation: there are a number of ways of teaching a patient to relax. The aim is for the patient to be able to control tension when necessary. It is essential that patients put it into practice during treatment sessions as well as during 'homework';

distraction: patients are taught to occupy themselves mentally when in anxiety provoking situations. Simple but prolonged mental tasks are best, such as counting things;

controlling thoughts: patients can learn to recognize that frightening thoughts are usually illogical and exaggerated ways of perceiving the situation. They can then replace the frightening thought with a more logical one;

controlling panic: a combination of relaxation, distraction and thought control will help the patient deal with particular crises.
- Deal with avoidance by encouraging the patient to gradually increase their exposure to anxiety provoking situations or sensations.
- Increase confidence by reviewing progress, discussing how particular strategies have helped, getting back to activities which may have been abandoned due to anxiety.

A case: an example of anxiety management training
A 41-year-old married salesman, complaining of chest pain and neck stiffness. He feared he had severe cardiovascular disease. Episodes of chest pain were accompanied by autonomic symptoms of anxiety and on investigation his cardiovascular system was normal. He had lost confidence in his work, e.g. using the telephone and talking with his manager, and in his social and married life. He ensured he was never left alone.

Treatment plan and homework tasks
Session 1. Detailed behavioural assessment followed by an explanation of the causes and mechanisms of anxiety and the rationale for treatment. The patient starts keeping a diary of his anxiety.
Session 2. Start relaxation training which continues as homework.
Session 3. Start combating avoidance: the patient starts to increase his use of the telephone, to increase the amount of contact with his boss and to be more open with his wife. He keeps a record of his success and finds his anxiety and his chest pain are not as bad as he feared.
Session 4. The patient has noticed that he undermines his self-confidence by self-critical thoughts. He practises spotting illogical self-critical thoughts, noting them in his diary and deliberately looking for more rational attitudes.
Session 5. A review of progress and reasons for success allows the patient to understand more about the nature of his disorder and the ways in which he can help himself. Homework tasks continue.
Session 6. Discussion of how to deal with setbacks when they occur and how to resist relapse.

What is the outcome for patients with neuroses?

Prognosis is worse when the initial symptoms are severe, social problems are present which are likely to persist, the patient lacks social support and friendships and when the patient's personality is abnormal. Neuroses related to temporary events in people of robust personality are likely to improve quickly. There is an increased incidence of suicide in neurotic patients over the general population. It should be noted that there are differences in outcome between the different neurotic syndromes, obsessional neurosis having the worst prognosis.

The differentiated neurotic syndromes

Anxiety states

Anxiety states are the most common neurotic syndromes. They consist of a combination of physical and psychological manifestations of anxiety, not attributable to real danger, which occur either in attacks or as a persisting state. There is no systematic pattern of avoidance. Other neurotic features, such as obsessional or hysterical symptoms, may be present but do not dominate the clinical picture.

The main symptoms and signs of anxiety are summarized in Fig. 7.3 with accompanying illustrations of their contribu-

tion to onset. Special features of anxiety states in the elderly are covered on p. 165.

Specific points to look for in the assessment of anxiety

Depression
A deliberate enquiry about depressive symptoms must be made of every anxious patient and checked with an informant. If the depressive syndrome is present this requires treatment as a priority. Neurotic symptoms commonly improve with the depression.

Drugs or alcohol
Anxiety may be a symptom of withdrawal, but may also be a cause of alcohol or substance abuse. It is not possible to make an adequate assessment of anxiety symptoms until 2 or 3 weeks after the patient is thoroughly detoxified. This would also apply to patients taking large dose of minor tranquillizers for whom the initial task must be to withdraw them from their drugs as far as possible.

Physical illness
Most patients with anxiety are concerned about their health and anxiety symptoms may mimic a large number of physical illnesses. Physical examination and adequate routine investigations are mandatory in patients with anxiety states. Consider physical causes particularly if there is no obvious psychological precipitant and when the personality is normal. Remember to exclude thyrotoxicosis, phaeochromocytoma, hypoglycaemia and asthma.

Fig. 7.3 Main symptoms and signs of anxiety

Symptoms and signs of anxiety

Psychological
- Feeling of fearful anticipation.
- Irritability.
- Restlessness.
- Worrying (often about symptoms).
- Poor concentration.

Physical
- Appearance of furrowed brow, tense, tremulous, restless.
- Gastrointestinal symptoms of dry mouth, lump in throat, difficulty swallowing, frequent or loose bowel motions, butterflies.
- Respiratory symptoms of tightness in chest, difficulty inhaling, breathlessness, respiratory alkalosis.
- Cardiovascular symptoms of palpitations, precordial discomfort.
- Central nervous symptoms of blurring of vision, prickling sensations, dizziness (not rotational).
- Musculoskeletal symptoms of ache or tension in the scalp, neck or shoulders.
- Sleep is disturbed by difficulty getting to sleep, followed by restless sleep with frightening dreams.
- Appetite is often disturbed with the patient preferring sweets and snacks to their normal meals.

Any of these symptoms may be the presenting complaint, particularly in general practice. Patients may deny having an anxious mood.

The onset of anxiety states

Two cases illustrating the ways in which preceding stress, physical symptoms and fearful thought content can be associated at the onset.

Case 1

A 32-year-old woman whose father had recently died during cardiac surgery. She had just had extensive building work to her house completed. She experienced sudden onset of symptoms while tidying the house and noticed breathlessness, palpitations, sweating, dry mouth, dizziness, weakness and tingling of peripheries. She began repeatedly to fear that she was having heart attacks with recurrence of these frightening symptoms, the episodes amounting to panic attacks. She began to avoid being anywhere alone as a result of these fears.

Case 2

A 46-year-old woman, under extra pressure at work, whose mother was ill and whose son was leaving home. She experienced pains in her head and shoulders, irritability and restlessness. She worried that symptoms would stop her making an effort and she would become 'a cabbage.' She did not develop panic attacks or a pattern of avoidance.

Schizophrenia

Anxiety may be the first symptom that is noticed.

What causes anxiety states?

Genetic

Anxiety states occur in about 2% of the general population and about 15% of the relatives of patients with anxiety. In a twin study 41% of MZ and 4% of DZ twin pairs were concordant for anxiety neurosis. This suggests that genetic predisposition is of considerable importance.

Psychoanalytic theories

Psychoanalytic theories describe the way the instinctual part of man conflicts with his social training and his conscience. It has been suggested that these conflicts, i.e. wanting to do something that you know you shouldn't, provide the psychic energy which is then released in the form of a neurosis. These ideas may provide a means of understanding the experiences of individual patients but their importance seems impossible to test.

Learning theories

Anxiety can be regarded as a fearful response which has become attached by conditioning to a stimulus which is not normally anxiety provoking. If a person becomes frightened by an experience or sensation (such as palpitations or breathlessness) or if he experiences frightening sensations in particular circumstances (such as on exertion or when at a height) anxiety may subsequently be provoked repeatedly by these physical symptoms or in these circumstances. Patients with severe anxiety give an account of such learning experiences, but those with milder disorders usually do not.

Learning theorists regard neuroticism, a stable feature of the individual's personality, as being related to an undue degree of lability of the autonomic nervous system which leads to a tendency to develop excessive anxiety, making the attachment of anxiety to inappropriate stimuli more likely.

How are anxiety states managed?

Psychological treatment

Support. Discussion and reassurance are often sufficient. Reassurance includes a clear explanation of the causes and nature of the patient's symptoms and the recognition that the patient's concerns about his symptoms have been appreciated. A clear plan of treatment is also reassuring.

Drugs (for more detailed discussion see Chapter 17). If drugs are to be used they should be only one component of a treatment plan in which the patient learns to solve the difficulties causing or maintaining anxiety. Drugs in use include:

- benzodiazepines: these are safe and effective anxiolytics but because of the risk of addiction they should be stopped after a few weeks;
- adrenoceptor antagonists: these are only useful in patients whose main concern is about palpitations;
- antidepressants: all types of antidepressant appear to have

---

Fig. 7.4 Graded exposure treatment

Rationale for exposure treatment

Severe anxiety has become strongly associated with particular everyday situations.

Fear of having symptoms causes anxiety, thereby provoking the very symptoms the patient fears and precipitating a panic attack.

Avoidance maintains the problem and makes it worse by:

- stopping the patient regaining self-confidence;
- giving only temporary relief from anxiety;
- spreading gradually to more and more situations;
- making it harder to face things eventually.

General components of exposure treatment

- Define problems and agree treatment targets.
- Patient to keep a diary of symptoms and of daily activities.
- Set homework which involves practice of anxiety management techniques and graded exposure.
- Identify strategies that have been helpful.
- Prepare for setbacks.

Specific components of graded exposure treatment: anxiety management training.

Learn to control symptoms using anxiety management techniques:

- relaxation;
- distraction;
- controlling thoughts;
- controlling panic.

Establish heirarchy of anxiety provoking situations.

Start with easiest and progress to harder situations.

Frequent, prolonged (>1½ hour) exposure sessions.

A case: an example of exposure treatment

History

A 23-year-old married woman with a child of 3 years presents complaining of attacks of palpitations, breathlessness and nausea over the previous month. She is pregnant, has recently moved house and faces considerable financial difficulty. The attacks occur most often in the supermarket, which she now avoids completely, but may also occur on the bus or when in other crowded public places. She avoids these situations unless she is accompanied by her husband. The physical examination proves normal as do all investigations.

Treatment

Session 1. With both the patient and her husband, discuss the nature and origin of anxiety symptoms and the rationale for exposure treatment. Establish aims of treatment and a heirarchy of anxiety provoking situations. Clarify the ways in which the husband can encourage and support the patient. The patient starts keeping a diary of symptoms and activities. Ideally her husband will attend all treatment sessions.

Session 2. Start relaxation training, which continues as homework.

Session 3. Review relaxation training, discuss and describe other anxiety management techniques, agree initial homework tasks for graded exposure practice.

Session 4. Review progress with anxiety management techniques. Agree further homework tasks for exposure practice.

Further sessions. Ensure that exposure practice is undertaken for all types of avoidance (shops, transport and crowds) so that withered confidence in one area will not generalize to other areas. Review progress, discuss the manner in which particular techniques may have helped and prepare for setbacks.

an anti-anxiety effect, even in the absence of depression. They are most effective in cases of severe anxiety with panic attacks. However their side-effects are often a cause of further anxiety, and relapse is common on withdrawal of the drug. The sedation they cause at night may be appreciated by patients with sleep disturbance.

What is the outcome for anxiety states?
Most anxiety states are brief and resolve spontaneously. If they last for more than a few months the outlook is poor. About 80% of anxiety states that last for longer than 6 months are still present 3 years later despite efforts at treatment. Brief depressive episodes occur repeatedly among many patients who have long-standing anxiety.

Phobic states

What are phobias?
Phobias are characterized by persistent and recurring irrational fears of a specific object, activity or situation which the subject tends to avoid. In most cases phobic patients recognize that they avoid situations because they anticipate overwhelming anxiety or some other strong emotion.

A number of fairly common disorders do not fit easily into these categories. For example, patients may have a fear of a particular illness, such as venereal disease or cancer, which may have the features of a phobia, including a pattern of avoidance. In the absence of avoidance these fears may be better understood as obsessional disorders.

Three features can therefore be identified in all phobias: anxiety symptoms; a recognizable pattern of situations that provoke anxiety; and avoidance of these situations.

Simple phobia
These are single non-social phobias not associated with leaving home. Patients characteristically complain of an unreasonable fear of a specific object or situation. These are commonly animals, particularly insects, reptiles or rodents, or they may be situations such as heights or thunderstorms. They are common in children and may persist into adult life.

Agoraphobia
The situations which provoke the greatest anxiety share the features of being far from home or from the help of a trusted person and of being in public view. Agoraphobia is usually associated with panic attacks. Patients commonly fear that they will have an attack of symptoms in which they may be seriously ill, do something foolish or be unable to control themselves. Usually there are multiple situations avoided including travelling, crowds, closed spaces, shops and heights. The more severe, the nearer to a place of safety the patient will stay and the more restricted their activities. In the most severe cases the patient may not be able to leave home at all. This pattern of avoidance inevitably also has a major effect on the families of patients.

Specific anxiety about vomiting in public or passing urine in public lavatories may lead to complicated patterns of avoidance and even difficulty in leaving home although this may be best described as a simple phobia because the term is not associated with panic but only with the avoidance of the event itself.

Social phobia
The symptoms of anxiety in social phobia are similar to those in other anxiety states but those features which might be visible to others, such as blushing, sweating and trembling, are more prominent. These patients are less likely to experience panic attacks than agoraphobics. The situations which provoke anxiety in social phobia share the characteristic that the person is, or feels, under observation by others. The more important the person who may be observing them and the more the patient has to do while being observed, the worse the situation. Typical situations avoided are eating in a public place, speaking in public or writing in front of others. Unlike the paranoid patient, the socially phobic patient does not feel persecuted and recognizes the excessive nature of his fear.

Social phobia will be distinguished from a personality disorder characterized by shyness and lack of self-confidence by having a recognizable time of onset and a more limited range of situations that cause anxiety.

Specific points to look for in the assessment of phobias
As with the anxiety states, and for the same reasons, it is essential that depression, drug or alcohol abuse and physical illness are excluded. In each case it is also important to develop some understanding of why avoidance has developed, for example has it been encouraged by a spouse. This will assist in planning a treatment which helps overcome avoidance.

What causes phobias?

The causes of avoidance
Avoidance itself will be due to a combination of factors which may include:
1 the severity of the attacks of anxiety: the more severe the attacks the more likely it is that the patient will develop a pattern of avoidance;
2 the circumstances in which the first attack has occurred: for example if it occurs in a shop, the patient may avoid shops whereas if the first attack occurs at home, it is less likely that a pattern of avoidance will develop;
3 the attitudes of family and friends: if others readily tolerate the restricted activities of the patient, avoidance will develop more readily;
4 aspects of the personality of the patient, such as their willingness to tolerate a restricted lifestyle or their ability to cope with adversity.

Causes of the specific syndromes

Agoraphobia. There is no evidence of genetic predisposition to agoraphobia, nor has any convincing evidence been found that particular early experiences are important. Agoraphobia usually develops in young adults. As with anxiety states, the first attack of anxiety commonly occurs in the setting of a stressful period in the patient's life. A small additional stress may then precipitate the first attack of anxiety symptoms.

Following one or more attacks the patient may anticipate another, particularly in situations where an attack has already occurred. The consequent anxiety about having a further attack will make another attack more likely and will encourage the development of avoidance. The situation in which the first attack occurs, such as in a shop, and the way the individual interprets the experience, largely determines the pattern of avoidance.

Social phobia. A social phobia may develop because of a combination of the circumstances in which the first attack of anxiety occurred (for example, a social setting) and a general lack of self-confidence in social encounters. The age of onset is similar to that for agoraphobia and onset is associated with recent stressful events.

Simple phobias. Starting in childhood, these may be learnt by imitation of parents or other children who are afraid. Others may be learnt from frightening events. There is some evidence that certain types of animal or insect are particularly likely to provoke a fearful response and that there is a particular readiness to react in this way in childhood.

How are phobias treated?

Behaviour therapy
Graded exposure treatment is the treatment of choice for phobic patients (Fig. 7.4). This procedure shares many features with anxiety management training, but lays special emphasis on controlling avoidance. Behaviour therapy is further discussed in Chapter 2, p. 26 and Chapter 18, p. 229.

Drugs
1 Anxiolytic drugs, such as benzodiazepines, can be useful very early in treatment to provide immediate relief while behaviour therapy is started.
2 Antidepressant drugs have been used to treat agoraphobic patients who have no current depressive illness. They have been shown to increase the benefit of exposure treatment but are less effective alone. There is a high incidence of patients dropping out of treatment because they cannot tolerate the side effects. There is also a high relapse rate when the drug is discontinued.

What is the outcome for phobias?
In most patients exposure treatments are effective in reducing phobias markedly and lastingly.
Indicators of a poor outcome are:
• poor motivation (best indicated by failing to attempt homework);
• significant degree of depression;
• continuing significant stresses;
• excessive consumption of alcohol or minor tranquillizers.

Obsessive–compulsive disorder
These are uncommon states in which the outstanding symptoms are of obsessional thoughts or compulsive behaviours. Obsessions are usually stereotyped, repetitive words, ideas, phrases, images or impulses which are generally accom-

---

Fig. 7.5 Obsessional thinking and compulsive rituals

Obsessional thinking
• Obsessional thoughts are usually unpleasant and attempts are usually made to exclude them. May be single words or phrases.
• Obsessional images are vividly imagined scenes of an often violent and disgusting kind.
• Obsessional ruminations are endless internal debates about everyday activities.
• Obsessional doubts concern actions which may not have been completed happily or safely.
• Obsessional impulses are urges to perform violent or embarrassing actions.

Compulsive rituals
• Repeated mental activities such as counting, naming objects, repeating words or phrases which may be meaningless.
• Repeated senseless behaviours (rituals, not tics or mannerisms) such as arranging clothes or objects, pacing in particular ways, gestures or postures.
• Some rituals have an understandable connection with associated obsessional thoughts such as washing hands or 'contaminated' objects, checking for satefy, repeating door locking.

---

panied by a sense of subjective compulsion. They have two important characteristics.
1 They are perceived by the patient as inappropriate or nonsensical.
2 They are seen as out of character but nonetheless coming from within the self as opposed to being due to external influences. These two features distinguish obsessive compulsive disorders from psychoses. Compulsions are repetitive, purposeful movements or actions which are usually performed in accordance with rules or in a stereotyped fashion. They share the same qualities as obsessions. Activities that are potentially pleasurable, such as eating, sexual behaviour, picking skin, etc., are not properly classified as obsessive–compulsive disorders.

An obsessional quality to thoughts or behaviour may accompany other illnesses, most commonly depression. Obsessive compulsive disorder can only be diagnosed in the absence of depression.

Features of obsessive–compulsive neuroses (Fig. 7.5)

Anxiety
Rituals commonly reduce anxiety for a while, but may increase it. The degree of anxiety experienced by obsessional patients may be considerably lower than in other neuroses. Patients often describe discomfort or dissatisfaction rather than anxiety.

What are the causes of obsessive–compulsive disorder?
Very little is known. The following factors deserve consideration.
• *Genetic.* Obsessional disorders occur in 5–7% of the parents of obsessional patients. This rate is higher than the general population. Numbers are too small to allow satisfactory twin studies.

- *Organic factors.* Obsessional symptoms were frequent in patients after the epidemic of encephalitis lethargica in the 1920s. However, in most obsessional patients there is no convincing evidence of disease of the central nervous system.
- *Early experience.* It is uncertain whether early experience, such as imitative learning, plays a part in causing obsessional neurosis.
- *Learning theory.* Some obsessional rituals are the equivalent of avoidance responses. The patient may fear that failure to carry out the ritual will lead to some unpleasant consequence. Some rituals, however, lead to an increase in anxiety and cannot be understood in this way.
- *Psychoanalytic theory.* Freud suggested that obsessive compulsive disorders result from repressed impulses of an aggressive or sexual nature. This idea is consistent with patients' frequent concerns over excretory functions and dirt.

It is impossible to draw any general conclusions about the origins of these disorders. In each individual case it may be possible to understand the onset of the disorder in terms of one or more of these factors.

Specific points in the assessment of obsessive–compulsive disorders

- *Depression.* Most obsessional symptoms occur as part of a depressive illness. This is particularly likely in patients who have obsessional traits in their premorbid personality. In such cases antidepressant treatment is indicated.
- *Schizophrenia.* Obsessional thoughts may be hard to distinguish from delusions. Careful assessment will indicate whether the patient recognizes the inappropriate nature of their thoughts and their origin within himself. If this remains uncertain, evidence of other symptoms of schizophrenia should be sought.
- *Obsessional personality disorders.* These can be distinguished from obsessive compulsive disorders by the absence of any recognizable time of onset and the lifelong history of marked obsessional behaviour.

How are obsessive–compulsive disorders treated?

Untreated obsessional neuroses often run a fluctuating course with long periods of remission. The effects of treatment are often disappointing. A thorough search for depression should be made to ensure that this readily treatable condition is not missed. Explanation and reassurance that the obsessional thoughts are not an early sign of madness which may lead to the destruction of the personality is useful for both the patient and his family. The patient's family may be involved in the patient's rituals and they will need to be involved in treatment.

Drugs

Anxiolytic drugs can be used to give immediate relief in the short term. Antidepressants have been tried but are probably not helpful in the absence of depressive symptoms.

Behaviour therapy

About two-thirds of patients with obsessional rituals improve if they can be persuaded and helped to resist the urge to carry them out ('response prevention'). Anxiety management training will help the patient to cope with the anxiety this generates. When rituals are reduced the accompanying obsessional thoughts usually improve as well. This approach is not readily applicable to patients whose obsessional rituals are in the form of thoughts rather than actions. In these circumstances patients may try to distract themselves in order not to carry out the mental ritual (see also Chapter 18, p. 229).

Psychotherapy

Support may be helpful and joint interviews with the spouse may be indicated when marital problems are caused by or are aggravating the symptoms. Exploratory/interpretative psychotherapy does not help and encouraging introspection may be harmful in these patients.

Psychosurgery

Psychosurgery may lead to a striking reduction in tension and distress. Because of its uncertain outcome and its risks of irreversible side effects psychosurgery should only be considered when a very severe disabling illness has persisted for many years and all other treatments have failed (see also p. 222).

Fig. 7.6 Hysteria

Mental symptoms (DSM-III-R: dissociative disorders)
- *Amnesia*: typically starts suddenly, long periods of life are forgotten, sometimes even personal identity.
- *Fugue*: similar to amnesia but in addition the patient wanders away from his usual surroundings.
- *Hysterical pseudodementia*: simple tests of memory are answered wrongly but in a way which suggests that the correct answer is known.
- *Multiple personalities*: sudden alternation between two patterns of behaviour, each of which is forgotten when the other is present. The 'new' personality usually contrasts strongly with the normal personality.
- *Hysterical psychosis*: these usually lack a number of features of true epileptic seizures, for example lack of unconsciousness, an unusual pattern of movements, lack of physical consequences of seizure such as incontinence, lack of EEG abnormality.
- *Hysterical psychosis*: represents the patient's idea of madness.

Physical symptoms (DSM-III-R: conversion disorders)
- *Disorders of movement*: paralysis, disorders of gait, tremor, aphonia or mutism (true aphonia excluded if patient can still phonate on coughing).
- *Disorders of sensation*: anaesthesiae, paraesthesiae, hyperaesthesiae, pain, deafness and blindness. Gastrointestinal symptoms: flatulence, regurgitation.

Note
- The severity of hysterical physical disorders varies from moderate (e.g. a limp) to severe (e.g. widespread paralysis).
- Patients with diagnosed physical illness may present hysterical symptoms (e.g. epileptic seizures + hysterical seizures).
- Patients diagnosed as having a hysterical disorder may also develop a physical illness.

Hysteria

What is hysteria?

Hysteria is a mental disorder in which motives, of which the patient seems unaware, produce restriction of the field of consciousness, loss of memory or dramatic personality change (DSM-III-R: dissociation disorder), or disturbances of motor or sensory function (DSM-III-R: conversion disorder) (Fig. 7.6). The symptoms seem to have a psychological advantage or symbolic value. In hysteria, therefore, there are symptoms and signs of disease in the absence of pathology, produced unconsciously and without any overactivity of the sympathetic nervous system. Since physical pathology can rarely be excluded completely when the patient is first seen the diagnosis of hysteria must be provisional when first made. Patients with hysteria are uncommon in psychiatric practice, although they are much more frequently seen in general practice. The low referral rate may be due to uncertainty about the diagnosis or a low expectation of effective treatment.

Hysterical symptoms may accompany other psychiatric disorders. In these cases the diagnosis is of the other psychiatric disorder, the syndrome of hysteria referring only to those cases where no other disorder is present.

Hysteria must be distinguished from histrionic personality disorder which refers to a lifelong pattern of behaviour (Chapter 9). Such people do not have an increased tendency to develop hysterical symptoms.

Common to all hysterical symptoms are three features.

1 Symptoms correspond to the patient's degree of understanding about illness and about anatomy and physiology. Unless they are clinically trained, there are usually obvious discrepancies between the hysterical signs and symptoms and those of organic disease.

2 The patient usually gains some advantage from their symptoms ('secondary gain').

3 The patient may be unconcerned by his symptoms ('belle indifference') in spite of showing exaggerated emotional reactions in others ways.

Note: do not rely heavily on evidence of secondary gain or belle indifference in diagnosing hysteria: many disabled people make the most of their disabilities and some will occasionally exploit them; some disabled people are not as distressed by their disability as one might expect.

Social and cultural variations

Hysteria presents in forms which are consistent with the patient's culture and experience.

1 **Epidemic hysteria:** hysteria can spread within a group. Symptoms of fainting and dizziness are common in such outbreaks.

2 **Latah:** found among women in Malaysia who show echolalia (repeating interviewer's words), echopraxia (repeating interviewer's movements) and other evidence of excessive compliance.

3 **Amok:** found among men in Malaysia who initially brood, then become violent. Amnesia is usually claimed afterwards.

Special features in the assessment of patients with hysteria – or how to avoid making mistakes in diagnosis

The diagnosis can be mistaken in three ways.

1 The symptoms are of a physical disease which has not yet been detected.

2 Undiscovered neurological disease may 'release' hysterical symptoms in some unknown way.

3 Genuine physical disease may stimulate hysterical elaboration of symptoms in vulnerable personalities.

To avoid these pitfalls the exact form of the symptoms and signs must be established and carefully compared with those arising from known diseases. Organic diseases of the central nervous system prove the most difficult to exclude. When hysteria is diagnosed, a mistake will be less likely if there is clear evidence of a precipitating stress and of secondary gain, and if the patient is under 40 years old.

Differential diagnosis

Once physical illness and other major psychiatric disorders have been excluded, two other conditions should be considered.

1 **Histrionic personality disorder** may lead to an exaggeration of physical symptoms and a dramatization of illness. In this case there will be a lifelong history of such behaviour.

2 **Malingering** is difficult to sustain and will be exposed by discrete and prolonged observation.

What causes hysteria?

Psychoanalytic theories

These propose that hysterical patients suffer from the effects of emotionally charged ideas lodged in their subconscious at some time in the past. When failure of the repression of these ideas threatens, possibly because of the demands of current stress, psychic energy is released and is discharged in the form of hysterical symptoms.

Genetics

There is no convincing evidence for a genetic aetiology.

A reflex mechanism

Hysterical symptoms may be seen as reflex reactions to protect the nervous system from excessive stress. They could then be prolonged if the patient finds them useful or by force of habit. These ideas have not been substantiated.

How is hysteria treated?

Immediate management involves reassurance and the suggestion of recovery, combined with resolution of any stressful circumstances that provoked the reaction. If the disorder has lasted more than a few weeks the approach involves minimizing the factors which reinforce or reward the behaviour and encouraging normal behaviour. It is useful to explain that the disability is caused by a psychological not physical process and that effort can overcome it. Attention should then be focused on the problems which provoked the disorder.

Abreaction has been used successfully to treat acute hysterical neuroses in soldiers in war-time. Under hypnosis or the effect of intravenous barbiturates the patient is encouraged to relive the stressful events which provoked the hysteria and to express the accompanying emotions. This approach is used uncommonly in civilian life.

Exploratory psychotherapy has been used frequently in

hysterical neurosis. There are many anecdotal reports of successful treatment but no controlled studies of its effectiveness.

What is the outcome for hysteria?

There have been many anecdotal reports of a good response to treatment, especially in those with disorders of recent onset which are clearly related to severe stress. There have been no systematic studies of response to treatment and clinical experience suggests that the outcome is frequently poor.

Syndromes related to the neuroses

Depersonalization syndrome

Depersonalization is a fairly common symptom of a number of syndromes. A primary depersonalization syndrome is rare. The patient describes feeling detached from the world and unreal, with dulled emotions and mechanical actions. The feeling is experienced as extremely unpleasant. The condition is most common in women. Onset is often in adolescence or early adult life. The disorder may persist for years with periods of remission. Anxiolytic medication may be helpful but support and encouragement may be all that can usefully be offered.

Munchausen syndrome

These patients present themselves at hospitals with dramatic symptoms which seem to require urgent attention or powerful analgesics. The symptoms and signs are produced deliberately and the patient usually makes an effort to deceive over personal details and previous admissions. The behaviour suggests a severe disorder of personality.

Hypochondriasis

The patient's concern for their health is excessive and is not justified. It may co-exist with actual physical disorder. Hypochondriasis occurs commonly in a variety of mental disorders but particularly in depression and anxiety states. There is little evidence that it exists at all as a separate neurotic syndrome in its own right. In those rare cases where primary hypochondriacal neurosis is diagnosed, treatment is limited to support and avoidance of continuous discussion of the patient's symptoms. Any new symptoms must always be evaluated thoroughly because even hypochondriacal patients may develop actual physical illness.

QUESTIONS

1 Discuss the value of the current system of classification of the neuroses (a) from the point of view of the psychiatrist and (b) from the point of view of the general practitioner. How might treatment approaches differ in these two settings?
2 (a) List the most important features of the syndrome of obsessive–compulsive disorder. (b) Describe the main features of the treatment of obsessive–compulsive disorder.
3 (a) List the principal features that are common to the various manifestations of hysteria. (b) Outline the steps in management of a 15-year-old who presents with paralysis of the right leg for which no cause can be found after extensive neurological examination.
4 A 23-year-old woman is referred to the out-patient department with a 9-month history of increasing difficulty in going into crowded shops, using public transport and leaving home. (a) List five specific aspects which are important for assessment. (b) Describe the principal types of treatment that may be useful in this type of problem.
5 Discuss the relative merits of psychological and drug treatments in the neuroses.

FURTHER READING

Gelder M.G., Gath D. & Mayou R. (1989) *Oxford Texbook of Psychiatry*, Chapters 6 and 7, Neurosis. Oxford University Press, Oxford.

8
Eating Disorders

Fact sheet

Definition

The term eating disorders refers to anorexia nervosa and bulimia nervosa and their variants. These disorders have in common a characteristic set of extreme concerns about shape and weight. Most of their clinical features may be regarded as secondary to these concerns.

Clinical presentation

Anorexia nervosa

- Characteristic overconcern about shape and weight (as in bulimia nervosa).
- Active maintenance of an unduly low weight (e.g. at least 15% below the expected weight for the person's age, height and sex) achieved mainly by strict dieting and excessive exercising and, in a minority, self-induced vomiting.
- Amenorrhoea (in post-menarchal females not taking an oral contraceptive).
- Depressive, anxiety and obsessional symptoms.
- Social withdrawal.
- Physical effects of starvation.

Bulimia nervosa

- Characteristic overconcern about shape and weight (as in anorexia nervosa).
- Normal body weight (in most cases).
- Frequent bulimic episodes ('binges'). These involve the consumption of unusually large amounts of food, given the circumstances, and loss of control at the time.
- Use of extreme behaviour to control shape and weight.
- Depressive and anxiety symptoms and, in a minority, substance abuse.
- Impaired interpersonal functioning.
- Electrolyte disturbance in those who vomit frequently or abuse large quantities of laxatives or diuretics.

Distribution

- Both disorders are largely confined to Western countries in which thinness for women is considered attractive.
- Anorexia nervosa mainly affects adolescent girls and young adult women. About 10% of cases are male. Amongst adolescent girls the prevalence rate is between 0.2 and 1.1%. The incidence rate is between 0.24 and 14.6 per 100 000 female population per annum. It is thought to have increased over recent decades. Cases from upper socio-economic groups are over-represented.
- Bulimia nervosa mainly affects women in their twenties. Male cases are rare. Amongst women aged between 16 and 35 years the prevalence rate is between 1 and 2%. Most cases have not come to medical attention. The incidence is not known. It is likely to have increased over recent decades. More even social class distribution than anorexia nervosa.

Aetiology

Predisposing factors include being an adolescent or young adult female in certain Western societies; dieting; a family history of eating disorders, obesity, affective disorder and substance abuse; a personal history of these disorders; premorbid low self-esteem and perfectionism. Maintaining factors include the physical and psychological effects of starvation; development of the characteristic extreme concerns about shape and weight; rewards of maintaining strict self-control; and secondary effects on others.

Assessment

Patients may present with some feature of the eating disorder (e.g. loss of control over eating), or they may present indirectly complaining of an associated physical or psychiatric feature (e.g. infertility, depression). A history should be taken from the patient and, if possible, an informant. No physical tests are required to make either diagnosis. Severity of associated psychiatric symptoms must be assessed. Patients with anorexia nervosa need a thorough assessment of their physical state. Patients who vomit frequently or abuse large quantities of laxatives or diuretics should have their electrolytes checked.

Management

Anorexia nervosa

Two aspects to treatment: establishing healthy eating habits and a healthy weight, and removing factors that have been maintaining the disorder. Engaging the patient in treatment can be difficult. Education is important. It is essential to establish the need for weight gain. With most patients, weight gain can be achieved on an out-patient basis, but full or partial hospitalization may be required. Two forms of psychotherapy are most widely used to supplement the weight restoration regime: psychoeducational and supportive counselling, and family therapy. Drugs have a limited role.

Bulimia nervosa

Great majority of patients may be managed on an out-patient basis. A specific form of cognitive behaviour therapy is the treatment of choice.

Prognosis

Anorexia nervosa

Varied outcome. Significant mortality rate. Long history and late onset are predictors of a poor outcome. Some patients develop bulimia nervosa.

Bulimia nervosa

No information on long-term outcome. In short-term, majority respond well to cognitive behaviour therapy. Low self-esteem predicts a poor outcome.

Introduction

The term eating disorders is used to refer to anorexia nervosa and bulimia nervosa, and their variants. These two disorders share many features and it is not uncommon for people to move from one disorder to the other, particularly from anorexia nervosa to bulimia nervosa. Together, the two disorders are a major source of psychiatric morbidity amongst young women.

Anorexia nervosa has long been recognized with particularly good descriptions being published in the UK and France in the last century. In contrast, the first series of patients with bulimia nervosa was published as recently as 1979.

Diagnostic criteria

Three features are required to make a diagnosis of anorexia nervosa. The first is the presence of certain characteristic extreme concerns about shape and weight. These are sometimes described as the 'core psychopathology' and they are pathognomonic of anorexia nervosa and bulimia nervosa. Various expressions have been used to describe them, including the 'relentless pursuit of thinness' and a 'morbid fear of fatness'. It is important to note that these concerns are far more intense than the dissatisfaction with shape and weight experienced by many young women today. The second diagnostic feature is the active maintenance of an unduly low weight. The definition of what constitutes low varies: a widely used threshold is being at least 15% below the expected weight for the person's age, height and sex. The low weight is achieved by a variety of means, including strict dieting or fasting, excessive exercising and, in some, by self-induced vomiting. Laxatives and diuretics may also be abused, and those with diabetes mellitus may underuse or omit insulin. The third diagnostic feature is amenorrhoea (in post-menarchal females who are not taking an oral contraceptive).

Three features are also required to make a diagnosis of bulimia nervosa. The first is the presence of attitudes to shape and weight similar to those found in anorexia nervosa. The second feature is frequent bulimic episodes. By definition, these 'binges' involve the consumption of unusually large amounts of food, given the circumstances, and loss of control at the time. The third feature is the use of extreme behaviour to control shape and weight. This behaviour resembles that used by patients with anorexia nervosa, although self-induced vomiting and laxative or diuretic misuse are much more common.

The great majority of people who meet the three diagnostic criteria for bulimia nervosa have a weight in the normal range. However, there are some who are significantly underweight and may be eligible for the diagnosis of anorexia nervosa. In practice both diagnoses are not given: instead, the diagnosis of anorexia nervosa trumps that of bulimia nervosa.

The diagnostic criteria for anorexia nervosa and bulimia nervosa are summarized in Fig. 8.1, and the relationship

---

Fig. 8.1 Diagnostic criteria for anorexia nervosa and bulimia nervosa

Anorexia nervosa
- Characteristic extreme concerns about shape and weight.
- Active maintenance of a low weight.
- Amenorrhoea.

Bulimia nervosa
- Characteristic extreme concerns about shape and weight.
- Frequent episodes of bulimia ('binges').
- Extreme methods of weight control.

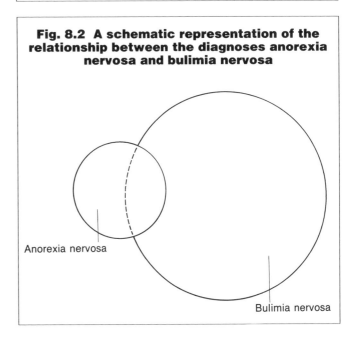

Fig. 8.2 A schematic representation of the relationship between the diagnoses anorexia nervosa and bulimia nervosa

Anorexia nervosa

Bulimia nervosa

---

between the two diagnostic categories is represented schematically in Fig. 8.2.

Distribution

Anorexia nervosa is largely confined to women aged between 10 and 30 years and to Western countries in which thinness for women is considered attractive. Estimates of the incidence of the disorder range from 0.24 to 14.6 per 100 000 female population per annum and it seems that the incidence has increased in recent decades. Estimates of the prevalence of the disorder amongst adolescent girls, the group most at risk, range from 0.2 to 1.1%. Anorexia nervosa is rarely encountered among men (less than 10% of cases are male) and it is uncommon among non-whites. The social class distribution seems to be uneven with cases from upper socio-economic groups being over-represented.

Bulimia nervosa is more common than anorexia nervosa. Amongst young women (aged 16–35 years) in the UK and North America the prevalence rate is between 1 and 2%. Most cases have not come to medical attention. Whilst there are no satisfactory data on the incidence of bulimia nervosa, it seems that the disorder has become more common over the past 25 years. In all countries in which anorexia nervosa is found, there has been a dramatic upsurge in the number of cases of bulimia nervosa: from being viewed as an unusual variant of anorexia nervosa, it is now the most common eating disorder encountered in psychiatric practice. Patients with bulimia nervosa are on average somewhat older than those with anorexia nervosa, most presenting in their twenties, and they have a broader social class distribution. The disorder is rarely seen in men.

Anorexia nervosa

Development of the disorder
The onset of anorexia nervosa is usually in adolescence, although prepubertal cases are encountered (see also p. 191). Occasionally the disorder does not begin until adulthood. Often it starts as normal adolescent dieting which then gets out of control. As the dieting intensifies, weight falls and the physiological and psychological effects of starvation develop. Additional methods of controlling shape and weight may be adopted at any stage. The characteristic over-concern about shape and weight is often not present at the outset.

Clinical features

Specific psychopathology
The weight loss is mainly achieved through a severe reduction in food intake. The amount consumed may be very small and some patients fast at times. Typically the range of foods eaten is restricted with foods viewed as fattening being avoided. Except in long-standing cases, appetite persists and for this reason the term 'anorexia' is not appropriate. Frequent intense exercising is common and adds to the weight loss. Self-induced vomiting and the misuse of laxatives and diuretics may also be practised, particularly by the sub-group of patients who occasionally lose control over eating.

Accompanying the disturbed eating habits is the so-called body image disturbance. This takes various forms. It may include a perceptual component such that all, or parts, of the body are seen as larger than their true size, and an attitudinal component characterized by an intense dislike of the body or parts of it. Neither feature improves as weight is lost: indeed, both tend to get worse.

General psychopathology
Depressed mood, lability of mood and irritability are common. In more chronic cases there may be hopelessness and thoughts of suicide. Anxiety symptoms, usually related to eating, are also prominent. Outside interests decline as weight is lost and social withdrawal may be marked. Obsessional symptoms are frequently present and often these focus on eating. There is preoccupation with thoughts about food, eating, shape and weight, and concentration may be impaired.

Physical health
Anorexia nervosa is associated with many physical abnormalities and their significance has been the subject of much interest. Earlier this century the disorder was mistakenly

attributed to pituitary insufficiency, and more recently, and again probably mistakenly, it has been suggested that there is an underlying primary hypothalamic disorder. The main argument for such a disorder rests upon two observations: first, in a small proportion of patients, menstruation ceases prior to weight loss; and second, restoration of a healthy weight is not always accompanied by the resumption of regular menstruation. However, in both instances it is likely that the underlying endocrine disturbance is secondary to abnormalities in eating.

Symptoms and signs. Many patients with anorexia nervosa have no physical complaints. However, systematic enquiry often reveals heightened sensitivity to cold and a variety of gastrointestinal symptoms including constipation, fullness after eating, bloatedness and vague abdominal pains. Other symptoms include restlessness, lack of energy, low sexual

---

Fig. 8.3 Anorexia nervosa: findings on physical examination

- Emaciation and low body weight.
- Short stature and failure of breast development (in those with a prepubertal onset).
- Axillary and pubic hair present and no breast atrophy (unlike hypopituitarism).
- Fine downy lanugo hair on the back, arms and side of face.
- Dry skin.
- Cold hands and feet.
- Dependent oedema.
- Low blood pressure and pulse.

Fig. 8.4 Anorexia nervosa: findings on investigation

Endocrine
- Low LH, follicle stimulating hormone and oestradiol levels.
- Immature pattern of LH release.
- LH response to LHRH is reduced.
- Low T3 and T4.
- Raised growth hormone and cortisol levels.

Haematological
- Mild neutropaenia.
- Normocytic normochromic anaemia.
- Low ESR.

Other metabolic abnormalities
- Hypercholesterolaemia.
- Increased serum β-carotene.
- Hypoglycaemia (may present atypically).
- Electrolyte disturbance (in those who vomit frequently or misuse large quantities of laxatives or diuretics).

Other findings
- Enlargement of the cortical sulci and cisternes, and dilatation of the ventricles ('pseudoatrophy').
- Osteopaenia and osteoporotic fractures.
- Delayed gastric emptying and prolonged gastrointestinal transit time.

ESR, erythrocyte sedimentation rate; LH, luteinizing hormone; LHRH, LH-releasing hormone.

appetite and early morning wakening. In post-menarchal females who are not taking an oral contraceptive, amenorrhoea is by definition present. Occasionally patients complain of infertility. The findings on examination are listed in Fig. 8.3.

Findings on investigation. These are listed in Fig. 8.4. Many of the abnormalities have been reproduced in experimental studies of the physiological effects of dieting and are reversed by the restoration of healthy eating habits and a normal weight.

Aetiology

Predisposing factors

Dieting appears to be a general vulnerability factor. It is a frequent precursor of anorexia nervosa and bulimia nervosa, and the two disorders seem to be largely confined to countries in which dieting is common among young women. However, whilst many young women diet, few develop an eating disorder. Therefore other aetiological factors must operate, some of which may interact with dieting.

A variety of risk factors have been implicated. These include premorbid obesity (25% of patients with anorexia nervosa and 40% of patients with bulimia nervosa have been overweight prior to the onset of the eating disorder), and long-standing low self-esteem and perfectionism. The parents often report that as children these individuals were exceptionally compliant and well behaved. Factors within the family are also relevant. There is an increased rate of eating disorders and affective disorders in these patients' families. However, there appears to be no cross-transmission in that the rate of eating disorders amongst the relatives of those with affective disorders is not raised. The observation that communication between family members is often disturbed is difficult to interpret since it has not been established whether the disturbance precedes or follows the development of the eating disorder.

Maintaining factors

As food intake decreases and weight is lost, there are secondary effects, some of which perpetuate the disorder. For example, delayed gastric emptying results in fullness even after eating small amounts, and social withdrawal isolates the person from his or her peers. Those who have been overweight are often understandably pleased with the weight loss and at first they may be complimented on it. There may also be gratifying secondary effects within the family. A case study is given opposite.

Assessment

Few patients with anorexia nervosa refer themselves for treatment. Usually they are persuaded to seek help by concerned relatives or friends and as a consequence they often attend somewhat reluctantly.

Careful history-taking from both the patient and, if at all possible, an informant will make the diagnosis clear. It will be evident that the weight loss has been self-induced and is associated with the characteristic core psychopathology. No physical tests are required to make the diagnosis, and unless

Case 1: a case of anorexia nervosa

The patient was 17 years old and in her last year at school. She lived at home with her parents. On their insistence she saw the family doctor on account of her weight loss – she had lost almost 20 kg over the previous 6 months. She reported that she had felt 'fat' for some years, but had only decided to do something about it following an adverse comment at school. At first she followed a diet that she had found in a magazine but more recently she had set her own diet to increase the rate of weight loss. She was attempting to eat no more than 2520 kJ (600 kcal) daily. She had ceased to eat with the family. As well as dieting, she exercised heavily. Each morning she would do an hour of exercise before leaving the house. She also jogged to school rather than taking the bus. She did not practise self-induced vomiting, nor did she abuse laxatives. She said that she felt fat, and she was particularly concerned about the shape of her stomach. The idea of gaining weight terrified her. She had been amenorrhoeic for 4 months.

There was no medical or psychiatric history of note in the family. Both her parents were doctors and her elder brother was at university. Her childhood had been unremarkable. Menarche was at age 13 years. Until recently she had done well at school. She was afraid that she might not succeed at getting into university. She had no close friends and had never had a boyfriend.

The family doctor found it hard to establish rapport. She decided that it would be best to see the patient again the following day when she had more time. At the second interview she broached the subject of anorexia nervosa, recommended a paperback on the subject, and asked if she might see the patient's parents.

So began a 6-month period of treatment involving a 2-month admission to the local psychiatric hospital followed by nutritional counselling and individual and family psychotherapy.

there are positive reasons to suspect another physical condition, no tests are required to exclude other medical disorders. Excluding the presence of co-existing depressive disorder can be difficult since depressive symptoms are a known consequence of semi-starvation. To make this diagnosis it may be necessary to wait until body weight has been restored. It is more straightforward deciding that a depressive disorder is not the sole diagnosis since the core psychopathology of anorexia nervosa is not present in depression and the weight loss is rarely self-induced.

Some patients present complaining of features associated with anorexia nervosa rather than the disorder itself. For example, they may present with gastrointestinal symptoms, amenorrhoea or infertility, or with depressive or obsessional features. However, once the weight loss has been identified, and it has been recognized to be self-induced, the diagnosis should become clear.

Whilst physical tests are not required for diagnostic purposes, all patients with anorexia nervosa should have a thorough physical examination and whatever investigations are indicated on the basis of the findings. The electrolytes should be checked of all those who frequently vomit or misuse significant quantities of laxatives or diuretics.

Management

Patients with anorexia nervosa vary. Some present with short histories and are willing and able to change, whilst others have an entrenched disorder and resist all attempts to help them.

In principle, there are two aspects to treatment. One is establishing healthy eating habits and a normal weight, and the second is the removal of those factors which have been maintaining the disorder. Both are essential. The normalization of eating habits and weight is mainly achieved though a combination of common sense advice and nutritional counselling. This may be achieved on an in-patient, day-patient or out-patient basis. Addressing the factors that have been maintaining the eating disorder generally involves the use of more specialized treatments such as family therapy or cognitive behaviour therapy. Both these treatments require training and are best conducted on an out-patient basis.

Drugs have a limited role. Short-acting minor tranquillizers may occasionally be used to lessen the anxiety some patients experience prior to eating, and if depressive symptoms persist following weight restoration, antidepressant drugs should be prescribed. Occasionally it is appropriate to use drugs to stimulate the resumption of regular menstruation. Tube feeding and intravenous hyperalimentation are rarely indicated.

The initial phase of treatment
There are four aspects to this phase of treatment.
- *Forming a collaborative therapeutic relationship.* This is especially important in patients who are reluctant attenders.
- *Educating the patient.* Patients need to learn about the clinical features of anorexia nervosa, the factors relevant to its development and maintenance, and the importance of weight gain. Certain popular books may be recommended.
- *Agreeing that there is a need for weight gain.* A major goal is to establish the need for weight gain. In doing so, it is important to emphasize that weight restoration is only one part of treatment, albeit a necessary one.
- *Deciding upon the treatment setting.* Most patients with anorexia nervosa may be managed exclusively on an out-patient basis. Some need an initial period of day-patient or in-patient treatment followed by out-patient care. Out-patient treatment is not appropriate if the patient's physical health is a cause for concern, if the weight loss is rapid, or if the patient is depressed and at risk of suicide. Partial or full hospitalization is also indicated if no progress is being made with out-patient care.

Not infrequently, in-patient treatment is indicated, but the patient does not want to be admitted. Under these circumstances, unless immediate hospitalization is essential, two options are available: either management on a day-patient basis or a brief trial of out-patient treatment. A small number of patients refuse admission even though their life is in danger. In such cases compulsory hospitalization must be considered.

In-patient treatment
Admission may be to a general or psychiatric hospital. In either case it is a great advantage if the ward staff are experienced in the management of these patients. Weight restoration may be achieved in either setting, but with a psychiatric admission it is easier to add the other forms of treatment needed to maximize the chance that progress will be maintained following discharge.

Within a few days of admission, patients should be introduced to the consumption of regular meals and snacks; and, if possible, by the end of 2 weeks these should be of a normal quantity and composition, consisting of about 8400 kJ (2000 kcal) a day. A target rate of weight gain of about 1 kg per week should be set, with the patient and staff monitoring progress each morning. Since between 12 600 and 21 000 kJ (3000 and 5000 kcal) a day are likely to be required to achieve this rate of weight gain, the meals and snacks will need to be supplemented. It is preferable to add energy-rich drinks rather than more food, since medically sanctioned overeating runs counter to the goal of helping patients establish healthy eating habits, and in addition it carries the risk of acute gastric dilatation.

The goal weight range should be one which does not necessitate dieting and one at which normal physiological functioning is restored. Once patients enter this range, the energy-rich drinks should be phased out, leaving them consuming a diet sufficient to maintain their weight. At this stage they should be given full control over their eating and they should be encouraged to shop, cook and eat out with friends and family. Unless considerable effort is put into this phase of treatment, there is a considerable risk of relapse following discharge.

Running concurrently with weight restoration should be other forms of therapy. At first, straightforward support is often best, but once the patient's mental state begins to improve, more specific procedures may be introduced, including cognitive behavioural interventions and family therapy.

With an in-patient regime of this type, body weight is usually restored to a healthy range within 2–3 months and the patient discharged 2–4 weeks later. The transition from in-patient to out-patient care needs to be carefully planned.

Day-patient treatment
There is increasing interest in the use of day-patient treatment in place of full hospitalization for all but the most ill patients. A comprehensive treatment programme can be provided, including supervized eating and weight gain, whilst patients remain based in their usual social environment. The hope is that day-patient treatment will be found to be associated with a reduced risk of relapse following discharge.

Out-patient treatment
This may be the sole form of treatment or it may follow a period of in-patient or day-patient care. Various approaches are used, including simple support and encouragement, a specific form of cognitive behaviour therapy, and various forms of family therapy. There has been so little research on the overall management of anorexia nervosa that few specific recommendations can be made. It is important to involve the family when treating young patients.

Course and outcome
For some, anorexia nervosa is a relatively benign self-limiting disorder; for others, about a quarter, it may lead to death or chronic disability. Few consistent predictors of outcome have been identified, the exceptions being a long history and late onset both of which are associated with a poor prognosis.

The presence of a low body weight, bulimic episodes, self-induced vomiting or laxative abuse, and a history of premorbid psychosocial problems, also tends to be associated with a poor outcome.

Whilst at least half the patients recover in terms of their weight and menstrual function, the disturbed attitudes to shape and weight often persist and eating habits may remain disturbed. Up to a quarter of the patients develop bulimia nervosa. Standardized mortality ratios have been reported between 1.36 and 6.01, the deaths being either a direct result of medical complications or due to suicide. The most recent follow-up studies have been obtaining lower mortality figures suggesting that the rate is falling. The outcome in males appears to be essentially the same as that in females.

Bulimia nervosa

Clinical features

Specific psychopathology
Anorexia nervosa and bulimia nervosa have very similar clinical features. The patients share the same extreme concerns about shape and weight and engage in the same methods of weight control. However, there are two features which distinguish patients with bulimia nervosa from those with anorexia nervosa: first, the body weight of most patients is in the normal range; and second, there are frequent bulimic episodes. These 'binges' are a source of great shame, they tend to be kept secret and, in the majority of cases, they are followed by self-induced vomiting or the taking of laxatives. They vary greatly in size: on average, they involve the consumption of about 8400 kJ (2000 kcal). Since the proportion of carbohydrate eaten is unremarkable, the popular term 'carbohydrate craving' is misleading. Between bulimic episodes, the patients restrict their food intake in much the same way as patients with anorexia nervosa. Figure 8.5 shows a monitoring sheet illustrating the eating habits of a typical patient.

General psychopathology
Depressive and anxiety symptoms are prominent, more so than in anorexia nervosa. A significant minority also have problems with alcohol or drugs. Interpersonal functioning is often impaired with there being difficulty initiating and maintaining close relationships.

Physical health
Symptoms and signs. The majority of patients have few physical complaints. Those most commonly encountered are irregular or absent menstruation, weakness and lethargy, vague abdominal pains and toothache. On examination, appearance is usually unremarkable. Salivary gland enlargement may be present: typically, this involves the parotids and gives the patient's face a slightly rounded appearance. The pathophysiology of the salivary gland enlargement is not understood. In those who vomit there may be calluses on the dorsum of the dominant hand (Russell's sign) due to the fingers being used to stimulate the gag reflex. Also, there may be significant erosion of the dental enamel particularly on the lingual surface of the upper front teeth. A minority

Fig. 8.5 A monitoring sheet illustrating the eating habits of a patient with bulimia nervosa

B, bulimic episodes ('binges'); V/L, vomiting or laxative use; *, episodes of eating viewed by the patient as excessive.

of patients, particularly those who take large quantities of laxatives or diuretics, have intermittent peripheral or facial oedema.

Findings on investigation. Of most importance is the electrolyte disturbance which is encountered in about half those who vomit or take laxatives or diuretics. Metabolic alkalosis, hypochloraemia and hypokalaemia are the most common abnormalities and they may account for the weakness and tiredness experienced by some patients. Clinically serious electrolyte disturbance is not often encountered and rarely does it merit direct treatment: instead, it is better to focus on the treatment of the eating disorder itself. Endocrine abnormalities may be present. These resemble those found in anorexia nervosa but are not as severe.

Aetiology
Many patients with bulimia nervosa give a history of disturbed eating stretching back into adolescence, and about a third have previously fulfilled diagnostic criteria for anorexia nervosa. Most of the remainder started with an anorexia

Case 2: a case of bulimia nervosa

The patient was a 24-year-old hairdresser. She presented to her family doctor complaining of depression. At first he thought that she had a depressive disorder and he recommended that she take an antidepressant drug. His suspicions were raised when the patient burst into tears on hearing that the drug could result in weight gain. He asked if she was concerned about her weight. This enquiry led to her divulging a 5-year history of eating problems, starting with an anorexia nervosa-like picture. For the past 3 years she had been overeating and vomiting several times each day and on occasions she had also taken large quantities of laxatives. She said that she was 'completely out of control' – she couldn't stop eating and she was preoccupied with her shape. She said that she knew that she looked normal but insisted that she was 'fat underneath'. She described repeatedly weighing herself.

In addition to the problems with eating, she had significant depressive and anxiety symptoms. She also drank excessively at times. Her relationships were problematic: she was having an affair with her employer, and whilst she realized that this relationship had no future, she felt unable to give it up. She had no confidants and reported that she found it difficult making friends, particularly with women.

Both her parents were dead. Her father had died from a heart attack when she was aged 4. Her mother had committed suicide 1 year earlier in the context of a long-standing depressive disorder. Her childhood had been disrupted by the death of her father and periods when her mother was severely depressed. She thought that she had underachieved at school. She had chosen hairdressing as a career since she was interested in fashion and design.

The family doctor made a diagnosis of bulimia nervosa. He took blood to check her electrolytes and referred her to a local psychiatrist.

nervosa-like picture although the weight loss was not of sufficient severity to allow the diagnosis to be made. Given this sequence of events, and the fact that the two conditions are so similar, it may be assumed that most factors of relevance to the aetiology of anorexia nervosa are also relevant to the aetiology of bulimia nervosa. Nevertheless, it seems that some factors preferentially increase the risk of developing bulimia nervosa. These include vulnerability to obesity, affective disorder and substance abuse, the rates of all three disorders being raised in the relatives of these patients. A history of sexual abuse predating the onset of the eating disorder is given by about a quarter of these patients. This rate is higher than that amongst matched subjects in the general population but no higher than that amongst young women with other psychiatric disorders. Sexual abuse is therefore not a specific risk factor for the development of the disorder. A case study is given above.

Assessment

Most patients with bulimia nervosa are ashamed of their eating habits and have kept them secret for many years. Like those with anorexia nervosa, they may present complaining of features associated with the disorder rather than the disorder itself. For example, they may present with gastro-intestinal or gynaecological symptoms, depression or substance abuse. Under these circumstances making the correct diagnosis can be difficult since there are rarely indications of the eating disorder.

Most patients who present with bulimia nervosa complain of loss of control over eating. Assessment is relatively straightforward and the diagnosis can be made with little difficulty. As with anorexia nervosa, no physical tests are needed to make the diagnosis. However, the electrolytes should be checked of all those who frequently vomit or misuse large quantities of laxatives or diuretics.

Management

The great majority of patients may be managed on an out-patient basis. Full or partial hospitalization is indicated under four unusual circumstances:
- if the patient is either too depressed to be managed as an out-patient or there is a risk of suicide;
- if the patient's physical health is a cause for concern;
- if the patient is in the first trimester of pregnancy since there is some evidence that the spontaneous abortion rate may be high;
- if the eating disorder proves refractory to out-patient care. If hospitalization is indicated, it should be brief and regarded as a preliminary to out-patient care.

With regard to out-patient treatment, the most effective treatment is a specific form of cognitive behaviour therapy. This is a specialized psychological treatment which aims to modify not only the disturbed eating habits but also the disturbed attitudes to shape and weight. It usually involves about 20 sessions over 5 months and results in substantial improvement in all aspects of the psychopathology. The techniques used include the following: the daily self-monitoring of relevant thoughts and behaviour; education about eating, shape and weight; the use of self-control procedures to help establish a pattern of regular eating; the gradual introduction of avoided foods into the patient's diet; and so-called cognitive restructuring procedures designed to identify and challenge problematic thoughts and attitudes.

Some patients respond to less intensive interventions and self-help manuals probably have a role. A 'stepped care' approach to management has been proposed in which treatments are provided sequentially according to need. This approach involves a simple intervention being used initially and more complex ones only if the patient fails to respond.

Antidepressant drugs are the only pharmacological treatment to have shown promise. They result in a decline in the frequency of overeating and an improvement in mood, but the effect is not as great as that seen with cognitive behaviour therapy and, more importantly, it is usually transitory. Appetite suppressants have no beneficial effect.

Course and outcome

As yet little is known about the course of bulimia nervosa. Many of the cases identified in community surveys appear to be relatively benign in that they are shortlived. In contrast, patients who are referred for treatment often have long histories with previously unsuccessful attempts to help them. Over half these cases respond well to cognitive behaviour therapy with the changes being maintained for at least the following year. Low self-esteem is a predictor of poor treatment response. There have been no studies of long-term outcome.

Atypical eating disorders

In addition to anorexia nervosa and bulimia nervosa, various 'atypical eating disorders' are encountered. These have not been well characterized. Most common are disorders resembling anorexia nervosa or bulimia nervosa but not quite meeting their diagnostic criteria. In addition, there are people with eating problems distinct from anorexia nervosa and bulimia nervosa. For example, there are those who vomit when anxious, and people who have difficulty eating or swallowing in public. Both these groups should be classed as having an anxiety disorder and treated accordingly. There is another group who stop eating as a way of bringing attention to themselves. Such people generally have major personality difficulties.

Finally, a note about obesity. Obesity is not an eating disorder: it is a condition of excess body fat, and genetic factors contribute substantially to its aetiology. Recently it has been recognized that a sub-group of the obese have an eating disorder in which there are recurrent bouts of overeating similar to those seen in bulimia nervosa. However, in the great majority of cases there is no associated extreme weight-control behaviour, nor are there concerns about shape and weight of the type present in anorexia nervosa and bulimia nervosa. Therefore the diagnosis of bulimia nervosa cannot be given. These people have high levels of depressive and anxiety symptoms and respond poorly to conventional forms of treatment.

ACKNOWLEDGEMENTS

CGF holds a Wellcome Trust Senior Lectureship and PJH is a Nuffield Medical Fellow. This chapter is based in part on a chapter in the *Oxford Textbook of Medicine*, Third Edition, edited by D. Weatherall, J.G.G. Leddingham and D.A. Warrell (Oxford University Press, Oxford).

READING FOR PATIENTS
AND THEIR FAMILIES

Cooper P.J. (1993) *Bulimia Nervosa: a Guide to Recovery*. Robinson, London.
Palmer R.L. (1988) *Anorexia nervosa*. 2nd Edition. Penguin, London.

FURTHER READING

Andersen A.E. (1990) *Males with Eating Disorders*. Brunner/Mazel, New York.
Fairburn C.G., Marcus M.D. & Wilson G.T. (1993) Cognitive behaviour therapy for binge eating and bulimia nervosa: a comprehensive treatment manual. In: Fairburn C.G. & Wilson G.T. (eds) *Binge Eating: Nature, Assessment and Treatment*, pp. 361–404. Guilford, New York.
Garner D.M. & Garfinkel P.E. (eds) (1985) *Handbook of Psychotherapy for Anorexia Nervosa and Bulimia Nervosa*. Guilford, New York.
Hsu L.K.G. (1990) *Eating Disorders*. Guilford, New York.
Russell G.F.M. (1992) Anorexia nervosa of early onset and its impact on puberty. In: Cooper P.J. & Stein A. (eds) *Feeding Problems and Eating Disorders in Children and Adolescents*, pp. 85–111. Harwood Academic Publishers, Chur, Switzerland.

9
The Personality Disorders

Fact sheet

Definition
Deeply engrained, maladaptive patterns of behaviour generally recognizable by adolescence or earlier and continuing through most of life.

Classification (see Fig. 9.1)

Presentation
Personality disorder presents because of:
- chance association with physical or mental illness;
- consequences of behaviour: e.g. work or marital difficulties, injury or intoxication;
- psychological complaint, e.g. tension, loneliness, etc.

Diagnosis
- Abnormal behaviour since adolescence either persistent regardless of external events or provoked by minor stress.
- Confirmed by informants.

Differential diagnosis
- Marked personality traits (too mild to be called personality disorder).
- Chronic mental illness.
- Acute stress reactions.
- Conduct disorder as a developmental phase.
- Acute brain syndromes.
- Mental impairment.
- Intoxication.
- Diagnosis most difficult when history is incoherent or inadequate and informants are lacking.

Aetiology
- Largely unknown.
- Inherited personality traits.
- ? disrupted or severely disturbed relationships in childhood.
- ? learned behaviour.

Distribution
- Lifetime prevalence between 2 and 3%.
- Male/female frequency probably similar.

Associated factors
- Crime.
- Substance abuse.
- Suicide/self-injury.

Assessment
Depends on detailed account of personal history and past behaviour. This can only be reliably obtained from other informants.

Management
- Drugs usually unhelpful.
- Problem-orientated management.
- Therapeutic community.
- Consider needs of family.

Outcome
- Little convincing evidence of effectiveness of treatment.
- Abnormal behaviour continues but is expressed with less energy with age.

What are personality disorders?

The concept of personality disorder can be understood as a medical model of severe social maladjustment. Social maladjustment, or deviance, does not equate with disease or illness unless it is a consequence of, for example, brain damage. Personality disorders, and milder personality problems, frequently accompany medical and psychiatric illnesses. Treating medically alone without regard to the influence of personality can lead to serious management problems. It is important to appreciate and take account of maladaptive patterns of behaviour in order to avoid such difficulties.

Psychiatrists also attempt to help people with personality disorders even though there is no evidence of disease. There is commonly an expectation of medical intervention by patients, relatives and society and psychiatry offers help for such problems. Although many are uneasy about it, personality disorders have come to be treated as psychiatric illnesses in their own right.

The first part of this chapter covers aspects of personality disorders in general. Because of the importance of sociopathic personality disorder in clinical practice, the second part of the chapter deals with this particular personality disorder in detail.

Definition

'Personality' refers to enduring qualities of an individual shown in ways of behaving in a wide variety of circumstances. The word 'disorder' refers to the degree and frequency with which maladaptive behaviour occurs. Distinguishing marked personality traits from personality disorder is not usually a helpful exercise, being only a matter of degree and being highly subject to the attitudes and experience of the person making the assessment. The term 'personality disorder' is usually reserved for only the most severe and persistent forms of disturbed behaviour.

Some people, who are otherwise normal, have inherited or acquired a vulnerability to develop neurotic illness in response to stressful events (see Chapter 7 on neuroses) and are described as having a vulnerable personality. Such people have normal (but vulnerable) personalities if their behaviour has not been severely and continuously abnormal before the neurotic illness developed. In personality disorders maladaptive behaviour occurs even in the absence of significantly stressful events.

The distinction of maladaptive behaviour due to personality disorder from that due to illness depends on the duration of the behaviour. If behaviour has always been maladaptive, it is a personality disorder. If there has been a change from normal to abnormal, it is an illness.

It is impossible to find entirely satisfactory criteria to distinguish normal from abnormal behaviour. Statistical criteria have been used to quantify variations in aspects of personality and behaviour, using a cut-off score to identify abnormality. These are of value in research but are not useful in clinical work with individual patients. In general, a social criterion is used, which defines maladaptive behaviour as behaviour which causes the individual or others to suffer.

This clearly has a more arbitrary cut-off and is based on the assessor's subjective impression of what is normal or abnormal.

Classification of personality disorders

ICD-10 offers a number of categories of personality disorder which are listed and briefly described below. Apart, perhaps, from sociopathic personality disorder such categories are not particularly useful. Any individual will present with a unique variety of problems which cannot be described adequately using a single diagnostic label. It is more useful in clinical work to describe the main features of the abnormal behaviour of that individual, which may include components of several of the personality disorders described in ICD-10. Such information is more likely to assist in predicting future difficulties and deciding appropriate ways of helping (Fig. 9.1).

Fig. 9.1 Personality disorders classified in ICD-10 (draft) (indicating comparable categories in DSM-III-R)

- *Paranoid (paranoid in DSM-III-R):* sensitive, suspicious and unforgiving. Excessive tendency to self-importance and self-reference. Combative and tenacious, assuming the same behaviour and attitudes in others.
- *Schizoid (schizoid and schizotypal in DSM-III-R):* lack of warmth and pleasure, detached, isolated, solitary, shy. May develop eccentricities.
- *Dyssocial (antisocial in DSM-III-R):* callous unconcern for others, irresponsible, irritable, aggressive. Lacks guilt and does not learn from punishment. Incapable of maintaining relationships.
- *Emotionally unstable (impulsive or borderline) (borderline in DSM-III-R):* emotionally unstable, impulsive with outbursts of anger. Borderline type includes disturbed or unstable self-image, aims or sexual preferences, associated with repeated self-injury.
- *Histrionic (histrionic and narcissistic in DSM-III-R):* self-dramatization with exaggerated shallow and labile emotions, suggestible, egocentric, easily hurt, craves attention and excitement.
- *Anankastic (obsessive and compulsive in DSM-III-R):* indecisive and cautious, excessively perfectionistic, conscientious and scrupulous. Rigid and stubborn. Vulnerable to unwanted intensive thoughts and impulses.
- *Anxious (avoidant in DSM-III-R):* tension and apprehension, feels insecure and inferior. Over sensitive to rejection and criticism. Need for security leads to restricted lifestyle.
- *Dependent (dependent in DSM-III-R):* subordination and compliance with others. Feels helpless and incompetent. Fears abandonment, needs reassurance.
- (DSM-III-R includes *passive aggressive type* categorized by various types of passive resistance to any demands).

Note. 'Immature' and 'inadequate' are frequently used terms which are both better avoided. They do not correspond to any particular ICD-10 categories and are often used pejoratively. It is better to try to define the ways in which the person's behaviour is inadequate or immature. Describing the person's problems in a more precise way is likely to lead to a more constructive approach to management.

What are the causes of personality disorders?

Little is known about the causes of variation in either normal or disordered personalities. However, there is a small amount of knowledge and there are a number of hypotheses which should be considered.

Genetic influences

There is convincing evidence, derived from observing the behaviour of babies, that a number of general aspects of behaviour can be inherited. Aspects of personality which can be identified early in infancy and which appear to persist into later years include:

1 a tendency to withdraw in the face of novelty;
2 slow adaptability to change;
3 high intensity of emotional reactions;
4 irregularity of biological function (sleep, elimination, etc.);
5 predominant negative mood (crying, fussy, etc.).

It is likely that more complex aspects of personality can also be inherited. When personality test scores of adult monozygotic twins are compared, the scores of those brought up apart are as similar as those reared together, suggesting a substantial genetic influence.

Relation to mental illness

It has been suggested that some disorders of personality (such as cycloid and schizoid personalities) may be partial expressions of a mental illness (manic depression or schizophrenia respectively). There is no convincing evidence to support this, but if it is so, the partial expression may take a quite different form from the full expression of the illness. In the examples above, there is no evidence that people with such personality disorders are particularly prone to such illnesses. On the other hand the children of patients with schizophrenia have been shown to have an increased incidence of anti-social behaviour and neuroses but not schizoid personality. The relatives of patients with manic depressive illness cannot be distinguished from the relatives of patients with unipolar depression. The one notable connection between mental illness and personality is that depression will frequently exacerbate personality traits. An example of this is the development of obsessional symptoms in people with obsessional traits following the onset of depression.

Psychoanalytic theories

It has been supposed that crucial stages of development must be passed through successfully if personality is to develop normally. Predictions have been made about the specific effects of failure at particular stages. For example, it was proposed that a failure to develop normally at the 'anal' stage would predispose this person to obsessional traits. Such an explanation for a personality disorder may be of help to patients or relatives by making their difficulties seem understandable. Unfortunately, psychoanalytic hypotheses are very imprecise and are difficult to test.

Early experiences

Considerable attention has been given to the effects of maternal or parental deprivation as a cause of sociopathic personality. This is discussed below. There is no convincing evidence that this form of deprivation causes other kinds of personality disorder. It is worth noting that if personality traits are inherited the parents and families of people with personality disorders are likely to be abnormal too, leading to disturbing early experiences to complicate the life of the individual with the personality disorder.

Assessment of personality disorders

The patient is rarely able to give a full account of their behaviour and assessment relies heavily on information obtained from other informants such as relatives, partners or employers and from other agencies such as probation officers and social workers. Observation of behaviour in a hospital setting many not be an accurate guide to the patient's normal behaviour. It is necessary to obtain a detailed account of the person's behaviour in the past and under a wide range of circumstances.

Rather than assigning a category to the personality, it is more useful to describe the main features of the person's behaviour in the descriptive terms used by ICD-10 or DSM-III (see Fig. 9.1). A description should include an assessment of strengths as well as weaknesses because it may be possible to build on the former whilst reducing the effects of the latter.

Particular attention needs to be paid to identifying circumstances that provoke undesirable behaviour. This may indicate practical ways of reducing the frequency of the behaviour.

Presentation of personality disorders

In the context of acute medical or psychiatric assessment it is often impossible to identify the presence of personality disorder, particularly when there is no knowledge about the patient's past behaviour. However, some behaviours are much more likely to be associated with personality disorder than others. These would include repeated self-injury or fighting, illegal drug misuse, alcohol dependence and eating disorders.

The presence of a personality disorder will become increasingly apparent with continued contact with the patient. Clinicians should be particularly sensitive to this possibility if they find themselves making unusual arrangements with the patient with regard to access arrangements, personal contacts, treatment approaches, etc. It is because personality disorders frequently go undetected but lead to serious distortions of the relationship between patient and clinician, sometimes putting both at risk, that all clinicians should receive supervision and be open to comment on any such abnormal relationships.

Treatment of personality disorders

General approaches to treatment
Engaging the patient in treatment requires a balance between accessibility, which allows the patient satisfactory access to care, and clear boundaries to the service on offer which protect the therapist both physically and emotionally. The clinician needs to be clear about which of the patient's problems are due to illness and are their responsibility to treat and which are not and are the responsibility of the patient to manage. On the whole, the role of the clinician is to inform, advise and create opportunities for the patient to change their behaviour.

The Mental Health Act (1983)
The Act only allows compulsory assessment (Section 2) or treatment (Section 3) of patients with 'psychopathic disorder', a sub-group of people with dyssocial or antisocial personality disorder. Treatment under Section 3 can only be justified if it is 'likely to alleviate or prevent a deterioration of his condition.'

Medication
There is little place for medication in the treatment of personality disorder. However, there is some evidence of a reduction in the difficulties of those with severe impulsive disorders of a borderline type using low doses of major tranquillizers.

Psychotherapy
Analysis of current behaviour provides the starting point for psychotherapy. Clarifying the ways a person relates to others, understands his and their feelings and copes with difficulties leads on to encouraging him to make necessary changes. Individual and group psychotherapies for those with personality problems are discussed in Chapter 18 with supportive psychotherapy of particular value to vulnerable patients.

Particular personality types may present particular difficulties in psychotherapy. For example, patients with hysterical personality disorders may make heavy demands on the therapist for extra time, medication and reassurance, or may create emotionally difficult situations by being seductive, aggressive or anxiety provoking in other ways. A patient with a schizoid personality disorder may drop out of treatment quickly, or remain detached from it and reluctant to be engaged emotionally. Psychotherapy with severely personality disordered patients is at best a slow process and often fails.

A problem-orientated approach
For the majority, support and supervision are often the most effective help that can be offered. The aims of such an approach would be to help the patient to avoid or better manage situations that provoke unwanted behaviour and to build on whatever strengths he may have. As with other behavioural treatments, the therapist should try to establish an alliance with the patient in which an 'experimental' approach is taken in attempting to find ways of achieving these goals. Cooperation is much more likely to be achieved when the patient is experiencing some set-back or difficulty. If no progress is made it will be necessary to decide whether further sessions are pointless because the patient is incapable, at that time, of benefiting, or whether further support is going to prevent the accumulation of additional problems and therefore be worthwhile.

Family therapy
It may be more helpful to try and influence the environment in which the patient lives than to change the patient's personality. Family therapy may help families to change their behaviour in a way that reduces triggers for abnormal behaviour in the patient. Clearer communications and more effective problem solving are probably the most useful changes. Families will benefit from a clearer understanding of the origin and nature of the disorder and of what will not help as much as from knowing what may help.

What is the outcome for personality disorders?

People with abnormal personalities appear to experience and cause less suffering as they get older. Most of the evidence for this comes from observation of those with sociopathic personality. There is no apparent change in the nature of the abnormal personality over time, but the abnormal behaviour is expressed with less energy and vigour with age.

Sociopathic personality disorder

The term 'psychopathic' personality is not useful because there is confusion about whether it refers to all those with disordered personalities or only those who are sociopathic. Asocial or antisocial personality disorder are terms equivalent to sociopathic personality disorder. Sociopathic disorder is also referred to extensively with reference to the Mental Health Act (1983), which still uses the term psychopathic disorder (Chapter 25, p. 316).

What is sociopathic personality disorder?
The essential features of this disorder are: failure to make loving relationships, impulsive actions, lack of guilt and failure to learn from adverse experiences. The failure to make loving relationships may lead to the person forming only brief, shallow relationships, or, in the most extreme form, may lead to cruel or degrading behaviour to others. Impulsiveness will lead to instability in most areas of life, particularly in work, marriage, the care of children, financial circumstances and the use of drugs and alcohol. The combination of personality features frequently leads to criminal behaviour, usually of a petty nature, but may include acts of

violence or sexual deviations (see Chapter 23, p. 293 and Chapter 24, p. 301). In addition, suicide is more common in this group (Chapter 19, p. 246).

Presentation of sociopathic personality disorder

A family history of sociopathic personality disorder is common. People with violent, antisocial personalities frequently report punitive, alcoholic parents and a history of rejection early in life. Childhood cruelty to animals is common.

A case example

A man of 18 was referred for psychiatric assessment by his GP. His main problems were persistent *lying* and an *inability to engage in any constructive activity or retain a job*. His referral was precipitated by an episode in which he *indecently assaulted a 6-year-old girl*.

His *difficulties had become apparent at the age of 7 when his parents were divorced*. He was *bullied* at school but was also a *disruptive influence* and was moved to a special boarding school. His mother reported that he *never established any friendships* although he described having some 'mates'. His mother described *episodes of deliberate cruelty* to animals.

His mother found him *very like his father* who was violent towards her, was also prone to lie continuously and was very unreliable in his behaviour. The patient had some of his father's mannerisms although they had not met for many years.

Although he was not being prosecuted for the sexual assault his family had requested an assessment because they feared that he would get into more serious trouble unless there was a change in his behaviour.

Individuals may present for medical attention as a result of:
1 physical illness;
2 the consequences of their behaviour, such as injury or intoxication;
3 psychological complaints, for example of tension, depression or loneliness;
4 a request for psychiatric assessment by a court.

What causes sociopathic personality disorder?

Genetic cause

Several studies have indicated that criminal behaviour is linked to some inherited component. In one study of 13 MZ twins 10 were concordant for criminal behaviour, whilst of 17 DZ twins of the same sex only two were concordant. In another study of 33 MZ twins 22 were concordant, whilst of 23 DZ twins only three were concordant for criminal behaviour. However, although these findings are suggestive of an inherited component, criminal behaviour is defined by the law and does not correspond directly with the criteria for sociopathic personality disorder. In a study of adoptees whose parents were identified as having a sociopathic personality disorder and who were separated from their parents at birth, 22% were diagnosed as having a sociopathic personality disorder. None of a group of controls, born of normal parents, had this diagnosis. These data suggest that an inherited component plays an important part in the development of a sociopathic personality disorder.

Chromosomal abnormalities

XYY karyotype was thought to be associated with abnormally aggressive behaviour. However, it has been shown to occur more frequently in the general population than was thought and cannot, alone, be sufficient to cause aggressive behaviour.

Cerebral pathology

A comparison of the electroencephalogram (EEG) recordings of men who had been habitually aggressive with those of a group who had had only a single outburst of violence, showed that 57% of the habitually aggressive group had abnormal EEGs (having excluded cases with mental subnormality, epilepsy and head injury). Only 12% of the comparison group showed abnormalities. Abnormalities were most common in the anterior temporal region. It has been suggested that these abnormalities might predispose to aggressive behaviour which is then precipitated by stressful events.

The effects of upbringing

It has been suggested that separation of a young child from its mother leads to the development of antisocial behaviour and a failure to form close relationships. It is now recognized that the effects of separation are very variable. Causes of separation will include antisocial personality in one or both parents, and these traits may be inherited by the child rather than *caused* by the separation. There is no evidence, at present, to prove that early separation, on its own, is an important cause of sociopathic personality disorder.

Learning theory

There are four ways in which antisocial behaviour might be learned:
1 a person may learn normally but learn antisocial behaviour from an antisocial family;
2 he may not learn appropriate behaviour because he is not presented with a consistent structure of rules;
3 antisocial behaviour may be learned because it is an effective way of coping with other difficulties;
4 the person may have a disordered ability to learn.
This last possibility is of particular interest, but does not account for the clear ability among those with sociopathic personality disorder to learn other behaviours and social skills normally.

Special features in the assessment of sociopathic personality disorders

The patient is often being assessed at the request of another person, for example the patient's family, their social worker or solicitor. Lack of cooperation is common but motivation can be encouraged. The extent to which the patient can be compelled to accept treatment under the powers of the Mental Health Act depends on the danger he presents to himself or others and on the degree to which the patient is likely to respond to treatment (see also Chapter 25).

The needs of partners and families must be considered independently of the individual's decision regarding treatment. They may be more in need of help and better able to benefit from it.

A simple behavioural analysis is helpful, with the main

aim being to identify triggers for undesirable behaviour and reasons for previous periods of desirable behaviour.

How are sociopathic personality disorders managed?

General principles

1 At an early stage, identify the features which are of particular importance such as triggers for dangerous behaviour, outbursts or other disturbed behaviour.

2 The patient remains responsible for his behaviour and its consequences.

3 The therapist offers support and help in achieving progress but the limits of what will be tolerated by the therapist and of what he will do **for** the patient (rather than done **by** the patient) must be clear. Such limits should be generous enough to allow the patient at least a reasonable chance of remaining in therapy, but not so generous that the therapist loses control of therapy.

4 Do not expect reliability, honesty, gratitude, regular attendance or warm rapport.

5 The therapist should obtain support from colleagues for his opinions about dangerousness, potentional for change and suitability for particular treatments at the outset and during crises.

6 Limit the number of people involved in managing the patient to one or two if possible.

7 Be suspicious of dramatic improvement.

Problems in management

1 Fluctuating rapport will demand different ways of responding to the patient at different times, sometimes requiring informality, sometimes careful detachment.

2 Evidence of depressive illness must be sought when patients complain of being helpless or hopeless. If found, this would be an indication for antidepressant medication. Encouragement and maintaining contact may otherwise be all that can be offered.

3 Repeated overdoses or self-mutilation require routine referral for physical management and firm adherence to previously agreed goals.

4 Admission to hospital only transfers the disruptive behaviour to a different place, encouraging avoidance of problems in future and causing difficulties to vulnerable inpatients.

Particular approaches to treatment

1 **Therapeutic community.** Management in a therapeutic community is of particular relevance in sociopathic personality disorder. It provides a setting in which social relearning can take place with patients accepting responsibility for their behaviour and its consequences. An important underlying principle is that people will learn more from a peer group than from those in a position of authority over them. In the therapeutic community, while staff retain overall control and responsibility, patients play a key part in formulating and enforcing the rules of the community. Patients live and work together, meeting regularly for group discussions where their behaviour and feelings are examined. Change is attempted by members of the community who, having similar difficulties, can both support others and present them with the evidence of their disordered behaviour. No controlled study of the value of this treatment has been carried out. Follow-up studies have reported improvement rates of between 40 and 60% (see also p. 236).

2 **Social care.** Family support may be all that can be achieved. With violent patients, estimating the risk to sexual partners and family members is a priority, as they may need urgent warning.

3 **Identifying specific problems** which have a remedy is occasionally helpful. For example: literacy tuition may improve self-esteem and work prospects; medical support may assist in arranging rehousing and deduction of rent and other bills at source; correction of physical abnormalities may improve self-esteem and social behaviour.

What is the outcome for sociopathic personality disorders?

There is some evidence that antisocial people over the age of 45 present fewer problems of aggressive behaviour, although their problems with personal relationships tend to persist. It has been shown that people with persistent antisocial behaviour in early adult life show improvement in later follow-up in terms of having fewer arrests or contacts with social agencies. Amongst offenders with sociopathic personalities whose first offences involved physical aggression, subsequent offences tended not be a consequence of aggression.

QUESTIONS

1 Sociopathic personality disorder has been called 'moral insanity'. Discuss the concept that personality disorders are illnesses.

2 A 19-year-old man has been accused of sexually assaulting a 13-year-old girl. His IQ is normal and he has no symptoms of mental illness. However, his family suggests that he has a personality disorder and needs treatment. Outline the procedure for assessment. List the management options available.

3 Outline the theories concerning the origins of personality disorders.

4 People with personality disorders rarely refer themselves directly to a psychiatrist for treatment. How might this affect attempts at treatment. What can the therapist do to make therapy more likely to be successful?

5 List the types of personality disorder described in ICD-10. What relationship do personality disorders have with the mental illnesses of similar name (viz. hysterical personality disorder/hysteria)?

FURTHER READING

Cleckley H. (1941) *The Mask of Sanity*. Henry Kimpton, London. [A source of case histories.]

Gelder M.G., Gath D. & Mayou R. (1993) *Oxford Textbook of Psychiatry*, Chapter 5, Personality disorder. Oxford University Press, Oxford. [A comprehensive review.]

Main T. (1957) The ailment. *Br. J. Med. Psychol.* **30**, 129–45. [An important discussion of the management problems presented by certain kinds of 'difficult' patient.]

Tyrer P. *et al.* (1983) Relationship between neurosis and personality disorder. *Br. J. Psychiatr.* **42**, 404–8.

Whiteley J.S. (1970) The psychopath and his treatment. *Br. J. Hosp. Med.* **3**, 263–70. [A review of sociopathic personality disorders.]

10
Substance Abuse

Fact sheet

Definition

Substance abuse is diagnosed when the use of any drug causes serious problems to the user, his or her family or society. **At-risk consumption** is diagnosed when an individual is at risk of developing such problems in the future as a result of the amounts he or she is consuming at present. **Addiction** is diagnosed if there is regular intoxication, uncontrollable craving, tolerance, dependence and detrimental consequences.

Substance abuse and any subsequent addiction is usually subdivided into abuse of alcohol and abuse of other drugs, of which the most important is probably narcotic abuse.

Alcohol abuse

Clinical presentation

- *Early stages*: history of heavy consumption may be the only sign. The early alcoholic may be asymptomatic or may present with social difficulties (e.g. marital disharmony or problems at work), or clinical symptoms such as frequent gastrointestinal problems, depression or anxiety, or alcohol-withdrawal symptoms such as tremor.
- *Chronic stage*: diagnosis is usually obvious. Alcohol withdrawal symptoms are severe, and there is progressive physical, social and mental deterioration, sometimes with descent into skid-row behaviour.

Diagnosis

A detailed alcohol consumption history should be part of any routine history taking. Clinical suspicions should be aroused in particularly high-risk groups, for example certain occupational groups and patients with known related medical or social problems.

Certain special investigations may confirm the diagnosis, for example liver function tests, MCV and gamma-GT.

Distribution

- Worldwide: Scotland, Ireland, America, France and Italy have a high incidence compared to countries like Holland.
- Sex: commoner in men.
- Occupational: commoner in alcohol-related industries such as catering, brewing or distilling.
- Prevalence in UK: 1–2% of the population have established alcohol problems. At-risk consumers are probably as common as 5–10% of the population.

Factors associated with alcohol problems

- Per capita consumption of alcohol.
- Stress, crises and major negative life-events.

Aetiological factors

Probably multifactorial; suggested causation models are: biological factors; psychoanalytic factors; behavioural factors; sociocultural factors; and genetic factors.

Main differential diagnosis

May mimic almost any medical or psychiatric condition.

Management

- Identification of patient.
- Helping the patient to acknowledge the problem.
- Controlled drinking programme *or* abstinence with withdrawal.
- Support and follow-up.

Prognosis

Very variable. Prognosis is much better if there is a good premorbid personality, and a stable family and occupational life.

Syndromes showing some of the features of alcohol abuse

Other drug abuse.

Narcotic abuse

Clinical presentation

Hallmark is physical dependence and tolerance. The most common clinical presentation is therefore with symptoms of withdrawal, which include agitation, pupillary dilation and abdominal cramps with diarrhoea and vomiting.

Diagnosis

- Observation of clinical features of withdrawal.
- Presence of needle-marks.
- Presence of opiates in urine.

Factors associated with narcotic abuse

Increased risk of death due to:
- overdose and poisoning;
- violence.

Factors associated with intravenous injections, e.g. hepatitis, infective endocarditis, HIV.

Annual death-rate of approximately 1:100 addicts.

Aetiological factors

Largely unknown. Opiate use usually diminishes with age.

Management

- Out-patient methadone substitution for maintenance *or* withdrawal, or admission for withdrawal.
- Psychotherapeutic support and follow-up, preferably in a specialized residential centre or therapeutic community.

Other commonly abused drugs

- Cannabis.
- Amphetamines.
- Cocaine.
- Barbiturates.
- Solvent abuse.
- Hallucinogens, e.g. LSD.

What is substance abuse and addiction?

There is a considerable difference between substance abuse and substance addiction, and it is important to remember that most people who abuse drugs do not become addicted to them, and indeed often come to no harm. Addiction of course is a different matter and usually results in some harm.

To make a diagnosis of addiction, it should be possible to demonstrate regular intoxication, uncontrollable craving, tolerance, dependence and detrimental effects (Fig. 10.1).

Both abuse and any subsequent addiction are usually subdivided into abuse of alcohol and abuse of other drugs. Abuse of other drugs can be further subdivided into opiate abuse and non-narcotic abuse (Fig. 10.2).

Fig. 10.1 WHO criteria for addiction to a drug

1 Periodic or chronic intoxication.
2 Overwhelming compulsion to take the drug and obtain it by any means.
3 Tendency to increase the dose because of tolerance.
4 Psychological and usually physical dependence.
5 Detrimental result to individual and society.

Fig. 10.2 Types of substance abuse

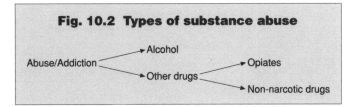

Alcohol abuse

Ethyl alcohol is a central nervous system depressant which is commonly used socially to promote relaxation and pleasure. The distinction between use and abuse is obviously not always easy, and a further distinction should be made between established abuse of alcohol and hazardous or at-risk consumption.

The World Health Organization in 1976 further subdivided alcoholism into alcohol-related disabilities and the alcohol dependence syndrome. An alcohol-related disability may be any damage suffered as a result of alcohol ingestion, whilst the alcohol dependence syndrome is an overwhelming psychological compulsion to take alcohol with subsequent loss of control. Alcohol-related disabilities and the alcohol dependence syndrome will, of course, often co-exist (Fig. 10.3).

Hazardous or at-risk alcohol consumption is a different concept, which attempts to identify individuals who may as yet show no signs or symptoms of alcohol-related disabilities, but who may be at risk of developing these disabilities in the future as a result of the amount of alcohol which they are consuming in the present.

Fig. 10.3 WHO definition of alcoholism

Alcohol-related disability: an impairment in the physical, mental or social functioning of an individual, of such nature that it may be reasonably inferred that alcohol is part of the causal nexus.

Alcohol dependence syndrome: a state, psychic and usually physical, resulting from taking alcohol, and characterized by behavioural and other responses that always include a compulsion to take alcohol on a continuous or periodic basis in order to experience its psychic effects or to avoid the discomfort of its absence.

Fig. 10.4

1 standard unit of alcohol
equals
½ pint of beer or cider
equals
1 single measure of spirit
equals
7.9 g or 1 centilitre of alcohol

The most popular quantitative measurement of consumption nowadays is the standard unit of alcohol, which is equivalent to $\frac{1}{2}$ pint of ordinary beer or cider, a single measure of spirits, a glass of sherry, or a glass of wine and contains 7.9 g or 1 centilitre of alcohol (Fig. 10.4). The Royal Colleges of Psychiatrists, Physicians and General Practitioners and the Health Education Council advise consumption of below 21 units per week in men, and 14 units per week in women and describe a consumption of over 50 units per week in men and 35 units per week in women as harmful.

Epidemiology and prevalence of alcohol abuse

Methods of estimating epidemiology and prevalence include direct and indirect methods (Fig. 10.5). The most accurate method is direct measurement by general population survey. A random survey of 2000 adults in the general population in England and Wales was carried out by Wilson for the DHSS in 1978, and showed that 6% of men and 1% of women were drinking above 50 units of alcohol per week, and this rose to 13% of men and 4% of women in the 18–24 age group (Fig. 10.6). In 1990, the Health Education Council carried out a survey which showed that 24% of men and 9% of women in the 18–24 age group were drinking over the recommended levels of 21 units per week in men and 14 units per week in women. This is likely to mean that several million people in

Fig. 10.5 Methods for estimating prevalence

1 Direct measurement, i.e. general population.
2 Indirect measurement, i.e. prevalence figures are derived indirectly from other measurements, e.g. from per capita consumption, from the number of deaths from cirrhosis or other alcohol-related conditions, or from attendance figures for alcohol problems at GPs, hospitals and social agencies.

this country are at risk of developing alcohol-related problems, and at least 1–2% of the population, that is approximately three-quarters of a million people, have established alcohol problems. Alcoholism is therefore believed to be the third major health hazard after heart disease and cancer.

Indirect methods of estimating prevalence are unsatisfactory because they almost always provide a gross underestimate; most alcoholics escape the statistics involved. For example, it is well known that general practitioners only diagnose one in 10 alcoholics under their care, and hospital doctors, including psychiatrists, also frequently miss the diagnosis.

How is alcohol abuse diagnosed?
One of the most obvious reasons for missing the early alcoholic is that he or she is often asymptomatic, may not have symptoms of dependence, is largely unaware of the dangers to his health, and his appearance and social status may not conform to the popular stereotype of the alcoholic as a down and out vagrant.

The most obvious way of recognizing alcohol abuse, especially in the early stages, is to ask the patient in detail how much they drink, which many doctors are embarrassed to do, or do not bother to do as they do not believe they will get a truthful answer. In fact it seems that tactful questioning on the lines of the quantity–frequency questionnaire is inoffensive and produces surprisingly accurate replies, and should be a part of any routine history taking (Fig. 10.7). The quantity–frequency questionnaire basically asks how many times a week the individual drinks beer, e.g. he may reply three times a week, and then how much beer is actually drunk when he does drink beer, for example he may reply three pints. This will tell you that the individual is consuming 18 units of alcohol of beer each week, and the questions are then repeated for wine and spirits. Alterna-

tively, or in addition, if the answers seem very high, one can go through a typical drinking day, or the previous week's consumption.

Suspicion should be aroused in particularly high-risk groups, for example certain occupational groups, patients with known related medical problems, patients with marital and social problems, patients with histories of repeated accidents, patients presenting with withdrawal symptoms, patients frequently requesting time off work or requests for medical certificates, and patients with associated psychiatric problems, particularly suicidal ideas (Fig. 10.8 and pp. 246, 249).

If the alcohol abuse has progressed to the stage of physical addiction or dependence, then the diagnosis can be confirmed by the presence of withdrawal symptoms, such as morning shakes, nausea and vomiting, etc., all abolished by a drink first thing in the morning (the 'hair of a dog' or 'eye-opener').

Most sophisticated aids to diagnosis include questionnaires such as the 'CAGE' (see p. 148) and investigations such as liver function tests, MCV and gamma-GT. These, however, are not always reliable, and are not real substitutes for a clinical diagnosis.

Once chronic alcoholism has become established, there is usually no problem with diagnosis. There is progressive deterioration with serious physical and mental symptoms, malnutrition and sometimes descent into 'skid row' behaviour. For an account of alcohol abuse in the elderly, see p. 165.

Aetiology: what do we know about the causation of alcohol abuse?
The aetiology of alcoholism is almost certainly multifactorial, but five main causation models are commonly described: biological, psychoanalytic, behavioural, sociocultural and genetic. These will be dealt with in turn.

Biological theories
This model postulates a variety of biological causes to explain physiological dependence on alcohol, but at present there is little conclusive evidence to support it.

Psychoanalytic theories
These theories postulate unconscious psychological reasons, originating in early life experience, for alcohol misuse. Freud, for example, suggested that alcoholism was related to the oral stage of development, whereby painful reality is denied and pleasure obtained by immediate oral gratification, in other words drinking.

Fig. 10.7 Example of quantity–frequency questionnaire

Beverage	No. of times/ week consumed	Average amount consumed each time	Standard unit equivalent
Beer	3	3 pints	18
Wine	3	3 glasses	9
Spirits	7	1 double	14
Total weekly consumption in units			41

Fig. 10.9 Effects and complications of alcohol misuse

Psychological

Effect on mood
- Acute, e.g. sedation and intoxication effects such as euphoria/dysphoria, aggression.
- Chronic effects, e.g. anxiety, depression.

Effect on cognitive function
- Acute intoxication, e.g. diminished judgement and memory, disinhibition.
- Chronic, e.g. alcoholic dementia.

Psychological dependence on alcohol
- Craving.
- Loss of control.

Psychiatric effects
For example depression, suicide (p. 246) sexual problems, anxiety, paranoia, morbid jealousy, hallucinations, DTs, dementia and the Wernicke–Korsakoff syndrome.

Social
- Relaxation of inhibition.
- Marital complications.
- Occupational complications.
- Legal complications.
- Increased accidents.
- Violence (p. 301).

Medical

Alcohol abuse can cause a large variety of medical complications, and in fact it has been estimated that 20% of all hospital beds are occupied by people with alcohol-related diseases which include:
- hepatitis and cirrhosis;
- pancreatitis;
- peptic ulcers and gastritis;
- peripheral neuritis;
- myopathies;
- heart failure and cardiomyopathies;
- fits;
- TB;
- weight problems;
- Mallory–Weiss syndrome;
- DTs;
- Wernicke–Korsakoff syndrome;
- alcoholic dementia;
- other rare neuropsychiatric complications, e.g. cerebellar degeneration, optic atrophy.

These psychoanalytic theories are very interesting, but they are very hard to prove or disprove. Psychologists have also tried to define an 'alcoholic personality', but all attempts to do so scientifically have failed. The most commonly proposed personality trait is anxiety, with subsequent self-sedation with alcohol.

Behavioural theories

Learning theory proposes that alcoholism is a conditioned behavioural response, which associates drinking with a positive rewarding experience, since it temporarily reduces anxiety and conflict in the short term. The guilt, misery, sickness and punishment that occur in the long term can be alleviated by further drinking, and this maladaptive behaviour is positively reinforced and a vicious circle is set up (Fig. 10.10). The important point about learning theory is that what is learned can in theory be unlearned, but in practice behavioural approaches including aversive conditioning and Antabuse do not seem to work very well.

Transactional analysis is another behavioural theory which views alcoholism as a series of transactions designed to obtain a personal advantage. For example a patient's partner may collude with the drinking behaviour because it gives them power or freedom, or hides their own deficiencies. It may even keep a failing marriage going. However, it is probable that such transactions maintain the drinking behaviour, rather than causing it in the first place.

Fig. 10.10 Maladaptive behaviour in alcohol abuse

Short-term positive experiences

Alcohol use

Long-term negative experiences

Sociocultural theories

These propose that a high incidence of alcoholism results from a combination of social conditions and cheap easily available alcohol. Important sociocultural factors appear to be race, religion, economic factors, occupational factors, sexual and marital status, stress and life-events such as grief (p. 272).

Genetic theories

It has been known for centuries that alcoholism tends to run in families.

> *'Drunken women bring forth children like themselves.'* (Aristotle)
> *'One drunkard begets another.'* (Plato)

It was apparent for some time that 25% of close male relatives and 5–10% of close female relatives of alcoholics are themselves alcoholics, compared to a general population prevalence of 3–5% in males and 0.1% in female. However, it was not clear whether this familial incidence was due to genetic or environmental factors, and twin and adoption studies were carried out to determine this, and on the whole have come down on the side of genetic factors.

Twin studies generally show a significantly higher concordance rate for drinking behaviour among male monozygotic twins than among dizygotic twins. Adoption studies also confirm the importance of genetic factors since they have mostly found that sons of alcoholics are almost four times more likely to become alcoholic themselves than the sons of non-alcoholics, irrespective of whether they are brought up by their alcoholic biological parents or by non-alcoholic foster parents.

However, it is not clear whether it is a biological factor or a psychiatric factor, such as personality traits or depressive tendencies, which is being transmitted and rendering the individual vulnerable.

In conclusion the precise aetiology of alcohol misuse is far from clear, but would seem to be unlikely to be explained by just one of the above models. It is likely that several factors interact, and are of varying importance in different patients.

The prevention of alcohol misuse

The prevention of alcohol misuse may be attempted in two broad ways: prescriptive and restrictive (Fig. 10.11)

Prescriptive prevention depends fundamentally on prescribing alcohol education for primary care workers, specialists and the general public to improve their awareness of alcohol-related problems. Alcohol education may improve primary prevention, and also secondary prevention by early identification and treatment, as has already been discussed.

Restrictive measures of prevention on the other hand involves Government policies, and can mostly be subdivided into restriction of availability and restriction of advertising. Restriction of availability may include such things as reducing the number of places where alcohol may be obtained (for example the number of licensed restaurants in an area or even banning the sale of alcohol in Government buildings such as NHS hospitals), restricting the number of hours in which alcohol can be bought, general restriction such as forbidding any level of alcohol in the blood when driving, and restriction of availability of alcohol by raising taxes and making it more expensive. It is no secret that the price of alcohol has fallen in recent years, relative to rising wages and inflation.

Whether these preventive stratagems are likely to work is not clear as yet. Large alcohol education campaigns, as were carried out in the north-east of England, do not seem to have made any appreciable impact on consumption. In addition it would appear from the Scandinavian countries that attempts to make alcohol more expensive and more difficult to obtain resulted in a large increase in illegal distilling.

Preventive measures in alcohol misuse are of course very important, but it would appear that more research is needed at the moment to make them effective.

Treatment of alcohol abuse

There is no magic cure for alcoholism, and treatment can only be successful if the patient is motivated and cooperative.

The basic steps in treatment are set out in Fig. 10.12.

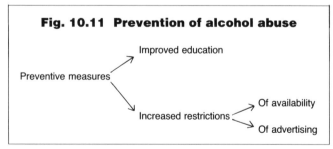

Fig. 10.11 Prevention of alcohol abuse

Preventive measures → Improved education

Preventive measures → Increased restrictions → Of availability

Increased restrictions → Of advertising

Fig. 10.12 Treatment of alcoholism— four stages

1 Identification of patient.
2 Helping the patient to acknowledge the problem.
3 Controlled drinking programme *or* abstinence with withdrawal.
4 Support and follow-up.

Controlled drinking versus abstinence

Once the patient has been identified and the problem has been acknowledged, both of which can be very difficult, the next stage is to decide whether to advise a reduction in consumption or total abstinence. Reducing consumption is called controlled drinking, and may be appropriate in early alcohol misuse, particularly if there are no clear symptoms of physical or psychological dependence. For the established alcoholic, particularly if withdrawal symptoms are present, abstinence appears to be the only practical aim.

Controlled drinking programme

The patient should first be advised of the likely serious consequence of his/her drinking, and a realistic drinking goal should then be agreed, for example two or three pints of beer two or three times a week. The patient should then be asked to keep a diary of alcohol intake, and the circumstances in which failure occurs, and an appointment is made for the following week. At this new appointment the consumption diary is reviewed, and should help in elucidating danger periods, for example passing the local pub on the way home from work. It may be necessary for the patient's lifestyle to be altered, for example finding another way home to avoid the pub.

New interests should be encouraged to avoid the previous drinking circumstances, and it is very important to involve the family. The patient should be reviewed weekly or fortnightly for the first few weeks, and then monthly for about a year. The patient should be told to report a relapse at once, and should be encouraged to take personal responsibility for his/her alcohol consumption.

Abstinence programme

If the patient has established alcohol problems, is experiencing withdrawal symptoms or has failed in the controlled drinking programme, then total abstinence should be advised.

If physical dependence is present, abstinence will result in acute alcohol withdrawal symptoms, which are chiefly symptoms of sympathetic overactivity and psychological discomfort and which usually manifest themselves within a few hours of abstinence (Fig. 10.13).

However, uncomplicated alcohol withdrawal is a short self-limiting condition, and can be undertaken on an in-patient or out-patient basis (Fig. 10.14).

The treatment of the withdrawal syndrome is symptomatic, and the mainstay of management is sedation with chlormethiazole or benzodiazepines to diminish the unpleasant withdrawal symptoms. The dosage prescribed depends on

---

Fig. 10.13 Alcohol withdrawal symptoms

1 Psychological symptoms, e.g. anxiety, restlessness.
2 Tremor.
3 Sweating.
4 Gastrointestinal symptoms, e.g. anorexia, nausea.
5 Tachycardia.
6 Fits.
7 Psychotic phenomena, e.g. hallucinations, paranoia disorientation and full-blown DTs.

the severity of the symptoms, and a reducing course of one week or less should be prescribed. If home detoxification is embarked on, only 2 days' supply of tranquillizers at a time should be prescribed, and it is best if the patient is visited at home in the first 48 hours, either by the GP or by an experienced community psychiatric nurse. The patient should be warned of the danger of taking alcohol and tranquillizers together, particularly chlormethiazole.

Vitamin supplements, especially the B complex, are also often indicated, especially if there is a history of malnutrition, since a shortage of thiamine may cause peripheral neuropathies or even the Wernicke–Korsakoff syndrome.

Complications of withdrawal

The two commonest complications are severe systemic disturbance, and fits, and they may occasionally be fatal. In these cases, which must always be managed in hospital, the patient should be more heavily sedated, and careful nursing care should be carried out including regular measurement of pulse, blood pressure and temperature, correction of fluid and electrolyte disturbance, and examination for infection and associated conditions such as pancreatitis and unsuspected injuries such as subdural haematoma. Fits are usually treated with an anticonvulsant such as carbamazepine, phenytoin or phenobarbitone.

The most common causes of death are convulsions, hypovolaemic shock, circulatory collapse or pulmonary complications.

The two urgent medical complications of alcohol abuse which are most commonly managed by psychiatrists are delirium tremens and the Wernicke–Korsakoff syndrome, since prominent psychiatric disturbance occurs in both conditions. Both are potentially life-threatening conditions.

Delirium tremens

Delirium tremens is, as its name suggests, a state of delirium resulting from alcohol withdrawal. It usually occurs 2 or more days after the last drink has been taken, and the usual signs and symptoms of delirium, such as confusion, disorientation, agitation, paranoia and visual and tactile hallucinations, occur. In addition there is usually a marked tremor, as usually occurs in severe alcohol withdrawal. The condition may be complicated by fits, hyperthermia, dehydration and electrolyte disturbance possibly with hypovolaemic shock, and pulmonary complications, all of which may be fatal.

Treatment consists of sedation with chlormethiazole or benzodiazepines (anticonvulsants if fits occur), correction of fluid and electrolyte imbalance and good nursing care as with any delirious patient so that associated conditions such as pulmonary complications are identified and treated early.

Wernicke–Korsakoff syndrome

Wernicke's encephalopathy was first described by Wernicke in 1881. The basic pathology is haemorrhage into the midbrain, secondary to vitamin B_1 or thiamine deficiency. It occurs most commonly in alcoholics, but can occur in any condition causing nutritional deficiencies.

The onset occurs over the course of a few days with a mild delirium, that is drowsiness and confusion, as well as ataxia and nystagmus, ophthalmoplegia and usually polyneuropathy.

Unless the patient is treated urgently with intramuscular thiamine, the patient may lapse into stupor and die or may progress to Korsakoff's syndrome, in which the haemorrhage extends further into the diencephalon and cerebellum with irreversible and severe amnesia, often with secondary confabulation. There may be some response to thiamine in 20% of cases.

Support and follow-up

To be effective, any treatment of alcohol abuse must include some measure of understanding of why the patient has turned to alcohol. It is of course very difficult to pinpoint reasons for drinking, but it would appear that the majority of alcoholics drink as a means of escape from painful experiences and discomfort, which may include depression, anxiety, boredom, frustration, guilt, shame, difficult responsibilities, unsatisfactory social circumstances, general stress and more subtle personality characteristics such as feelings of inadequacy and inferiority and an inability to be assertive (Fig. 10.15). Once this pattern has been established, it may continue even after the original precipitant has been resolved, either to combat withdrawal symptoms or as a learnt reaction to certain behavioural cues such as passing by the pub.

Once the main reason for drinking has been identified, then appropriate measures should be carried out to help the patient preferably on an out-patient basis. These measures may include counselling, supportive psychotherapy, group therapy, family/marital therapy (Chapter 18); treatment of associated psychiatric or physical problems such as depression or anxiety; and environmental manipulation if this seems appropriate, for example career or financial advice or help with housing or other social problems.

The patient may also be encouraged to remain abstinent if he is followed up regularly, and attend specialist organizations such as Alcoholics Anonymous, day centres or dry

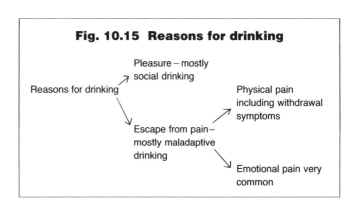

Fig. 10.15 Reasons for drinking

Reasons for drinking
→ Pleasure – mostly social drinking
→ Escape from pain – mostly maladaptive drinking
→ Physical pain including withdrawal symptoms
→ Emotional pain very common

hostels. Sometimes it is also appropriate to use drugs such as Antabuse (disulfiram) or Abstem (citrated calcium carbimide) to encourage abstinence, but the patient must be reasonably responsible and motivated as fatal interaction with alcohol may occur. These drugs impair the breakdown of alcohol in the liver by inhibiting acetaldehyde dehydrogenase, and alcohol breakdown stops at the acetaldehyde stage. Therefore if alcohol is taken within 3 days of taking these drugs, acetaldehyde will accumulate and cause vasodilatation with flushing, headaches, nausea, vomiting, hypotension and possibly death. Occasionally Antabuse implants which last up to 6 months, are used, but their efficacy has been disputed.

Case 1

Robert is a 35-year-old man who *frequently presented to his GP* with complaints such as *dyspepsia* and *gastritis* and *low back-pain*. He looked very *anxious*, and questioning elicited that he had *numerous social problems* including debts and problems at work. In addition his *wife had been threatening to leave him*

He was treated with benzodiazepines and returned to the surgery a fortnight later requesting a further sickness certificate. On this occasion the GP noticed a *smell of alcohol*, and enquired about Robert's alcohol intake.

Robert then admitted to drinking at least six pints of beer each night in the pub. He was *spending most of his money on alcohol* and became *aggressive* when drunk which was causing *problems with his wife*. He was often *unable to perform properly at work* because of hangovers, especially after the weekend.

He requested help with his drinking and was referred to his local Community Alcohol Team.

Case 2

Stephen is a 50-year-old company director who was *admitted to hospital* for investigation of his *anorexia* and *loss of weight*.

A gastroscopy was set up for the day after admission, and he was noted to be very *shaky* and *anxious* in the morning. Gastroscopy revealed nothing abnormal apart from evidence of *gastritis*, but by the evening he apeared *very shaky, unwell* and *slightly confused*. The night-staff became alarmed when he accused them of trying to kill him and said he could see faces in the curtain.

The medical registrar felt this was a psychiatric problem, and called the psychiatrist, who diagnosed *delirium tremens*. Stephen's family confirmed that he drank two bottles of wine a day with meals but were astonished by the diagnosis since he never appeared drunk, and he had been drinking this amount for years. His admission to hospital was the first time in several years that he had not had his customary two bottles of wine.

Prognosis

As might be expected, prognosis is much better if there is a good premorbid personality, and if the patient's family and occupational life have not yet been completely disrupted.

Drug abuse

A drug in this context is taken to mean a substance which alters psychic perception and reality. The classification of such drugs is, as already stated, conventionally sub-divided into alcohol and other drugs, and the latter is usually further sub-divided into narcotic and non-narcotic drugs. However, there are various other ways of classifying drugs, for example prescribed and non-prescribed, legal and illegal, etc.

Following guidance from the WHO Expert Committee on Drugs, the term 'drug dependence' is generally preferred to 'drug addiction'. WHO have defined drug dependence as a state arising from the repeated administration of a drug on a periodic or continuous basis. This state is therefore obviously very variable, but habitual use and psychic dependence are almost invariably present although physical symptoms of dependence may be absent.

Drug dependence: a state arising from the repeated administration of a drug on a periodic or continuing basis. (WHO)

Epidemiology and prevalence of drug misuse

As with alcohol, the epidemiology of drug misuse can be estimated directly or indirectly. The direct method involves a survey of the population and is generally more accurate, particularly with 'soft' drugs such as cannabis. A survey carried out in Britain by Mott in 1982 revealed that 5% of the population admitted to having ever used cannabis, but a similar study carried out in Scotland by Plant *et al.* (1985) showed that in the area which they studied, by the age of 20, 33% of men had tried cannabis, 6% have tried amphetamines and 5% have tried solvents. Experience with other illicit drugs was very rare, and regular or harmful abuse of any of the drugs was also rare.

Indirect methods of measuring prevalence include per capita consumption and mortality figures, and may be more accurate for drugs such as heroin but even then it is very difficult to be precise. The Office of Health Economics (1992) gives the official number of addicts in the UK as 17 000, but the true figures may be as much as five times that figure, i.e. closer to 85 000. Women are believed to make up approximately 30% of that number.

The Royal College of Psychiatrists quotes mortality figures of 159 deaths in Britain in 1983 resulting from drug misuse, 77 from the inhalation of glue and other solvents and 82 from the misuse of opiates and other illicit drugs. In 1986, there were 130 deaths in England and Wales associated with controlled drug misuse (OPCS, 1988).

The total heroin consumption in the UK in 1982 was estimated to be around 1500 kg.

HIV risk and drug injecting behaviour

Injecting drug users are now known to be at high risk of HIV if needles are shared or dirty needles are used. There is an important preventative role in terms of education particularly for heroin and cocaine users, for example by encouraging smoking or free-basing instead of injecting. There is also a strong argument for the provision of free needles.

The prevention of drug misuse

Preventative strategies should include primary and secondary prevention. Primary prevention involves preventing a disease from affecting a healthy population, and this is mainly by drug education and drug control measures. In the producer countries, this should include crop substitution advice as well as law enforcement.

In the UK, law enforcement is aimed at importers, users and dealers. The point of entry is obviously important, and Customs and Excise play an important part. However, paradoxically legalizing drugs is often proposed as a preventive strategy. Some of the arguments behind this proposal are that law enforcement is very expensive, and it may be more cost-effective to spend the same amount of money on other aspects of prevention. In addition, legalizing drugs will result in a decrease in their street-price, which may deter producers and dealers and theoretically should also result in a decrease in drug-related crime such as theft.

Secondary prevention means the prevention of complications in patients who already have a disease. In this context it involves mainly drug education, early identification and treatment. Treatment should obviously be aimed at abstinence, but harm minimization must be attempted in those users who cannot achieve abstinence. This includes advice on how to reduce harm, a needle exchange scheme providing free needles and syringes, easy access to contraceptives to prevent unprotected sex, and all attempts to reduce injecting behaviour which may include methadone maintenance programmes. In addition harm minimization must also obviously include the medical treatment of serious complications such as psychosis, acute intoxication, overdose and hepatitis.

Narcotic drug abuse (Fig. 10.16)

Narcotic drugs or opiates are themselves usually subdivided into three groups:

- opium;
- opium alkaloids, e.g. morphine, codeine;
- synthetic opioids, e.g. methadone, heroin.

Opium

Opium is Greek for juice, and is so-called because it is derived from the exudate of the seed-capsule of the poppy, *Papaver somniferum*. The origins of its use and abuse are lost in antiquity, but both the use and the abuse of opium itself is widespread in the 20th century.

Opium alkaloids

The two most important opium alkaloids are morphine and codeine, both of which are of considerable medical use in the treatment of pain. In addition codeine is also used in the treatment of cough and diarrhoea. Both morphine and codeine are not infrequently abused, most commonly by patients for whom they were originally prescribed or indeed by physicians or paramedical staff who have relatively easy access to them.

Synthetic opioids

The most important group of opiates in the addiction field are the synthetic opioids, and the most important of these are methadone and the semi-synthetic opioid heroin.

Heroin is the most widely abused of all the opiates. Most of it originates in the Indian sub-continent. Ironically it was originally introduced by Bayer in 1898 as a non-addictive cough suppressant. There are three ways of taking the drug: injecting, snorting and 'chasing the dragon' which is the inhalation of heated heroin.

Methadone was synthesized in Germany during the Second World War. It is similar to heroin, but differs in two important properties: (a) it is effective orally; and (b) tolerance is relatively slow to develop. Its main use is in treating heroin addicts.

Fig. 10.16 Narcotic drug abuse

Effect of opiate use
- Hallmark is *physical dependence* and tolerance.
- Euphoria.
- Analgesia.
- Drowsiness.
- Respiratory depression.
- Gastrointestinal spasm and constipation.
- Nausea and vomiting.
- Fits.
- Pupillary constriction.
- Skin effects: flushing, warmth, itching.

Many of these effects can be counteracted by the opiate antagonist nalorphine.

Causes of death from opiate abuse
- Overdose or poisoning – may be deliberate or may be associated with inexperience or loss of tolerance.
- Violence.
- Factors associated with intravenous injection, e.g. hepatitis, HIV, infective endocarditis.

Diagnosis of opiate abuse
1 Presence of needle-marks.
2 Presence of opiates in urine.
3 Signs and symptoms of withdrawal:
  - restlessness, insomnia, agitation;
  - yawning;
  - abdominal cramps with diarrhoea and vomiting;
  - muscle cramps and twitching;
  - pupillary dilation;
  - goose-flesh and sweating;
  - rhinorrhoea and lacrimation;
  - tachycardia;
  - pyrexia.

NB. Symptoms tend to peak at the second or third day. They may mimic an upper respiratory tract infection.

Opiate poisoning
Coma occurs with a decrease in pulse, respiration, blood pressure and temperature.

Treatment of poisoning
- Gastric lavage if the drug has been ingested.
- Artificial respiration if respiratory arrest occurs.
- Intravenous naloxone.

Treatment of heroin addiction

The two most popular methods of treating heroin addicts is either out-patient methadone substitution and maintenance, or hospital admission for withdrawal.

1 *Out-patient methadone maintenance.* Substitution of methadone for heroin has proved popular in addicts who are unwilling to withdraw from heroin completely. It has the advantage that methadone is safer than heroin, it keeps the addict away from the drug sub-culture and its association with crime, and it establishes a rapport with the addict which can be used to encourage withdrawal. However, it maintains an opiate addiction, albeit of a safer kind, and it is therefore tending to lose popularity.

2 *In-patient admission for withdrawal.* This is probably now the treatment of choice. Heroin can either be stopped without any alternative medication ('cold turkey'), or more commonly methadone linctus is substituted for heroin and withdrawn over a week or two. Withdrawal is unpleasant, but is self-limiting and is usually free from complications. In fact the DHSS has recently recommended that low dose, highly motivated addicts can be withdrawn on an out-patient basis by experienced practitioners.

Following withdrawal, it is very important that psychotherapeutic support is maintained for several months, preferably in a specialized residential centre or therapeutic community, and after that through organizations such as Narcotics Anonymous.

Non-narcotic drug abuse

Non-narcotic drugs which are commonly abused can be categorized into sedatives, stimulants and hallucinogens, and drugs within any of these groups usually share several common properties (Fig. 10.17).

Sedative misuse

These drugs, like alcohol, are CNS depressants and several of the symptoms of abuse and withdrawal will be seen to be similar. Sedative misuse is by far the most common of all drug abuse, and the three most commonly abused sedative drugs, apart from alcohol, are barbiturates, benzodiazepines and solvents (Fig. 10.17).

Barbiturates

The barbiturate group of drugs were introduced in 1903. They are sedative drugs and their properties, and hence symptoms of abuse, are very typical of the sedative group of drugs (see Fig. 10.18). Chronic abusers, however, are often asymptomatic apart from slightly slurred speech. The diagnosis is confirmed by urinary screening for the drugs

---

Fig. 10.17 Non-narcotic drug abuse

Sedatives, e.g.
- alcohol;
- barbiturates;
- benzodiazepines;
- solvents.

Stimulants, e.g.
- amphetamine;
- cocaine.

Hallucinogens, e.g.
- cannabis;
- LSD.

Fig. 10.18 Properties of sedative group of drugs

1 *General CNS depressant action*, causing drowsiness and depression of neuromuscular activity, like incoordination, ataxia, nystagmus, diplopia, strabismus, slurred speech and coma. Hence commonly used as tranquillizers, hypnotics and anaesthetics.
2 *Psychological and physical dependence*: withdrawal symptoms often include psychological symptoms such as anxiety, tremor, rebound insomnia, fits and delirium.
3 *Tolerance*.

---

involving paper chromatography and ultraviolet spectrophotometry, and supported by evidence of withdrawal symptoms which once again are very similar to withdrawal symptoms, seen in alcohol dependence and other sedative dependence.

It must be emphasized that barbiturates are very dangerous drugs, and are a common cause of death in suicide and accidental poisoning including children. Accidental poisoning is common because as tolerance is marked, addicts are often regularly taking near-lethal doses. It is obviously important that such patients are withdrawn from barbiturates as a matter or urgency.

Treatment and management. Addicts should always be withdrawn from barbiturates in hospital, because of the risk of death. The patient is given a dose of pentobarbital or phenobarbital equivalent to their normal daily dose and this is reduced by approximately 10% a day, or less if signs and symptoms of withdrawal become apparent. Following withdrawal, it is important that support and follow-up is maintained.

Treatment of poisoning includes gastric lavage or using activated charcoal to reduce absorption, the correction of fluid and electrolyte inbalance (usually dehydration), and forced alkaline diuresis with intravenous sodium bicarbonate to increase elimination.

Benzodiazepines

Benzodiazepines are commonly prescribed (often on repeat prescription) and commonly abused. It is said that one person in 50 in the UK, that is well over a million Britons, take them regularly chiefly for their hypnotic or anxiolytic effects. About 10% of regular users are addicted.

Benzodiazepines share many of the properties of other sedative drugs, including drowsiness, tolerance and psychological and physical dependence with withdrawal symptoms which include anxiety, rebound insomnia, anorexia, sweating and fits. The clinical picture can be distinguished from a simple anxiety state by the presence of increased sensitivity to sensory perceptions, including hearing, light, and touch. Dependence can occur after only a few weeks of use, and the withdrawal symptoms usually start within a few days of stopping the drugs, and may persist for several weeks (see also p. 221).

Benzodiazepines are relatively safe drugs, even in overdose, but the withdrawal syndrome may be dangerous, and for this reason patients taking very large amounts of diazepam or its equivalent should be withdrawn from the drug in hospital. In addition, as with alcohol, patients with a past history of fits or delirium should also be withdrawn from the drug in hospital.

The treatment of benzodiazepine dependence includes withdrawal from the drug gradually over a period of weeks and months. If withdrawal symptoms occur, then the drug should be withdrawn even more slowly because of the danger of fits, which may occur several weeks after withdrawal. Clonidine and propranolol may help withdrawal symptoms, but any epileptogenic drugs should be avoided.

As the cause of benzodiazepine dependence is mainly iatrogenic, it is obviously important from a preventive point of view to educate doctors about the danger of addiction. It is also important to emphasize that benzodiazepines should not be given on repeat prescriptions partly because of the danger of dependence and partly because many of these legally prescribed drugs find their way onto the black market.

In addition, benzodiazepines appear to be implicated in approximately 40% of all self-poisoning. The effects of poisoning, as expected, include dizziness, uncoordination, ataxia, slurred speech and possibly coma, but death is rare.

Solvents

The commonest form of solvent abuse is glue-sniffing for it's toluene content, usually occurring in children and young teenagers. It can either be sniffed directly from the container or from a plastic bag held over the nose. Less common forms of solvent abuse are paint-stripping fluid, lighter fluid containing butane, petrol, typewriter correction fluid, shoe polish and various aerosols such as hair spray.

Once again several of the properties of sedative drugs are evident, including euphoria and disinhibition, dizziness, drowsiness, slurred speech, ataxia and sometimes hallucinations. Tolerance is marked as is psychological dependence, but unlike the other sedative drugs, physical dependence with withdrawal symptoms does not seem to occur. Symptoms which should arouse suspicion of glue-sniffing include sores on the lower half of the face sometimes associated with persistent headache, sore throat and runny nose, smell of glue, loss of appetite and weight, wooziness and 'drunken' behaviour.

Glue-sniffing is a dangerous and common activity, and can sometimes be fatal. There are over 100 deaths a year from solvent abuse (Fig. 10.19). The treatment of poisoning is supportive.

It has been estimated that 10% of secondary school children try sniffing, usually in their early teens, but only 1–3% become long-term users. Most of these solvents are cheap and easy to obtain. However, since 1985 the Intoxicating Substance Supply Act makes it an offence to supply a person under 18 with a substance which one has reason to believe would be used to achieve intoxication.

Stimulant abuse

This group of drugs have a characteristic euphoric alerting effect. The two most commonly abused stimulants are amphetamines and cocaine. Formal treatment of the withdrawal state is not usually necessary with stimulants since physical dependence is not dramatic.

Amphetamines

The amphetamine group of drugs may be taken as tablets, inhaled or injected intravenously. Their current medical indications are minimal.

The effects and corresponding withdrawal symptoms of amphetamines are shown in Fig. 10.20, although it should be noted that physical dependence is not usually dramatic. It is important to note the similarity of amphetamine psychosis to schizophrenia. It is distinguished from schizophrenia by the fact that symptoms usually disappear spontaneously within 2 weeks. The diagnosis of amphetamine abuse can also be confirmed by screening the urine using paper chromatography, within 48 hours of use. Psychosis should be treated in hospital. Sedation with neuroleptic drugs may be necessary. Following recovery, attempts should be made to encourage the patient to discontinue amphetamine abuse. Overdosage of amphetamines can be fatal (Fig. 10.21).

Over the last 10 years the synthetic derivative of amphetamines *ecstasy* has also been widely misused, particularly as a 'party' drug at 'rave parties'. Fits, collapse, hyperpyrexia, renal failure and death may follow, and psychological effects such as paranoia and hallucinations may also occur. With regular use there is trismus of the jaw, anorexia and weight loss, fatigue, jaundice and depression. Tolerance also occurs.

Cocaine

Cocaine is an alkaloid derived from the leaves of the tree *Erythroxylon coca*, which grows in South America, where it has been used for its stimulant effect for many centuries (Fig. 10.24). It can be ingested, sniffed, smoked or injected. In Victorian times it was commonly and openly used and was also at one time included in small quantities in some

---

Fig. 10.20 Amphetamines

Effects	Withdrawal symptoms
Alerting effect	Fatigue and drowsiness
Euphorant effect	Dysphoria, depression, anxiety
Anorexia	Extreme hunger
Amphetamine psychosis	Disorientation and confusion
Pallor, tremor and hypertension	Headache, sweating, cramps and
Tolerance and dependence	feelings of hot and cold

Fig. 10.19 Causes of death from glue-sniffing

1 Direct toxic effect on hepatorenal system, brain and bone marrow.
2 Bronchial spasm with cardiorespiratory arrest.
3 Poisoning with coma and cardiorespiratory failure.
4 Asphyxiation with plastic bag.
5 Trauma and other violent deaths while intoxicated.

Fig. 10.21 Amphetamines: causes of death

Acute poisoning	Associated with its intravenous use
Hyperpyrexia	Hepatitis
Coma	Lung abscess
Cardiovascular shock	Endocarditis
Fits	AIDS

cola drinks. Its euphoric effects are very similar to those of amphetamines, and similarly tolerance and dependence occur. Tolerance can be very marked, and often the dosage required to produce the required psychological effect is not much less than the toxic dose. The treatment of acute poisoning is short-acting intravenous barbiturates.

In the 1980s a new form of cocaine arrived on the market, which has been described as one of the most pleasurable and addictive drugs and which has also been blamed for a wave of violence in America. This was *crack*, which was discovered accidentally when the hydrochloride molecule was removed from cocaine hydrochloride to enable it to be smoked rather than snorted. The name crack comes from the sound made when it is smoked. It achieves its effects in seconds and is said to be the most powerful stimulant of all. It is, however, followed by a profoundly acute depression and anxiety, and it is the intense craving for more to alleviate these effects which is believed to be responsible for the violent crimes which seem to be associated with it. There is therefore some evidence that crack induces a psychological addiction, but it is still unclear whether there is any physiological dependence.

Hallucinogen abuse

This group of drugs, which as expected, share many properties, include cannabis, *d*-lysergic acid diethylamide (LSD), phencyclidine hydrochloride (PCP or 'angel dust'), and mescaline, a naturally occurring plant extract. There are no medical indications for their use at present (Fig. 10.23).

By far the most commonly abused hallucinogen is cannabis, with approximately three-quarters of a million regular users in Britain. The origins of its use are lost in antiquity. Cannabis is the name given to drugs derived from the hemp

plant *Cannabis sativa* and the most common of these drug preparations are marijuana, ganja and hashish in order of increasing potency.

The treatment of drug abuse

Drug addiction treatment services usually consist of a network of services operating at community, district and regional levels. Community services consist of those services offered by general practitioners, and depending on the area services may also be provided by voluntary organizations and community drug teams. The Department of Health has for many years encouraged general practitioners to look after addicts on their lists, and one of the functions of community drug teams is to support the general practitioners in doing this. One of the most important roles of the general practitioner is to identify and engage the addict, and then embark on treatment or refer on to specialized services.

The community drugs team is a group of professionals in the drugs field, often including doctors, nurses, social workers, psychologists and probation offficers, who are based in the community. Their role is to support primary care workers in the identification and treatment of addicts, and also to offer an assessment, counselling and detoxification service. Their work may also include health promotion, needle exchange clinics, etc., as well as links with voluntary organizations such as Narcotics Anonymous and other self-help groups.

Patients presenting particularly difficult problems will be referred on to district services which are usually hospital-based. The vast majority of these patients are narcotic abusers. These are usually referred to an out-patient clinic in the first instance where an attempt may be made at out-patient detoxification. If this fails or if the patient is unwilling to attempt detoxification, methadone maintenance may be offered. However the patient may be willing to attempt in-patient detoxification in the local in-patient unit.

Many areas also have the back-up of a regional unit to whom a small number of patients may be referred for specialized advice and intensive treatment which will usually address many aspects of the addict's life such as personal relationships, and so on.

In the treatment of drug addiction, it is important to appreciate that it is not usually possible to treat the addiction in isolation, and the patient's personality, background and environment must all be taken into account. A comprehensive assessment is therefore very important, and there should be access to specialized therapies such as family therapy if necessary. In addition the patient should be prepared for difficulties he or she is likely to encounter following treatment to prevent relapse, and after-care should be arranged, which will usually include follow-up and referral to organizations such as Narcotics Anonymous.

Ethical issues and addiction

Particularly difficult ethical issues exist in relation to the addictions where there is serious doubt about the existence of a disease concept. This is relatively unusual in the practice of medicine and raises special issues with regard to treatment. The area is further complicated by legal issues as the use of most drugs causing dependence is illegal. Finally,

Fig. 10.24 Ethical issues and substance misuse

- Problems relating to definition, i.e. is addiction a disease?
- Problems relating to advertising of alcohol and tobacco and other economic issues.
- Problems relating to marketing, e.g. many commonly abused substances were first introduced by pharmaceutical companies unaware of their addictive potential.
- Problems relating to harm minimization strategies, e.g. methadone maintenance maintains addiction and in addition prescribed methadone often finds its way onto the open market.
- Problems relating to legal issues, e.g. should drugs be legalized? Drug enforcement policies are often justified on the grounds that drug misuse imposes costs on non-users such as health care, drug-related crime such as theft, lost production, etc.

there are many economic issues to consider particularly with legal drugs such as alcohol and tobacco which provide a very large number of people with jobs and are a considerable source of revenue to the government (see Fig. 10.24).

Conclusion

In conclusion, the incidence of substance abuse and addiction is high, and is a major source of morbidity and mortality both in Britain and throughout the world. In Britain there has been an encouraging reduction in nicotine abuse, but the abuse of alcohol and other drugs remains high. Public concern and public money is often directed at illicit drug misuse, and this is indeed a serious problem, but it is important to remember that it is the legal drug alcohol which is most widely used in our society and which numerically causes most harm in terms of social problems, morbidity and mortality. It is also important that treatment strategies are not over-emphasized at the expense of preventative strategies, and that methods of encouraging prevention continue to be explored and implemented.

QUESTIONS

1 Discuss the problems of alcohol-related harm, to include medical, psychiatric and social factors.

2 A 58-year-old divorced man with a long history of alcohol misuse is referred from the Accident and Emergency Department. On examination he is shaky and disorientated, and complains of seeing insects on his bed. Discuss the management.

3 Discuss the concept of drug addiction with particular reference to the World Health Organization criteria. Illustrate your answer with examples.

FURTHER READING

Raistrick D.S. & Davidson R. (1985) *Alcoholism and Drug Addiction.* Churchill Livingstone, Edinburgh. [An excellent basic book on the problems of alcoholism and drug addiction.]

Royal College of Psychiatrists (1986) *Alcohol – Our Favourite Drug.* Tavistock Publications, London. [This report from the Royal College of Psychiatrists deals with the effects of alcohol, alcohol dependence and alcohol-related disabilities, as well as the causes of drinking and its prevention and treatment.]

Royal College of Psychiatrists (1987) *Drug Scenes.* Gaskell, London. [Another report from the Royal College of Psychiatrists, this time dealing with drugs other than alcohol.]

NATIONAL BODIES IN THE FIELD OF THE ADDICTIONS

Alcohol Concern, 275 Grays Inn Road, London WC1X 8QF (tel: 071-833-3471).

Standing Committee on Drug Abuse (SCODA), 1–4 Hatton Place, Hatton Gardens, London EC1N 8ND (tel: 071-351-6794).

Narcotics Anonymous, PO Box 417, London SW10 0PS.

Alcoholics Anonymous, 11 Redcliffe Gardens, London SW10 (tel: 071-352-3001). Councils on Alcoholism, local branches throughout the UK.

11
Organic Psychiatric Disorders

Fact sheet

Diagnosis of bodily disease in psychiatry
Diagnostic clues to the presence of underlying bodily disease in patients presenting psychiatrically may be found in the initial history, mental state examination and physical examination, in special tests, and in the subsequent course of the patient's disorder. The most important of these clues are organic symptoms in the mental state examination, especially impairments of cognitive function. Most of the other clues may seem obvious, *but* they are often overlooked. These clues are set out here in the order in which they are likely to appear clinically.

History
1 *Presenting complaints*. These may point to impairment of cognitive function (e.g. memory problems).
2 *History of presenting complaint*. Look for aetiological factors:
- positive – history of physical factors (e.g. head injury, fits);
- negative – absence of history of physical or psychological factors (which of course may co-exist).
3 *Past and current medical history*. Look especially for:
- serious physical illness, accident or operation;
- medication, including recent changes.
4 *Family history* of organic disorder, especially dementia or general medical conditions.
5 *Personality*:
- unexplained change;
- frontal lobe disinhibition.
6 *Personal history*. Employment history, etc., may give background for assessment of present intellectual level.

Mental state examination
Appearance/behaviour:
- uncharacteristic anomalies suggesting cognitive impairment;
- restricted scope of activity, repetitive behaviour, perseveration;
- associated neurological signs.

Speech. As for appearance/behaviour; look especially for perseveration, and/or word finding and naming difficulties.

Thought content:
- impoverishment of thought content;
- concrete thinking.

Delusions. Organic delusions are:
- poorly elaborated;
- not well sustained;
- lack emotional intensity.

Hallucinations. Organic hallucinations are:
- visual;
- formed;
- coloured;
- moving;
- often show size distortion.

They are more troublesome in the evening.

Cognitive functions. These are most important of all, especially:
- clouding of consciousness – a mild global impairment of cognitive functioning. This is characteristic of an acute organic state;
- disturbed orientation for time, place and person. Time disorientation, including disturbed recall of the sequence of recent events, is often the first sign of clouding of consciousness;
- memory – recent. Defective short-term memory is often the first sign of a chronic organic state. Assessed clinically using the 'name and address' test;
- memory – remote. Assess loss of general information;
- concentration. Disturbed in its own right and/or may impair performance on other tests. Use 'serial sevens' or other similar test;
- general intelligence. Look for overall decline and verbal-performance discrepancy (where this is relevant it is normally assessed by a clinical psychologist).

Physical examination
Physical signs must be looked for, and not ignored if they are found. In particular, look for signs that others may have missed, e.g. unilateral anosmia.

Special tests
Laboratory/X-ray, etc:
- simple screen if indicated;
- otherwise as per suspected underlying disorder.

Clinical psychology:
- IQ testing;
- memory tests.

Course and outcome
Even if no organic clues at initial presentation, the possibility of underlying bodily disease should be reviewed carefully if the patient fails to improve, or their condition deteriorates or changes in any other way.

Introduction

This chapter will be concerned with the diagnosis of bodily disease presenting psychiatrically.

Bodily diseases (cerebral tumour, diabetes, thyrotoxicosis, pneumonia, syphilis, etc.), although often associated with psychiatric symptoms, less commonly actually present psychiatrically. Usually the psychiatric symptoms are secondary. It is therefore important not to over-diagnose such conditions, rushing into pointless examinations, tests, and so on. But it is also important not to **under**-diagnose them. Everyone's nightmare is to miss the (rare) patient presenting with, say, depression who turns out to have a cerebral tumour. But it is more often important clinically to detect the patient whose depression is symptomatic of anaemia, for example, or the first sign of an early dementia.

What is needed, then, is a balance between over-diagnosis and under-diagnosis. It is this balance that this chapter is intended to help you to achieve.

The most direct clinical clues to possible underlying organic disease are often in the **mental state examination**. Certain particular psychiatric symptoms, especially (but not only) disturbances of cognitive function, point strongly to organic pathology. Thus, much of this chapter will be taken up with describing these 'organic' symptoms and the 'organic states' defined by them. However, since functional symptoms may also (though less commonly) be produced by organic pathology, we will also be considering what other organic clues may be present in:

1 the **history**;
2 the **physical examination**;
3 the results of **special tests**;
4 the **course** of the patient's disorder.

Details of a number of particular organic psychiatric conditions, including aspects of their aetiology and treatment, will be found in other chapters; notably, substance abuse in Chapter 10, confusional states and other psychiatric symptoms of general medical conditions in Chapter 12, the dementias in Chapter 13, and epilepsy in Chapter 14.

Organic states

In physical medicine the patient's symptoms often point both to particular bodily parts or systems and to particular pathologies. Central chest pain, for example, radiating to the neck and down the left arm, points to ischaemic disease of the heart. Organic psychiatric symptoms on the other hand, are on the whole non-specific. Exceptions include Wernicke's encephalopathy in alcoholism (Chapter 10), and the frontal lobe syndrome (Fig. 11.1). But in general, whatever the pathology, and whether it is localized (cerebral tumour, stroke) or generalized (metabolic disorders, infections), the psychiatric symptoms will be much the same. It is as though the brain, at least in its higher functions, has only this limited 'organic repertoire' of ways of responding to the gross pathology of most bodily diseases.

However, there is one feature of the underlying pathology which does make a consistent difference to the psychiatric

---

Fig. 11.1 Frontal lobe syndrome

The frontal lobe syndrome is one of the few localizing syndromes in psychiatry. It is a syndrome of disinhibition due to frontal lobe (or occasionally to anterior temporal or parietal lobe) damage.

Disinhibition is shown by over-familiarity and tactlessness in dealing with others, over-talkativeness, and childish jokes and pranks. The patient may show disregard for the feelings of others. He may become involved in minor delinquencies, and commit sexual indiscretions. His mood is characteristically one of fatuous euphoria. Concentration is impaired. Orientation, memory and general intelligence are usually normal. He is likely to seem cheerfully unaware of the embarrassment and difficulties he is causing.

Head injury and meningioma are common causes. Unilateral anosmia may be the only hard sign of the latter, though extension of the lesion to adjacent structures may produce other neurological signs.

Other less common presentations of frontal lobe damage include a slowly developing retarded depression, incontinence of urine with apparent unconcern, and stupor (see also 'depressive stupor', Chapter 6).

---

symptoms, viz. its rate of progression. Rapidly developing pathology tends to produce different symptoms from slowly developing pathology. Hence **acute and chronic organic states** are distinguished clinically, though in practice the picture is often mixed. We will be noting some of the differences between the symptoms of acute and chronic states later in this chapter. They are summarized in Fig. 11.5.

Organic symptoms

Organic psychiatric symptoms may be found in any part of the mental state examination. The most important (because they are the most common and specific) are disturbances in the cognitive functions – orientation, memory, attention and intelligence. These symptoms will thus be considered first.

Disturbances of cognitive function

Organic states, such as toxic confusional states and dementias, are not difficult to diagnose once they are well established. The trick, however, is to be able to identify them at the earliest possible stage, so that appropriate treatment can be started and (where possible) permanent damage avoided. For this, careful testing of the cognitive functions is essential.

First, two general points about cognitive function testing.
1 It is especially important here to remember all the points of good clinical practice outlined in Chapter 3. In particular, remember that most patients will be anxious about their performance, and anxiety is by far the most common cause of spuriously abnormal cognitive function test results. So anything you can do to reduce the patient's anxiety will help to produce meaningful results.
2 As with any other clinical testing, in general medicine as well as psychiatry, practice is essential. To stand any chance of identifying a disturbance of cognitive function at a usefully early stage, you need to have practised these tests on as wide as possible a range of both functional and organic patients.

Orientation

Orientation is tested in three modalities: time, place and person. A patient is fully oriented if he knows what time it is, where he is, and who the people around him are.

Testing orientation for time

1 Ask the patient what time it is. An easy enough test, certainly. But interpreting the results may not be. First, because orientation in time is a matter of degree, minor inaccuracies are the norm and there is no sharp cut-off between normal and abnormal. Second, because disorientation for time is not necessarily a sign of organic impairment. Ordinary distress, or being in unfamiliar surroundings (as in hospital), is enough to cause a greater or lesser degree of disorientation. Organic disorientation is likely to be more profound than non-organic, but, again, the difference is one of degree. So, if the patient knows clearly what time it is, well and good. But if not, further testing is indicated.

2 Ask the patient the day of the week and the date. Again, minor inaccuracies are not necessarily significant. Uncertainties about the exact day of the month, for example, are normal. On the other hand, getting the year wrong is probably a sign not just of disorientation but of organic disorientation.

3 Find out if the patient knows qualitatively where he is in time. A patient who is merely distressed, even if he is further disorientated by being in unfamiliar surroundings, is unlikely to have lost track of time to the point where he no longer knows even qualitatively where he is in time. Thus, if you get equivocally abnormal results on 1 and 2 above, it is useful to go on to ask the patient: e.g. if it is morning, afternoon or evening; if it is before or after lunch; if it is early or late in the year; and so on. Inaccurate responses to questions of this kind could well be an indication of organic disorientation.

4 Check that the patient's recollection of the sequence of recent events is accurate. This aspect of orientation in time is especially useful clinically. One's recollection of the sequence of recent events, over the last few hours or so, is normally highly stable. Thus, although not always present, even minor inaccuracies in a patient's recall of this sequence are likely to be a sign of organic, rather than merely of functional, disorientation. It is true that patients with memory disorders (see below) may sometimes show similar inaccuracies. But usually they miss out events rather than recalling them in the wrong order, and memory disorders, anyway, are another symptom of organic damage. This area of testing is of course one in which the reports of 'other witnesses' are crucial (Chapter 3, p. 37).

Testing orientation for place

Ask the patient where he is. Orientation for place, like that for time, is a matter of degree. There is unlikely to be any significance in the patient being uncertain, say, of the name of the hospital he is in, or of the exact department. But if he is mistaken about the general nature of where he is – if he thinks he is at home or in his office – he is likely to be organically impaired.

Testing orientation for person

See if the patient knows who you and who other people around him are. What is important here, analogously with orientation for time and place, is not people's names, but their general status. Does the patient know that you are a medical student (or doctor); or does he think you are his employer, or the bank manager, or someone from his past? One obvious problem here is to distinguish disorientation from delusion. But this depends on interpreting what the patient says in the light of his history and mental state as a whole. (All clinical testing is of course context dependent.)

Memory (Fig. 11.2)

Clinically, memory is tested as recent (or short term) and remote (or long term). Recent memory is to do with new learning; it is the ability to retain and recall new information. Remote memory is what it says; it is the ability to recall memories laid down a long time ago.

Testing recent memory

The best test of recent memory is the name and address test. Essentially, you give the patient a name and address to remember and see if he can recall it after an interval of a few minutes. However, the details of how the test is performed are important. You can think of it in seven stages.

Fig. 11.2 Memory disorders

Apart from some special syndromes (e.g. alcoholic blackouts, Chapter 10), most memory disorders fall into one of four main groups:

Pure amnesic syndrome
This is a syndrome of pure short-term memory loss. It occurs with bilateral hippocampal lobe damage due, e.g., to:
1 carbon monoxide intoxication;
2 herpes encephalitis;
3 bilateral posterior cerebral artery thrombosis.
   Occasional iatrogenic cases have occurred following temporal lobectomy for epilepsy.

Korsakoff's syndrome
In this syndrome short-term memory loss is associated with confabulation (see Chapter 10, p. 121). The anatomical lesion is also more extensive, a number of mid-line structures as well as the temporal lobes being involved.
   Besides alcoholism, this syndrome may be caused by:
1 any other cause of thiamine deficiency, e.g. starvation, hyperemesis gravidarum, gastric disease and liver disease;
2 any other cause of deep mid-line damage, e.g. pituitary tumours and craniopharyngioma, tuberculous meningitis, head injury, etc.

Dementia
In dementia, there are widespread disturbances not only of both recent and remote memory but also of other cognitive functions, and the pathological lesions are correspondingly widespread.

Hysterical amnesia
Like all hysterical symptoms (Chapter 7, p. 93), hysterical memory loss is diagnosed partly by the absence of evidence of organic pathology, partly by the presence of evidence of functional pathology. Many memory disorders (e.g. after head injury) show mixed organic and functional features.

1 **Explain to the patient that you are now going to give him a name and address to remember and that you will want to see how much of it he can recall after about 5 minutes.** Explanation is essential – to remember anything you need to be motivated to remember it. Be careful, however, not to raise the patient's anxieties unnecessarily. It is important to explain what you are doing in neutral terms; make it part of your 'routine patter'; and don't use terms like 'easy', 'simple' or 'little' in describing it – nobody wants to feel they may fail an easy test!

2 **Choose a name and address to suit the patient.** Some people use a standard name and address. But this is a mistake for two reasons. First, because it may contain mnemonic clues for a particular patient (e.g. the road name may be the name of his road, or it may rhyme with it) and this test is a test of **new** learning. Second, it is often important to repeat the test more than once: with an anxious patient, for example, you may want to start with a short and simple name and address (to give them confidence) before trying a more demanding one; similarly, if you get equivocal results with a first test, you may need to repeat it with other names and addresses of varying difficulty. A name and address of average difficulty would be 'Mr Dennis Quiley, 43, New Addington Street, Lincoln'. But this is given here just as an example.

3 **Write down your chosen name and address.** In psychiatry, you should of course write down all your clinical findings at the time you make them, this being the only reliable way to produce vivid, accurate and complete clinical records. This is especially important here. You might forget the name and address after 5 minutes (especially if busy). It also helps to reduce the patient's anxiety.

4 **Read out the name and address to the patient.** It is usually best to read it through in one go. Read steadily and clearly and without special emphasis.

5 **Ask the patient to repeat it.** This is necessary to ensure (a) that the patient has heard it correctly (he may be deaf), and (b) that it has been registered in his immediate memory store.

6 **Introduce distracting material.** Even with an advanced dementia, a patient may be able to keep quite complicated and lengthy material in his head by simply repeating it over and over to himself. To test short-term memory, the name and address thus has first to be displaced from the immediate memory store, and then later recalled. Simple repetition, even if sustained over several minutes, is not enough. At this stage, therefore, you should go on to the other tests of cognitive function (to be described). Completing these should take about 5 minutes after which you can return to stage 7.

7 **Retest – after about 5 minutes.** Ask the patient how much of the original name and address he can remember. Write down, or mark clearly on the original name and address, exactly what the patient is able to recall.

As with other tests of cognitive function, minor inaccuracies in recall are not likely to be significant. However, if in doubt, test further. In this connection a number of other tests of recent memory are sometimes used, e.g. the 'Babcock sentence' (see Fig. 11.3). However, these are on the whole not as useful as further name and address tests (as mentioned in stage 2, above).

Testing remote memory

1 **Explore the patient's general knowledge.** Everyday information – about recent history, local geography and the like – is in long-term memory store. The conventional tests of remote or long-term memory thus involve seeing if the patient knows, say, six major towns, the dates of the Second World War, four prime ministers, etc. Unlike recent memory testing, it is helpful in testing remote memory to have your own standard list of about 10 items – it has been shown that long lists produce no more information than short lists, and they fatigue the patient.

2 **Explore the patient's personal knowledge.** General knowledge varies widely with culture, education, intelligence, etc., and in addition to your standard questions it may be helpful to explore the patient's knowledge in an area familiar to him, e.g. if he is a gardener, see how many different kinds of flower he can name.

Concentration

Concentration is the capacity for sustained attention. It is tested both in its own right (since it is impaired, *inter alia*, in organic states) and because normal concentration is a condition of adequate performance in any other test.

Testing concentration

1 **The 'serial sevens' test.** Ask the patient to take sevens away from a hundred until he gets down to nought, going as quickly as he reasonable can without making mistakes. Write down what he says as he says it, marking any errors. Record the number of errors and the time taken.

Fig. 11.3 Other cognitive function tests

A great many different cognitive function tests are described besides the main ones outlined in this chapter. Two which you may come across (see text) are:

The Babcock sentence

This is sometimes used as a test of recent memory. It is a more or less nonsensical sentence which is repeated to the patient until they can remember it correctly. After an interval, in which distracting material is introduced, they are then asked to see how much of it they can recall. Both the number of initial repetitions required, and the number of words correctly recalled after the interval, are recorded.

The sentence reads 'The one thing a nation needs in order to be rich and great is a large secure supply of wood.'

Digit span

In this test the patient is asked to repeat after the examiner a random list of numbers of varying length, either forwards ('the forward digit span') or backwards ('the reverse digit span'). The results are given as the numbers of digits which can be recalled forwards and backwards respectively.

Although sometimes described as a test of memory, the forward digit span has been shown to be commonly unimpaired even in an advanced dementia. For this reason, however, it is sometimes useful in assessing possible hysterical amnesia: the hysterical patient, though not showing signs of an advanced dementia, may nonetheless be unable to do even a simple digit span. The reverse digit span is more useful as a test of concentration than of memory.

Fig. 11.4 Clinical psychological testing

Clinical testing of the cognitive functions is sometimes supplemented by more formal and extensive testing by a clinical psychologist. This is especially helpful in two areas.

General intelligence (IQ)

Various IQ tests are employed, e.g. the Weschler adult intelligence scale (the WAIS). In all these tests a variety of standard questions are given, the scores being referred to a normalized scale (i.e. the average value being set at 100). Two main subscales of IQ are defined, verbal and performance. Verbal IQ is concerned with language function; performance IQ with arithmetic and visuo-spatial functions.

In dementia there is a fall in full-scale IQ. This may be difficult to assess at an early stage since it has to be judged against previous academic and employment achievements. More useful is 'verbal-performance' discrepancy; verbal IQ is more dependent than performance IQ on long established skills and is therefore relatively **protected** in an early dementia. A performance IQ more than 20 points below verbal IQ may be significant.

Memory

There are many tests of new learning, e.g. the paired associate learning test, which can sometimes give a useful quantitative estimate of memory impairment.

Other tests

A number of tests are available both for specific areas of damage (e.g. frontal lobe damage) and for dementia.

All of the above tests may be useful in equivocal cases. However, their particular value is for slowly developing conditions where retesting is required after an interval. Quantitative changes in cognitive function are far more reliably measured by tests of this kind than by clinical testing and may be diagnostically crucial.

2 Other tests. If 'serial sevens' is too difficult (mathematically) for the patient, or if you want to start with a simpler test (to boost their confidence), try 'serial fives', or just 'fives from thirty', or the days of the week or the months of the year backwards.

The point of all these tests is that they cannot be done automatically but require concentration. Counting forwards, or reciting the days of the week forwards, could be done parrot-fashion.

Intelligence

Other than from the history, intelligence is not normally tested at the bed- (or desk-) side. There are clinical tests available, but if IQ testing is important it is probably better done as a special test by a clinical psychologist (see Fig. 11.4).

Cognitive function in acute and chronic organic states
(Fig. 11.5)

In well-established organic states, e.g. in an advanced dementia or in a severe toxic confusional state, all of the cognitive functions are likely to be impaired together, often grossly so. It is at an earlier stage that the differences between an acute and chronic organic state, noted in Fig. 11.5, may be apparent. Thus, in a chronic organic state (as in a dementia), the first change is most often impairment of memory, especially **short-term memory**. In an acute organic state on the other hand (as in a toxic confusional state), there may well be a mild global impairment of cognitive functioning right from the start. This is called **clouding of consciousness**. It is the first slip away from full consciousness towards semi-coma, and it may be shown by a variety of non-specific symptoms such as reduced awareness of the environment, odd and inconsistent behaviour, suspiciousness and irritability. However, the most likely specific symptom at an early stage of an acute organic state is a disturbance in **orientation, especially for time**, rather than in memory. Careful testing of

Fig. 11.5 Acute and chronic organic states

An organic state is a mental state in which one or more organic symptoms are present. Organic states, although pointing to underlying bodily pathology, are thus defined, like most other psychiatric diseases, symptomatically (see Chapter 1). Organic symptoms vary with the rate of progression of the underlying pathology. Often the clinical picture is mixed. However, the main features of acute and chronic states may be summarized thus.

	Acute	Chronic
Clinical examples	Confusional states, e.g. sedative overdose, hypoglycaemia.	Dementias.
Early warning symptoms (see text)	Clouding of consciousness, shown especially by disorientation, especially for time.	Disorder of memory, especially of recent memory.
Well developed syndrome	Marked clouding of consciousness with disorientation for time, place and person; impaired concentration and memory (if testable). Reduced awareness of and responsiveness to the environment. Odd behaviour, disorganized and inconsistent. Appearance often dishevelled and frightened (especially if deluded or experiencing hallucinations). May show specific signs of underlying pathology.	Severe impairment of all cognitive functions; deep amnesia, short and long term; grossly defective orientation, attention and IQ. Behaviour often muddled and inappropriate. Appearance unkempt (if unattended) – unwashed, poor nutrition, oddities of dress. Mood may reflect delusions and/or hallucinations (e.g. depression, suspiciousness). Associated neurological and general medical signs often present.

The aetiology of organic states is summarized in Fig. 11.7. The assessment and management of acute organic states is described in Chapter 12, and of chronic organic states in Chapter 13. (NB. The term 'organic' is sometimes also used as an aetiological term indicating *any* symptom known to be *due* to bodily pathology; see Chapter 1.)

these functions in particular, therefore, of short-term memory and of orientation for time, is essential to the early diagnosis of organic states.

Other organic symptoms

Apart from cognitive function testing, organic symptoms may be detected in other parts of the mental state examination. These symptoms, although also pointing to underlying bodily disease, are not as specific as impairments of cognitive function in this respect. Nonetheless, they are often diagnostically important, especially when the results of cognitive function testing are normal or equivocal.

There are a great many of these symptoms. Only the more common and clinically useful will be described here. They will be considered under the relevant headings of the mental state examination.

Appearance and behaviour

Anomalies in the patient's appearance and behaviour (if uncharacteristic of them) may point to organic impairment, e.g. frequently leaving pans to boil dry or forgetting to dress properly, in an early dementia, or, sometimes, minor delinquency (such as shoplifting) in a confusional state. Rather more specific are anomalies that reflect the patient's failing intellectual powers, in particular the following points.

1 Restriction of activity. The patient may restrict his activities to an increasingly limited area within which he is able to cope ('shrinkage of the milieu'). He avoids new and unfamiliar situations. Within his safe area he may become excessive orderly, while outside this area he slips into chaos. This is called 'organic orderliness' – superficially it may resemble obsessional orderliness.

2 Repetitive activity. Because of the progressively restricted scope of his activities, and because of memory impairment, the content of the patient's activities is impoverished. He will often repeat things that he has done several times, apparently without any awareness of what he is doing (unlike the obsessional of course).

3 Perseveration. This is a particular kind of repetitive activity. It is an inability to stop one thing and move on to the next. What is observed behaviourally is that the patient keeps repeating the last part of his current activity, e.g. when doing up a row of buttons he may continue to attempt to button the last in the row instead of stopping and going on to something else. Perseveration, although not always present, is a diagnostically useful organic symptom since it is qualitatively (not just quantitatively) different from normal.

Besides these behavioural anomalies, there will often be associated neurological symptoms. An important early sign of diffuse cerebral damage is the appearance of **stereotypies** – frequently repeated, apparently purposeless, small scale, voluntary movements, e.g. plucking at the bed clothes, or touching one's cheek repeatedly, etc. (see also Physical Examination below).

Speech

Speech, like behaviour, may show a variety of more or less non-specific anomalies together with:

1 restriction of content;

2 difficulty **finding words** and **naming objects**;

3 reduced fluency;

4 repetition;

5 perseveration.

The last, in speech, is especially striking when it occurs. Again, be alert to any neurological abnormalities.

Thought content

The content of the patient's thoughts, like their behaviour and speech, reflects the decline in their intellectual functions in being **impoverished**. They may also show 'concrete thinking', i.e. an inability to abstract the sense of what is said from its literal meaning. This can be tested by asking the patient to explain the meaning of a common proverb.

Mood

Organic mood change, so-called, is an impoverishment of mood. The patient's emotional responses lack depth and are poorly sustained. Besides this general impoverishment, they may show more specific changes, e.g.:

1 emotional incontinence: excessive laughing or crying initiated by trivial stimuli and then continuing unchecked;

2 threshold effects: no apparent response up to a level of stimulation and then a sudden excessive reaction;

3 incongruous emotion: failure to respond to significant stimuli, but excessive response to trivial stimuli;

4 catastrophic reaction: a sudden explosive outburst of rage and distress often prompted by the recognition of failing powers – this may be the first signal of early organic impairment, e.g. if such a reaction occurs during cognitive function testing. All these symptoms are characteristic more of chronic than of acute organic states. In acute states, the predominant emotion is commonly **bewilderment** verging on fear (or actual terror, as in delirium tremens).

Delusions

Organic delusions are characterized by their form. They are poor quality delusions, a product of combined intellectual and emotional impoverishment. Unlike functional delusions, they are:

1 poorly sustained, coming and going in a few hours or days;

2 simple rather than elaborate;

3 lacking in emotional intensity.

They have no characteristic content, though they are often of persecution or of loss.

Hallucinations

Where organic delusions are poor quality delusions, **organic hallucinations** are good quality hallucinations. Think of the flying pink elephants of music-hall 'DTs' for a useful paradigm. Organic hallucinations are:

- visual;
- formed, being of people, animals and things;
- coloured;
- moving;
- often show size distortion (e.g. Lilliputian figures).

A further feature is that they are often more troublesome to the patient in the evening or in other conditions of low illumination.

Other organic clues

Clues to bodily disease both in the history and in the physical examination may be important diagnostically, especially in the early cases with which we are particularly concerned here. Both kinds of clue are obvious enough. But, perhaps for this reason, both kinds of clue are all too often overlooked.

History

There may well be clear indications in the history of **impaired cognitive functioning**, e.g. memory difficulties, episodes of confusion, etc. However, the history alone is not to be relied upon in this respect. Often in an early organic state, there are no such direct indications. Conversely, patients with functional disorders, especially depression, will often complain of memory difficulties even though their memory is functioning normally as judged by clinical testing.

Presenting complaints

Apart from complaints related to impaired cognitive functioning (which may often be reported by relatives rather than by the patient themselves), these are non-specific.

History of presenting complaints

Look for **aetiological factors**. These may be:
1 positive, i.e. organic factors such as head injury, fits (see also Fig. 11.6), influenza, etc., related to the onset of symptoms;

2 negative, i.e. an apparent absence of aetiological factors, functional or organic. In the latter case the 'hidden variable' may be unrecognized bodily disease. Note, however, that the presence of functional aetiological factors (e.g. stress) certainly does not exclude the possibility of organic pathology.

Past medical history

Ask especially about past or current history of **physical illness, accidents** or **operations**, and **medication including any recent changes**.

Family history

Check for **relevant family history**, e.g. of dementia, or of general medical disorders such as heart disease, diabetes and epilepsy.

Personality

There may be unexplained changes in personality, often of a non-specific nature, but sometimes including evidence of disinhibition suggestive of the frontal lobe syndrome (see Fig. 11.1). Besides personality, enquire also about **alcohol consumption** and **illicit drug use**.

Personal history

The main significance of the patient's personal history in this context is to provide a background of educational and academic attainment against which their current level of intellectual functioning can be assessed (Fig. 11.4).

Fig. 11.6 Differential diagnosis of epilepsy

Although epilepsy has traditionally been associated with mental disorder, it is important to recognize that a large majority of epileptics are free from psychiatric difficulties. However, epilepsy is important in psychiatry (see also p. 302, Fig. 24.1):
1 because a fit or other epileptic phenomenon may point to organic pathology (see text);
2 for its social and psychological complications in some cases (see Chapter 12, p. 146);
3 in the differential diagnosis of a number of psychiatric disorders.

    This last is a large topic; see, for example, Lishman (1987) Chapter 7, for a full discussion. The essential point to remember is that even with modern ambulatory EEG recording methods the diagnosis of epilepsy still depends first and foremost on careful clinical observation. In this figure, some of the more important clinical features of epilepsy are given, together with its principal psychiatric differential diagnoses.

Epilepsy
Paroxysmal (i.e. 'fits')
Key features: a disturbance of behaviour and/or awareness that is:
- **repeated**;
- **stereotyped** in form, showing the same progression of symptoms;
- of **sudden onset**;
- **spontaneous** and usually **rapid** in resolution.
Unconsciousness, self-injury and incontinence are common but not invariable.

Note that other causes of ictal phenomena must be excluded, e.g. syncope, Stokes–Adams attacks, aortic stenosis, hypoglycaemia, transient cerebral ischaemic attacks, etc.

States of longer duration (i.e. automatism, fugues)
These conditions are similar to paroxysmal epileptic phenomena except that they are of longer duration and less stereotyped in form. The patient may show quite complex, organized activity, but there is usually evidence of **reduced level of consciousness**, e.g. impaired awareness of surroundings and a degree of incoordination of movement.
(Epilepsy is also discussed in Chapter 14, p. 177, as a common complication of mental handicap.)

Psychiatric differential diagnosis
Hysterical fits (which, like epilepsy, may point to organic pathology – see Case 1, p. 137); **panic attacks** (but note that emotion and/or overbreathing may provoke epilepsy); **schizophrenia** (first rank symptoms may occur in the aura of temporal lobe epilepsy, but are repeated and stereotyped).
Psychogenic fugue (especially hysterical or depressive); **other causes of clouding of consciousness** (see text); **somnambulism** (epileptic automatism is sometimes confined to sleep).
Aggressive outbursts (aggression as an epileptic phenomenon shows the general features of epilepsy and is unprovoked and motiveless).

Fig. 11.7 Aetiology of organic states

Almost any general medical or surgical condition affecting the brain may produce organic symptoms. The following is a summary of some of the more important.

- *Degenerative disorders*: arteriosclerotic dementia, Alzheimer's, Pick's, Huntington's, Creutzfeldt–Jakob, normal pressure hydrocephalus, multiple sclerosis.
- *Space-occupying lesions*: cerebral tumour – primary or secondary, subdural haematoma.
- *Trauma*: concussion, post-traumatic dementia.
- *Infections*: pneumonia, septicaemia, meningitis, general paresis, chronic meningo-vascular syphilis, subacute and chronic encephalitis, AIDS.
- *Vascular lesions*: cerebral arteriosclerosis, stroke, subdural and subarachnoid haemorrhage. Heart disease. Cranial arteritis.
- *Epilepsy*: 'epileptic dementia', petit mal, postictal states, automatism.
- *Metabolic disorders*: uraemia, liver disorder, remote effects of carcinoma, renal dialysis.
- *Endocrine disorders*: myxoedema, Addison's disease, hypopituitarism, hypo- and hyperparathyroidism, hypoglycaemia.
- *Intoxication*, short- and long-term effects: drunkenness, 'alcoholic dementia' and Korsakoff's psychosis; drug intoxication or overdose; industrial intoxication. Withdrawal syndromes.
- *Anoxia*: anaemia, post-anaesthesia, congestive cardiac failure, chronic pulmonary disease, carbon-monoxide poisoning.
- *Vitamin lack*: lack of thiamine, nicotinic acid, B_{12}, folic acid.

Acute organic states are generally caused by rapidly developing pathology, chronic organic states by slowly developing pathology (see Fig. 11.5) (see also pp. 158–161; the dementias).

Physical examination

In psychiatry, as in physical medicine, if there is any suggestion of possible unrecognized bodily disease, a careful **physical** and **neurological** examination is indicated. Even if someone else has already done a 'physical', your own examination will still be necessary. This is because you will often be looking for different things. In the neurological examination, for example, careful testing of the sense of smell may reveal unilateral anosmia, which may be the only hard sign of a frontal lobe meningioma.

Special tests

The extent of laboratory, X-ray and other special tests is of course governed by the clinical indications in a given case. A simple screen of investigations (blood count, ESR, urea and electrolytes, liver function tests, blood sugar, and chest X-ray) is worth doing if physical disease is suspected on general grounds but there are no specific indications of what may be wrong. This list may be extended if it is wished to exclude potentially remediable causes of dementia (see Chapter 13). A list of some of the more important causes of organic states is given in Fig. 11.7.

Course and outcome

Even if there is nothing to suggest organic pathology in the initial presentation, a patient whose condition (a) fails to improve when it should, (b) deteriorates or (c) changes unexpectedly in any other way, should be **reviewed** with this possibility in mind. One of the most common causes of failure

---

Case 1

Mrs A.B., a 60-year-old housewife. Admitted as an in-patient with *hysterical paralysis of her right arm*. Initial mental state and physical examination showed no abnormalities other than *minor depressive symptoms* including *loss of interest and fatigue*. Her husband confirmed these symptoms and added that she had become *irritable and complaining, especially about the cold*. A few days after admission she complained one evening that she had seen mice in the kitchen. This occurred again the following night (but there were no mice there) and she became *increasingly agitated*. At this stage a review of her physical condition and cognitive functions revealed possible *early short-term memory loss*, and she was found to have *low thyroxin*.

Diagnosis: dementia secondary to myxoedema.

Note: (a) possible organic hallucinations (seeing mice) prompted review of physical condition, though (b) hysterical conditions should always raise the possibility of an early dementia in older age-groups.

Case 2

Mr W.B., a 35-year-old bank employee. Brought to casualty by the police on a Saturday afternoon and said to be *'behaving oddly' after being arrested for minor shoplifting*. Seemed *bemused* by what had happened, but gave an apparently clear account of events during the day up to the time that he entered the shop. Physical examination showed no abnormalities. His wife said that he had not been on 'good form' recently, but attributed this to pressure of work. However, *on checking his story of events of the day, it was found that he had recalled them in the wrong temporal sequence*. Further testing showed *glycosuria*.

Diagnosis: acute organic state secondary to hypoglycaemia (temporarily relieved by a cup of sweet tea he had been given by the police).

Note: (a) the importance of careful testing for time disorientation, especially sequence of recent events, (b) his wife's (natural) tendency to ascribe his recent ill-health to stress, in the absence of recognized physical disease.

Case 3

Mr J.D., a 55-year-old labourer. Brought to casualty by the warden of a hostel where he was living. Said to be *confused and aggressive*. His *breath smelt of alcohol* and he was *uncooperative*. The warden confirmed that he was a *heavy drinker* but said that he thought he had *not been drinking that evening*. A (necessarily limited) *physical examination showed no abnormalities*, and blood and urine samples were obtained. It was agreed that he would be kept in for observation overnight. By the next morning, although he no longer smelt of alcohol, *he was still confused. Neurological examination at this stage showed a slow reacting pupil and an extensor-plantar response.*

Diagnosis: subdural haematoma.

Note: (a) this patient might easily have been sent home as a 'drunk', (b) multiple diagnoses (alcoholism plus subdural) are not uncommon in organic psychiatry, (c) the atypical presentation – history neither of head injury nor of fluctuating level of consciousness, both probably obscured by alcoholism.

to respond to antidepressants, for example, is unrecognized bodily disease. Deterioration in cognitive functioning over a period of time is particularly suggestive here – hence the need for meticulous testing and recording of these functions in the initial assessment of the patient.

QUESTIONS

1 Define 'organic symptom' and 'organic state'.

2 What is the earliest symptom likely to be in (a) an acute organic state, (b) a chronic organic state?

3 How may information from people other than the patient help in detecting time disorientation?

4 Does a history of stress (or other functional aetiological factor) associated with the onset of a psychiatric illness exclude the presence of organic aetiological factors? If not, why not?

5 If there are no organic clues in the history, mental state examination, physical examination and special tests, what else may point to underlying bodily disease?

FURTHER READING

Hunter R. *et al.* (1968) Three cases of frontal tumour presenting psychiatrically. *Br. Med. J.* **3**, 9–16. [This paper describes three cases of frontal meningioma which were missed respectively for 3, 25 and 43 years. It is a cautionary tale!]

Lishman W.A. (1987) *Organic Psychiatry*, 2nd Edition. Blackwell Scientific Publications, Oxford. [This is the main reference book for organic psychiatry. Although a large textbook it is easily readable. Introductory chapters contain details of all the various organic symptoms and discussions of aetiology and pathology. Further chapters cover the main topics of importance in organic psychiatry: alcoholism, cerebral tumour, head injury, vascular disorders, endocrine diseases, etc.]

Minsky L. (1933) The mental symptoms associated with 58 cases of cerebral tumour. *J. Neurol. Psychopathol* **13**, 330–43. [This is a review of the features of patients presenting psychiatrically who turned out to have cerebral tumours. The findings illustrate all the important points about why organic pathology is sometimes missed in patients presenting with psychiatric symptoms.]

Morris R.G. (1991) Cognition and ageing. In: Jacoby R. & Oppenheimer C. (eds) *Psychiatry in the Elderly*, Oxford, Oxford University Press, Chapter 3. [A useful review of recent work on the cognitive changes which occur in normal ageing and dementia.]

Ron M.A., Toone B.K., Garralda M.E. & Lishman W.A. (1979) Diagnostic accuracy in presenile dementia. *Br. J. Psychiatr.* **134**, 161–8. [A follow-up study of patients diagnosed as having dementia. It shows that the diagnosis is less reliable than had previously been thought. In 31% of patients the diagnosis proved to be mistaken at 5–15 year follow-up. The most commonly missed differential diagnosis was depression.]

III
SPECIAL GROUPS

12
Psychiatric Problems in General Practice and Hospital

Fact sheet

Nature and classification of disorders

Family and hospital doctors may encounter the whole range of psychiatric disorders, but in particular those resulting from or associated with physical disorders.

Psychiatric disorders can present with physical symptoms, as in the case of minor affective disorders, neuroses, personality disorders, major affective disorders, factitious disorders, alcohol and drug abuse, eating disorders and sexual problems.

Physical disorders can cause psychological symptoms, e.g. organic brain syndromes, systemic disorders with CNS manifestations, as a result of diagnosis, treatment and course of a physical illness, and following childbirth.

Psychiatric and physical conditions can sometimes occur together without a causal link, and psychiatric disorders can sometimes present to physicians without any physical symptoms.

Disorders of special interest to GPs and hospital doctors

- *Minor affective disorders*: mild and usually transient disturbances of mood, which are usually related to personal and social difficulties. They are very common in general practice.
- *Major affective disorders*: less common than the above, but important to recognize both in general practice and hospital.
- *Factitious disorders*: rare, but often difficult to treat, often seen in casualty departments. The patient simulates physical or mental illness to obtain treatment and admission.
- *Alcohol abuse*: particularly common in hospital patients, but also in general practice, where it is often missed.
- *Eating disorders*: common in general and hospital practice. The main types are anorexia nervosa, bulimia, and obesity.
- *Organic brain disorders*: acute (delirium) and chronic (dementia) are common in hospital patients.
- *Affective and other disorders*: resulting from the investigation, diagnosis, medical and surgical treatment, and outcome of physical disease.
- *Puerperal disorders*: puerperal psychoses are the most severe, although they respond well to treatment. Other disorders are post-partum blues, and post-partum depression.

Epidemiology of psychiatric disorders in general practice

About 30% of patients attending their GPs may be suffering from psychiatric disorders, often together with physical symptoms. Women present to their doctors with such problems more often than men, and the proportion tends to increase with age in both sexes.

GPs fail to identify about 30% of those who attend with psychiatric disorders.

Epidemiology of psychiatric disorders in the general hospital

About 30% of patients attending general out-patients may be suffering from psychiatric disorders, especially in patients with chronic and disabling conditions.

Of all general in-patients, about 30% suffer from affective disorders, although the condition tends to be severe in only half of them. Organic brain disorders are common, especially in older patients or in those severely ill. Alcohol abuse is present in about 20% of those admitted to general hospital. Deliberate self-poisoning or self-injury are common reasons for admission to hospital.

Affective disorders and alcohol abuse are often missed in the general hospital.

A significant proportion of patients seen in casualty departments suffer psychiatric disorders, in particular alcohol and drug abuse, neurotic disorders, and personality problems.

Causes of psychiatric disorders

The same factors as in conditions occurring in psychiatric settings, but with the added influence of physical disorder, its treatment, and course.

Management of psychiatric disorders

Prevention

Adequate information and advice concerning investigation, diagnosis and treatment of physical disorders will reduce the risk of adverse psychological reactions.

Assessment

Attention must be paid to the possibility of psychological problems, and symptoms should be evaluated carefully.

Management in general practice

Careful assessment of the symptoms and problems should lead to a decision as to whether to refer to a psychiatrist or treat in general practice. Only 5% of patients with psychiatric disorders are usually referred on to the specialist. Explanation and advice, reassurance, counselling aimed at family and social problems and cautious use of medication are usually effective.

Management in the general hospital

Psychological, social and physical methods of treatment as in the case of general practice patients are usually effective.

Outcome of psychiatric disorders

General practice psychiatric problems have good short-term outcome, with most patients recovering within 6 months to a year. General hospital patients with affective disorders also have a good outcome in the short term. Organic brain disorders have a poorer outcome. In the long term, general hospital patients with psychiatric disorders have a poorer physical outcome.

What types of psychological problems occur in general practice and hospital?

Psychiatric disorders are not just dealt with by psychiatrists, or seen only in psychiatric hospitals and clinics; patients attending their general practitioners and those under the care of hospital doctors often present with symptoms of psychological distress, and some may suffer frank psychiatric illness. It is, therefore, very important for those working in such medical settings to be aware of the possible presence of psychological problems in their patients, and to be able to assess their nature and severity, and take steps towards their effective management.

While the psychiatric disorders seen by family and hospital doctors cover the whole span of psychiatric illness, from minor stress reactions to major psychiatric conditions, there is, not surprisingly, a preponderance of psychiatric syndromes associated with physical disorders. The association between physical and psychiatric symptoms can be complex and may raise important issues about aetiology, some of which will be discussed in this chapter.

Classification and presentation of psychiatric disorders

As in the case of other disorders, it is possible to classify psychiatric syndromes in different ways, for example by reference to their symptoms, or by considering their likely aetiology. In practice, it is not uncommon to use both types of models of classification simultaneously.

The following practical classification of psychological disorders in general and hospital practice will be used here (see also Fig. 12.1).

Fig. 12.1 Classification and presentation of psychiatric disorders in general practice and hospital

Psychiatric disorders presenting with physical symptoms
1 Minor affective disorders and adjustment reactions.
2 Neuroses: anxiety disorders; hysterical disorders; somatization disorders.
3 Personality disorders: histrionic; antisocial; dependent.
4 Major affective disorders: major depressive episode; dysthymic disorder.
5 Factitious disorders.
6 Alcohol abuse.
7 Eating disorders: anorexia; bulimia; obesity.
8 Sexual problems.

Physical disorders leading to psychological symptoms
1 Organic brain disorders.
2 Systemic disorders with CNS manifestations.
3 Impact of diagnosis, treatment and course of physical disorders.
4 Puerperal disorders.

Psychiatric and physical disorders presenting together without causal link

Psychiatric disorders without physical symptoms

Psychiatric disorders presenting with physical symptoms

Here the primary disorder is psychological, but the nature of the symptoms may prompt the person to seek help from the family doctor or hospital physician. The following conditions can present in this way: minor affective disorders with somatic symptoms of anxiety (palpitations, shortness of breath) or depression (tiredness, loss of appetite); adjustment reactions; neurotic disorders, such as anxiety states, hysterical disorders or somatization disorders; personality disorders; major affective disorders; factitious disorders; substance abuse, in particular alcohol; and other conditions, such as eating disorders and sexual problems.

Physical disorders leading to or causing psychological disorders

Primary brain disorders, such as a brain tumour or head injury, and physical disorders with CNS effects, such as endocrine abnormalities, can initially present with psychological symptoms alone, or together with physical symptoms.

Physical disorder can lead to psychological problems, even without the presence of brain pathology; for example, a person suffering from a severe and life-threatening condition could develop symptoms of depression or even a major depressive episode. Similarly, intensive medical or surgical treatment, especially if associated with disfigurement, can contribute to the development of psychological disorders.

Sometimes, physical events, like childbirth, can be associated with the onset of psychiatric illness, as in the case of the puerperal psychoses.

Physical and psychiatric disorders presenting together by chance, without a specific aetiological link between them.

Psychiatric disorders presenting without added or associated physical disorder.

Description of the main psychiatric syndromes

The first two groups of disorders will be considered below.

Psychiatric disorders presenting with physical symptoms

Minor affective disorders and adjustment reactions
The minor affective disorders are characterized by the presence of mood abnormalities, such as anxiety or depressive symptoms. In contrast with the major affective disorders (see Chapter 6), their symptomatology is mild and transient, and usually related to environmental difficulties, such as marital or employment problems. Adjustment reactions are conditions arising in previously healthy individuals in response to clear environmental stressors which have taken place over the previous days or weeks. Adjustment reactions go beyond what would be regarded as normal, and may present with a range of maladaptive responses, including symptoms of anxiety or depression, with emphasis on somatic symptoms, like palpitations, shortness of breath, headaches and other aches and pains, abdominal symptoms, etc.

The neuroses
These are discussed in detail in Chapter 7, and it should suffice to remind the reader here of the frequency of somatic symptoms in such neurotic conditions as the anxiety dis-

orders, dissociative (hysterical) disorders, and somatoform disorders.

Somatoform disorders are characterized by physical symptoms suggestive of an organic disorder, in the absence of demonstrable pathology. The symptoms are not produced by voluntary control, as they would be in the case of factitious disorders or malingering. They include somatization disorders, conversion (hysterical) disorders, hypochondriasis and psychogenic pain disorder. *Somatization disorders* are characterized by a history of multiple physical complaints starting before the age of 30, and including a wide array of symptoms affecting the gastrointestinal, cardiovascular, reproductive and other systems, in the absence of organic disease. *Conversion disorders* involve loss of physical functioning suggesting organic disease, in the absence of physical disorder, but where psychological stressors have played a part in the development of the symptoms. The patient is meanwhile not conscious of the associations between precipitants and symptoms, and is not intentionally producing them. *Hypochondriasis* is characterized by preoccupation with fears or beliefs of serious illness, often based on misinterpretation of physical sensations, in the absence of evidence of physical disorder. *Psychogenic (somatoform) pain disorder* consists of preoccupation with pain in the absence of organic pathology, or when organic pathology is present, concerns about pain appear to be out of keeping with the degree of physical disease.

Personality disorders

See Chapter 9 for discussion of this topic. Personality disorders characterized by histrionic, antisocial or dependent features are particularly likely to present to family and hospital doctors. Alcohol and drug abuse may be an added complication which leads to referral for medical attention (see Chapter 10).

Major affective disorders

Major depression and dysthymic disorders may present with somatic symptoms, such as loss of weight or appetite, lack of energy, hypochondriacal preoccupations, etc., and their recognition and accurate management may present a challenge to the clinician (see Chapter 6, p. 74).

Factitious disorders

Factitious disorders are characterized by symptoms which are produced deliberately, and are aimed at obtaining medical or surgical treatment and hospitalization. The symptoms are usually sugestive of somatic illness: the patient may simulate symptoms of physical disease, and cause self-mutilation or interfere with bodily functions or medical tests. Mental symptoms may also be simulated. The patient shows a persistent pattern of behaviour, and may travel from hospital to hospital, sometimes using a false name, to receive treatment. Usually the description of the problems is detailed and embellished with fantastical circumstances. The name of 'Munchausen syndrome' is used to describe this behaviour.

In contrast with other disorders such as malingering, which is understandable in terms of specific precipitants and motives, patients with factitious disorders appear to lack a specific reason for their behaviour, beyond that of receiving medical care.

Alcohol abuse

Alcohol-related problems are not uncommon in general medical patients, whether they are the result of alcohol addiction or of problem drinking. Accidents at work, home, or on the road, gastric and hepatic disease, and unexplained bouts of ill-health may be suggestive of alcohol abuse (see Chapter 10).

Eating disorders

Anorexia nervosa, bulimia nervosa and obesity are the main eating disorders. They all commonly first present in general medical settings and are described in Chapter 8.

Sexual problems

Concerns about sexual functioning and specific sexual dysfunctions (erectile impotence, loss of interest in sex) are not uncommon in general and hospital practice, and in particular in gynaecology and infertility clinics, where sexual dysfunctions such as vaginismus or impotence leading to non-consumation may be encountered. See Chapter 23 for discussion of the assessment and management of sexual problems.

Fig. 12.2 Acute organic brain disorder

1 Clouding of consciousness, with altered orientation and concentration.
2 Perceptual abnormalities, such as illusions and hallucinations.
3 Memory impairment, especially for recent events.
4 Impairment of thinking and speech with incoherence.
5 Abnormalities of psychomotor activities, with agitation or retardation.
6 Development over hours or days, and with daily fluctuations.
7 Evidence of organic disorder.

Epidemiology
Up to 30% of patients in medical or surgical beds develop acute organic disorders, the highest prevalence occurring in intensive care units. Older patients are more likely to develop such disorders.

Aetiological aspects
Almost any brain or systemic disorder can lead to an acute organic syndrome, and so careful screening and investigation is required to establish the cause.

Management
The physical cause of the disorder needs to be identified and treated. In addition, symptomatic measures can be of help, for example, the patient should be nursed in a well-lit and quiet room and stimulation should be kept to a minimum. Physical methods of treatment can be of help, in particular major tranquillizers such as haloperidol.

Course and prognosis
Acute organic brain syndromes are transient, and the majority last about 1 week. Outcome will depend on the nature of the aetiology of the disorder, and in general full recovery is the rule.

Examples of physical disorder leading to psychological problems

Case 1: depression following mastectomy

Karen was a 46-year-old librarian, married and with two grown-up children, who was admitted to hospital one week after she had consulted her GP after she *discovered a lump in her breast*. After the necessary investigations had been carried out, she had surgery, and she knew of the possibility of malignancy. When she came round after surgery, she realized *she had had a mastectomy and the house surgeon explained that she had cancer*.

Her initial reaction had been one of disbelief and shock. She had been very busy at work and looking forward to a holiday, and she found it difficult to take in the events of the previous week. She *hardly slept* during the following days, and found it *difficult to talk to her husband or the children* about her feelings. They had all been supportive, but she knew her husband was distressed, and had also avoided talking about her illness. Karen found herself *bursting into tears* when one of the nurses asked how she felt, but she had *avoided further discussion* so as not to upset or embarrass the nurse.

After discharge home, she saw her GP, a female doctor, who made the point of asking how she felt and how the family was coping. Karen found this intrusive, and dismissed the doctor's questions by insisting on an early return to work, which took place 3 weeks later. On returning to work, Karen found it *difficult to talk to colleagues about her illness*, and was irritated by people who kept bringing up the subject. She *began to feel anxious* when she read in the papers or saw on TV anything related to cancer, but at the same time, felt drawn to such news, and searched the papers for articles on the subject.

At the end of the first month after her operation, she *started to feel tired and tearful*, and *her appetite had deteriorated*. She had *lost interest in her appearance*, and *had not been out socially*. She had *not managed to examine her scar*, and *had not allowed her husband to look at it*, or touch her. She was particularly anxious in case her husband should wish to have sex, whilst at the same time felt disappointed that he had not made any moves towards comforting her. Karen was now thinking about giving up her job, and in the last few days she had started to *fantasize about how she could kill herself*.

The situation continued to deteriorate over the next 6 weeks, until she saw her doctor again to ask for a sickness certificate as she *did not feel capable of going to work*. This time, she responded to the doctor's questions, and *agreed to talk to her husband about how she was feeling*, and to come back to the surgery with him in a few days' time. Over the next 3 months, she saw her doctor fortnightly, sometimes alone, and sometimes with her husband. The meetings were usually short, but after discussion in the doctor's presence, she felt usually more cheerful, and he was also more forthcoming. *Gradually, she began to feel more confident*, and he started to show physical affection, but without sexual contact. After some *advice from her doctor on breast prostheses*, she obtained one, and made plans once more for the postponed holiday. The holiday was helpful in that Karen and her husband had time to themselves. She returned to work afterwards, and the relationship with her husband continued to improve.

Case 2

Alison was a 27-year-old woman who was admitted voluntarily to a psychiatric in-patient unit together with her 8-week-old baby daughter Kate, after she had become *depressed and was unable to look after the baby*.

The pregnancy, which was her first, had not been planned, but Alison and her husband Tony had soon accepted the fact, and welcomed the prospect of starting a family. Alison had a full-time job as laboratory technician, and she had not made a decision yet as to whether to return to work. Her husband was a police officer, and they had been in the area for 2 years.

There had been *no problems during pregnancy*, and *delivery was uneventful*, and Alison returned home after 4 days. Her mother had come to stay initially for a couple of weeks, but had in fact stayed until Alison was admitted to hospital. At first, there had been no difficulties, but after 10 days or so, Alison began to complain of *tiredness* and of *loss of appetite*, and her mother started to take a more active part in looking after the baby. By the end of the third week, Alison was *tearful and unhappy*, and she *had started to worry about the baby's health*. Alison's husband was beginning to feel that her mother was perhaps taking over the care of the baby, and there had been some arguments between him and his mother-in-law, which had upset Alison. A week later, Alison mentioned this to her GP, with whom she had a good relationship, and she found this of some help. However, *she was now convinced that it had been a mistake to have a baby, she lacked confidence in her ability to look after Kate*, and was very concerned about the baby's development. Alison had *lost a good deal of weight, was not eating*, and she was *waking up early in the morning, even when the baby did not need feeding*. Her GP thought that she needed antidepressants, but Alison refused medication, as she was breast feeding, and she did not wish to take any drugs. The doctor arranged to see her 10 days later, when the situation had deteriorated further, and at this stage, Alison *accepted medication*, after discussion with her husband. However, when she was seen again a few days later, the only improvement was in her insomnia, but *she was now convinced that the baby was ill and losing weight, in spite of evidence to the contrary. She felt the baby was going to die as a result of her own behaviour towards her mother, and she had stopped eating and drinking*. She needed prompting to hold the baby and to look after her own appearance, and she was pale and tearful. At that point she was *admitted to hospital*.

On admission, Alison was found to be suffering from a *severe depressive disorder*, with marked somatic features, such as *retardation, early waking* and *loss of weight and appetite*. Her *mood was much worse in the morning*, and improved during the day. She had *delusional beliefs* about the health of the baby consistent with her depression.

She was *treated first with antidepressant drugs in higher doses to those prescribed by her GP*, and *after a week she agreed to receive ECT*. After four treatments, her mood had improved markedly, and after a further four she was able to have weekend leave, and she was discharged a few days later. During her admission, the baby had stayed with her, under close nursing supervision. As Alison improved, she took a more active part in the care of the baby, and by the time she went home, she was fully responsible for her care.

She *continued to take antidepressants for another 6 months*, during which time she and her husband were seen together as out-patients, and the risks of further episodes were discussed.

Two years later, Alison and Tony discussed with the GP their wish to have another child. During her pregnancy and after delivery her mood was monitored by her doctor, and no difficulties developed. *Three years later, and following her father's death, Alison had a depressive episode* which required treatment with antidepressants as an out-patient.

Physical disorders leading to psychological symptoms

Organic brain disorders and systemic disorders with CNS symptoms

Acute and chronic organic states, whether due to primary disorder of the brain or systemic conditions, may present with florid psychological symptoms, as discussed in Chapter 11, p. 134, and careful assessment of the clinical features and aetiology will be needed before planning treatment (Fig. 12.2).

Impact of diagnosis, course and treatment of physical disorder

Patients confronted with the knowledge that they suffer a potentially serious disorder are likely to show in the short term, signs of distress, fear, tearfulness, and other forms of mood disturbance. Their relatives may experience similar difficulties. Such reactions should be regarded as normal, but sometimes their severity and prolonged course may suggest that the patient is suffering from a formal psychiatric disorder, and is in need of more specialized help. Many factors will contribute to determine whether a patient is going to cope well or badly with the diagnosis of a particular disorder. For example, the seriousness of the illness, the degree of uncertainty involved in its future course, and the nature of the treatment and its side effects; the patient's previous experience of similar illness, personally or in relatives, the person's ability to cope with adversity; and the nature of the supports and social problems that confront the patient now (Case 1).

HIV infection illustrates clearly the way in which a physical disorder can be associated with psychosocial problems as well as neuropsychiatric syndromes (Fig. 12.3).

Chronic disorders such as diabetes or epilepsy may cause especial problems, because of the need for constant medication and monitoring. Young patients, in particular, may find it difficult to come to terms with their condition, and this may lead to non-compliance with treatment, and in turn, to increasing physical deterioration.

Treatments which involve unpleasant side effects, such as vomiting, pains, etc., or disfigurement and mutilation, as in the case of mastectomy or amputation, are much more likely to be associated with psychological distress and disorder.

Patients with terminal illness and their relatives face especial difficulties, which are discussed in Chapter 2.

Puerperal disorders

Three types of psychiatric syndromes may follow childbirth. *Maternity blues.* This is a common (present in more than half of births), transient and mild disorder, characterized by symptoms of depression, anxiety, irritability, and subjective complaints of impaired concentration. The syndrome usually takes place within the first week post-delivery, and does not require specific treatment, beyond reassurance and support. Its aetiology is not well understood, although hormonal changes are assumed to play a significant part.

Puerperal psychosis. Between 1 and 2 women/1000 births develop a major psychiatric disorder following childbirth which requires hospitalization. The condition usually devel-

ops during the first 4 weeks after delivery.

Clinically, the most common syndrome is that of a major affective disorder, usually with marked depressive symptoms, although mania is not uncommon. Schizophrenic syndromes can also develop, as well as mixed disorders, with affective and schizophrenic symptoms. Puerperal psychoses are clinically similar to other psychoses not arising after childbirth, and they are generally not regarded as a distinct disease entity.

The treatment depends on the clinical picture, so that ECT, antidepressants and major tranquillizers may be used. It is desirable to keep the mother and baby together, and especial facilities may be required for their adequate nursing. It is also important to assess whether the baby is at risk of harm or neglect in the short term as a result of the mother's condition, and to take the necessary precautions.

The short-term outcome is good, the larger majority of patients recovering within 3 months. In the long term, about one in five tends to experience similar problems in further pregnancies, and about half suffer depression unrelated to childbirth (Case 2).

Post-partum depression. Depressive syndromes of mild to moderate severity affect about one in ten women after childbirth, and they usually start within a few weeks of delivery. Depression after childbirth does not appear to be different from other depressive syndromes unrelated to pregnancy, and their treatment and outcome is consistent with this (see Chapter 6, p. 81 for details). Prescribing in pregnancy and the puerperium is covered on p. 222.

Presentation and recognition of psychiatric disorders in general practice and hospital

Psychiatric disorders in general practice

How common is it?

A significant proportion of patients seen in general practice present with psychological problems. It has been estimated, for example, that in one year as many as 14% of registered patients will consult for largely psychological conditions. This means about 280 patients/year for each 2000 registered patients. In addition, many more will present with psychological disorders in association with physical conditions.

Not all individuals who are experiencing psychological problems in the community will consult their family doctors, and some studies have suggested that only about a third of such individuals actually take steps towards seeking medical help. A variety of factors contribute to visiting the surgery, such as the severity of psychological distress, the presence of chronic physical conditions, and lack of social supports or employment. See Chapter 16, for further discussion of the various levels of care and the factors associated with their provision.

About one-third of all patients consulting their family doctors have been shown to suffer from psychiatric disorders. In about half of these cases, the disorders are mild, and this means that a family doctor would expect to find that one in every six patients coming to the surgery presents with significant psychological symptoms, whether with physical problems or alone.

What psychiatric syndromes are seen in general practice?

The large majority of psychiatric disorders in general practice are minor affective disorders and adjustment reactions, presenting with symptoms of anxiety (about 40% of psychiatric disorders) or depression (about 30%), with much smaller proportions for organic brain disorders, major affective disorders, and schizophrenia. Psychological problems in general practice are usually associated with social difficulties, such as marital and family problems, financial and employment stress, and social isolation.

Recognition of psychiatric disorders in general practice

There is evidence that family doctors identify a significant proportion of patients with psychiatric disorders. Some studies suggest a figure of as many as two-thirds, although there will be differences between doctors, and also between disorders. For example, alcohol abuse may be harder to recognize than a severe anxiety state, and there is also the suggestion that depression is often missed.

It has been shown that patients whose psychiatric disorders are known to their GPs, have a better short-term psychological outcome, presumably because the doctors act on their knowledge, and take steps to manage the disorder. It is, therefore, important to be able to recognize the range of problems likely to present in general practice.

Accurate recognition of psychiatric disorders in general practice can be enhanced by the following guidelines.

1 Think about the possibility of psychological problems; they are common, and they often present with physical disorders.

2 Most psychiatric problems in general practice do not require intensive or specialized and complex treatments; listening to the patient, and giving information and advice may be all that is needed in most cases.

3 Develop a style of interview that allows the patient to express concerns or anxieties, and remember to ask questions about psychological functioning, in particular about depression and anxiety, and to explore the patient's social circumstances. Be prepared to follow leads.

4 Become familiar with the psychiatric resources in your area, so that you can seek advice about further management or referral to the appropriate services.

Psychiatric disorders in the general hospital

Out-patient clinics

A significant proportion of patients attending general hospital out-patient clinics suffer psychiatric disorders. In the majority of cases, the psychiatric disorder is related to the main physical problem, but, in some cases, the psychological problems are independent of physical disease, or are even primary. Clinics dealing with potentially severe disorders (such as heart disease), chronic conditions (such as epilepsy and diabetes), and conditions with marked social impairment (such as chronic renal failure and multiple sclerosis) are likely to have a larger share of patients with significant psychological symptoms.

The course of some common disorders can be influenced by psychological factors, which may play a part in their onset, likelihood of relapse, degree of recovery and compliance with treatment. Examples of conditions where psychological factors can be important include: asthma, hypertension, myocardial infarction, ulcerative colitis, premenstrual tension, and peptic ulcer.

As in the case of general practice patients, accurate recognition of the presence of psychological disturbance in general out-patients will depend on the doctors' awareness of the possibility of such problems, and their willingness to initiate adequate management.

General hospital in-patients

What are the psychological problems, and how common are they?

Psychiatric disorders are common in general hospital patients, and they are usually associated with physical disease.

The most frequently encountered are affective disorders (minor affective disorders, adjustment reactions, and major affective disorders). Some degree of affective disturbance can be detected in about 30% of medical patients, although moderate and severe forms probably amount to only half this figure.

Organic brain disorders, either acute (confusional states) or chronic (dementia), are common in older patients, and they may present important diagnostic and management problems.

A history of alcohol abuse is present in about 20% of patients admitted to the general hospital, but doctors often fail to recognize the problem.

Deliberate self-poisoning and self-injury are frequent reasons for admission to the general hospital. The assessment of these patients is discussed in Chapter 19, p. 252.

Recognition of psychological problems in the general hospital

It is essential for the doctors to be aware of the possibility of psychological problems, in particular when the history, the nature and severity of the physical condition, and the patient's response, are suggestive of the presence of problems.

It is important to evaluate the patient's mood, and to ask the necessary questions to establish whether there is persistent low mood and other symptoms of severe depression, or to what extent the patient's symptoms are an understandable and normal reaction to the physical problems (see Chapter 6, p. 81, for the assessment of affective disorders). Some studies have suggested that as many as half of the cases of depression are missed by hospital doctors.

It is also important to be familiar with the clinical assessment of the cognitive state, so as to be able to recognize the presence of cognitive impairment suggestive of an organic brain syndrome (see Chapters 11 and 13).

Finally, the identification of alcohol abuse can be facilitated by considering this possibility in patients with gastric and hepatic disease, those involved in accidents (at work, at home, on the road), and in patients with acute organic syndromes. Once a likely patient has been identified, the interviewer should try to establish the quantity and type of alcohol habitually consumed, the psychological, physical and social consequences of alcohol, and the presence of signs of addiction (see Chapter 10).

The use of questionnaires could be of value in the screening for possible alcohol abuse. The CAGE questionnaire is often used, in view of its easy administration (Fig. 12.4).

Accident and emergency departments

About 30% of patients attending emergency departments have been found to be suffering from psychiatric disorders. They include those referred to hospital following deliberate self-harm, and patients suffering from the consequences of alcohol or drug abuse. Patients with neurotic disorders, such as anxiety states, panic disorder, hypochondriasis or hysterical disorders, may seek urgent medical help. Patients with factitious disorders, and those with a range of personality disorders can become regular attenders. Occasionally,

---

Fig. 12.4 The CAGE questionnaire for the screening of alcohol abuse

C = Have you ever felt you should **C**ut down on your drinking?
A = Have people **A**nnoyed you by criticizing your drinking?
G = Have you ever felt **G**uilty about your drinking?
E = Have you ever had a drink first thing in the morning to steady your nerves (**E**ye opener)?

Affirmative answers to any two or more questions are strongly suggestive of alcohol abuse.

---

schizophrenic patients may be seen in casualty as a result of self-inflicted injury or self-mutilation.

Identification of psychological problems and their careful evaluation is especially important in casualty departments, so that patients suffering from severe psychiatric disorders, in particular those at risk to themselves or to others, can be given prompt help.

What are the causes of the psychological problems seen in general practice and hospital?

Psychiatric disorders seen in non-psychiatric settings are likely to be influenced by the same aetiological factors as those seen in patients referred to the psychiatric services. They are, up to a point, the same kind of patients, but with a generally milder range of symptoms in the case of those seen in non-psychiatric settings.

It is an interesting and intriguing fact that psychological and physical problems occur together more often than would be expected, and this is true when looking at patients referred to either general hospitals or the psychiatric services. The reasons for this association are complex. For example:
1 psychological disturbance could lead to physical disease, either as a direct result of it, or as an indirect consequence of the disorder;
2 physical disorder could lead to psychological disorder, either by direct effects on the CNS, or indirectly, as a result of fears about outcome, disability, etc.;
3 the association may be due to chance;
4 both types of disorder may be the result of shared vulnerability.

The possible influence of psychological factors in the development of physical disorders has been the subject of considerable interest to psychiatrists over the years. During the first half of this century, the focus of attention was what was known as 'psychosomatic disorders', which included a range of conditions of uncertain aetiology, such as peptic ulcer, ulcerative colitis, asthma and eczema. A variety of theories were put forward suggesting an association between personality and specific disorders, as well as advocating the use of psychotherapeutic techniques for the treatment of these conditions. 'Psychosomatic medicine' was largely derived from psychoanalytic theories, and lacked an empirical and scientific basis. However, one positive effect of this school of thought has been its drawing attention once more to the interaction between psychological and physical disorders.

It could be argued that all physical disorders, and not just a particular group of conditions, should be regarded as psychosomatic, in that, to some degree, psychological factors can play a part in their development, impact and consequences, and eventual outcome.

Precipitants

The precipitants of psychiatric disorder in general practice and hospital are often related to the development of symptoms of physical illness, its investigation and treatment. The nature of the physical condition, and in particular its severity, likely consequences in terms of degree of interference with life, disability, disfigurement, pain, etc., will affect the risk of psychological problems. As in the case of disorders presenting to psychiatrists, a wide range of life events, including psychological and social stresses, may contribute to the disorder. The physical disorder itself may cause psychological symptoms directly, and this can also be the result of the treatment given.

Predisposing factors

The previous personality and demographic characteristics may influence the probability of psychological problems in patients with physical disorders. For example, individuals who take pride in their physical appearance or fitness may find it particularly hard to cope with illness, and those who coped badly with adversity in the past may lack the resources to deal with the current problems. Young people may find it more difficult to face serious illness, and as a result develop affective disorders, whilst older patients may be more likely to suffer organic brain syndromes.

The nature of the person's social supports is likely to be relevant. Those who are socially isolated, or experiencing marital, financial, or employment difficulties are at greater risk of psychological disturbance.

Maintaining factors

The course of the physical condition will be important: prolonged and painful illnesses, or those where the medical or surgical treatment has unpleasant side effects will be associated with a greater risk of psychological problems. Uncertainty about outcome, and concern about the impact on relatives will be important factors. The nature of the care given by members of the medical or surgical team may also be relevant; early recognition of the psychological problems and adequate management will reduce the risk of persistent problems.

How should psychiatric disorders in general practice and hospital be managed?

Prevention

This is particularly important in the case of patients admitted to the general hospital. As was discussed earlier, coming into hospital is usually a stressful experience, especially when the process of investigation of physical symptoms, uncertainty of diagnosis or the prospect of painful treatments are added. It is therefore not surprising that some patients become depressed or anxious as a result of hospitalization.

However, the doctors, nurses, and other staff involved in the patient's care can do much to minimize the adverse effects of admission. For example, by being aware of the patient's anxieties and worries, by making sure that any investigations or clinical procedures are explained to the patient, and by being prepared to answer questions about the patient's condition.

Breaking bad news to patients and their relatives is usually difficult, both for the patient and for the doctor, but it is important not to add to the distress by making sure that the right moment is chosen for the disclosure, by allowing sufficient time and privacy, and by being prepared to answer the patient's questions. It is also important to learn to cope with the patient's distress or tears, without running away, patronizing the patient, or calling the psychiatrist!

Assessment

The first step in the assessment of psychiatric disorder in the general hospital or general practice is to be prepared to recognize its existence. As was discussed earlier, psychological problems are not uncommon in these patients, and the patient may not necessarily be aware of the nature of the problem.

It is important to include some routine questions about anxiety and depression, alcohol consumption and family relations during the interview with or clerking of the patient. It is often useful to ask relatives or others who are in close contact with the patient.

In the case of hospitalized patients, the nurses' observations are usually invaluable. Many patients find it easier to confide in the nurses, and they may express anxieties or concerns that they would not disclose to the doctors. Similarly, the nurses' reports of the patient's behaviour may be extremely helpful in the diagnosis of organic brain disorders.

The objectives of assessment are listed in Fig. 12.5.

The process of establishing the presence of a psychiatric disorder is covered elsewhere. When considering the likely causes, in particular when dealing with patients in hospital, it is very important to be aware of the possible direct effects of physical illness or its treatment, as for example in the case of acute brain disorders.

The decision as to whether to ask for a psychiatric opinion, either to help with the assessment of the problem, or to give

---

Fig. 12.5 Aims of the assessment of psychological problems in general hospital and practice

1 **Is there a psychiatric disorder**, or is this an understandable reaction to the circumstances?
If there is a disorder:
- what is it?
- what is its severity?

2 **What are the causes of the disorder?** In particular, what psychological, physical and social factors may be relevant?

3 **Is there a need for treatment of the disorder?**
If so:
- what kind of treatment would be indicated (psychological, physical, social)?
- who should be involved? In particular, is referral to a psychiatrist indicated?

advice about or take over management is likely to be influenced by many factors, apart from the actual psychiatric disorder. GPs and hospital doctors vary in their degree of confidence in the management of psychiatric problems, and this will affect referral rates. The nature of the local psychiatric services and their availability will also be a relevant factor.

In recent years, there has been a move towards the development of closer links between psychiatrists and family and hospital doctors. Many general hospitals now have easy access to psychiatric teams for the assessment and management of psychological problems. Two main types of work are involved: (a) consultation work, where the psychiatrist is asked to see the patient and perhaps take over management; and (b) liaison work, where the psychiatrist meets regularly with physicians and nurses to discuss difficulties with patients, and where the aim is to enhance the ability of the medical team to deal with psychological problems. There are similar schemes in general practice.

Management

Management of psychological problems in general practice

The large majority of psychiatric problems identified in general practice are managed by the GP; only about 5% of such patients are usually referred to psychiatrists, and those referred tend to be suffering from serious and severe disorders, such as schizophrenia, manic disorders or suicidal depression, or to have conditions known to respond to specialized treatments, such as agoraphobia.

Treatment in general practice will depend on the nature of the condition, and it is likely to include a variety of psychological, physical and social measures.

Much can be achieved by giving basic explanation and advice about the nature of the symptoms, their causes, and the likely outcome. In the case of minor affective disorders of recent onset, which are very common in general practice, there is good evidence that such basic counselling is as effective as anxiolytic drugs and more acceptable to patients, while being no more time consuming than the prescribing of medication (Fig. 12.6).

In the case of more persistent disorders, further psychological help may be needed, in the form of problem-solving counselling, relaxation training or other such techniques (see Chapter 18, p. 229, and also Chapter 7, p. 88).

Social factors are usually relevant, and it may be necessary to provide practical advice, counsel the partner or other family members, or consider referral to a marriage guidance counsellor.

If medication is to be used, it is essential to establish that drugs are indicated and likely to be effective. Not all patients with anxiety symptoms need anxiolytic drugs, and not all patients with depressive symptoms are likely to benefit from antidepressants. Psychotropic drugs should be reserved for patients suffering from persistent, severe, and well-defined disorders, and, in the case of anxiolytics, they should be used for a limited period of time (no more than 2 weeks), and in parallel with efforts to deal with the causes of the disorder (see Chapter 17, p. 220).

Fig. 12.6 Basic counselling in general practice

What brings the patient to the surgery?
- What symptoms does the patient complain of?
- What family and other problems does the patient face?
- Why does the patient come at this particular moment?
- Can a psychiatric or physical diagnosis be made?
- Would a problem list be more useful?

Feedback to the patient
- Explain the nature and significance of symptoms and problems.
- If psychological factors are important make sure you do not make the patient feel you dismiss the problems as 'in the mind', as opposed to 'real but produced through mental mechanisms'.
- Reassure the patient: the symptoms are not unusual, they do not indicate serious illness, and they are likely to improve, provided the right action is taken by patient and doctor.
- Encourage patient to ask questions and comment on your views.

What to do next
- Does the patient have any suggestions as to what to do next?
- Explore the causes further, and start to tackle each problem/symptom/cause at a time.
- Give symptomatic advice: distraction, relaxation, exercise.
- Encourage patient to communicate with partner, relatives, friends.
- Offer to see patient with partner and other family members.
- Suggest involvement of other agencies: voluntary groups, marriage guidance, social services, specialist services.
- Discuss whether further appointment is appropriate.
- Agree on specific tasks before next meeting.

Patients with somatoform disorders, in particular those with somatization disorders and hypochondriasis, are not uncommon in general practice. Whilst some are easy to manage by simple explanation and minimal reassurance, many develop chronic difficulties which are much harder to manage. It is in the nature of such disorders that they tend to respond in the short term to physical examination, clinical tests and reassurance, but remission tends not to be long lasting, the patient soon returning for further tests and reassurance. One important obstacle is the patient's reluctance to regard his or her symptoms as related to psychological factors, rather than organic disease. Management should include clear and unambiguous provision of information, together with explanation of the mechanisms through which the symptoms arise. In more severe cases, cognitive–behavioural techniques can be effective, and they will include the identification of cues to thoughts of illness, together with discontinuation of reassurance and further clinical tests or procedures.

Management of psychological problems in the general hospital

Much of what has been said above about general practice patients is applicable to the general hospital setting.

Conversion disorder (hysterical neurosis) is sometimes seen in the general hospital. Such a diagnosis should be made with great caution, as there is a good deal of evidence that many patients so labelled are subsequently found to be suffering from severe physical disorder which had not been adequately investigated. Co-existence of both physical and psychological syndromes is not uncommon, and the psychological assessment and provision of information and reassurance as well as advice for more specific psychosocial difficulties may be very effective in such cases.

As regards psychological management, hospital teams sometimes divide their roles amongst its members, so that medical social workers, nurses, or health advisors may develop a special interest in dealing with psychological problems. Successful examples of this include work with patients after mastectomy or amputation of limbs, and counselling in sexually transmitted disorders. Some such schemes include a liaison psychiatrist, as described above.

Psychotropic drugs also have a place in the treatment of psychiatric disorders, especially in acute brain syndromes, where antipsychotics like haloperidol, can be very effective (see Chapter 17, p. 213). Insomnia can be a distressing symptom in hospital, and it needs to be carefully evaluated before starting drug treatment, as it could be a symptom of severe depression, as well as a normal reaction to pain or discomfort. If hypnotic drugs are to be used, this should be for a limited period of time, and the patient should not be sent home on the drugs if at all possible.

The management of terminal illness and death raises special problems for patients and relatives, but also for the staff looking after them. These are discussed in Chapters 21 and 22.

What is the outcome of psychiatric disorders in general practice and hospital?

The outcome of the disorder will naturally depend on the nature of the particular condition, and the relevant chapters should be referred to for information. However, it is possible to make some general comments about the outcome of common disorders seen in general practice and hospital.

The outcome of psychiatric disorders in general practice

Most psychiatric problems seen in general practice tend to recover in the relatively short term. For example, about two-thirds of new cases recover within 6 months, and about 75% within a year. Chronic disorders, not surprisingly, run a less favourable course, and only about 50% tend to recover within a year. Patients who are given anxiolytic drugs when they first consult their doctors are more likely to go on taking them for months, compared with those patients not given medication at the outset.

Patients who develop chronic psychiatric disorders are more likely to have suffered more severe psychiatric symptoms at the time when they first consulted their doctors, and to have had a past history of psychiatric difficulties. They may also suffer from chronic physical ill-health, and have persistent family and social difficulties.

The outcome of psychiatric disorders in the general hospital

As far as it is known, the affective disorders seen in the general hospital have an outcome similar to the problems seen in general practice, so that most patients recover within a few months. Persistent psychiatric disorder is associated with a past history of poor coping, with chronic physical problems, and with the absence of supportive relatives and friends. Medical patients who suffer significant psychiatric disorder appear to have greater mortality in the long term.

The outcome of organic brain disorders will depend on their aetiology and underlying pathology, and their outcome appears to be worse than for the affective disorders.

QUESTIONS

1 What differential diagnoses would you consider in the case of a 42-year-old man who arrives in casualty in an agitated state, and suffering from palpitations, tremor and disorientation?

2 What advice would you give to the mother of a 17-year-old girl who comes to the surgery worried about her daughter's intense dieting?

3 How would you manage a 70-year-old man, admitted to hospital following a chest infection, who becomes agitated in the middle of the night, and accuses the nurses of trying to poison him?

4 How would you manage a 26-year-old woman who becomes acutely distressed and tearful 4 days after the birth of her first baby?

5 How would you treat a 45-year-old married women who comes to your surgery complaining of irritability, tension and difficulty doing the shopping?

6 How would you deal with a 37-year-old married man who has been found to have acute leukaemia, and who asks you not to tell his wife what is wrong with him?

FURTHER READING

Catalan J. (1990) Psychiatric manifestations of HIV disease. *Baillière's Clin. Gastroenterol.* **4**, 547–62.

Catalan J. & Gath D. (1985) Benzodiazepines in general practice: time for a decision. *Br. Med. J.* **290**, 1374–6. [A critical review of benzodiazepines.]

Gelder M., Gath D. & Mayou R. (1980) *Oxford Textbook of Psychiatry.* 2nd Edition. Oxford University Press, Oxford. [Clear, concise and comprehensive.]

Goldberg D. & Huxley P. (1980) *Mental Illness in the Community— The Pathway to Psychiatric Care.* Tavistock Publications, London. [A thorough review of mental disorders in general practice, including issues such as hidden morbidity and factors affecting referral.]

Kaplan H.I. & Sadock B.J. (1983) *Modern Synopsis of Comprehensive Textbook of Psychiatry/IV.* 4th Edition. Williams & Wilkins, Baltimore.

Lader M.H. (ed.) (1983) *Mental Disorders and Somatic Illness. Handbook of Psychiatry 2.* Cambridge University Press, Cambridge. [A comprehensive up-to-date review.]

Lishman W.A. (1987) *Organic Psychiatry— The Psychological Consequences of Cerebral Disorder.* 2nd Edition. Blackwell Scientific Publications, Oxford.

Loyd G. (1991) *Textbook of General Hospital Psychiatry.* Churchill Lvingstone, London.

13
The Psychiatry of Old Age

Fact sheet

Demography

In 1981, 18% of the population of England and Wales were of pensionable age (9 million people). Numbers of older people have increased throughout this century:

- in 1901, 0.4% of the population was over 75 years old;
- in 1981, 6% of the population was over 75 years old (3 million people);
- in 1981, 0.5% of the population was over 85 years old;
- by 2021, 1.1% of the population will be over 85 years old (an increase of 120%).

Two-thirds of the over-75s are women; two-thirds of these women are widows. One-third of all pensioners live alone.

Presentation of psychiatric problems

Emergency presentation
Is usually due to:

- physical illness; } leading to acute
- effects of medication; } confusional state
- breakdown of the support system;
- major change of environment;
- paranoid illness (primary or secondary), hypomania;
- attempted suicide.

Non-emergency presentation
May occur in:

- moderate or mild depression;
- moderate or mild dementia;
- multiple handicaps gradually intensifying;
- neuroses (anxiety and hypochondriasis especially);
- alcoholism.

Many problems arise out of an *interaction* between the patient and his circumstances.

Essential elements in assessment

- *Preliminary information* about the *context* of the referral: the people involved and the social environment of the patient. See the patient *at home* if possible.
- *From the patient*: the patient's view of the problem, systematic assessment of *mental state*, *physical health* and different aspects of *cognition*.
- *From the informant*: *history* of the onset and development of illness, nature of the *current problems*.
- *Investigation* focused on potentially treatable illness.

Essential elements in management

- Identify all factors contributing to the problem.
- Distinguish unalterable and modifiable factors.
- Cooperation between different agencies.

- Keyworker responsible for coordination of all interventions, monitoring and follow-up.
- Management plan which is adaptable to changing levels of disability and of resilience of carers.

The dementias

- Prevalence increases with age: roughly 6% at age 70–80; 20% in over-80s.
- Commonest causes are Alzheimer's disease and cerebrovascular pathology.
- Important to identify the rare cases of treatable dementia.
- Management focuses on accurate diagnosis; information and advice on other sources of help; measures to maintain optimal general health and least burden of 'added disability'; provision of appropriate types of care; support to carers (family and professional).

Depression

- Very common: 8–14% of over-65s have symptoms deserving medical intervention and 1–2% of over-65s have depression severe enough for hospital treatment.
- Often unrecognized or untreated (or social support given instead of medication).
- Association with physical illness.
- Relapse is common: need for long courses of treatment, good follow-up and surveillance of medication.

Paranoid states

- Primary and secondary paranoid states.
- Association with: sensory impairment, socially isolated personality; also with depressive illness and dementia.
- Responsive to medication.

Other psychiatric conditions

- Anxiety states, agoraphobia, hypochondriasis.
- Adjustment reactions.
- Family pathology: the old person as the 'identified patient'.
- Alcoholism and other dependencies.

Physical disabilities in old age

- 4% of over-65s living at home are **bedfast or housebound**; (in the over-85s, the proportion is 20%).
- 30–40% of the over-65s at home have **hearing difficulties**.
- 5% of the over-80s are registered **blind**; there are probably as many again who are not registered but equally disabled.
- In the over-75s, 16% of women and 8% of men have regular episodes of **urinary incontinence**.

Introduction

Numbers

The number and the proportion of old people in our population are increasing; the greatest increase is amongst the very old. In 1951 there were 271 people aged 100 and over; by 1971 there were 2320. Women outnumber men in the higher age-groups: in the age-group 65–74 women form 54% of the total; in the age-group 85 and over, they make up 80%.

The major reason for this increase is not the prolongation of elderly lives now, but the saving of young lives at the beginning of this century. In Fig. 13.1 you will see that in 1911 life-expectancy for those who were **already** 65 was only slightly less than it is for 65-year-olds now; it was the average life-expectancy **at birth** that was so much less than now.

Living arrangements (Fig. 13.2)

Most old people live alone or with another person of similar age. Half the women over 65 are widows. One-third of old people have no surviving children, or never had any. About 5% of older people live in institutions – the same proportion as at the beginning of the century.

One-quarter of all pensioners (about 2 million people) need to claim Income Support to make ends meet. Two-thirds of their income is spent on fuel and food (compared to one-quarter of the income in an average household). Half the pensioner households have no telephone. Nine-tenths of pensioners living alone have no car. Twelve per cent of homes occupied by the elderly have only an outside toilet.

Special considerations in old age

Mental illness

The principles of psychiatric **diagnosis** and **treatment** are the same in older people as at any age, but there are special features of old age that influence the **presentation** and **management** of mental illnesses. These are discussed later in the chapter.

The patient (Fig. 13.3)

It is common for old people to have many disabilities at the same time, and the co-existence of physical and mental illness can make either of them harder to diagnose or to treat, as with depression in a setting of chronic pain, or a fractured femur in a patient with dementia. Psychiatric approaches are

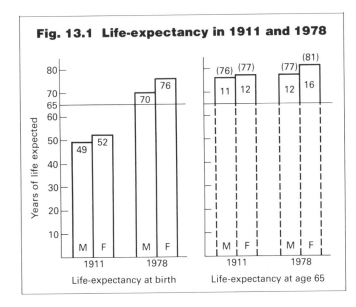

Fig. 13.1 Life-expectancy in 1911 and 1978

Years of life expected

Life-expectancy at birth
- 1911: M 49, F 52
- 1978: M 70, F 76

Life-expectancy at age 65
- 1911: M (76) 11, F (77) 12
- 1978: M (77) 12, F (81) 16

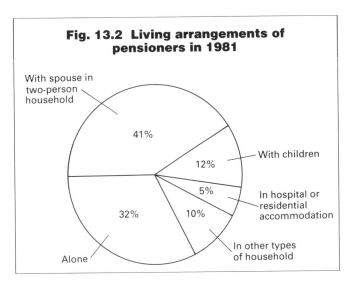

Fig. 13.2 Living arrangements of pensioners in 1981

- With spouse in two-person household 41%
- With children 12%
- In hospital or residential accommodation 5%
- In other types of household 10%
- Alone 32%

Fig. 13.3 Special considerations in old age

The patient
- Multiple illnesses (medical and psychiatric).
- Multiple problems (social, financial, family).
- Communication difficulty, sensory impairment.
- Need for collateral sources of information.
- Vulnerability to drug side effects.
- Atypical presentation of disease.
- Misidentifying treatable illness as normal ageing.

The social context
- Marginal status in society.
- Social isolation; enforced closeness.
- Threats to autonomy and unwelcome dependence on help.
- Constraints of institutional life.
- Interdependence of services for the elderly.
- Inequalities in the provision of services.

Ethical and legal issues
- Accepting risks.
- Conflicts of interest between patients and carers.
- Who speaks for the patient unable to speak for himself?
- The Mental Health Act (1983): compulsory admissions, treatment of the patient unable to consent.
- Finances: payment for care or legacies to children? Court of Protection, Enduring Power of Attorney.
- Research with cognitively impaired patients.
- Nearness of death: what makes a life worth living? What is 'death with dignity'?

most handicapped by those disabilities that limit communication: sensory impairment, especially deafness; language disorder, as with dysphasia following a stroke; and dementia itself. Thus in old age psychiatric diagnosis is often crucially dependent on collateral sources of information, such as relatives or nurses. Illnesses in old people are often compounded by other problems, such as financial hardship, poor housing or loneliness. Metabolic changes with old age make people more vulnerable to drug side effects; but they are also vulnerable to the opposite danger of undertreatment by too-cautious prescribing. Treatable illnesses in old people may be missed because the presentation of the illness is unusual, with the classical syndromes appearing in bizarre, fragmented or muted forms; and tolerant carers may overlook important symptoms, accepting them as an inevitable part of ageing, instead of seeking skilled help.

The social context (Fig. 13.3)

Articulate and forceful old people are now challenging the perception of their age-group as marginal to society, unproductive, content to receive such help as society chooses to offer. But for too many old people reality is still a matter of harsh choices within a narrow range of options. A widow struggling against loneliness as her friends die one by one may have no choice but to give up the flat in which all her married life was spent, to move into an old people's home, sharing a bedroom and sitting at table with companions she would not freely have chosen. For a proudly independent man, disabled by a stroke, to be bathed and dressed by a cheery care assistant who calls him Dad may be a heavy price to pay for remaining in his own home.

The social context also influences the help that psychiatric teams can offer; behaviour that is harmless in an old person on their own (collecting and hoarding small objects of no value, for example) can cause havoc in a residential home. Because the interests of the elderly cross many administrative boundaries, psychogeriatric teams spend much time in working and planning with social services, housing authorities, voluntary bodies and primary care. This interdependence is echoed within the psychogeriatric team itself, where colleagues in different disciplines must all learn something of the other's trade, and must know when to call on each particular skill. Lastly, most psychogeriatricians hold that responsibility to individual patients also entails a responsibility for advocacy on their behalf, to try and achieve a more equitable distribution of resources towards older people.

Ethical and legal issues (Fig. 13.3)

When old people need help, benevolent helpers may be tempted to take over their lives more than is needed. The danger is greater when the helpers' motives are not so pure, and their own interests are involved in the outcome of the help they are giving. (These interests may be financial or emotional, fear of blame, the wish to safeguard a job, to settle old scores or to placate others.) When old people put themselves at risk, or refuse help – whether through choice or confusion – does intervention diminish their lives more than the risk warranted? In families caring for an elderly relative, the network of old emotional ties and current finan-

---

Fig. 13.4 Legal powers

Enduring Power of Attorney
Power of Attorney is a legal arrangement (through a solicitor) by which one person empowers another to manage his affairs. If the person granting the power becomes mentally incapable, the power lapses. **The Enduring Powers of Attorney Act (1985)** now enables Powers of Attorney to be created which will survive any subsequent mental incapacity of the donor. (The donor must still be capable at the time of creating the power. When he becomes incapacitated, the EPA must be registered with the Court of Protection.)

Court of Protection
The Court of Protection is concerned with the protection of the property of people not capable (because of mental disorder) of managing their own affairs. Application to the Court is made through a solicitor, supported by evidence from a registered medical practitioner, and the Court will then appoint a Receiver (who may be a relative) to act on the patient's behalf. The procedure can be slow and expensive, but it is the only legal way in which a mentally incapable person's affairs can be managed, if he has not created an Enduring Power of Attorney while he was well. 'The Court has no concern with a person's medical management.'

---

cial obligations may not be operating to the old person's benefit – should the professionals step in? Legal means exist for dealing with some of these issues: the Mental Health Act (see Chapter 25), the Court of Protection and Enduring Power of Attorney (see Fig. 13.4).

Old people tend to have a more realistic view of death than the young, and for many it is not a frightening prospect. Given the opportunity, they may express clear views on their own choices between an earlier death or a distressful treatment. On the other hand, patients with dementia, although incurably ill and unable to tell us what their own choice would be, often do not seem as distressed by their condition as their carers are. Concern about the quality and dignity of demented peoples' lives may generate ethical debate. Do such debates serve merely to cloak the difficulty **we** have in providing enough good and dignified care for these people?

Older people: psychiatric assessment

Presentation

The common psychiatric illnesses of old age tend to develop relatively slowly (dementia more so than depression). Under favourable circumstances, when patients or relatives become aware in good time that there is a problem, and bring it to the general practitioner, he can respond himself or refer to a specialist without particular haste. Where psychogeriatric services are well established, this process of early awareness and timely referral is actively encouraged. However, many referrals also come to psychogeriatric teams for urgent help in a **crisis**, and this usually has to do with factors additional to the psychiatric condition itself. **Physical illness** may precipitate a crisis by adding an acute delirium to a pre-existing mild dementia, or by imposing hospital care on a person just maintaining their grasp of reality at home. A **system of support** for an old person may break down because of sudden illness in the carer, or in someone for whom the carer feels even more responsible than for the old person, or because the carer has been struggling too long with a task beyond her strength, and can't drive herself any harder. A **person living on their own** may be managing, just short of serious risks or self-neglect, unaware that they need help or that there is any help to be had, until the situation comes to the notice of a concerned person who makes the judgement that the situation ought not to be as it is, and demands action. If this demand comes from someone who also feels uncomfortable about not having noticed sooner, or done more to help, the demand for action is likely to be stronger in proportion to the sense of guilt. Relatives who live at a distance from the old person and can only visit occasionally are more likely to make hasty interventions of this kind, and

they may also bring the old person home with them immediately, and find that they do not know how to cope with the situation that results.

The process of assessment
A wide range of factors may precipitate the referral of an old person for medical help, and further factors influence the choice of psychiatric (rather than geriatric, perhaps) referral. The **response** to the referral must take account of the whole system (the patient, the carers, their beliefs and assumptions) in order to intervene in the right place. Diagnosis of any illness at the centre of the problem is the first duty of the doctor, but it is embedded in the broader process of assessment, which may also entail a judgement at an early stage as to whether other professionals should be involved from the start.

Thus assessment begins even before the patient has been seen. Whenever possible, information is collected from any

---

Fig. 13.5 The first three steps in assessment

1 The context
Collect information if time permits:
- to understand reasons for the referral;
- to decide where to see the patient (preferably at home);
- to identify a suitable informant;
- to decide whether assessment should be done jointly with another agency (e.g. social worker);
- to clarify what information you will need to gather from the informant and the patient.

2 Seeing the patient
The home
- Dangers and assets of the home (busy road, unprotected fires, steep stairs).
- Home as the record of the patient's history and personality (photographs, pets, handiwork, comforts).
- Evidence of illness (unused rooms, decaying food, whisky bottles).
- Neighbours, fellow-residents, staff (angry, indifferent, anxious, caring).

The patient
- Follow general principles, but modify the structure of the interview to suit the patient, if concentration is poor, or they are quickly exhausted, or irritated by certain questions.
- General health; physical handicaps (sight, hearing, mobility).
- Clear or clouded consciousness?
- Cognitive state (use evidence from whole interview, as well as specific tests: see pp. 131–137).
- Altered mood (look especially for depressive thinking).
- Clues to abnormal beliefs or perceptions.
- Insight.
- Check what medication the patient has.

3 History from the informant
- Onset and course of the problem (be specific about details).
- Past history of the patient.
- Possible causative factors (alcohol, bereavement, trauma, family history, family stress).
- Current physical illnesses.
- Current prescribed or self-administered medication.
- What exactly is the problem now?
- What is the *informant's* interpretation of the problem?

Fig. 13.6 Further steps in assessment
(starting from the most essential and the least costly or distressing)

Physical examination
Sometimes best done separately under good conditions, perhaps at doctor's surgery or day hospital rather than patient's house.

Look for:
- causes (e.g. chest infection in acute confusion, signs of alcohol abuse);
- complications (e.g. dehydration, burns, bruises);
- additional disabilities (e.g. arthritis, Parkinson's disease).

Routine laboratory investigation

Intervention with monitoring
e.g. diagnostic trial of antidepressant medication, or introduction of home help. Monitoring of the intervention is essential. One person (often the community psychiatric nurse) takes responsibility for this.

Admission for assessment
Day care or in-patient care.

Advantages
- Skilled observation over long periods of time.
- Access to specialist input (e.g. occupational therapist, geriatrician).
- Freedom of action for the patient, in an environment tolerant of odd behaviour, with stable and predictable timetable, and variety of activities and levels of sociability.

Disadvantages
Upsetting removal from familiar surroundings. May take the problem away temporarily, without necessarily solving it.

Special tests of mental function
Where presentation is atypical or the cognitive problem is hard to define (e.g. dementia presenting early with 'frontal' features).

Special investigations
- Such as CT scan or EEG.
- As a rule, indicated only on specific clinical grounds, e.g. if the clinical picture is atypical, or to exclude a possible treatable cause of dementia (normal pressure hydrocephalus, subdural haematoma).

people already involved, to give the context to the referral, so that the questions become clear and the interview with the patient can be carried out in the most informative way. The next step is to see the patient. Ideally this should be done in the patient's home, where he will feel most secure, where the truest picture of what has been happening is likely to be seen, and where a great deal of vital information can be gleaned from the details of the patient's living arrangements (see Fig. 13.5). An independent interview with an informant should **never** be omitted. Where there is no obvious person close to the patient to fill that role, the necessary information can often be pieced together from a number of sources, such as neighbours or a distant relative, as well as the various professional contacts.

By this stage a provisonal formulation of the problem can usually be made, and any additional steps in assessment planned (Fig. 13.6).

Illnesses of old age

We shall now discuss two important classes of illness in old age, the dementias and affective disorders, and then briefly consider the special features of other psychiatric conditions when they present in late life.

The dementias

Definition
'Dementia' is not the name of a single disease, but a generic term covering numerous conditions that have certain clinical features in common. The characteristics of a dementing illness are:
1 impairment of several aspects of cognition at the same time (or 'global intellectual impairment');
2 preservation of clear consciousness.
If consciousness is impaired, the condition is defined as an **acute confusional state** (or acute brain syndrome) (see p. 134) rather than dementia. Features which used to be regarded as part of the definition of dementia, but for clarity are best omitted from it, are irreversibility of the condition, and aetiology.

Thus, the syndrome of dementia is recognized by its clinical features. However, the *causes* of dementing illnesses are categorized in terms of their pathology, and this usually means that a definite diagnosis in a given case of dementia has to await post-mortem examination.

The commonest pathological cause (found at post-mortem in about 60% of patients dying in hospital with a diagnosis in life of 'dementia') is Alzheimer's disease. Next in frequency is cerebrovascular pathology (found in about 20% of such autopsies as a sole cause, and in another 10% in combination with Alzheimer's changes). Dementia associated with Parkinson's disease is increasingly being recognized. Other causes are much less common, but as some are potentially treatable, clinical vigilance is directed towards detecting those few treatable causes (Fig. 13.7).

Diagnosis
It is worth emphasizing again that the diagnosis of dementia is made on clinical grounds, and that (except in very early cases) it is not usually difficult to make, providing that the evidence is properly looked for. But where doctors fail to speak to an informant, or base their examination of the patient's mental state on a social conversation, without systematically testing cognitive function, they may not recognize dementia where it is present, or may wrongly suspect it where a different psychiatric condition is occurring.

The main conditions to be **distinguished** from dementia are:
1 acute confusional state (acute organic brain syndrome);
2 affective disorder (usually depression, but also hypomania and mixed states);
3 specific neurological syndromes (e.g. dysphasia following a stroke, pure amnesic syndromes);
4 lifelong low intelligence, especially when compounded by poor physical health and social deprivation.
Evidence from the informant is needed especially on the onset and time-course of the illness, and the current range of problems experienced. Examination of cognitive function should at a minimum include tests of orientation, remote memory, and registration and recall of new (simple) information; and should make some estimation of the use of language, abstract thought and visuo-spatial skills. Several short tests of mental function are available. The Mini-Mental State Examination is quick and acceptable to most patients, and is widely used (see Fig. 13.8). Further information on cognitive testing of organic states can be found in Chapter 11, pp. 131–137.

Information gathered from the patient and the informant will go some way towards suggesting the **cause** of the dementia. As yet, there is no specific diagnostic test for either Alzheimer's disease or multi-infarct dementia, and in life both these diagnoses are made presumptively, awaiting confirmation after death. Where the history, examination of the patient or routine laboratory investigations suggest the possibility of one of the rare causes of dementia, further specific investigation is warranted.

Management – general principles
Alzheimer's disease (in common with most of the other dementias) is as yet an untreatable condition, and one in which the erosion of the patient's intellectual and emotional reserves leaves him progressively more dependent on others to provide an appropriately 'prosthetic' environment for him. The responsibility for creating such supportive environments is shared amongst many separately administered bodies with different philosophies, time-scales and sources of funding. Only when these agencies work well together can the responsibility towards the sufferer from dementia be properly fulfilled, by providing a pattern of care at the level of intensity suited to his needs at each stage of the illness until death. This ideal is only rarely approached, alas. The chance of attaining it is greatest where there are family members who have the will and the strength to act as the backbone of the care. Then the professional input can be concentrated on helping the family members, by offering a shared understanding of the illness, emotional support, time

Fig. 13.7 Common and rare causes of the dementia syndrome

Common causes

	Alzheimer's disease	*Multi-infarct dementia*
Distribution	• Prevalence rises with age. Rare before age 65 (0.1%) Found in 6% of 70–80 year olds, 20% of over-80s. • Commoner in women. • High incidence in Down's syndrome.	• Commoner in men than women. • In men under 80, probably commoner than Alzheimer's disease.
Aetiology	• Genetic predisposition. • Cause otherwise unknown.	• Cerebrovascular disease.
Onset and progression	• Onset insidious. • Progression gradual.	• Abrupt onset, often with episode of confusion which partly remits. • Stepwise progession.
Clinical features	• Memory and orientation usually affected early. • Dyspraxia and dysphasia associated with worse prognosis. • Social competence often preserved initially.	• Patchy cognitive impairment; some faculties well preserved. • Insight often retained, and depression likely. • History of hypertension, focal neurological signs, and fluctuating severity may be found.
Prognosis	• Very variable, but roughly 7-year survival from diagnosis (depends on age).	• Roughly 5-year survival from diagnosis. • Treatment of hypertension does not cure dementia, but may prevent progression.
Pathology	• Neurofibrillary tangles. • Senile plaques. • Deficit of cholinergic transmitter system. • Other neurotransmitters also affected (mainly in younger patients).	

Rare causes

Potentially treatable or preventable causes	*Untreatable causes*
• Alcoholic dementia. • Normal-pressure hydrocephalus. • Chronic subdural haematoma. • Benign tumour (e.g. frontal meningioma). • Thyroid deficiency, B_{12} deficiency. • Cerebral trauma (e.g. in boxers – 'dementia pugilistica'). • Neurosyphilis. • Cerebral anoxia (e.g. after cardiac arrest).	• Parkinson's disease, cortical Lewy body disease. • Pick's disease. • Huntington's chorea. • Creutzfeld–Jakob disease. • Multiple sclerosis. • Malignant tumour (e.g. cerebral metastases). • HIV dementia.

and space away from the task of caring in a reliable routine, immediate response in crises, and partnership in planning each step into the future.

Where specific problems arise in the care of a patient with a dementing illness, it is helpful to think of the clinical picture as the combined result of:

1 the kind of person the patient is (the premorbid personality and intellect);

2 the distribution and severity of the pathological process in the brain, and the specific handicaps arising from that;

3 the response of the patient to the illness (emotional reactions and coping strategies);

4 the effect on the patient of other people's reactions. With such a framework, it becomes easier to understand the origins of problems for which help is being sought, and to determine what kinds of intervention might help with them. In the next section, we look at some ways of tackling the problems associated with dementing illnesses (Fig. 13.9).

Common problems in dementing illnesses

The loss of insight that often occurs in a dementing illness means that problems are experienced less by patients than by the people looking after them. Therefore offers of help must take the carers into account as much as the patients. Much help of a general kind can be given by relieving stress on the patient, relieving stress on the carer, and by altering the environment; but sometimes specific solutions to particular problems are needed, and often carers themselves show the greatest ingenuity in finding these. Mutually supportive groups (such as the Alzheimer's Disease Society) enable such information to be shared.

Ways of relieving stress on the patient

1 Illness: treat any additional illness or disability energetically.

2 Environment: make the patient's environment as consistent and predictable as possible, with clear cues to place and time; reinforce the comprehensibility of the environment at every natural opportunity (introduce yourself by name,

Fig. 13.8 The 'Mini-mental state examination' (see Folstein et al., 1975)

Orientation	Score
1 Can you tell me what	
year it is?	1
season?	1
date?	1
day?	1
month?	1
2 Can you tell me where we are?	
what town (or village)?	1
what street (or hospital)?	1
what house (or ward)?	1
what county?	1
what country?	1

Registration

3 'I would like you to remember three things for me. The three things are . . . (name three objects, taking 1 second to say each)'. Then ask the patient all three, after you have said them. Give one point for each correct answer. Then repeat the three objects until the patient can repeat them all. 'Now please keep remembering those three, and I will ask you about them later'. — 3

Attention and calculation

4 Serial sevens. Give one point for each correct answer. Stop after five answers. Alternative: spell 'WORLD' backwards. — 5

Recall

5 Ask for the names of the three objects learned in question 3. Give one point for each correct answer. — 3

Language	Score
6 Point to a pencil and a watch, say 'Can you tell me what that is called?'	2
7 Ask the patient to repeat 'No ifs, ands, or buts'.	1
8 Ask the patient to follow a three-stage command: 'Please take this piece of paper in your right hand, fold it in half, and put it on the floor'.	3
9 Ask the patient to read and follow the written command: 'CLOSE YOUR EYES'. (Write the command in large clear capitals.)	1
10 Ask the patient to write a sentence of his or her choice. (To score correct, the sentence must contain a subject and a verb. Spelling mistakes do not matter.)	1
11 Draw the design below and ask the patient to copy it. (Draw it with side of 1.5 cm at least. To score correct, each pentagon must have 5 sides and the intersecting sides must form a quadrangle.)	1

TOTAL = 30

Cut off point for probable cognitive impairment is 24.

---

address the patient by name, explain where you are, etc.).
3 Activity: give the patient access to enjoyable activity, tailored to his competence: return to areas of expertise (e.g. recollecting the past) as a break from the demands of present difficulties.
4 Communication: adapt communication strategies to the abilities of the patient. Language may be more impaired than sensitivity to emotional and non-verbal communications, and messages that are meaningless in a literal sense (e.g. 'I want to go home', when the patient **is** at home) can be understood emotionally ('I feel insecure'). Reinforce words with gesture, avoid ambiguity and distraction, and keep sentences simple.
5 Memory: impaired memory can be turned to good account: if a patient is upset by a task (such as dressing), experienced carers will withdraw for a minute or two; as the memory of the upset fades, the task can be resumed.

Ways of relieving stress on the carers
1 Information: this must make sense to the carer within the framework of **their** understanding of what is happening. Listen to what the carer says to you, so that you neither overload with unwanted detail, nor assume more understanding than the carer yet has.
2 Misconceptions: carers find it hard to judge how much of the patient's behaviour can be attributed to the disease, and are often hurt by what they see as deliberately unkind or obstinate behaviour. Help carers to understand the cognitive difficulties in a more detached way.

3 Caring for themselves: carers need to be encouraged to preserve some time free for themselves, to take adequate food and rest, to maintain their own interests and to keep up their friendships. Feelings of guilt, duty to the patient, or sheer exhaustion make it difficult for carers to see the sense in these recommendations.
4 Support and sharing: this includes sharing of day-to-day practical tasks (with help from a care assistant, day centre, etc.), and sharing of the emotional burden. Local relatives' support groups and national organizations (Association of Carers, Age Concern, Alzheimer's Disease Society, etc.) can play an important part in this.

Altering the environment
1 Practical modifications: low-level light to guide the way to the bathroom, door catches to prevent wandering onto a busy road, storage heaters instead of coal fire.
2 The social environment: explanations to neighbours, negotiation with local shopkeepers to control shopping sprees; introduction to day care.
3 Move to a different place: including admission to hospital, to local authority or private home, where more care is available. Moves need not always be permanent: regular relief admissions can interrupt an escalation of problems at home, with the beneficial effects lasting for a substantial period after the return.

Fig. 13.9 Specific problems

Problem	Possible solutions	Problem	Possible solutions
Forgets medication	Calendar box; neighbour or care assistant sets out medication.	Disinhibition of sexual behaviour	Encourage open discussion of problem among carers, so that they can give clear unembarrassed cues to patient at the time to orient him to the social context (e.g. encourage masturbation in private rather than public rooms).
Forgets familiar people	Explain to the people; show them how to introduce themselves naturally.		
Forgets he repeats himself	Help carer to introduce distraction, give carer relief.	Shouting	Try to find the cause (e.g. deafness, pain), if no cause found, try to reward silence with caring attention, and refrain from rewarding shouting. But apparently causeless shouting is one of the most difficult problems in dementia.
Emotional reactions to disability: clinging, anger, stubborn adherence to familiar routines, catastrophic reaction	Reduce stresses on patient, introduce change very gradually, preferably through one trusted person. Introduction to supportive, friendly environment (e.g. day care) is often very helpful, once patient can be brought to go.		
Wandering outside the house	Accept the risk; alternative daytime activity; change the door catches.	**Problems in the carer**	
Night-time restlessness	Reduce daytime boredom, avoid too-early bedtime, maintain clear diurnal rhythm in household, provide commode for nocturnal micturition, careful medication (not benzodiazepine).	When the carer: • is too frail, ill, or dies; • is also demented; • is depressed; • has other problems, competing family loyalties; • dislikes and resents the patient; • feels unskilled or unsupported; • worries about the effect of the patient on other people (fellow-residents, children); • is 'locked in' to caring and can't let go or accept help.	These require major changes in the situation, through substantial help coming into the home, or a move (partial or complete) of the patient out of the home, and effective support to the carer over the long term.
Financial incompetence	Arrange to draw pension (as appointee), discuss with local shops and banks, Enduring Power of Attorney, Court of Protection.		
Aggression	Try and work out causes: if driven by paranoid ideas, treat with medication; if not, understand antecedents if possible, and counsel carer accordingly.		
Incontinence	Reduce obstacles to continence (difficulty in getting out of chair or walking, awkward geography of house, complicated clothing, constipation). Regular reminders or actual taking to toilet. Pads often confuse a potentially continent patient, avoid them if possible.		

The affective disorders

Depression

It is widely assumed that 'psychiatric illness in old age' is virtually synonymous with dementia. In fact the affective disorders, depression in particular, contribute up to half the workload of a comprehensive psychogeriatric service. Depression in old age is very common, very distressing and sometimes lethal, but very treatable. It demands the same vigilance and commitment from hospital and community services as do the dementias. Earlier in this century, almost any psychological symptoms in old age were regarded as a sign of organic brain disease, and the herald of an inevitable dementia. But in the 1950s, the pioneering epidemiological studies of Roth and his colleagues in Newcastle showed that affective disorder and dementia were clearly distinguishable categories of disease on grounds of their natural history and prognosis, both for recovery and for survival.

Prevalence figures for depression in old age depend on the method of study and the definition of depression used. As a rough guide, 10% of the over-65s in a community will have signs of depression severe enough to warrant medical attention. Among older old people living in residential care (a selected population), between 30 and 50% may be depressed. Sadly, many cases of depression are not recognized by their doctors, or, if they are, they are not treated effectively, although other psychoactive drugs (such as benzodiazepines for insomnia) may have been prescribed.

Suicide is commoner in old age than in youth, while attempted suicide is less common. Important risk factors are unrecognized depression, social isolation (especially

Fig. 13.10 Difficulties in diagnosing depression

Misleading symptoms	May be mistaken for:
Agitation	Anxiety, difficult personality
Hypochondriacal fears	Neurotic disorder, difficult personality
Retardation	Dementia
Delusions	Schizophrenia
Cognitive slowing and poor concentration	Dementia

Depression present but camouflaged by:	Hidden signs of depression
Physical illness	Biological features (sleep, appetite, etc.)
Understandable stresses	Pathological mood change and depressive cognitions seem 'reasonable in the circumstances'
Difficult premorbid personality	Onset of novel symptoms is masked
	Self-report is discounted

if recent, as for example following bereavement), fear of physical illness (real or illusory), and alcohol dependence. Men are at greater risk than women.

Recognition of depression in old age may be difficult because of an unusual pattern of symptoms, or because the setting in which the depression occurs is camouflaging the typical symptoms (Fig. 13.10).

Nevertheless the **principles of diagnosis and management** of depression are unaffected by the age of the patient. The most valuable information, as with younger patients, is to be found in the history, the biological features and the content of thinking (see also pp. 74–80).

Aetiology

A family history of affective disorder is somewhat less common in late-onset depression than in younger patients. There is a clear statistical association between physical illness and depression, but the link between the two is complex, probably involving both the biological and the social effects of illness. Major life events (especially in poor social circumstances, and in the absence of close relationships) are as important in precipitating depression in the old as in the young.

Treatment

Psychological and physical methods of treatment are equally important, and can successfully be combined.

Support

Formal analytic psychotherapy is not recommended, but support informed both by psychotherapeutic principles and by practical common sense is essential. Relatives also need support to help the patient through a depressive illness. Sometimes marital or family therapy is indicated. Cogni-

tive therapy has also successfully been used in old age depression.

Medication

All medication must be started at a low dose, with careful monitoring, and should then be built up gradually until the medication is effective, or side effects prevent further increases. The ultimate dose reached **may** be as high in old as in young people, but beware of precipitating a toxic confusional state. Standard tricyclics may be used; dothiepin is useful where anticholinergic side effects are troublesome; mianserin or lofepramine are safer where cardiotoxicity is a risk. Trazodone is often well-tolerated and can have a useful sedative effect. The place of SSRI's in old age depression is not yet clear: they may precipitate agitation and anxiety. (See Chapter 17 for further discussion of medication, including p. 222.) Lithium is as valuable in the old as in the young for prophylaxis of manic-depressive disorder or recurrent depression, but the risk of side effects is greater. The combination of diuretics with lithium is dangerous without very close supervision of the blood level. Depressive symptoms in the setting of a known dementing illness present great problems in diagnosis and management; toxic side effects of medication can occur at quite low doses. Trazodone may prove to be the safest drug so far in these circumstances, but where the evidence for a depressive illness is strong, ECT may be the best treatment option.

ECT

The safest and most effective treatment of depression in old age. However, it still carries alarming overtones for patients and their relatives, and so tends to be reserved for urgent treatment of severely depressed people, where risk of suicide or dehydration does not permit delay (see pp. 211–213).

Prognosis

The chances of recovery from an episode of depression are good, but there is a high risk of relapse. Only about a third of those who recover remain well over a 3-year follow-up, and the remainder of the patients run a relapsing or chronic course. This is worse than in younger depressives, but in them also it has been recognized that the risk of relapse is high. There is now good evidence that antidepressant treatment should be maintained for at least 2 years, and perhaps for life.

In old age depression, mortality is increased by comparison with non-depressed people of the same age: there is a greater excess of deaths from cardiovascular disease than from other causes. There is some evidence that there may be organic brain changes associated with ageing (different from the changes responsible for dementing illnesses) that are causally related both to depression and to the greater mortality associated with depression in old age.

Mania and hypomania

New onset of manic illness in old age is rare, but many patients with onset of manic-depressive illness in their younger years will continue to have manic as well as depressive episodes as they grow older.

As in depression, the presentation may be atypical. Mania

with thought disorder and pressure of speech, but without overactivity, can resemble dementia or an acute confusional state. Mixed mood states quite commonly occur, with elements of irritability, pessimism, expansiveness and psychotic thinking all occurring simultaneously.

There is an association with physical illness, and underlying causes (such as trauma or infective illness) must be carefully looked for. Pick's disease can present with a hypomanic-like episode.

Treatment is with neuroleptics as with younger patients (but the risks of Parkinsonian side effects and of tardive dyskinesia are greater. Haloperidol is effective as an acute treatment but caution is needed because its long half-life increases the risk of toxicity markedly in the longer term). Lithium may be used as an acute treatment as well as prophylactically.

Other psychiatric conditions

Paranoid states
Both primary and secondary paranoid states (see also Chapter 5, p. 69) can present in old age. One in 10 new admissions in the over-65s to psychiatric hospitals are for paranoid illness, and these include both primary paranoid states and late-onset schizophrenia with paranoid features. A primary paranoid state in old age is sometimes called 'late paraphrenia'. This term refers to 'a well-organized system of paranoid delusions with or without auditory hallucinations existing in the setting of a well-preserved personality and affective response' (Roth).

Secondary paranoid features are often seen in depression, mania, acute confusional states, and dementia (particularly Alzheimer's disease, often early in the disease).

The content of the delusions in a primary paranoid state in old age is often more believable than in young patients, and it may be important to check whether the 'delusional belief' is in fact true. Outside the territory of the delusional belief the patient's social behaviour and day-to-day competence may be little affected. In other cases the persecutory delusions may cause the patient to sabotage the very relationships on which she depends for support.

Primary paranoid states in old age are commoner in women, in the presence of sensory (especially hearing) impairment, and in those with long-standing personality traits of aloofness, withdrawal or suspiciousness. A family history of schizophrenia may be found although not as commonly as in young paranoid patients. The illness usually responds well to medication but, where insight is lost, treatment may need to be started under the Mental Health Act, and be continued with depot medication. Sometimes compliance with medication is erratic due to forgetfulness rather than to resistance, and then pimozide or trifluoperazine can be useful drugs, taken as a single daily dose under the supervision of, say, a home help or a day centre.

Anxiety states
As in younger patients, pathological anxiety can present in a variety of forms: as generalized anxiety, with or without panic attacks, as agoraphobia or a specific phobia, and (probably more commonly than in young people) as hypochondriasis. Apparent onset of an anxiety state in old age may in fact be a new episode in a long-standing recurrent illness; or it may be the manifestation of a lifelong vulnerability that has been revealed by the loss of a protective relationship, for example by the death of a husband. The differential diagnosis of pathological anxiety in old age is from agitated depression, toxic confusional state, withdrawal state (from alcohol or benzodiazepines), and physical illness (such as a cardiac arrhythmia). It is particularly important to make the diagnosis correctly, since each of these conditions requires a different, specific, method of treatment, and none of them will be helped by the unthinking prescription of tranquillizers.

The principles of treatment are the same as with younger patients. Behavioural and cognitive methods can be very successful, but they are likely to need more therapist hours, over a longer period, than with young patients. Benzodiazepines should be avoided even more than in young people, because of the risks of dependence and confusion associated with their use; although in occasional cases the benefits of a low steady dose of benzodiazepine may outweigh the disadvantages.

Alcohol abuse
The prevalence of alcoholism among older people in the community is quoted as 2–10%. This includes many with onset earlier in life (though many alcoholics will have died before reaching 65). For about 10% of elderly alcoholics the problem began after 65, often in response to some environmental stress such as bereavement or retirement, especially where there was unrecognized depression. Presentation may be indirect, by the non-drinking spouse or another relative of the alcoholic becoming ill. Sometimes the presentation is as an emergency, through withdrawal symptoms, delirium tremens (for example after admission to hospital following injury), or Wernicke's encephalopathy. Alcoholism may, alternatively, be recognized as the underlying cause of a different psychiatric condition such as dementia. Abstinence may be easier to achieve than in the young alcoholic, especially where the previous personality was good or where a major change in social circumstances (such as a move into residential care) relieves some of the factors that originally led to or maintained the drinking.

Adjustment reactions
Psychological symptoms occurring in direct relation to major stress occur in old age as at any other, and the frequency of stressful events (especially losses) is greater in old age. Considering the many kinds of loss that old people bear (loss of spouse, home, social role, independence, physical health) the surprising fact is that so many old people cope so well.

Family and relationship problems
As in child psychiatric practice, the old person can become the 'identified patient' in what is really a family problem. (Institutions – residential homes or hospital wards – can act just like families in this respect.) Problems arise when families, especially those with young members, dutifully take a

Case 1

Mr N., a 69-year-old widower, gave up his part-time job in a local garage because he felt he was no longer up to it. He repeatedly consulted his GP with complaints of dyspepsia and constipation, and was afraid that he had cancer; the worry was waking him at night. Eventually the GP referred him for gastroscopy, but the next day he took an overdose of his sleeping tablets. Assessment in hospital revealed that he was unshakeably convinced that his alimentary canal was blocked with cancer, and he refused food and fluids.

A course of ECT was recommended to him, to which he passively agreed. His daughter and son-in-law, believing that he had an irrecoverable illness, put up his house for sale so as to raise funds for him to go into a nursing home. Only firm advice persuaded them to put off the sale.

Giving up activities usually enjoyed, self-criticism, constipation, insomnia, fear of physical illness, tiresome and demanding behaviour can all be features of depression.

Suicide in the elderly is often preceded by contact with a doctor and the prescription of psychotropic medication.

ECT is particularly indicated where delay in the treatment of depression would be dangerous.

Relatives may assume that any psychological symptom in the old is the herald of dementia, and may make hasty decisions without consulting the old person.

Case 2

Mr K., an 82-year-old married man, was admitted to a surgical ward for a transurethral prostatectomy. Postoperatively he was restless and anxious, with rambling speech; he was disoriented, and suspicious of the nurses, though his wife's presence reassured him. With antibiotics for his chest infection, the acute state settled. When interviewed, his wife said that Mr K. had been having difficulty with his memory for 2 years. If he went out he was oblivious of danger, and easily got lost. He often wet himself, but refused to wash or to change.

She had not told her GP feeling it was just his age. She wanted to go on looking after him, but was 85 herself, and afraid that she might die suddenly, leaving him helpless. A discharge plan was worked out, which included home help and day care on the psychogeriatric

Signs of an acute confusional state.

This history and the absence of evidence for any other cause of dementia made the diagnosis of Alzheimer's disease most likely. A relatively mild episode of delirium can bring an unsuspected dementia to light.

Many cases of dementia are unknown to their GPs.

Much of the care of frail elderly people falls on the shoulders of other frail people. Good coordination between hospital, GP, and community services is vital

Case 3

A general practitioner requested an urgent visit to a 76-year-old lady, Mrs B. The psycho-geriatrician arrived to find a patient stuporose, a furious son-in-law, and an exhausted and tearful daughter. With difficulty, the doctor pieced together the story. When Mrs B.'s husband died, her daughter felt bound to bring her to live with her family. Things went wrong from the start. Mrs B. made constant demands on her daughter, criticized her son-in-law, and was resented by her two teenage grandsons. There were frequent rows, and Mrs B. became tearful and withdrawn. The GP prescribed an antidepressant for her, but over the next few days she became agitated and confused. Following an emergency call to the GP she was given an injection of chlorpromazine. Next day Mrs B. was barely rousable, and the son-in-law

A 'something must be done' referral, with little background information.

Major change in living arrangements can lead to adjustment problems; death of a protective spouse may bring to light unsuspected mental illness.

A patient with cognitive impairment is particularly at risk from the side effects of medication.

Escalation of the toxic confusional state by addition of another drug with its own side effects.

With ECT, followed by dothiepin, he made a full recovery, though he remained a rather solitary, uncommunicative man, keeping his distance from family and friends because he was afraid they despised him as a 'looney'. The dothiepin was tailed off after 6 months, but at the next visit by the CPN he was again convinced that he had cancer.

The dothiepin was restarted, and the CPN helped Mr N. to discuss his fears with his family. They responded warmly, and with their support he began to attend a lunch club in the village and to help out occasionally at the garage.

Personality factors may be important in maintaining illness.

Do not forget the stigma of mental illness, especially among the elderly who grew up in the era of permanent commitment to asylums.

Relapse of depression is common in old age, and good follow-up is essential.

Psychotherapeutic work, especially with the family, and pharmacotherapy should complement each other.

ward; a commode was provided for Mr K. to use at night. With his prostatic problems relieved, Mr K. was now dry provided his wife reminded him to use the toilet at regular intervals. The following summer Mr K. was admitted for 2 weeks while Mrs K. visited an old friend; and over the following year the frequency of the relief admissions was increased. As Mrs K. became frailer she asked for Mr K. to be considered for residential care. On a trial admission to a small nursing home he was well liked and seemed happy, and he was offered a permanent place.

Six months later Mr K. developed a chest infection. After careful discussion with Mrs K. and the staff of the home, the GP decided not to prescribe antibiotics, and Mr K. died peacefully 3 days later.

in making a discharge plan work.

Incontinence can have multiple causes, and remedying one may solve the problem.

Support systems for demented patients need to be flexible and capable of changing to meet increasing needs.

Dilemmas concerning 'letting die' and 'striving to keep alive' have to be thought out afresh for each patient, jointly with those concerned with him. (Withholding antibiotics does not always lead to death of course.)

demanded she be 'taken away'. At this point the psycho-geriatrician was called in.

He explained that he would bring Mrs B. into hospital for a short assessment admission, and that he would plan the future together with the family when the assessment was completed. With all medication stopped, Mrs B. emerged as a sociable person, with moderate cognitive impairment, who quickly became anxious if intellectual demands were made on her. Their own strain relieved, the family were keen to have her home again. The CPN visited weekly to help the family involve Mrs B. without overwhelming her, and without neglecting their own needs.

When the first encounter with psychiatric services is in crisis, giving clear and realistic information is especially important.

Caring for an elderly relative at home is a difficult task and needs as much help from the professions as do the elderly living on their own.

parent into their home and only realize the implications later; or when old enmities within a family are played out as power shifts from one generation to the next; or when the old person uses a financial hold (such as ownership of the house or hopes of inheritance) over the family; or when the family together are under some particular pressure or conflict of responsibility arising from outside.

QUESTIONS

1 You are a houseman working on a surgical ward. The nurses tell you that 80-year-old Mrs N. is unmanageable at night, and ask you to prescribe 'something to calm her down'. How do you assess and manage the problem?

2 An enthusiastic Head of Home is appointed to the local authority ('Part III') home in your area. She invites you (a local GP) to give a series of seminars to the care staff on psychiatric problems in old age. What ideas would you especially want to get across to the care staff?

3 At the same home, the staff ask you to see Mr E., a well-liked resident who has recently become surly and irritable. They suspect that he is depressed. What evidence for this diagnosis will you look for?

4 You are the duty social worker in a small town. A middle-aged single woman comes into your office in tears. Her mother came to live with her 3 years ago when she was widowed: now the daughter cannot cope. 'I promised father that I would look after mother when he died, but we never got on before, and now I'm afraid that I will really hit her.' How can you help her? What other sources of help can you turn to?

5 You are a community psychiatric nurse, and regularly visit a voluntary day centre for the elderly. The organizer is upset because Mr B., a new attender, has made suggestive remarks to one of the volunteers, and tried to embrace one of the ladies attending the centre. What can you do to help?

FURTHER READING

Folstein M.F., Folstein S.E. & McHugh P.R. (1975) 'Mini-mental state.' A practical method for grading the cognitive state of patients for the clinician. *J. Psychiatr. Res.* **12**, 189–98.

Jacques A. (1988) *Understanding Dementia.* Churchill Livingstone, Edinburgh. [Excellent account of many aspects of dementia, with a problem-solving approach to management.]

Jacoby R. & Oppenheimer C. (eds) (1991) *Psychiatry in the Elderly.* Oxford University Press, Oxford. [A multiauthor textbook covering the basic sciences (neuropathology, psychology, etc.), clinical syndromes, and practical interventions relevant to old age psychiatry.]

Mace N.L., Rabins P.V. & Castleton B.A. (1985) *The Thirty-Six Hour Day.* Hodder & Stoughton with Age Concern. [The British version of an American book written for relatives, which all professionals should read for its practical wisdom and insight.]

Mahendra B. (1984) *Dementia.* MTP Press Ltd, Lancaster. [Deals with subject of dementia in depth and with enthusiasm, with much interesting detail (including a chapter on famous people who became demented).]

Murphy E. (ed) (1986) *Affective Disorders in the Elderly.* Churchill Livingstone, Edinburgh. [Survery of present knowledge in this important field, where many questions await further research.]

Wattis J. & Church M. (1986) *Practical Psychiatry of Old Age.* Croom Helm, Beckenham, Kent. [A concise, clear and eminently practical book; especially good on psychological aspects.]

USEFUL ADDRESSES

Age Concern, Astral House, 1268 London Road, London SW16 4ER (tel: 081-679-8000).

Carers' National Association, 20–25 Glass House Yard, London EC1A 4JS (tel: 071-490-8818).

Alzheimer's Disease Society, Gordon House, 10 Greencoat Place, London SW1P 1PH (tel: 071-306-0606).

14
Learning Disability

Fact sheet

Definition
A condition of arrested or incomplete development of the mind, which is especially characterized by impairment of skills manifested during the developmental period, and contributing to the overall level of intelligence, i.e. cognitive, language, motor and social abilities.

Classification
The assessment of intellectual level should be based on whatever information is available.
1 Clinical findings.
2 Adaptive behaviour.
3 Psychometric test: (a) profound, IQ 0–20; (b) severe, IQ 20–35; (c) moderate, IQ 35–50; (d) mild, IQ 50–70.

Epidemiology
Prevalence rates:
- profound: 1 in 2000 population;
- severe and moderate: 1 in 300 population;
- mild: 1 in 70 population.

Historical and contemporary perspectives
- Mental Health Act 1959.
- Education Acts 1971 and 1981.
- Disabled Persons Act 1986.
- Care in the Community 1990.
- Children Act 1989.

Presentation and diagnosis
- *At birth* if a clinical syndrome is present which is invariably associated with an intellectual impairment.
- *In infancy*, through recognition of a delay in development. The greater the degree of disability the earlier the diagnosis.
- *At school age* with learning difficulties.
- *As an adult* reacting under stress with emotional ill-health and social difficulties in relationships, day-to-day tasks, etc.

Aetiology

Genetic conditions
- Single abnormal gene.
- Chromosome abnormalities.
- Multi-factorial.

Environmental
- Infections.
- Trauma.
- Asphyxia.
- Toxins.
- Tumours.

Assessment
1 Medical investigations.
2 Consideration of factors influencing development.
3 Multi-professional assessment.
4 Shared action planning and care management.
5 Review of plans.
6 Re-assessment at life transition points: (a) school-age; (b) leaving school; (c) leaving further education; (d) leaving home.

Services

Helping families and carers
- Involving parents, carers and the disabled person as partners.
- Allocating time for the expression of anxieties and disappointment.
- Assessment and action in the interest of the person's total living environment.

Helping a person learn social independence and interaction skills
- Establishing communications and a positive relationship.
- Breaking down each skill to be taught into components.
- Teaching each step in natural sequence.

Presentation of associated medical conditions
1 Dependent on recognition by parents and carers: (a) unusual or out-of-character behaviour; (b) unusual appearance.
2 Associated conditions: epilepsy, 30–70% risk.

Presentation of associated psychiatric disorders
- Majority of people do not have a psychiatric disorder, their behaviour is consistent with their intellectual impairment.
- Psychiatric disorder does occur in approximately 30% of people with a moderate or severe learning disability.
- A change of conduct or behaviour is the commonest presentation.
- Significant numbers have recognizable disorders of mood, neurotic reactions to stress or organic disorders.
- A firm diagnosis of schizophrenia is only possible in those people with sufficient language.

Behavioural analysis and treatment of distressing behaviour
1 Eliminate medical cause for behavioural change.
2 Evaluate effect of recent life events or changes in relationships.
3 Analysis of patterns of behaviour: (a) antecedents; (b) behavioural description of problem; (c) consequent events which may be reinforcing and maintaining the behaviour.
4 Plan of care: (a) list of activities the person likes and ways of communicating; (b) description of each goal to be achieved in given time; (c) method to be used; (d) review of success or failure of the care plan; (e) replan for same goal or new goal.

Services for people with learning disability
- Community learning disability team.
- Alternatives to parental care.

What is learning disability?

A person with significant intellectual impairment, resulting from a genetic disorder or arising during their development, has difficulty in learning and in attaining the standards for their age and cultural group in the following areas:

- communication;
- social skills;
- personal independence;
- self-sufficiency.

In this country 'learning disability' is the popular and official term for this condition known internationally as mental retardation.

The definition of 'mental retardation' found in the tenth edition of the *International Classification of Diseases* (F70–F79) appears under the heading of mental disorders. The definition is as follows 'a condition of arrested or incomplete development of mind which is especially characterised by impairment of skills manifested during the developmental period, contributing to the overall level of intelligence, i.e. cognitive, language, motor, and social abilities'. The level of intellectual functioning is determined by assessment with a general intelligence test and significantly below average performance is defined by a standard score (e.g. IQ) more that two standard deviations from the mean (e.g. IQ 70).

However, the IQ should not be applied rigidly and assessment of the person's level of functioning should be based on clinical evidence of adaptive behaviour as well as psychometric tests.

'Intelligence is not a unitary characteristic but is assessed on the basis of a large number of different more-or-less specific skills'. People may show severe impairments in one particular area, e.g. language, or a particular higher skill in another area, e.g. visuo-spatial tasks. This presents a problem in deciding on the severity or overall level of learning disability.

The affected person may learn some or none of the necessary skills for living unsupported and the amount they achieve will ultimately determine the severity of their handicap.

How is learning disability classified?

The World Health Organization (1968) uses the following terms:

- *Profound handicap.* Those people who require total care to maintain life (IQ 0–20).
- *Severe handicap.* People who will develop sufficient self-care skills to wash, dress, feed and keep continent but may have insufficient language to be understood by strangers. They require social support from family and or trained staff working alongside, enabling them to form relationships and enhance their feelings of self-worth through learning new things and achieving some control over their own lives (IQ 20–35).
- *Moderate handicap.* People who will achieve success in personal hygiene, develop sufficient language to be able to communicate their wishes and choices, participate in everyday living tasks and leisure pursuits, to their own and others'

satisfaction and pleasure. As adults they require the stimulus of family, friends or paid care person to maintain their skills and to enable them to participate in community life (IQ 35–50).

- *Mild handicap.* A large number of children known to have learning difficulties in academic subjects and to have intelligence quotients two or three standard deviations from the mean adapt to work and marriage as adults and are not subsequently identified as different from the rest of the population (IQ 50–70).

Learning disability prevalence rates

- *Profound handicap*: 1 person in 2000.
- *Severe and moderate handicap*: 3 persons in 1000.
- *Mild handicap*: varies according to the case-finding methods used. Studies of whole populations reveal a peak in numbers identified around age 14 at 14 per 1000.

Fig. 14.1 Historical perspectives

Since the 17th century our society has recognized some people as being 'stupid', unable to learn like others, being different in both appearance and behaviour and having a condition which originates in childhood and persists throughout life. The term idiot, imbecile and moron are in use today as descriptions of incomprehensible behaviour and are applied in a derogatory manner. At one point in history the terms idiot, imbecile and feeble-minded person were recognized terms in the field of education. The Education Acts 1870 and 1899 were attempting to distinguish between those people who could benefit from education and those who could not but who may respond to 'training'. Society was also interested in separating those who were from birth considered unlikely to be able to guard against common dangers and support themselves as adults, from lunatics who became unable to do so later in life. People thus identified could under the law be detained in registered hospitals or institutions for care. The categories were defined in the Mental Deficiency Act of 1913.

The legislation was accompanied by the widely held belief that mental defectives were a danger to society because they were potential criminals, immoral, usually the carriers of venereal diseases, and the women had many children all of whom were as defective as themselves. These are myths but at the time society adopted the policy of 'segregation' to prevent mentally defective people reproducing and increasing these undesirable elements in the population.

People were 'certified as mentally deficient' and 'put away' in recognized institutions. Within the institution segregation of male from female was a further assurance of non-reproduction. These institutions grew in numbers and in size (as large as 2000 places) and society lost sight of the original reasons for promoting them, preferring to consider their provision was necessary in the interest of the handicapped people who must surely wish 'to live with their own kind'. The 1945 Health Act brought these institutions into the hospital service and doctors and nurses were established as the carers and treatment givers.

The 1959 Mental Health Act introduced the concept of **subnormality** and **severe subnormality**. These were defined as a **'condition of arrested or incomplete development of mind'**. There was discussion before the Act became law on whether the 'intelligence quotient' or 'mental age' as measured by psychometric tests should be included as a criteria for the detaining of a person under this section. The medical establishment recommended its exclusion as they considered people with dull–normal and even normal intellect may have characteristics from early youth of an underdeveloped mind resulting in failure to achieve normal social behaviour.

Continued on p. 170

After the Mental Health Act, 1959, the vast majority of people detained in hospitals became 'voluntary patients' and very few have been admitted compulsorily for treatment from that time unless they have a diagnosed mental illness.

In the 1960s social policies started to change towards people with disabilities. North American and Scandinavian countries reduced the size of their institutions. Results of research in this country in the mid-1960s on the care of mentally retarded children (the Brookland Experiment) acted as stimulus to change. A small group of children were taken out of a large hospital and lived in a small family-type unit. Their developmental progress was significantly quicker than a matched control group of similar children left in the large hospital.

In 1969 'The Ely Report', an inquiry into care received by people in a large hospital led to a government white paper published in **1971** called **'Better Services for the Mentally Handicapped'**. Health and local authorities have used the policy statements and requirements predicted in this document as a basis for planning and operating present services. The Government set up a National Development Group to promote good practices. Although this was disbanded there remains a National Development Team whose remit is to visit district health authorities and local authority Social Services departments by invitation and encourage joint planning between them and modern care practices throughout the UK.

The 1971 and 1981 Education Acts have set the scene for the future provision by making it a statutory requirement for all handicapped children whatever the severity of the disability to receive education from the age of 2–19 years.

If a child is ascertained as having **special educational needs**, a multidisciplinary assessment involving the parents, followed by a written statement of the requirements must be undertaken and reviewed at least annually.

The Mental Health Act 1983 definition excludes a person with a learning disability from being compulsorily detained in hospital, except under the short order Section 2, 4, or 136, 137, unless they suffer from **'mental impairment'** which is defined as **'severe or significant impairment of intelligence and social functioning associated with abnormally aggressive or seriously irresponsible conduct on the part of the person concerned'**.

The Royal Society for Mentally Handicapped Children and Adults (MENCAP) promoted the view that learning disability is not a mental disorder but a socially defined disability.

The Children Act 1989 states children with disabilities should be given the same rights and access to services as all other children.

In 1991 Stephen Dorrell, a health minister, in a speech to MENCAP said that there was national agreement to use the term 'learning disability' instead of 'mental handicap'. People with intellectual impairments who can articulate their views do not like the work 'mental'. They wish to avoid all labelling and be accepted by society as people with individual special needs.

Diagnosis and assessment

Presentation and diagnosis

A prediction that a person will have a special educational needs can be made at birth or even prenatally if there is clinical evidence of a condition invariably associated with an impairment of cognitive, language, motor and social abilities, i.e. Down's syndrome.

Those children who do not have an obvious physical or physiological abnormality at birth will come to the attention through delay in reaching their developmental milestones. The greater the severity of their mental retardation the earlier the diagnosis will be made. Most mildly disabled children will reach school age before their difficulties become apparent. They are slow to grasp the fundamentals of reading, writing and calculating. If the teacher refers to the school psychological service their intellectual impairment will be revealed on the administration of psychometric tests.

There are a few people with mild learning disability not ascertained as children as having a significant intellectual impairment who are referred to the learning disability services as adults either because they are reacting to stress with unadaptive behaviours or they have a diagnosable mental illness which has been unrecognized.

Causation

A **mild learning disability** will be determined by several interacting factors, i.e. genetic, educational, social and environmental. It is rare to find a specific underlying medical condition but a considerable number of mildly learning disabled people will have signs of neurological damage and a significant number will have associated demographic features of social deprivation, i.e. poor housing, overcrowding and generally poor health.

In about two-thirds of **moderately** or **severely** learning disabled people, it is possible to diagnose a specific pathological condition known to impair intellectual function.

Medical investigations

The diagnosing of a biomedical condition underlying an intellectual impairment will usually be undertaken by a paediatric assessment centre. A careful history followed by physical examination and investigations should be done as shown in Fig. 14.2. The medical investigation of all children and adults with an intellectual impairment should be undertaken.

1 To ensure that any biomedical pathology which is causing abnormal development of the individual is diagnosed and if possible treated, so ameliorating its impact.

2 To give parents wherever possible an explanation of the cause of the intellectual impairment.

3 To diagnose any condition which may be genetic in origin, so enabling family members to receive genetic counselling on the risks of their offspring being affected.

4 To mount a programme for prenatal diagnosis for future pregnancies, if this is possible for the condition concerned, and the parents so wish.

Assessment

The overall aims are to assess the numerous factors which may be influencing the development of a child (or adult) using the expertise of different disciplines and through co-ordinating their findings to generate an **individual planned programme** for clinical, therapeutic and educational management.

The objectives of assessment are the following.

1 To diagnose any biomedical cause for the handicap which could be treated or ameliorated.

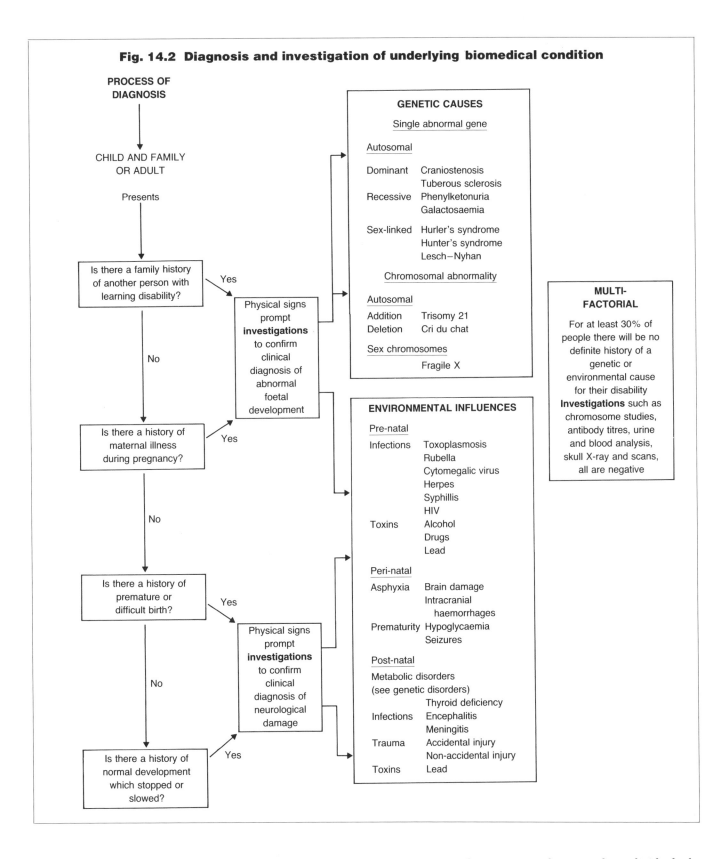

Fig. 14.2 Diagnosis and investigation of underlying biomedical condition

PROCESS OF DIAGNOSIS

CHILD AND FAMILY OR ADULT

Presents

Is there a family history of another person with learning disability? — Yes

No

Is there a history of maternal illness during pregnancy? — Yes

No

Is there a history of premature or difficult birth? — Yes

No

Is there a history of normal development which stopped or slowed? — Yes

Physical signs prompt **investigations** to confirm clinical diagnosis of abnormal foetal development

Physical signs prompt **investigations** to confirm clinical diagnosis of neurological damage

GENETIC CAUSES

Single abnormal gene

Autosomal

Dominant — Craniostenosis / Tuberous sclerosis
Recessive — Phenylketonuria / Galactosaemia
Sex-linked — Hurler's syndrome / Hunter's syndrome / Lesch–Nyhan

Chromosomal abnormality

Autosomal

Addition — Trisomy 21
Deletion — Cri du chat

Sex chromosomes — Fragile X

ENVIRONMENTAL INFLUENCES

Pre-natal

Infections — Toxoplasmosis / Rubella / Cytomegalic virus / Herpes / Syphillis / HIV
Toxins — Alcohol / Drugs / Lead

Peri-natal

Asphyxia — Brain damage / Intracranial haemorrhages
Prematurity — Hypoglycaemia / Seizures

Post-natal

Metabolic disorders (see genetic disorders) — Thyroid deficiency
Infections — Encephalitis / Meningitis
Trauma — Accidental injury / Non-accidental injury
Toxins — Lead

MULTI-FACTORIAL

For at least 30% of people there will be no definite history of a genetic or environmental cause for their disability **Investigations** such as chromosome studies, antibody titres, urine and blood analysis, skull X-ray and scans, all are negative

2 To ascertain any other medical condition which may interfere with learning such as visual/auditory impairments.
3 To assess degree of intellectual functioning.
4 To assess degree of developmental delay.
5 To assess the person's emotional development.
6 To assess the family's needs for support.

7 To examine the interaction between the individual, the immediate environment, education and social settings and to assess the strengths and weaknesses of the whole support system.
8 To construct a plan of care in the form of an individual planned programme.

Fig. 14.3 Clinical features of the two most common syndromes

Down's syndrome
First described by Down in 1866. The report of the extra chromosome being present was by Lejeune in 1959. Frequency is 1 in 600 births.

Physical features
- Eyes have upward and outward slant.
- There are epicanthal folds.
- The palpebral fissure is oblique.
- White patches on the edge of the iris. Brushfield spots.
- Head is small and occiput is flattened.
- Ears small and low set.
- Legs and arms short, hands broad and flat and the little fingers have a single crease; 50% of people have a single palm crease.
- At birth babies are hypotonic but this reduces later.

Accompanying potentially disabling conditions:
- 80–90% have a hearing loss;
- 30–40% heart defect;
- 0–4% congenital duodenal atresia;
- 4–8% cataract or keratoconus.

Increased risk of following disorders:
- leukaemia;
- thyroid dysfunction;
- Alzheimer's disease.

Fragile X chromosome
Described in 1969 by Lubs. Fragile site on the long arm of the X chromosome. Accounts for approximately 30% of all learning disability. Affects 1 in 600 males. Fewer women are affected and rarely have physical features.

Physical features
All of the following are only present in 50% of affected men:
- elongated faces;
- large and prominent ears;
- macro-orchidism.

Accompanying abnormalities
- Speech and language delay.
- Hyperactivity.
- Autistic features.
- Increased risk of psychiatric disorder.

Fig. 14.4 Assessment of a child with developmental problems

1 Diagnosis of any factors which have caused the mental impairment (paediatrician).

2 Explanation and clarification with parents of diagnosis and medical prognosis (paediatrician, general practitioner, health visitor).

3 Multidisciplinary assessment of child and family needs
Child:
- associated medical conditions (paediatrician);
- sensory impairments (audiometrist, ENT surgeon, optomotrist, ophthalmic surgeon);
- physical disabilities (physiotherapist, orthopaedic surgeon);
- feeding and communication (speech and language therapist);
- dietary needs (dietician);
- intellectual impairment and educational needs (educational psychologist and teacher);
- emotional and social behaviour (clinical psychologist);
- symptoms of emotional illness (child psychiatrist).
Family:
- social circumstances and emotional health of family (social worker);
- symptoms of emotional illness (psychiatrist).

4 Family/child service requirements: case conference to decide which services required to enable learning and maximum potential development of child to be achieved and secondary handicaps prevented (community child/health doctor, educational psychologist, social worker, teacher).

5 Individual programme plan
- written with *parents as partners*
- identification of appropriate keyworker or case coordinator (health visitor, paediatric nurse, teacher counsellor, community nurse registered in learning disability, general practitioner, or any of the former).

6 Regular review built into plans for care and treatment and education. Re-assessment at life transition points:
- pre-school–school;
- junior school–senior school;
- school–further education;
- education setting–work/occupation;
- family care–own home.

Individual planned programmes

To be successful the parents or carers and the person with the disability need to be involved in the formulation of the priorities for treatment and be encouraged to participate as partners with the professional in the implementation of the agreed programme. A named professional should be chosen as the programme coordinator usually the keyworker and regular review of the plan should take place.

There are certain critical points in the lifecycle when the multidisciplinary review should be called. These are when major choices have to be made.
1 Special or usual nursery school.
2 Neighbourhood school or special school.
3 Secondary education.
4 Further education (statutory review of someone with special educational needs takes place at $13\frac{1}{2}$ years of age).
5 Leaving home.
6 Day occupational/work placement.

Parental and family reaction

Families describe their response to the news of their child's intellectual impairment as 'shock at the tragedy', both for themselves at the loss of their expected 'complete child' and for the child, who is unlikely to experience or achieve success as measured by our society. Following the shock of the news there follows a 'reality crisis' resulting from the practical problems of organizing the family's daily life around the extra demands made on the parents by a disabled child. Family life will be affected at every stage thereafter.

The establishing of a marital partnership, followed by adjustment to being parents and the arrival of the first child is stressful. The joy of the baby's birth and the excitement and speculation about its future will compensate. Pride in announcing the new member and showing them off to relatives and friends are accepted and expected happenings. If, however, the baby is physically different, the perfect person of whom there were high hopes is taken away. They are lost and are to be replaced by a child whom people pity rather than admire, who is an embarrassment rather than someone to be proud of. Feelings of not being able to cope are present in all new parents but will be reinforced because of the uncertainty over how the baby will develop.

After being told the news, whether the diagnosis is made at birth or if it is made later, parents will mourn the loss of the imagined perfect person before they can accept the real one.

Case 1

Family care and a plan for life. Sarah is the youngest of a family of four children. Her mother recognized there was something abnormal about her baby's appearance at the time of her birth but none of the staff in the maternity suite made any comment, so she kept her anxieties to herself. Later the same day her husband came back to see her, saying they had an appointment with the consultant paediatrician. Both parents were asked into a private office to see the consultant; the senior nurse was also present. They were asked if they had noticed anything unusual about the baby. The consultant pointed out the physical features which indicated to him that this baby was likely to have *Down's syndrome.*

The manner in which parents are told the news of their child's disability will depend on the personal style of the doctor and the certainty of the diagnosis.

There followed an exchange and clarification on how the baby may develop. Emphasis was on the *similarity to other babies but with the added dimension of a delay in acquiring skills,* rather than the differences. A brief mention was made of the *help which could be expected* from the health, education and local authority services and from contact with other parents of children with Down's syndrome. The interview closed with the consultant pointing out that the senior nurse would be available during the rest of the day to continue the discussion and answer queries about what had been said. The consultant could be contacted by telephone if required and would return the next day in any case to see them.

The initial shock and distress when the parents are told of their baby's disability prevents them concentrating on the contents of the initial interview.

The parents were put in touch with the Down's Syndrome Society. They received a visit from another parent whom they found very supportive.

A variety of feelings are experienced by the parents at this time. There is a sense of grief and loss – the hopes for the expected child are taken away by the news. The usual feelings of protectiveness towards the helpless baby may mingle with revulsion at the stigmatizing physical appearance.

Sarah was *assessed at the paediatric centre* and her health visitor was chosen to be the keyworker for the family to ensure *a coordinated treatment programme and regular reviews of her progress.* A teacher/counsellor employed by the education authority visited and adjustments were made within the family so teaching time could be given to Sarah, particularly focused on communication.

Feelings of inadequacy and uncertainty about how to 'cope' are relieved for the parents by being given practical tasks to help their child develop. The aim is for them to achieve a sense of competency in their own abilities to teach self-help skills.

Sarah went to a *special play group,* then the *nursery class of a special school* and remained in the same school until aged 11. She then moved to the *local comprehensive school to a 'special needs class'.* She attained a reading age equivalent to an 8-year-old; an ability to calculate at the level of a 4-year-old. She and classmates participated in art classes, cookery and other practical subjects with others of their age and mixed at social times (lunch and break) with the rest of the school. She was then a student at a College of Further Education. The curriculum was aimed at teaching her hygiene, care of her clothes, the use of public transport, shopping, preparing simple 'survival' meals, use of the telephone and how to summon help in an emergency, etc. She concentrated for long periods and was pleased when she achieved.

The policy in education of segregation and specialization has changed over the last decade to one of integration into the usual educational institutions. The individual teaching programmes provide for participation in the ordinary school curriculum.

After leaving college at 19, Sarah became a trainee in a small business which packed stationery. She is one of three disabled people employed by the firm. She is able to learn quite complicated tasks providing they are taught in stages.

Sarah has a girlfriend with whom she spends an evening a week but she oftens states she wants a boyfriend. Her *disabilities in language remain* and strangers have difficulty in understanding her. She is friendly and will try to engage people in conversation. Her *family are concerned about the dangers of exploitation* and particularly by the thought of her having a sexual relationship resulting in pregnancy.

Physical pubertal changes in people with Down's syndrome are usually later for both sexes. Fertility is reduced but achieved by females, not having been reported in males. The fundamental desire for an emotional attachment to another person, including a sexual need, is always developed.

Her family feel she is capable of learning new social and living skills and despite their feelings of protectiveness would wish her to eventually move into her own home. However, they are certain she will *need support and supervision by themselves or paid carers for the rest of her life* despite her emotional adjustment, her independence in self-care skills and her way of life.

Parents with pre-school children

The pre-school years are filled with hard physical work, washing, feeding, dressing, keeping young people occupied and it is usual for one parent to take more of the burden. Parents of a disabled child may not see any progress in self-care and feel this time is stretching away into the future. Professional staff may be suggesting 'early intervention' programmes which encourage and teach parents how to help their child. The parents have the dilemma of apportioning time to all the family members and any special sessions may overload them and reinforce their feelings of not coping. Most parents of young children try to have a baby-sitting arrangement so they can have time off, but friends and family may not feel very comfortable in looking after a disabled child and therefore parents' time alone together may be limited.

Parents with schoolchildren

The choosing of a school and anticipation of joining with other families in school activities and in watching the social and academic achievements of their child will be very different for parents, particularly when the choice has to be made for special education in a segregated school. However, it may be a relatively peaceful time for the family once the school has been accepted by their child and themselves.

Parents with adolescent children

Puberty brings the worry of choice of secondary school and the realization that the usual growth in independence is not going to happen. Parents will be confronted by their adolescent children on many issues including attitudes to sex but for the disabled adolescent daughter or son there will be an ambivalence wishing them to do things that others do but also wanting to protect them from exploitation and/or hurt feelings over broken relationships. There will be the strong wish to deny this child has sexual feelings and is growing into an adult.

This is the time when there appears no end to the dependence as there may be nowhere to go, no work and few if any leisure activities which are acceptable and accepting of people with a disability.

Older parents

If their son or daughter remains with them, they will be denied the chance to renew their own relationship at the 'empty nest stage' and to develop new interests and activities. They may keep the disabled person dependent on them until they in turn become old and dependent on others.

Provision of services

Helping families and carers

Families who have been asked to look back at their experiences since first hearing the news of their child's impairment are usually agreed that professional staff, doctors, nurses, social workers, teachers, etc., will achieve greater cooperation and success when conducting interviews and treatment programmes if they are aware of the following.

1 Time given by the professional person to the family or carers during which they are enabled to ask questions about the affected development of their child is very valuable.

2 Honest admission of not knowing the answer followed by an **expressed willingness to find out** enhances the professional's image.

3 Acknowledgement to parents and care workers that they are the experts in the person's behaviour patterns will give them confidence to report unusual or 'out of character behaviour' which can then receive early attention.

4 Taking care to demonstrate that the same thoroughness is being taken in a physical examination, an investigative procedure and/or treatment as for any other member of society, will allay usually unexpressed fears that standards are being altered because the person has 'learning disability' and therefore 'devalued' in the eyes of the professional.

5 Recognition of parents and care workers as partners and their inclusion in all decisions over therapy and 'care programmes' is more likely to lead to successful outcome.

6 Parents hope for **empathic understanding** of their inner feelings about their child's disability. Consequently the professional should repeatedly **create opportunities** for their expression but **not demand** self-revelation.

7 At those times when the **emotional health of the whole family or care group has to be considered**, the professional person needs to take the initiative. One or more family or other group members may be overwhelmed by the stress of living with and caring for a disabled person. The functioning of the whole family or living group should be assessed as a total system and the professional in contact should judge if a period of relief from care may be in everyone's interest. This concept 'in the interest of the family or group as a whole' is not often appreciated by parents or carers **at the time** and they resist taking up offers of relief care because they feel it is 'giving up' or they are 'failing' their person with a disability. The professional then has to use his/her expertise in changing the family or care staff's perspective of the situation and encourage them to accept a sharing of the burden of care.

Finally, both family therapy, particularly of a supportive or restorative type and individual counselling have an important role in helping families and carers.

Helping the disabled person: self-care and social interaction skills

1 Most researchers agree babies and young children participating in organized **'early intervention programmes'** acquire skills quicker than those not receiving a specific programme. A considerable amount of time and energy has to be given by the parents or care person to such a structured teaching regime if it is to be effective.

2 Educationalists and parents are increasingly aware of the importance of their **interactions with the child being 'fun' for both**. Finding out what a person of any age likes and dislikes, what activities they will initiate for themselves and their particular rhythms over eating, sleeping, moods, etc., are the basis for any close relationship. Learning takes place most readily within a mutual positive teacher/pupil interaction.

3 Establishing communication with the disabled person is the first requirement if they are to learn about the world and satisfy even their most basic human wants and needs. Communication of wants and wishes starts with the realization by the person that if they do something, it is followed by something happening back, i.e., if they make a particular noise or gesture they get food or a social response from another person.

Many children and adults with cerebral damage have a far greater understanding of language than they are ever able to express because of physical articulation difficulties. Down's syndrome children have difficulty in articulation because of their relatively large tongue and the configuration of their mouth and palate. Hearing and visually impaired children are in most need of an 'alternative' or 'additional system' of communication. These systems have and are being developed, i.e. British sign language, Makaton, Bliss communication boards, computers, etc., but the fundamental learning of 'symbolic' meaning has to come first.

4 Initiation of exploratory and purposeful activity is diminished in people with an intellectual disability and they require others to stimulate them and constantly bring to their attention any interesting features of their environment or activity in which they are engaged. If left without teaching, training or prompting they will withdraw into their own inner world and indulge in ritualistic, purposeless activity. They need their families and or carers to help them participate and make sense of the world around them.

5 There has been considerable **research into the methods of teaching living skills**, such as communication, dressing, control of bladder and bowel, hygiene, etc., and the principles on which success has been based are those of **'operant conditioning'** and the breaking down of each skill into small steps, teaching each step separately but in a natural sequence. The usual teaching programme has the following stages:

- assessment with the person of their skills, personality, likes, dislikes, atc.;
- agreement with the person and or his/her carers on the priorities for the individual of learning a particular skill;
- listing of the objectives of the teaching programme including a written description of the skill to be taught;
- selecting who is to teach the skill;
- writing down the sequence of steps required and, using previous knowledge of that person's likes, the rewards to be given;
- implementing teaching of each step with desired behaviour followed by reward;
- monitoring the progress at every stage of the programme and adapting techniques accordingly;
- evaluation of the success of the programme and whether the objectives are achieved or not and if not, *why*.

General services

Invariably a person with a disability will need the help of several different professionals at various stages in their development. As these professionals will be employed by different authorities, i.e. health, social services, education, there is a need to bring them together to work as a team. Most districts have district handicap teams for children and also community learning disability teams which work along-side. Community paediatricians and child psychiatrists are usually members of the district handicap team and specialist psychiatrists are members of the community learning disability team.

The Community Learning Disability Team

The aims of this team are to ensure services are coordinated and available as near to the person, his family and/or care worker as is possible and practical. Team membership may include a nurse (trained in learning disability), social worker, doctor, psychologist, occupational, speech and physiotherapists giving all or part of their time to the activities of the team.

The numbers of individuals who constitute the team, their professional background and the size of the population they serve varies nationally. The team members will all have experience in working directly with people with a learning disability and their families and expect to also offer advice, information and practical help to doctors, nurses and therapists in the general health services, to residential, day and field social workers in social services and educationalists in schools and colleges.

A proportion of the team's work is given to assessing and treating those people with learning disability, their families or care persons who have special problems. These would only be a small minority of the people with a learning disability in the catchment area.

The work of the teams for adults may alter under the care in the community policies. Social services have been given the lead responsibility for identifying need and arranging services for people with learning disability. They will have to provide assessment and care management for those who meet the eligibility criteria. The practice of involving the person with a learning disability in their assessment has been the practice within the specialist health and social services for many years. The term 'shared action planning' describes the process.

Fig. 14.5 Role of a Community Learning Disability Team

1 To identify those people who have learning disability living in the catchment population, assess and register each person's current and future needs for service.

2 To document the local provision in terms of:
- family support and relief care;
- residential services;
- day-care centres;
- leisure activities;
- voluntary-run services;
- educational opportunities;
- work opportunities.

3 To make themselves available to be consulted by other professionals, the person with the learning disability and/or their families or carers.

4 To structure their internal organization so they are effective in:
- advertising their service;
- receiving and processing referrals;
- assessing a person's total needs through shared action planning;
- selecting the appropriate services with them;
- operating a specialist treatment programme when required.

Alternatives to parental care

The developmental needs of children require that they have a caring adult to relate to, whose attention is not shared with too many others and who will stimulate the child's interest in their surroundings, encouraging learning and independence.

Children

There are a few children with learning disability who live away from their family of origin. A child with learning disability, whose family is unable to care for them, will be treated like any other child under the Children Act 1989. Fostering is the ideal but if this proves difficult to arrange, a place will be provided either in a children's home or a residential school. This will depend on the age and needs of the individual child.

Families differ in the manner in which they cope with their handicapped child and the added work they entail. Although parents are often reluctant to subject their child to the experience of being away from them they sometimes recognize that for the general welfare of the whole family a periodic relief from care is required. The accessibility to the family and their satisfaction with the standard of the short-term relief service may influence the timing of their request for permanent alternative care and delay it for years. Various schemes exist, including the following:

Parent organized. Parents organize themselves into a mutual support group and run baby-sitting or holiday stays on a token exchange basis.

Linked foster family. Foster parents paid for by statutory services are linked with several families who negotiate periods of relief care for the handicapped child.

Staffed group homes. In some localities there is a short-term relief service based on a staffed house able to care for several children at any one time. The person-in-charge organizes the admissions and contracts with families to provide regular periods of relief care throughout the year and offer support and care during unforeseen crises.

Adolescents

The main developmental need for an adolescent is to prepare for leaving home as a competent adult. This should be catered for during their stay away from their family. The type of accommodation chosen, i.e. alternative family or peer-group living should provide the following:
- promotion of social interaction skills;
- creation of opportunities for choice;
- the handling of responsibility and risks.

These should be reflected in the operational policies of the agency running the service and be clearly understood by the families who participate.

At this stage many more families become aware of their inability to attend to the development of their other children because of the burden of physical care for a teenager with multiple handicaps or of the disruption to family life from someone with troublesome behaviour.

They either look for some relief care or ask for an increase if they are already receiving it. In organizing the services for those with extra special needs such as multiple physical and profound learning disability or physical frailty, it has to be remembered that they are not compatible with young people who are behaviourally disturbed, i.e. over-active and destructive. Fostering in a linked family or a stay in a staffed group home are the main possibilities.

Adults

It should be expected that a person with learning disability will live independently from the family when they reach adulthood. Some families prefer to care for the disabled person within their own home but others wish their son or daughter to be away from them. The options available are often very few and the amount of support and residential accommodation limited. Around **two-thirds of adults** with learning disability **live with their families** and attend day centres organized by social services. The following schemes may exist.

Health organized and funded. Specialist health services are provided for people who need the expertise of specifically trained doctors, nurses, therapists because of multiple or complex health-related problems such as profound life-threatening conditions, physical disabilities and or behaviour which is distressing or dangerous to the person or those around them. This expertise should be in the form of personnel supporting a person in ordinary accommodation in the community adapted to the person's needs.

Social services organized and funded. Hostels, staffed and unstaffed, houses for a small group, warden-controlled flats, lodgings in paid foster family, lodgings with a specially paid landlady.

Private or voluntary organized and funded agencies. Registered homes – large and small, warden-controlled special housing. Village communities run by charitable trusts.

Physical and psychiatric disorders

Physical illness

A person with a learning disability is at greater risk of physical and emotional ill-health than other people. It is particularly important to diagnose and treat physical disorders both to relieve the distress they cause, about which the person might not be able to communicate and to ensure that learning difficulties are not compounded.

Recognition that the person who cannot express themselves verbally is unwell will be made by those who know them on the basis of change in their usual behaviour. As with babies and infants, the doctor and patient have to rely on the observations and actions of parents or carers in seeking medical aid. It is important therefore that the general practitioner and parents and/or carers establish a mutual trusting relationship.

General medical conditions

General history taking and an enquiry of bodily functions may lead to a diagnosis but particular difficulties may be experienced in recognizing pain from the following:

- tooth decay;
- otitis media;
- joint disease;
- oesophageal reflux;
- dysmenorrhoea;
- migraine.

Epilepsy

The prevalence rate of a single epileptic seizure in the general population is 5% and in those with learning disability it is between 30 and 70% the risk increasing with the severity of the handicap.

There are two types of epileptic seizures which are difficult to diagnose in a person with a learning disability. A partial seizure may go undiagnosed as the outward signs are facial or limb movements which an untrained observer may associate with the learning disability; and an 'absence seizure' of under 3 seconds which causes subtle changes in behaviour unlikely to be recognized. This can be very serious if the absences occur in a series with very little time between each one. During an absence the person will be unable to respond to instructions and therefore unable to learn.

Aggression as part of a previously diagnosed seizure has been reported in many studies but it is very rare for it to be the presenting feature of epilepsy. The aggression associated with a seizure will characteristically be of acute onset, brief (under a minute) and be a series of purposeless movements of the limbs. It may occur particularly during the course of a partial seizure and the confusional state following a generalized seizure.

Close surveillance is required of the anti-epileptic medication prescribed for someone with a learning disability. This ensures the successful control of the seizures which may change over time, in frequency and/or type. It also ensures that the person is not suffering from the side effects of the medication. Reliance on maintaining drug blood levels within the therapeutic range is not sufficient as the individual responses to the same dose are so varied in people with a learning disability. Good record keeping by the parents or carers, who should have the reasons for doing so explained to them, is the best method of judging the least amount of medication to give satisfactory control. Mono rather than polypharmacy is the aim so the person's learning abilities are potentiated by the control of the seizures and not suppressed by the toxic effects of the medication.

Behaviour or conduct disorder

Behaviour disorders in a person with a learning disability may be defined as a disturbance of emotions, behaviours and relationships which are inconsistent with the person's intellectual impairment and are sufficiently intense and persistent to cause distress to the person or those caring for them. The majority of people who have mild, moderate, severe or profound mental retardation do *not* have a behaviour disorder. The behaviour patterns of some people may be linked to a biomedical condition. For example, self-injurious behaviour is one of the manifestations of an abnormal gene on the X chromosome which causes a deficiency in an enzyme needed for the metabolism of purine. The behaviour pattern is the same for each person affected. They severely damage the tissue of their lips and fingers through biting themselves (Lesch–Nyan syndrome).

The person with autism develops idiosyncratic communication patterns and routines which vary from person to person but they all have some behaviour patterns in common. These form the basis of their developmental disability. They do not attempt to direct the attention of another person to an object or event of interest either verbally or by pointing, nor do they monitor people's gaze so they do not learn to pay attention to things and events that others are watching. We do not know the biochemical mechanisms which form the basis for this behaviour pattern but there are two genetic conditions where the person has similar behaviours; these are fragile X syndrome and phenylketonuria. There is optimism that future research will provide new ways of preventing or treating the chemical imbalances which underlie the mental impairment and are producing the behavioural patterns which can be so disabling. Meanwhile, we have to assess the innate impairment and behaviours in the context of the person's relationships and environmental pressures, any of which may be causing them to react with an increased frequency and intensity of their usual behaviour pattern or be producing and maintaining new ones.

Assessment

This will be made on the basis of a history which will be dependent on the knowledge and observations of the family or carers, a mental state examination, physical examination and investigations which would include a behavioural analysis (see Fig. 14.6). It is important to establish if there have been any life changes which might have influenced the person's behaviour.

The degree of intellectual impairment should first be established and any underlying or associated medical condition diagnosed. The person with a mild disability will be able to give the interviewer an account of their previous history on which to base their assessments; however, reports from people who know the person can help give a fuller picture of their developmental history and of the manner in which they adapt their behaviour to different situations or cope with stress.

For those with a moderate or severe disability, the reports of their families or carers of their usual behaviour and unusual or 'out of character' behaviour will be of increased importance in both assessing their life skills and any underlying or associated medical conditions which may be having an impact on their functioning.

Careful notes should be made of changes of people present in the person's home or within their occupational group and of changes in their programme of activities. These changes can act as a 'trigger'. This event may not have been acknowledged by either the person or those around them as stressful.

Mental state examination

Those people with a severe or moderate learning disability will have difficulties in expressing their thoughts and communicating their feelings but should always be given an opportunity to do so. An interview should be conducted in familiar surroundings with encouragement to engage in an activity which encourages communication such as looking at photographs, etc. The person should be seen both in the presence of someone they know well who can interpret for them and alone. For those with a mild learning disability little adjustment to the usual examination is necessary except in the use of language which should be simplified and follow the lead of the person in the use of descriptive terms.

Treatment

For those people who have no identifiable physical or psychiatric disorder, behavioural therapy will be the treatment of choice. This requires there to be a detailed behavioural analysis. There first has to be a description of the particular piece of behaviour which is distressing and a careful study of why the behaviour is being maintained, i.e. what rewards does the behaviour elicit for the person and what prompts the behaviour. An analysis of the capacity the person has to learn a different behaviour to substitute for the one considered inappropriate should be undertaken and also a list made of things or activities the person finds rewarding so they can be used as reinforcers.

For most behaviour disorders the treatment will be an individual programme of behavioural modification. Group and individual psychotherapy programmes have been developed such as 'anger management' groups using role play and activity-based techniques.

Psychiatric disorder

People with learning disability suffer from genetically or biologically determined mental illness in the same way as other people but unless they are referred to a doctor or health professional who is trained to recognize the symptoms, the diagnosis may not be made. This is because depression and or mania may be *confused with a behaviour disorder* and unless specifically questioned, family and carers will not mention changes in appetite, sleep patterns, social activities or weight. The feeling of a general lowering of energy which depressed people describe can be difficult for the person to communicate and yet treatment and relief of suffering could be easily instigated.

Schizophrenia is more difficult to diagnose due to the need for language to express thoughts and ideas. However, with careful observation and history taking, fearfulness, sleep disorder and hallucinations can be elicited and most often a paranoid idea expressed or indicated by a person's actions.

People with Down's syndrome are at high risk of

Alzheimer's disease. The person will be observed to be losing the skills which they have attained, perhaps more withdrawn, and uninterested in activities which they have previously enjoyed. It is important to distinguish between dementia and a depressive illness because of the availability of treatment for the latter condition.

Like others, people with learning disability suffer from stress-related disorders. They may react to changes in their life situation with depression or an anxiety state. The cause of their reaction may be missed, such as the move away of a particular member of staff or physical ill-health and sometimes the intensity of the reaction seems to the carer to be out of proportion to the changes which have happened. Careful explanation and frequent reassurance helps the person readjust. Sometimes skilled counselling is needed.

The treatment for a diagnosed mental illness will be the same as for other people but there may be difficulty in obtaining informed consent from the person to treat (see below).

Legal framework, service principles and ethical issues

The Children Act 1989 provides a legal framework and safeguards for children with disabilities and draws together the social services department functions towards children ensuring those with disabilities receive the benefit of the social services' powers and duties which they have for all children whom they look after. The guidance and regulations volume 6 of the Children Act lists the principles on which services should be based.
- The **welfare of the child** should be **safeguarded** and **promoted** by those providing services.
- A primary aim should be to **promote access** for all children to the same **range of services**.
- Recognition of the importance of parents and families in children's lives.
- **Partnership between parents and local authorities** and other agencies.
- The **views of children and parents** should be sought and taken into account.

The Education Act 1981 and The Disabled Persons Act 1986 require the local authority social services departments to assess young people with disabilities at the time they leave school for a range of welfare services as outlined in the Chronically Sick and Disabled Persons Act 1970. At 18 the young person becomes an adult and if they have been assessed under the Education Act or the Children Act as 'in need' they will be covered by the provisions of the NHS and Community Care Act 1990 which includes assessment of their needs for continuing community care services as adults.

The Children Act states **all** children should be involved in planning their futures. Even children with a severe learning disability and/or very limited expressive language can communicate preferences if there are skilled people to listen to them. A child or young person under 18 years with or without disabilities has the right to refuse to submit to a medical, psychiatric examination or other assessment though this may be against the wishes of their parents, providing he or she is regarded as having sufficient understanding to make an informed decision. Since May 1984 courts have been able to appoint guardians *ad litem* to safeguard and promote the interests of the child in care proceedings. One aspect of this is advice to the court on whether the child has sufficient understanding to personally consent to an examination or assessment and the guardian *ad litem* is able to seek and present professional opinion on the child's capabilities. Guardians *ad litem* are appointed if a court is satisfied there is a conflict of interests between child and parents.

If the professional opinion is that a child of whatever age or disability is not of sufficient understanding to consent or refuse medical examination or procedures then under the law the decision would be taken for them in their best interest.

When the person becomes 18 and an adult the legal framework within which services are provided changes as there is no statutory duty on the local authority to make community services available. Although they have a duty to assess and offer **choice of services it is only within the resources available**.

The **assessment process** under the 1990 NHS and community care act is described in 'Caring for People – Community Care in the Next Decade and Beyond – Policy Guidance'. There are three processes.
- Assessment of the user's circumstances.
- Design of a 'care package' in agreement with users, carers and relevant agencies to meet the identified needs within the resources available, including help from willing and able carers.
- Implementation and monitoring of the agreed package; review of the outcomes for users and carers; and any necessary revision of service provision.

An important feature of the service is that it is **based on a 'needs led' approach.** The intention is to ensure that people are not fitted into existing services but that services are adapted to individual needs. Although social services departments have overall responsibility for coordination of the services required, the day-to-day management and provision of the services needed will often rest elsewhere. Packages of support can be put together using statutory, e.g. social services and health services, or the voluntary and independent sectors.

There has to be the closest liaison between health, adult education, employment services, social services and housing if the person with a learning disability is to receive sufficient support to enable them to take their place as a full citizen in society with the rights and responsibilities that implies. The principles the services should follow are summarized in a client's charter used by the Oxfordshire Learning Disability NHS Trust (Fig. 14.7).

The **involvement of an adult person with a learning disability in decision making is paramount**. Their dependency on others, such as their parents or paid carers makes it easy for people to treat them as children and not as adult citizens and capable of taking decisions for themselves. Consent

Fig. 14.7 Basic values underlying services for people with learning disability

- **Individuality**
Each person is entitled to be treated as an individual.
- **Status and respect**
Each person is entitled to be given the opportunity and support to present themselves with dignity, and to be treated with respect.
- **Choice**
Each person is entitled to be given the opportunity and support to make choices and be involved in decision making.
- **Continuity**
Each person is entitled to continuity and progression through the different stages of their life.
- **Relationships**
Each person is entitled to a network of friends, the opportunity and support to remain in contact with relatives and the opportunity to develop deeper relationships.
- **Community presence**
Each person is entitled to live as part of an ordinary community taking full advantage of the local facilities.
- **Competence**
Each person is entitled to opportunities to develop skills and support in minimizing their disability.
- **Health and comfort**
Each person is entitled to professional services aimed at maximizing physical and mental health, comfort and safety.
- **Representation**
Each person is entitled to an advocate or representative who is not in the employment of the service.
- **Professional service**
Each person is entitled to receive a professional service that identifies its aims and constantly monitors how well it meets those aims and addresses any shortcomings.

for non-urgent medical and surgical treatments have been sought from relatives and professional carers by doctors when they feel the person is incapable of decision making. **Good practice** would now ensure the person with a disability was **informed** about the need for **medical intervention and consent** obtained from them if at all possible. Under the present legislation, if the person is so severely mentally incapacitated they cannot make an informed decision, no one can give valid consent on their behalf. The medical profession is able to proceed without valid consent in an emergency, acting under common law – they would be negligent if they didn't act when the person's health and safety is endangered. In the case of a non-emergency medical condition and in other situations such as making significant life decisions, difficulties can arise. There are no arrangements for appointing a guardian *ad litem* for an adult with a disability whose capacity for decision making in particular circumstances is in question.

The social situations which arise are usually concerning the **person's autonomy**, for example **their safety and those of others** if they live in their own accommodation without supervision. There are risks of **possible exploitation** by others in the use of money or property and of physical or sexual abuse.

Most property and personal decision making for profound, severely and many moderately disabled people are made informally by parents and or paid support workers. In assessing need and planning care packages the involvement of all professional staff and support workers plus the parents of the person safeguards the person's best interest. Someone should try to find out from the disabled person **whom they would like to be involved**, particularly if the person themselves is not able to comprehend the situation and service issues sufficiently to make a valid decision. Staff may disagree with parents on what is in the best interest of the person or disagree with one another. Most people with a learning disability can decide who they wish to be present to help them make a decision over their future. Those people who are unable to communicate these wishes need to have someone to represent them. Parents would see themselves in this role but there are times when they may not be able to be objective and their own fears, feelings or emotional needs interfere with their decisions.

There are advocacy services available in most areas of the country. Advocates are usually volunteers who have undergone training in how to communicate with people with a severe learning disability, how to get to know them and be confident in speaking on their behalf.

The Law Commission has published a consultation paper – 'Mentally Incapacitated Adults and Decision Making' – which is concerned with people who have mental disability or disorder which is of such a degree that they are incapable of taking decisions for themselves. It is anticipated there will be new legislation based on this consultation.

The more severely disabled the person the greater the need for resources to support them and enable them to have the opportunities for living as a participating member of society. How finite resources are shared across people with learning disability is not always on the basis of need. Often those parents who are articulate and learn how to influence the system get the resources for their son and daughter although their assessed need may be less than some others. The same amount of resources could assist several people with a mild disability to get out and about and use community facilities but only help one person who is severely disabled and needs greater support to achieve the same activity.

There is also the dilemma of allocating resources to people whose quality of life in the eyes of society will never equal others whose lives may be saved if the resources were put into acute medicine and advanced technology. It is the same medical advances and technology which is improving the chances of life for very small premature babies who are at greater risk of intellectual impairment than other babies and which also keeps more people alive who are severely impaired and disabled.

QUESTIONS

1 A mother brings her 40-year-old son with Down's syndrome to you. She says that she is worried because he is sleeping during the day and has changed from being a very neat and tidy person to being careless about his dress and in the manner in which he eats. How would you investigate her concerns?

2 Miss A, aged 22, is brought to see you by the social worker who cares for her in the local hostel for people with learning disability. Miss A is waking early in the morning, going into the bathroom, turning on the taps and flooding the room. She washes her hands frequently during the day and gets very angry, hitting out, if someone tries to stop her. The social worker is asking you to prescribe a sedative. How would you manage the situation?

3 Miss K comes to see you as she is getting married and knows her future husband has a learning disabled brother and uncle. She is concerned about their baby being similarly affected. How do you advise her?

4 The parents of a young woman with a learning disability have asked their general practitioner if she could have a hysterectomy. They report they are fearful of her becoming pregnant because she would be unable to look after a child. They cite her inability to manage her menstruation as evidence of her dependency. They feel hysterectomy would remove two blocks to her achieving independence and be in her best interest. If you were the general practitioner, what would be your response?

FURTHER READING

Griffiths M. & Russell P. (eds) (1985) *Working Together with Mentally Handicapped Children.* Human Horizons Series. [This book considers the nature, cause and effect of the major handicapping conditions. It emphasizes the need for a partnership between parents and professionals. It is edited by a paediatrician and a parent and is aimed at a wide readership.]

Matson J.L. & Mulick J.A. (eds) (1991) *Handbook of Retardation.* Pergamon General Psychology Series. [Provides a broad overview and latest information on research philosophy and treatments in the USA, all of which are applicable to people in the UK.]

Reed Committee Report of the Official Working Group on Services for People with Special Needs – People with Learning Disabilities (Mental Handicap) or with Autism. Department of Health Home Office 1992. [This discusses the services for people with learning disability and contains information on the policies of health and social services.]

15
Children and Adolescents

Fact sheet

Definition
Child psychiatry deals with mental disorders in children and young persons. It differs from adult psychiatry in three important respects.
1 Some disorders represent a failure of normal development.
2 Behavioural symptoms as well as abnormalities of mental state are common findings in the clinical picture.
3 The clinical features of psychiatric syndromes will vary with the child's age.

Presentation and diagnoses
The main clinical presentations are:
1 *conduct disorders*: lying, stealing, destructiveness, bullying. Other features may include poor friendships and infrequently fire-setting (see p. 306);
2 *emotional disorders*: anxiety, fearfulness, sadness. Other features may include school refusal and somatic presentations, e.g. abdominal pain;
3 *failure of normal development*: encopresis and enuresis, poor speech and language development, disorders associated with poor physical development, e.g. clumsy children;
4 *hyperkinetic disorders*: marked restlessness, inattention and behaviour difficulties.

Neuropsychiatric presentation
Investigations for neurological disease should be considered in children with a history of **normal development** and absence of **adverse precipitating family and social factors** who present in the following ways.
1 Acute onsets of emotional or behavioural symptoms.
2 Deteriorating clinical signs and symptoms.
3 Any disorder which includes clouding of consciousness or abnormalities of the special senses.
4 Loss or deterioration of an already acquired developmental skill in either speech, language, visual or perceptual skill or other motor abilities.

Aetiology
Differential contributions will occur from:
1 defects, disorders and diseases of the CNS, e.g. neural tube defects, bacterial infections, trauma;
2 marital discord and family difficulties, e.g. violence at home;
3 psychiatric disorder in family members;
4 learning problems and school difficulties;
5 problems in making and/or keeping friends both in school and neighbourhood;
6 temperament and personality, e.g. irritability, impulsivity and attention difficulties.

Factors associated with childhood disorders
1 *Conduct disorders*:
  • commoner in boys;
  • commoner in disadvantaged families.
2 *Emotional disorders*:
  • equally common in boys and girl;
  • can occur in advantaged or disadvantaged families.

3 *Failures of normal development*:
  • commoner in boys;
  • usually associated with late maturation or CNS disease;
  • exacerbated adverse family and social factors.

Distribution
Exact rates of emotional and conduct disturbance/disorder in the community are unknown but are influenced by social and geographic factors. Thus between 5 and 20% of children are likely to develop behavioural or emotional disturbance before reaching adulthood, with the rates being greater in urban rather than rural environments.

Assessment
The following are important in assessment and examination
1 Different informants may give different information.
2 Individual psychiatric examination of the child.
3 Play is important in evaluating children under 8.
4 Parents interviewed separately, particularly mothers, are important sources of history taking.
5 Marital and family interviews are relevant in many cases.
6 School reports are important ways of obtaining information on educational achievement and social relations.
7 Siblings and peers can provide further important information on popularity and social relations.

Management
1 *The child*: brief problem-solving or explanatory psychotherapy; behavioural psychotherapy; play therapy (mainly for children under 8); groupwork; longer term psychotherapy; support casework; pharmacotherapy.
2 *The family*: family therapy; assessment of parenting abilities; support casework during child treatments.
3 *The environment*: reorganizing social and/or domestic arrangements; school-based interventions; use of residential services, e.g. psychiatric in-patients or social services placements; day units. Liaison with paediatrics and primary care.

Prognosis
1 In *conduct disorders*:
  • poor in long-standing disorders with ongoing adverse family hostility, parental criminality and chronic parental psychiatric disorder;
  • carries an increased risk (especially boys) for criminality and alcohol abuse into adulthood.
2 In *emotional disorders*:
  • generally good;
  • severe cases may continue to adult neuroses.
3 In *developmental disorders*:
  • age and development related. The majority of enuresis and encopresis being absent by late adolescence;
  • hyperkinetic children may show a change in their symptoms and a proportion will go on to develop personality difficulties and make a poor adjustment into adulthood;
  • children with speech and language delay at 3 are at risk for learning difficulties and behaviour problems by 8.

What is child psychiatry?

Child psychiatry is the branch of medicine that is concerned with the evaluation and treatment of children and adolescents with disturbances of mood, thoughts or behaviour. In many cases, children's symptoms arise in the context of disturbed family relations (hence the term child and family psychiatry is some clinics). For others, social disadvantage will play a contributory role in their disturbance.

A large proportion of children will not exhibit major psychiatric symptoms but will complain of, or have reported by others (parents, teachers), symptoms of anxiety, distress and socially handicapping or unwanted behaviour. Present estimates indicate that between 5 and 20% of all children will experience significant emotional distress or behavioural difficulties. Child psychiatrists require a firm knowledge of child development as well as adult psychiatry and it is helpful to be familiar with the 'basic sciences' of development including developmental psychology and neuroscience.

The majority of child psychiatrists work in hospital clinics and in community settings such as health centres and child guidance clinics. Many work in multidisciplinary teams with social workers, clinical or educational psychologists and community psychiatric nurses.

The majority of child mental health difficulties can be managed on an out-patient basis. There is, however, a significant number of cases that require day-patient and in-patient facilities. Most child psychiatric teams are district-based, serving a population of one child psychiatrist per 120 000 people. Day-patient services are often available in districts but in-patient facilities may be regional and serve up to four or five district services.

Child psychiatry has an important preventative role in child mental health and a major philosophy is identifying and promoting the best interests of the child.

The community role of child psychiatry promotes close links with primary care teams including health visitors and community psychiatric nurses. Prospects for the future include closer ties between community and hospital services, an emphasis on liaising with other child health facilities including paediatrics and school medical doctors as well as continuing research into service provision, treatment methods and aetiologies of psychiatric disorders of children and adolescents.

Causes and classification

Causes
It is unusual to find a single clear-cut cause for a childhood psychiatric disorder. Four main groups of factors may be considered as shown in Fig 15.1.

Interactions may occur between these factors, for example a child with a birth defect born to a family with chronic marital disharmony and financial difficulties has a greater risk of psychiatric disorder than a child with one of these factors alone.

Fig. 15.1 Aetiological factors in child psychiatric disorder

Constitutional factors
- Chromosomal abnormalities.
- Polygenic influences.

Physical factors
- Injury.
- Disease.
CNS damage increases risk fivefold.
Non-CNS chronic illness increases risk threefold.

Temperament
- Irregularity.
- Poor adaptability.
- High emotionality.

Environment
- Chronic marital disharmony.
- Violence in the family.
- Chronic persistent difficulties with family or friends.
- Acute stressful events.
- Learning difficulties.

Constitutional factors
Constitutional factors reflect those with which the child is born. The genetics of the common psychiatric disorders are as yet poorly understood. Chromosomal abnormalities may increase the risk of psychiatric disorder as a result of mental retardation or presence of specific syndromes, e.g. Down's syndrome or tuberose sclerosis. Polygenic influences may be particularly important and reflect a combination of genes which increase the probability of one disorder or another, e.g. infantile autism, childhood depression. Polygenic factors are also important for the development of intelligence, temperament and personality traits.

Physical disease and injuries
Physical diseases and injuries increase the risk of psychiatric disorder and may occur at any time from conception. Infections, bacterial or viral, at any time *in utero* or in early life can increase the risk of psychiatric disorder via influences on the neurodevelopment of the brain. Brain disease or damage may be caused by a variety of factors, hypoxia and birth injury being the two commonest. Brain-damaged children have an increased risk of psychiatric disorder, particularly behavioural problems. Children with definite evidence of brain damage have at least a fivefold increase in the risk of psychiatric disorder compared with the general population. Children with chronic physical handicaps not involving the brain have a threefold increase in the risk of psychiatric disorder. Important non-disease processes such as malnutrition, physical deprivation and non-accidental injury can result in brain damage and must be remembered.

Physical disease not necessarily affecting the brain may increase the risk of psychiatric disorder by impairing normal development. Thus children with physical handicaps and musculoskeletal diseases that are chronic have increased rates of psychiatric disorder and children with complex medical problems such as diabetes and asthma may show psychiatric disorders particularly in the presence of environmental stresses, a further example of interactions between causal factors.

Temperament
Studies on children's temperament have indicated that there are marked individual differences in children's temperaments as characterized by such reactions as irregularity of sleeping and eating, social withdrawal, poor adaptability to changing social circumstances and high emotionality. Children with difficult temperamental characteristics are more at risk from psychiatric disorder, often as a result of interactions with environmental factors.

Environmental factors
Social and family circumstances have been shown to be directly involved in causing child psychiatric disorder.

Of particular importance for the development of *conduct disorders* are:
1 chronic marital disharmony;
2 having a single parent;
3 paternal history of criminality;
4 children who have been taken into the care of the local authority through neglect or deprivation;
5 history of parental psychiatric disorder.
Often more than one child in the family is or has been conduct disordered.

For *emotional disorders* environmental factors are less clear, they appear more associated with:
1 problems within family relationships such as inadequate communication and trust between parents and siblings;
2 marital disharmony, particularly in the presence of overt hostility;
3 a history of depression in a parent.

Children are likely to produce emotional or behavioural symptoms in the presence of acute stressful events and schoolage children can develop depressive symptoms in the presence of recent bereavements. As the child develops increasing autonomy and increasingly widens his or her social experience, the availability, adequacy and intimacy of friendships becomes important in normal development. Their absence may increase the risk of psychiatric disorder at all ages. Reconstituted families are those where two adults form a new family and are bringing up children from previous relationships. Children from both reconstituted and single families may be at greater risk from both emotional and behavioural difficulties.

The classification of childhood psychiatric disorder
The classification of psychiatric disorder in childhood and adolescence is not entirely satisfactory. In part, this is because the ideal classification requires a considerable knowledge of the aetiology, clinical features, natural course and outcome of disease and at present knowledge is limited in many of these areas. However, advance has been made with the use of multi-axial systems. These allow the classification of a number of features, not just the signs and symptoms. In child psychiatry therefore, the five-axis scheme of the International Classification of Diseases is used (Fig. 15.2).

Fig. 15.2 International classification of childhood psychiatric disorder

Axis 1: *psychiatric syndrome*, definitions given by which a diagnosis (depression, hysteria, conduct disorder, etc.) is reached based on signs and symptoms obtained from parents and child (see also p. 14).
Axis 2: *specific delays in development*, which consist of speech and language difficulties, often identified as learning disorders and motor difficulties (in coordination and clumsiness).
Axis 3: *child's intellectual level* in form of IQ score: severely impaired, less than 50; moderately impaired, less than 70; no impairment, greater than 80; 70–80 is considered borderline and requires further careful evaluation.
Axis 4: *associated medical conditions* in any system (CNS, gastrointestinal, cardiovascular, etc.).
Axis 5: *abnormal psychosocial circumstances* to which the child is exposed. This axis refers to:
- descriptions of the family structure, i.e. one-parent family, living in care, number of children and adults in the household
- inferences about normal family function, i.e. discordant or hostile parental relations, hostile parent–child relations.

Axis 1 allows for diagnosis and each category is in theory mutually exclusive. Similarly so for axis 3 – intellectual level. Axis 2, however, can be coded to indicate none, one or more developmental delays and axis 5 similarly about psychosocial circumstances (clearly a child may be in one- or two-parent families and experience hostile relations). Axis 4 will code all medical diagnoses that the child has received.

The importance of a multi-axial system lies in being able to describe the child and his or her family in a broad and detailed descriptive manner which allows a formulation of all possible factors that contribute to the child's psychiatric disorder. It has been shown that this descriptive formulation is a better predictor of a child's eventual outcome than a diagnosis based simply on signs and symptoms.

The assessment procedure in child psychiatry

General principles
The assessment in child psychiatry can be divided into the following components.
1 Child interview.
2 Adult interview, including marital/parental interview.
3 Family interview.
A clinical decision must also be taken as to the timing and order of interviewing, i.e. some child psychiatrists prefer to interview the whole family at the first session, whereas for others interviewing the individual child and the parents separately is seen as the first interview. Psychiatric interviews in child psychiatry may be expected to take between 1 and $1\frac{1}{2}$ hours in the first instance.

A recommended procedure is as follows.
1 *Introductory interview*: all people who attend an interview are invited into the room where they are asked for their

understanding of why they have been referred and what problems brought them to the clinic. This constitutes an orientation exercise for the family and allows the psychiatrist to obtain an understanding of the parents' and child's comprehension of the referral and its merits and to clarify any questions family members may have about seeing a child psychiatrist. The psychiatrist then explains that all family members have an opportunity to be seen individually and there may be family sessions so that no one need feel that they have been reported on unfavourably.

2 *Further interviews*: the introductory family interview can then be halted to carry out individual interviews with parents and child. Alternatively, the orientation exercise can be extended into a more formal family interviewing method to collect factual information and to make further observations on family behaviour and interaction. It is probably important that the psychiatrist has an opportunity to see both child and parents on their own to obtain adequate mental states and personal histories.

The general principles of psychiatric interviewing are covered in Chapter 3. However, there are some specific issues pertinent to children that require clear elucidation.

The psychiatric interview
Children are more defensive and secretive than adults and the initial clinical interview must be structured to take account of this. Questions should begin with neutral topics that enquire about the child's likes and dislikes at home, school and with his or her peers. Emotional topics should be enquired about in a calm and collected manner as an anxious voice will result in a defensive and anxious child. In particular the time of onset, frequency and duration of signs and symptoms may require corroboration from another source such as a parent as children's cognitive development which includes their sense of time will influence the reliability of some of their reports.

Play
Non-verbal methods of assessment and interviewing are important in younger children and in those with limited verbal abilities. The use of play allows an assessment of development both in motor and psychological terms as indicated in the schema below. Play is an important medium for younger children to express their anxieties and concerns, and to provide their histories through description with materials rather than with words.

Social and educational enquiries
Assessment in child psychiatry is generally not limited just to the interview with the family. Social enquiry reports obtained by visits to the home and schools will often provide important information concerning educational progress and inter-personal relationships both in the classroom and in the immediate vicinity of the school. It is important to obtain parental permission to approach the school for a report. If parents decline, however, this must be respected. It is also important to consider assessment across time. In some cases more than one interview session may be required before arriving at a formulation, particularly in the case of children with communication difficulties, such as speech and language disorders or temperamentally shy and withdrawn children or where family members may be seen at home. Assessments should not be long drawn-out affairs, however, and adequate formulations can be made in the majority of cases attending a clinic within a $1\frac{1}{2}$-hour interview.

Formulation of a case
It is important to delineate the relationship between the environment, the child's stage of development and the disorder. The formulation should include a description of the child's physical appearance and an adequate description of development covering motor as well as psychological capacity. Duration and frequency of symptoms should be described and contributory and aetiological features outlined. Factors that may be protecting the child from either greater or different difficulties should also be emphasized. The formulation should include necessary investigations in the treatment plan, indicating how the psychiatrist intends to proceed.

Assessment in primary care settings
The child psychiatrist provides substantial time for the assessment of a new referral, at least $1\frac{1}{2}$ hours in most clinics and perhaps much longer in complex cases involving a number of other agencies (school, social services).

Time like this is generally not available to the general practitioner, health visitor or community nurse. In these circumstances a briefer history and examination is inevitable. Mothers or the main caretaker, should be viewed as the main informant. Present history should concentrate on the problem areas. Changes in frequency, duration and severity of behaviours previously noticed but not considered worrying should be recorded. Note carefully the development of new signs and/or symptoms including those that mother may perceive as problematic, or a sign of disorder (e.g. becoming quieter, social withdrawal or retiring to bed earlier than usual).

Talking to children or observing play can be difficult in a busy general surgery. If history from a mother suggests talking to the child may be required it is better to see him or her after school and at the end of surgery when a little more time may be available.

Observation of toddlers and young children at home by health visitors or community nurses can be markedly helpful in assessing problem areas. Primary care workers should have access via the telephone to discuss worries about children and families with the child psychiatry team. Many minor emotional and behavioural issues can be dealt with in this way with additional support given to the primary care team. Visits to the psychiatric clinic and liaison with child psychiatrists by the primary care workers may also alleviate the need for direct referral. Close working relationships between health care professionals can result in more efficient management of many child difficulties and identify more reliably those children who require specialist help.

Clinical presentations

This section will focus on the common disorders presenting to child psychiatry clinics. Reference will then be made to important but less common conditions. Figure 15.3 highlights the major syndromes.

Conduct disorder

Conduct disorder refers to children who present with abnormalities of behaviour characterized by aggression, stealing, lying, poor friendships and infrequently, fire-setting. Referral may be because of one or a multiplicity of these symptoms.

The environment plays an important part in the presentation and understanding of conduct disorders (see p. 185).

Stealing is the commonest and **fire-setting** (see also p. 306) the rarest presenting symptom. **Aggression** is more common in boys. The sex ratio of conduct disorders is three boys for every girl. Less well-defined behaviour problems in the pre-school child may persist as conduct disorder in middle childhood. Most cases of conduct disorder are relatively longstanding with duration of symptoms longer than 12 months. The reason for referral is often because the family can no longer cope with continuous difficulties in the home or antisocial activity has precipitated concern at school or in the community at large.

Children with severe and intractable symptoms can be considered as delinquent.

Temperament may be important. Children with conduct disorders, particularly boys, are often described as showing higher rates of impulsivity, overactivity and aggression prior to the onset of disorder. Some cases show considerable degrees of anxiety and depression. These emotional symptoms are less pervasive and severe than in true emotional disorders. Treatment and outcome are determined by behavioural rather than emotional symptoms in these cases.

The prognosis for conduct disorders depends on the severity, duration and setting of symptoms. Long-term prognosis is poor for children with severe conduct disorder. There is a strong association between severe conduct disorder and later

personality difficulties. Prognosis for relatively brief periods of difficult behaviour, particularly in cases where there are few family and temperamental risk factors, is much better. A case vignette shows an example (Case 1).

Emotional disorders

Emotional disorder is characterized by symptoms of anxiety, such as fearfulness, panic, phobias, and depression, such as misery, sadness, thoughts of hopelessness, apathy and loss of appetite.

The main emotional disorders to consider are stress reactions, anxiety states, hysteria, depression, obsessional disorders and eating disorders.

Stress reactions

Perhaps the commonest problem to present in primary care are children with acute onset symptoms, commonly of anxiety, as a result of a recent stressful life event that has occurred in the previous days or weeks. These reactions do not constitute psychiatric illness unless they persist for longer than 4 to 6 weeks or result in serious symptoms or disruptions of school and social life. Common examples will be hospitalizations, minor accidents in the home, house moves and birth of a sibling.

Stress reactions are influenced by a child's development. For example, being in hospital is more stressful for 2–3 year olds than 6–7 year olds. In adolescence common stresses relate to social relationships, both with the same and the opposite sex, such as loss of a best friend or boyfriend.

Because the majority of these stress reactions are self-limiting, support and reassurance to the family in primary care is the management of choice. Health visitors can play a major role in pre-school stress reactions by home visits and monitoring outcome. Educational psychologists and teachers with counselling experience provide important psychological support to social and exam stresses within schools.

Anxiety states

Anxiety states occur throughout childhood and adolescence but their presenting symptoms may change with development. With the pre-school child separation anxiety states are characterized by behavioural symptoms of excess dependency on the mother, failure to explore new environments and withdrawal from existing social contact. In many cases there is a concurrent anxiety depressive state in the mother. In the school-age child the emergence of more generalized anxiety disorders occurs in family and social circumstances, often with episodes of panic associated with palpitations, tachycardias and sweating. **Specific fears and phobias** may develop in this age-group, although they are relatively uncommon. These specific phobias are often focused on animals or in circumstances related to recent stressful events such as phobias about crossing the road following a road traffic accident. In later childhood and adolescence children suffering from anxiety symptoms may show greater social pathology with significant problems in social relationships and withdrawal from peer groups. Somatic symptoms such as abdominal pain, headaches and fluctuating aches and pains are quite common amongst anxious children of all ages.

Case 1: Conduct disorder

A 12-year-old boy was referred to the child psychiatry department from his general practitioner with a 6-month history of *stealing money* from his parents, regularly but intermittently. This symptom had been *associated with frequent and regular episodes of lying and occasional episodes of destructiveness* around the house. He had been caught *shoplifting* twice and received a severe caution from the police.

He refused to speak to the general practitioner and was *described as sullen and miserable* throughout that interview.

Both parents and the child attended the child psychiatry clinic. Family assessment revealed that they were all aware as to why they had come. There were differences of opinion concerning the need to attend. The father felt the boy required firm discipline, mother felt that this was not the right way and that he needed someone to talk to. A marital interview revealed an *unsatisfactory marriage* of 14 years' duration, with the *father paying little attention to family life* and preferring to concentrate on his own hobbies and interests. Over the past 12 months both the identified patient and his older brother had been complaining about their parents not paying them enough attention. This had been associated with a deterioration in the marriage.

The identified patient had been unplanned but wanted by his mother. He had attended school without any difficulties but was considered to be not very bright and had received *remedial education* for mathematics. His progress had been poor, although his attendance had been regular. His relationship with his brother was quite good. The brother was considered to be educationally below average and had had episodes of disturbed behaviour but regularly attended school.

The child was interviewed alone. Although initially defensive, he indicated that he was aware of his symptoms and knew that they caused problems for his

family. He felt that he had not intended to embark on a career of crime and was aware of the consequences. He *became tearful during the interview and angry*, particularly when discussing the quality of family life. He had few friends and no close friend. *He generally kept things to himself* and when he had troubles or worries he didn't share them with either his parents or his social group. He had no particular hobbies or interests and said he enjoyed playing computer games.

Physical examination was normal. He was on the *third centile for height*, and was in early puberty.

Formulation

A 12-year-old pubertal boy with a 6-month history of conduct disorder characterized by stealing, lying and one episode of antisocial behaviour associated with emotional symptoms. The referral was precipitated by the social consequences of shoplifting, an acute stress for the family and for the child in the presence of an ongoing series of difficulties. However, the symptoms revealed environmental factors:
1 *chronic marital disharmony*;
2 *poor family relationships*–both between parents and children, especially father and identified child;
3 *educational difficulties* of long-standing nature with secondary *social difficulties* in making friendships. Being small and having poor speech contributed to his poor socialization.

Treatment plan

Liaison with GP and School Services
1 **Discussion took place with GP and educational psychologist** who had seen him for learning difficulties in the school setting.

2 **School and social enquiry reports** from home and school visits with a social work colleague were obtained with parental permission, and the educational psychologist provided assessment of classroom and playroom behaviour obtained by direct observation.

Clinic treatment
Family therapy over four sessions took place to help clarify with the family the links between the child's symptoms and:
● chronic marital difficulties;
● parental disagreement over child management;
● poor social relations between father and son.
Initial goals of therapy would include increasing activities between father and son that both agreed on, and helping the patient discuss and explain his perception of family life, school and social difficulties.

Follow-up management
1 **A follow-up home visit** occurred 2 weeks after the end of treatment to discuss progress.
2 **A feedback session for the primary care team (GP, health visitor)** was arranged at the clinic and it was agreed that community based monitoring would continue for a further 6 months on a monthly basis with visits by the psychiatric social worker to the family concerning the maintenance of the goals established in the child psychiatry clinic.
3 **Revisit to school by child psychiatry team** to inform year tutor/head teacher and school doctor of outcome and to identify that monitoring will occur via the psychiatric social worker.

School refusal is a particular form of emotional disorder and must be discriminated from **truancy** which is an intentional desire not to attend school. School refusal occurs in children of any age but peaks at the age of 5 and in early adolescence. School refusal is associated with temperamental difficulties, episodes of anxiety, social withdrawal and shyness. A small proportion of later onset school refusers may have prominent signs of depression. School refusal may be associated with maternal depression and family difficulties. Occasionally school refusal is a result of school-based problems, although this is uncommon and when it occurs it is more likely in the adolescent who has acute social difficulties.

Hysteria

Hysteria occurs in childhood and presents with symptoms of the musculoskeletal system and CNS such as abnormal gait, visual disturbances, paraesthesiae and variable degrees of pain. Some children with hysteria are occasionally depressed, and many appear to be free from serious emotional or behavioural symptoms. Hysteria is rare under the age of 5. Missed organic diseases can occur at any age.

Depression

Depression in childhood is less common than anxiety disorders. Although many anxious children present with transient sadness and misery this does not constitute a diagnosis

Case 2: Emotional disorder

A 9-year-old boy was referred via the school medical officer with the GP's agreement to the child psychiatry clinic with a 3-month history of *increasing social withdrawal, poor concentration and sleeplessness*. He had recently shown *a reluctance to go to school* which prompted a visit from the general practitioner.

He was the youngest of two children, (he had a 16-year-old sister). They *lived with their mother who had separated from the father* 4 years previously. However, over the past 12 months the father had sought to regain the custody of his children, and the *relationship between the parents was poor*. There was a *family history of depression* on both sides of the family; the mother had been treated by a psychiatrist in the past. The boy had been a planned pregnancy and reached his developmental milestones within normal limits. He had no past medical or psychiatric history, had normal school attendance and was described as of at least average intelligence. The mother had *moved house 9 months before and this had resulted in a change of school and loss of friends.* The boy had not settled in his new school and had told his mother that he wanted to go back to their former house and his former school.

Psychiatric interview revealed a *distressed mother* who was uncertain of the outcome of the legal proceedings. She believed that her son was depressed as a result of marital and family problems. Psychiatric interview with the boy revealed *a child with persistent sadness and misery and poor rapport with gaze aversion* during the interview. He declared that he had become *anxious and worried about his mother* over the past few months but showed no hostility towards his father. He wished that the marriage had worked and that all the family would be able to live together, but he knew that this was not possible. He declared that he was unhappy with the new house although he was not worried particularly about his new school. He said he felt more *anxious about making friends* and pushed himself forward far less than previously, preferring his own company. He said that a few months previously he had been optimistic about the future but now he was less certain. He declared that he had *recently had thoughts of harming himself*.

Physical examination was normal and height and weight were on the fiftieth percentile. He was prepubertal.

His father came to the clinic and confirmed the marital and family history. He felt that if he was allowed to look after his son himself he would not be depressed and that his future would be brighter than if he stayed with his mother.

Formulation

A 9-year-old prepubertal boy with a recent history of emotional disorder, dominated by depression and characterized by social withdrawal, deteriorating concentration and sleeplessness. The referral was precipitated by extension of symptoms into the school setting.

The disorder occurred against a background of marital disharmony and recent stressful life events in school and home. Both these factors contributed to the aetiology. The family history of affective disorders suggested a genetic component.

Treatment plan

Liaison with referring doctor and school
Because the school doctor had initiated the referral he was contacted with parental permission and a school visit was made to discuss the recent problems with the school doctor, teacher and educational psychologist who provides specialist detail on school-based problems.

Social work assessment
Home visits were made by the social worker in the child psychiatry team to both parents and a joint parent interview to discuss their son's problems was arranged with the psychiatrist to take place in the clinic. Three sessions of joint parent work were agreed on to help organize acceptable access of the child to father and help both parents to put the interests of their son before their personal disagreements.

The legal officers and the court were informed of this work.

Clinic treatment
1 Individual psychotherapy for the boy, focusing on the association between alterations in social and family life and present thoughts and feelings.

2 A focused programme of increasing social activities and the explaining of the relationship between personal achievement and the lessening of feelings of hopelessness and helplessness would be planned with the therapist.
3 Support for the mother would be given when her son's symptoms would be explained to her. There would be **mother/child sessions** to explain the nature of the child's treatment and to encourage mother's participation. **Father** would be informed of progress and offered support as well.
4 Antidepressant medication would be considered if symptoms persisted or there was an increase in severity in spite of psychological treatment.

Monitoring progress in the community
The **educational psychologist** agreed to **monitor school progress** on a regular basis throughout treatment and for the subsequent 12 months. Monitoring would involve discussion with teachers on classroom behaviour and educational performance; and regular brief 15-minute conversations with the child to encourage participation in school life to the full.

Follow-up management
1 Follow-up consisted of monthly attendance at the clinic for 6 months. On three occasions the educational psychologist attended follow-up meetings.
2 Social workers attached to the divorce court monitored parental progress and the GP liaised closely with the school medical officer over general health issues, including vague or ill-formed physical symptoms suggestive of potential relapse.

At 18 months the child was symptom free and had settled into school but required some support in the clinic and in school as his parents had not resolved their legal dispute, and at times of court appearances the mother became anxious and the child became concerned for her.

Social work support to mother continued from the child psychiatry clinic and to father from social workers attached to the court.

---

of depression. Severe and persistent dysphoria and thoughts of hopelessness and helplessness are the commonest signs and symptoms in childhood depression. The vegetative or biological signs are less common but become more prevalent during adolescence. Depression is unusual before the age of 8 and increases markedly after puberty.

Suicide in middle childhood is rare. Attempted suicide is more common and it's prevalence is similar to depression in increasing markedly after puberty. Most cases of attempted suicide, however, are not depressed although care must be taken to evaluate all cases of deliberate self-harm especially in the prepubertal child. In the latter cases it is advisable that a psychiatric opinion be sought (see also p. 248).

Obsessional disorders

Obsessional disorders are a particularly severe form of anxiety neurosis. They arise in childhood at approximately 8 years of age, they are very persistent and may show a poor prognosis with a fluctuating course into adult life. There is often a family history of obsessional symptoms and depression. Obsessional neuroses are not to be confused with obsessional symptoms that arise in acute anxiety and occasionally in depressive episodes. Children are more prone to obsessional behaviours under these conditions, even in the absence of obsessional traits in their personalities.

Eating disorders

Eating disorders in childhood have different forms of presentation at different ages. In the pre-school child **food refusal** represents a form of negativistic behaviour and on its own should be seen as a feature of normal development as the child struggles with finding the balance between personal autonomy and parental control. If associated with sleeplessness, difficult behaviour and aggression, advice from a health visitor and GP should be sought. A small proportion of cases, especially in the presence of maternal psychiatric disorder may benefit from child psychiatry intervention.

In middle childhood **food fads** are common and may not reflect psychological difficulties. Some children can develop acute **food refusal** and in some of these cases depression should be considered.

Anorexia nervosa is a serious eating disorder of late childhood and adolescence (see also p. 100). The adolescent presents with characteristic features of avoidance of high calorie foods, carbohydrates and fats, distorted body image associated with excessive weight loss and denial of thinness. Amenorrhoea is invariably present. Both sexes can show delayed pubertal growth. Associated factors can include variable degrees of sadness, excessive exercise and a preoccupation with toys and objects of a younger child.

There may be a long history of eating difficulties from early childhood. Family disturbance is prominent in many cases often with covert reinforcements to maintain the adolescent in her condition. Aetiology is complex, reflecting family psychopathology, a failure to negotiate normal psychosexual development and failure in accepting personal autonomy. The initial management is the attainment of an adequate weight and normal diet. Altering body image and promoting mature personality traits are desirable treatment goals, but are often difficult to achieve.

The condition is increasing, and is significantly more common in girls. Boys generally present in adolescence and prepubertal cases younger than 12 of either sex should be carefully examined for the presence of uncommon physical conditions such as juvenile Crohn's disease or coeliac disease.

Bulimia nervosa is rare in childhood although serious cases of psychogenic vomiting occur. Bulimia with alternating episodes of binge eating and vomiting can be seen in early adolescence but appears at present to be mainly a disorder of older adolescents and young adults (see also p. 103).

There are continuities between childhood emotional disorder and adult neurosis. Depression and obsessional neuroses show a strong relationship between childhood and adulthood. Overall, neurotic symptoms in childhood increase the vulnerability for later forms of adult neurotic disorder but the associations are not clear-cut and the conditions by which some children may be at risk and others not are far from well understood.

Psychoses in childhood and adolescence

The major functional psychoses are less frequent in children than in adults and particularly uncommon in the prepubertal child. **Schizophrenia** and **manic depression** both occur and are generally associated with a family history of functional psychosis. The clinical manifestations and treatment are similar to adult patients and are described in Chapters 5 and 6.

In prepubertal children **organic brain disease** should be excluded, particularly tumours and temporal lobe epilepsy (see Chapter 11).

A rare group of disorders termed the **disintegrative psychoses** occur in children between 3 and 8 years of age. These disorders present with a deterioration of global development in an often previously well child. Loss of speech and language and episodes of confusion and disorientation are common presenting complaints. These children show a continuing deterioration with death often in early adolescence. A variety of rare metabolic disease infiltrating the brain are implicated although often aetiology is unknown.

Developmental syndromes

Disorders of speech and language can give rise to specific or pervasive disorders of development including associations with childhood psychoses. **Infantile autism** is a specific disorder characterized by failure of communication, poor socialization and lack of symbolic play. The disorder occurs across the full range of IQ but many are mentally handicapped.

Children with **difficulties in reading, writing and mathematical skills** may present to a child psychiatrist with emotional or conduct disorder. Some of these children will have a **developmental language disorder**. In these children delays in central nervous system development result in difficulties in processing language and in learning properly. Attention to the underlying learning difficulty is important and includes discussion with school as some children will require special education for their difficulties as well as attention to their presenting symptoms.

Enuresis

Enuresis is a disorder defined as the failure to obtain normal bladder control by day or night by the age of 5. Epidemiology has shown that between 5 and 15% of children are wet at night at 5 years of age. By the age of 7 rates of daytime and night-time wetting have fallen to 5% of the childhood population. The problem is more frequent in boys: Developmental immaturity of bladder physiology may be important in some cases. Psychological and social adversity may predispose the child to anxiety and subsequent enuresis. Factors already indicated in the 'at risk' section for psychiatric disorder should be noted. There is often a family history of enuresis and in some cases simple supportive measures are all that is required with advice to the mother about general toilet training which in some cases may not have been carried out correctly. In others there will be marked psychological difficulties requiring psychiatric treatment. The bell and pad together with out-patient family support is the most widely used treatment. This involves placing a pad between the bed-sheets connected to an alarm. When the child voids whilst sleeping the electrical circuit is closed and the alarm rings waking the child up who then proceeds to the toilet. This is an example of behaviour therapy in child psychiatry (see p. 26 and p. 229). Individual and family therapy may be important in some cases particularly if other emotional or behavioural difficulties are diagnosed.

Encopresis
Encopresis is defined as the passing of normal faeces in abnormal places. Most children have obtained adequate bowel function by the age of 4. In those children who have not obtained adequate bowel function by this age poor normal toilet training technique by parents must be excluded. For many children seen in the child psychiatry clinic, however, encopresis reflects serious emotional disorder and may be associated with abnormal toilet training often with parents who resort to harsh punitive methods. This disorder commonly presents in children between 4 and 7 years of age. Physical causes for soiling should be looked for as must the presence of mental handicap where delays in development are more common. Treatment is often aimed simultaneously at symptom removal and attention to underlying psychological difficulties in the child using individual or family interventions.

Hyperkinetic disorder
Hyperkinetic disorder is a developmental disorder characterized by pervasive restlessness, inactivity, poor attention and concentration. These children may present in the pre-school period with marked restlessness, inactivity and failure to respond to adequate parenting. More commonly, however, they present in the school period, with increasing signs of conduct disorder as a result of their failure to conform to the necessary rules of school and failure to learn adequately.

Problems with attention and concentration are found in children with conduct disorder and this group do not necessarily show signs of developmental difficulties. It is not yet clear if this symptomatic association constitutes a specific clinical entity. A case vignette is provided as an example (Case 3).

Emotional neglect
Emotional neglect can also result in significant emotional difficulties. These children have been little studied. Anec-dotally, there is a suggestion they may be at risk of depressive disorders in childhood and develop chronically poor self-esteem. The neglected child is characteristically 'hungry' for social and personal stimulation and can be non-discriminating in friendship-making, often attaching him- or herself quickly to strange adults and children. In early childhood many of these children present to paediatric clinics as 'failure to thrive' with a fall-off in expected height and/or weight for their age. Principles of management again rest on eliminating neglect and providing a facilitating environment for normal development.

These syndromes reflect an important area of child psychiatry, where the promotion of normal development may lower the risk of subsequent psychiatric disorder in both child- and adulthood.

Child maltreatment
Non-accidental injury (NAI) including **sexual abuse** is a serious risk factor for conduct and emotional disorder in childhood and a potential risk factor for emotional problems in adulthood.

Children particularly at risk are those born to parents who were themselves physically or sexually abused. There are a number of other well-documented maternal risk factors for non-accidental injury, including:
1 teenage pregnancy;
2 single parent;
3 admission to special care baby unit immediately after birth;
4 maternal psychiatric disorder.
Factors in the children, suggesting abuse include:
1 infants who become immobile in the presence of parents and other adults (frozen watchfulness of infancy);
2 children with repeated and apparently unconnected minor injuries and accidents over weeks or months;
3 children with persistent sexually precocious behaviour with peer group and adults and a knowledge of adult sexual behaviour.
The absence of these factors does not exclude NAI or sexual abuse. Children of all ages and all social classes may be NAI victims. A central aim of intervention is to prevent further abuse and facilitate normal development.

Multidisciplinary teamwork is essential in these cases where social workers have a significant role in assessment of family functioning and advocating the child's best interests often with the help of the courts. Further aspects of child maltreatment are covered in Chapter 24, p. 307.

Some issues of adolescence
Adolescence consists of the teenage years and reflects psychological and physical changes from child to adulthood. Surprisingly little is known about the developmental mechanisms which operate at this age. It is acknowledged, however, that adolescents have particular age-related problems.

Thus it is at this age that the individual asserts increasing autonomy, seeks a closer identification with peer groups and struggles with loosening family ties. Adolescence is a time of identification with particular sub-cultures and experimentation with differing life-styles. Increasing personal enquiry,

Case 3: Hyperkinetic disorder

A $3\frac{1}{2}$-year-old boy was referred to child psychiatry with a 6-month history of *temper tantrums, inattention and restlessness* at his nursery school. Teachers became worried that he *failed to make progress in comparison with the other children* in the class. He had *difficulties in making friends*. In discussing this with his parents they recalled that he had always been a handful at home, with numerous *accidents as a small child*, tripping upstairs, falling out of a chair, etc. The parents had been married for 5 years and had no difficulties although recent disagreements over their son's problems had resulted in some *marital tension*. He had been their first pregnancy and was an only child.

Parents and child were seen together in the clinic and throughout the first interview the *child was restless and inattentive. His play throughout was unconstructive and he moved from one object to another, failing to sustain his interest* in any of the age-appropriate toys available to him. His personal history indicated a *difficult labour and delivery*. Forceps had been used, and he had had a low Apgar score and had spent the first 72 hours of life in special care. He had had *problems in sucking* throughout the first few months of his life and had been a *poor sleeper*. Although he had reached his motor milestones within normal limits, he had always been shown to be somewhat *clumsy*, having difficulty in grasping toys adequately and could not produce fine motor movements. He had shown *little interest in books or reading* despite both his parents being of normal intelligence and many books being available to him. It was hoped that he would improve by going to nursery school but this had not been so.

Play interview with the child indicated *unconstructive play, increasing restlessness and inattention in the presence and absence of his mother*. He was no more responsive to the play worker than he was to his mother, he showed few creative ideas, he could not develop a story using toys and was content to knock toys down, knock over bricks and throw sand and water in an unconstructive manner.

Formulation

A $3\frac{1}{2}$-year-old boy with a history of perinatal adversity, clumsiness and school difficulties characterized by poor attention and concentration, marked restlessness and associated learning difficulties. The situation had resulted in marital tensions. The referral was a result of school difficulties. A preliminary diagnosis of the hyperkinetic disorder was made.

Treatment plan

Liaison with primary care and school services

1 Parent's permission for contacting school and primary care team was obtained. The health visitor was invited to the clinic and provided a report on her observations of his early development and was asked to assist in the overall management by monitoring progress at home and advising the mother on parenting skills with a difficult child.
2 Nursery school was visited and the child observed in the classroom and at play by the child psychiatrist and reports from school obtained.

Hospital investigations

It was decided to investigate him further in the hospital as follows.
1 **Paediatric neurology** as a day case to evaluate the extent of his physical handicap. He was clumsy throughout his day-patient attendance but neurological investigation revealed no structural central nervous system pathology. His EEG was described as immature with no specific abnormalities.
2 **Neuropsychology** to assess his language and development and intellectual ability. He was shown to be of average intelligence but with specific difficulties in word recognition which may lead to later reading difficulties.
3 **Developmental play** sessions to evaluate the extent of his functional abilities and the interaction between his physical and psychological skills. Assessments were carried out as a day-patient, the child attending the clinic with his mother on three occasions

and with both parents twice. In group play he was easily frustrated and aggressive and found difficulty in sharing games and toys. In individual play he was shown to be anxious of reading and learning materials and wary of making relationships with the play therapist.
The health visitor, schoolteacher and educational psychologist attended the clinic and watched an individual play session through a one-way screen.

The diagnosis of hyperkinesis was confirmed, associated with specific learning difficulties. Aetiology was probably a result of perinatal difficulties resulting in functional rather than structural cerebral damage.

Clinic and community-based treatment programme

1 It was agreed that the health visitor would liaise with the play therapist to encourage the mother to engage him with simple exercises to improve his confidence with motor and reading tasks.
2 **School** would concentrate where possible on more 'one to one' work.
3 **The family** would attend the clinic for play sessions together with child and parent counselling on a fortnightly basis for 3 months.

Follow-up management

1 **The health visitor** continued to liaise with the clinic and school. Although the family did not attend the clinic, **home visits and telephone communication** with a social worker from the psychiatric clinic continued until aged 5 when settling into ordinary school was achieved without difficulty.
2 **Learning difficulties** whilst diminished, persisted but were managed within mainstream education.

---

beginning the development of a permanent adult value system, and a sense of self-reliance and responsibility are all more apparent at this age.

It is not surprising, therefore, to find that adolescence also confers on the individual the increased risk of adult psychiatric disorders. Schizophrenia, manic depression and paranoid psychoses are all to be found in adolescents, although rarely in children.

Anorexia nervosa has previously been described and reflects uniquely the dilemma of adolescent development.

Furthermore, the use of drugs and alcohol become prevalent, in particular solvent abuse and use of marijuana, although increasingly heroin and cocaine (see Chapter 10).

Social, cultural and family factors all make a causal contribution to adolescent psychopathology. Some psychiatrists specialize exclusively in this age-group and many regions have developed specialist young people's or adolescent services. Figure 15.4 summarizes the major differences of development on psychopathology.

The outcome of psychiatric disorders in childhood and adolescence

It is important to recognize that as yet the natural course and outcome of the majority of disorders in childhood and adolescence is not fully understood.

Furthermore, outcome depends on a multiplicity of factors, in particular:
1 severity of disorder;
2 age and duration of onset;
3 the quality of family life;
4 the presence of overall disadvantage and scholastic achievement.

Finally, it should be noticed that the form and expression of symptoms can change with age. Both the short-term (months and first 1–2 years) and the long-term (adult adjustment) outcome are different for different disorders.

Developmental syndromes involving delays of normal development (encopresis, enuresis) generally have a good short- and long-term prognosis with nearly 100% of children well adjusted as adults. A very small percentage can remain with difficult and intractable symptoms well into late adolescence.

Developmental syndromes involving speech and language disorders have a prognosis associated with appropriate maturation of the central nervous system and the prevention of secondary psychological difficulties (e.g. development of selfesteem, family disharmony as a result of difficulties and adverse school pressures to achieve). Children with severe learning difficulties involving reading, writing and mathematical skills may have persisting difficulties as adults.

Infantile autism has a poor prognosis, the majority of children requiring extensive psychiatric support and remedial education throughout childhood. Some of these children are able to lead independent lives as adults but the majority require sheltered accommodation and substantial family or local authority supervision.

Hyperkinetic disorders have an outcome that may be more dependent on the presence of conduct symptoms and educational progress. In the absence of these difficulties, the prognosis is good in both the short and long term. The majority of cases, however, have persistent behavioural difficulties at home and school, although attentional difficulties diminish towards adolescence. A significant proportion with conduct disorder, perhaps 10–15%, develop significant antisocial traits as adults. These are almost entirely male and carry an increased risk of criminality and alcoholism in adult life.

Conduct disorders in general show a fluctuating and stormy short-term course with episodes of difficulty often related to persistent social and family disadvantage. There is no clear evidence yet on the outcome into adulthood. Conduct disorder that presents early tends to persist into middle childhood and early adolescence. Severe conduct disorder and delinquency in the presence of persisting social and family disadvantage has a poor outcome into adulthood with a characteristic 'cycle of disadvantage' with similar disturbances repeated in the next generation. Cases of acute onset occurring in previously well-adjusted children and families probably have a good short- and long-term outcome.

Emotional disorders have a good short-term outcome with appropriate intervention. **Obsessional states, severe depression** and rare cases of **hypomania** may persist into adulthood as episodic fluctuating disorders. Severe anxiety neurosis such as can be seen in intractable school refusal can also persist into adulthood, often as agoraphobia.

Outcome for functional psychoses in both the short and long term are similar to adulthood.

Child psychiatry and the law

Rights and responsibilities

In England and Wales the Children's Act 1989 consolidated the rights of children in law to achieve a better balance between adult duties to protect children and the need to allow parents to challenge state authority fairly and quickly. The new act is complex and there are many far reaching implications for children, parents and local authorities. Three core features need mentioning. Firstly, under the new law the welfare of the children must be the paramount consideration of the courts when making decisions. Secondly, the concept of parental responsibility has been introduced to replace that of parental rights emphasizing the duties and obligations of the parent rather than their possession of the child. The law increases the opportunities for children to be parties, separate from their parents, to legal proceedings concerning them. Thirdly, local authorities are charged with a duty to safeguard and promote the welfare of children in need. The law confers certain duties and responsibilities on local authorities to provide services for children and their families in relation to their new statutory obligations (this has not automatically resulted in an increase in resources for child and family care).

Consent to treatment and access to health records

Case law has clarified that children under 16 are capable of providing full consent to treatment. Children under 16 must therefore give their voluntary and continuing permission for receiving a particular treatment. If children are considered not competent under the law, (through mental impairment or mental illness) the consent of a parent or guardian is appropriate. Similarly, children who are mentally competent to give or withhold consent are competent to decide about access to records. If there is a conflict between the wishes of a parent or guardian and that of the child, the best interests of the child are paramount. Good practice is obtained through the involvement of children and parents in decision making about treatment and maintaining clear and concise records.

Aspects of treatment

Multidisciplinary teamwork

The assessment procedure in modern practice involves professionals from different disciplines. Psychiatrists, social workers, psychologists, nurses and psychotherapists may all contribute to different aspects of assessment and formulation depending often on local resources. Psychiatrists must evaluate children's mental states and formulate the case. Family interviewing, play assessments and overall or educational enquiries may be carried out by other members of the team.

Multifactorial aetiologies are common in child and adolescent psychiatry and require clear history taking and analysis of the presenting problems. Treatment follows on from this procedure and must involve:
1 the identification of treatment goals;
2 the focus of treatment;
3 the selection of appropriate treatments.

Child-focused treatments

Psychotherapy involves treating children's anxiety and feelings of depression and the ways in which children think about their symptoms and think about their lives. Individual and group methods are appropriate for school-age children and adolescents, often involving once to twice-weekly sessions for 6 to 12 weeks or longer. When children are receiving **individual** or **group** treatments, families may receive support from other professionals, often a social work team member. If this is adequately done, there is rarely a conflict of interests between the parental desire for information and the child's desire for occasional confidences to be kept.

Behavioural psychotherapy (see pp. 26 and 229–230) is particularly appropriate in many childhood disorders. This often involves helping children develop **wanted** behaviour rather than removing **unwanted** behaviour. Thus learning social skills or the attainment of bowel and bladder control using reward methods such as star charts or other tokens (including 'real rewards' such as pocket money) represent achieving desired behaviours.

Family therapy

Family therapy is an important treatment modality in child psychiatry (see also pp. 236–238, inc. Case 13). This involves meeting with all family members. Under these conditions the children's symptoms are seen as reflecting the family pathology and the whole family must be treated together, often to redefine more clearly the way in which families communicate, to understand the child's role in the family and to improve relationships. Family therapy is generally active, involving the setting of tasks and solving clearly identified problems. Specific issues for child psychiatrists lie in preventing children from getting lost in family therapy and not having enough space to give their own stories; and allowing young children with poor verbal communications the opportunity to use play, even in family sessions, to express how they feel and how they think about family life.

Drugs

Psychotropic drugs have a small but important part to play in child psychiatry. **Antidepressants** can be important in cases of severe childhood depression. Neuroleptic drugs are indicated in children who develop functional psychoses and **lithium** may be prescribed in a child who presents with acute hypomania. **Anxiolytics** such as benzodiazepines may have a place in acute panic and acute school refusal, but have no place in long-term treatment because of the increasing tolerance and risk of dependency. Amphetamine drugs, CNS stimulants, such as **methylphenidate** and **pemaline**, are of importance in some cases of the hyperkinetic disorder where they lower restlessness and improve inattention and concentration, particularly in the first few weeks of treatment.

In general, drug prescribing should be carried out under psychiatric supervision and generally requires the use of day-patient and in-patient facilities.

Accommodation

Residential treatment or childcare arrangements are sometimes indicated, and in a very small number of cases there is a need for secure accommodation for children who commit severe offences.

QUESTIONS

1 What diagnosis needs to be considered when a 9-year-old boy is described by his parents as markedly quieter over the last 3 months, showing no interest in his friends, failing in his schoolwork and off his food? What information will you want to confirm your diagnosis?

2 If a 4-year-old girl appears clumsy and subject to bad tempers at home and at school, can you reassure the parents that she will 'grow out of it' without further investigation? If not how would you investigate the probable cause of her behaviour and symptoms?

3 A 15-year-old boy has a 3-year history of persistent shoplifting, truancy and disorderly behaviour. What family background and social circumstances might you elicit at psychiatric interview? Is he at risk from adult psychiatric disorder and if so what in particular?

4 If a schoolteacher seeks advice on the telephone about a 6-year-old girl who is persistently lifting her dress, attempting to kiss boys and engaging in physical contact with male teachers what would you advise her to do? How might such children be interviewed to obtain a history of their recent experiences?

5 If a 12-year-old girl is dieting excessively, with consequent loss of weight over the last 6 months, would you agree with the point of view that this is likely to be 'no more than a food fad'? What other information would seek to refute this possibility?

FURTHER READING

Black D. & Cottrell D. (1993) *Seminars in Child and Adolescent Psychiatry*. Gaskell Press, Royal College of Psychiatrists, London. [A good readable introductory text to child and adolescent psychiatry.]

Graham P. (1991) *Child Psychiatry: A Developmental Approach*, 2nd Edition. Oxford University Press, Oxford. [A comprehensive and readable text for students and practitioners. Perhaps the best overview for practitioners.]

Hill P. (1989) *Adolescent Psychiatry*. Churchill Livingstone, Edinburgh. [A useful text focusing on a range of issues including adolescent development and psychiatric diagnosis.]

Rutter M. & Hersor L. (1985) *Child and Adolescent Psychiatry: Modern Approaches*. 2nd Edition. Blackwell Scientific Publications, Oxford. [A scholarly and thorough exposition of current thinking in child and adolescent psychiatry.]

Richman N. & Lansdown R. (1990) *Problems of Preschool Children*. John Wiley, Chichester. [A very good introduction to emotional and behavioural development and disorders in young children.]

IV
TREATMENT STRATEGIES

16
Mental Health Care Services

Fact sheet

Objectives of mental health services

1 To promote measures which improve mental well-being and prevent mental illness.

2 To provide accurate diagnosis and effective treatment of curable conditions.

3 To prevent unnecessary loss of functional ability and quality of life in those suffering from incurable mental disorders.

4 To support the care given by friends, family and voluntary groups.

5 To provide a service that is acceptable both to those affected by mental illness and their supporters.

6 To provide good quality accommodation for those whose mental disorder makes it impossible for them to live on their own or to find accommodation that they can afford.

7 To evaluate services regularly and provide feedback to the population served by those services.

8 To make the most effective and efficient use of resources.

Rank order of categories of disease, according to types of burden

Conditions which cause 50% of the total burden		% of total burden
In-patient days	*Mental illness*	31.31
	Mental handicap	15.19
	Cerebrovascular disease	4.86
Out-patient referrals	Neurological disorders	9.82
	Accidents and suicide	7.84
	Bone and joint disease (other than arthritis)	6.87
	Digestive disorders	6.72
	Skin diseases	5.90
	Urogenital disease	5.50
	Mental disorders	3.96
	Arthritis and rheumatism	3.72
GP consultations	Respiratory infections	16.03
	Mental disorders	7.73
	Bronchitis and asthma	5.07
	Skin diseases	4.84
	Accidents and suicide	4.63
	Digestive disorders	4.05
	Arthritis and rheumatism	3.99
	'Other heart disease'	3.06
	'Other bone and joint disease'	2.79
Days of sickness benefit	Bronchitis and asthma	11.46
	Mental disease	9.55
	Accidents and suicide	8.81
	Arthritis and rheumatism	7.22
	Respiratory infections	7.17
	Ischaemic heart disease	5.73
	Digestive disorders	5.73

Hospital admissions for mental illness (DHSS, 1978)

Disease	% of total
Parasuicide	35
Depression	13
Schizophrenia	10
Alcoholism	4
Drug dependency	1
Senile and presenile dementia	3
Other psychoses	5
Neurosis	7
Personality and behaviour disorders	6
Mental handicap	1
Others	15
Total	100

Annual consultation rates for mental diseases in general practice (RCGP/OPCS, 1974)

Disease	Annual consultation rates per 1000 general population
Anxiety	73
Depression	90
Psychoses	25
Psychosomatic	31
Others	100
Total	319

Decision making in mental health services

Type of decision	Corresponding level of decision making
1 'How much of my time should I give this patient?'	Every professional who works with people who suffer from mental illness.
2 'How many days of hospital care should we allocate to this patient?'	The consultant and other members of the team who know the patient on the ward
3 'Which group should have the money available for ward improvements – elderly patients with dementia or the younger patients with schizophrenia?'	The psychiatric unit general manager and the unit executive
4 'Which should have priority – the Psychiatric Hospital or the General Hospital?'	The District Health Authority
5 'Should we employ more social workers for mental illness or put more resources into the prevention of child abuse?'	The Social Services Committee
6 'Should we ask all Health Authorities to make care of elderly people their top priority or should other groups have priority?'	The Secretary of State for Health and Social Security
7 'Should we put more money into the Health Service or into housing?'	The Cabinet

Appendix
Current pattern of health care funding and staff

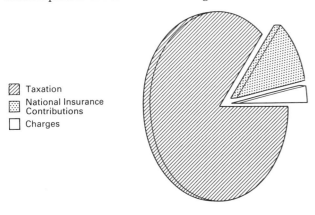

⊘ Taxation
⊡ National Insurance
  Contributions
☐ Charges

Health authority gross expenditure by service group

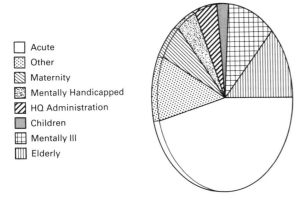

☐ Acute
⊡ Other
⊘ Maternity
⊞ Mentally Handicapped
⊘ HQ Administration
▦ Children
⊞ Mentally Ill
▥ Elderly

National Health Service directly employed staff in England

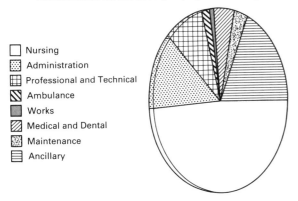

☐ Nursing
⊡ Administration
⊞ Professional and Technical
⊠ Ambulance
▦ Works
⊘ Medical and Dental
⊡ Maintenance
⊟ Ancillary

Mental health care

Psychiatric illness is usually considered in terms of its impact on the individual and his family but it is also a type of health problem which has a major impact on society as a whole, as the figures in the fact sheet demonstrate.

In this chapter we consider ways in which society meets this challenge.

The mental health of an individual is determined by two competing sets of forces. There are those which have an adverse effect on mental health and either lead to mental illness or prevent or slow down recovery. These factors are discussed in Chapter 2 which reviews the causes of mental illness. Ranged against these adverse factors is mental health care, a wide range of different types of care which prevent mental illness, promote recovery of mental health when illness occurs, and allows the individual with incurable or chronic mental health problems to cope with dignity.

Four types of care
A great deal of prominence has been given to community care in the last few years but the term 'community care' is confusing and unhelpful. It is usually used to mean the provision of professional services outside the main hospital setting with the implication that there are two types of care – hospital care and community care – as illustrated in Fig. 16.1.

However, this concept of community care is far too narrow and contains a number of anomalies. For example, the use of 'community' to mean outside hospital implies that a hospital service is not a community service, which is absurd.

Furthermore, much of the debate about care for people with mental illness has focused too much on professional care and it is more appropriate to think of four different types of care as demonstrated in Fig. 16.2.

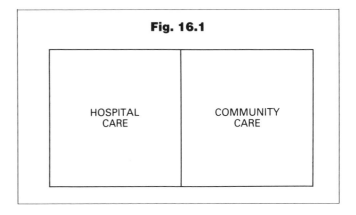

Fig. 16.1

HOSPITAL CARE

COMMUNITY CARE

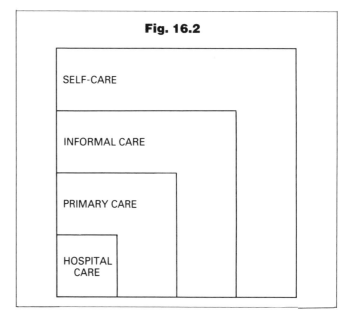

Fig. 16.2

SELF-CARE

INFORMAL CARE

PRIMARY CARE

HOSPITAL CARE

This figure demonstrates that the four different types of care are not necessarily mutually exclusive and that individuals are often receiving all four types of care, if not simultaneously at least during the course of a week (Case 1).

Case 1

Mary T. is aged 45 and single. She has been given a number of different diagnoses including schizophrenia and personality disorder, but does not conform to any classic diagnostic syndrome.

She lives in a small local authority flat and *her mother visits* her most days, in part to help her with the practicalities of life such as her rent rebate, in part to provide her with some company and to persuade her to keep attending the day hospital.

She visits her *general practitioner* frequently with a wide range of physical symptoms and is visited at home by a *psychiatric community nurse* if she does not attend the day hospital. She receives regular injections of a phenothiazine prescribed in an attempt to prevent her quarrelling with her neighbours yet again.

Self-care

Self-care is the most important type of care.

Preventive self-care

Some mental illnesses such as Alzheimer's disease and schizophrenia affect individuals no matter what their lifestyle or behaviour has been, but other disorders are not of this inevitable nature and appear to affect people whose ability to cope with life's challenges is less well developed. Some people can preserve their mental health more effectively than others, but the development of coping ability appears to relate largely to one's early life and attempts to provide people with a general ability to cope with life's challenges in a more resilient fashion, whether by assertiveness training or life skills training, have not so far been demonstrated as being effective in reducing the incidence of mental disorder.

It does appear, however, that people can be taught how to cope with specific problems if they are offered help soon after the problem has developed. For example, counselling and support, often by others who have faced the same problem as well as by professionals, can help people adversely affected by bereavement, violent crime, or the onset of a disabling disease, not simply by providing emotional support for them but also by providing skills which they can use to adapt successfully to their changed condition or circumstances.

Supportive self-care

Things people do for themselves often help them to cope with and solve psychological problems without professional intervention. Many people solve their own problems either by finding a way to cope when they are faced with a challenge or sometimes by chance, as demonstrated by Case 2.

Furthermore, when an individual is getting help from a doctor or some other professional they have to decide if they wish to accept the professional's advice, for example to take the medicine prescribed. Doing what the professional advises is usually called 'compliance', although 'consent' would probably be a more appropriate word as the term 'compliance' has connotations of weakness and passivity on the part of the person with the psychological problems.

Case 2

On her first day at kindergarten a 4-year-old girl became so upset as her mother prepared to leave that the *mother was forced to stay with her until the end of the school day*. The same thing happened every day thereafter. The situation soon grew into *a considerable stress for all concerned*, but all attempts at solving the problem failed. One morning *the mother was unable to drive the child to school and the father dropped her off* on his way to work. The child cried a little but soon calmed down. When the mother again took her to school on the following morning there was no relapse; the child remained calm and *the problem never recurred*.

The obvious question arises: what would have happened if the school psychologist had had a chance to start working on this problem? In all likelihood the case would have been diagnosed as a school phobia, and, depending on the psychologist's professional mythology, the dependency needs of the child, the overprotectiveness of the mother, the symbiotic aspects of their relationship, a marital conflict between the parents causing the child's behaviour problem could conceivably have become the object of therapy. If at age 21 the daughter had run into emotional difficulties of some kind or another, she would already have had a psychiatric record reaching all the way back into childhood, and this in turn would define her prognosis as worse than otherwise.

Patients are usually blamed for poor compliance but in most cases the person primarily responsible is the professional giving the advice, for studies of 'poor compliance'

Fig. 16.3 A short list of compliance-improving actions for busy practitioners

For all regimens
Information
1 Keep the prescription as simple as possible.
2 Give clear instructions on the exact treatment regimen, preferably written.

For long-term regimens
Reminders
3 Call if appointment missed.
4 Prescribe medication in concert with patient's daily schedule.
5 Stress importance of compliance at each visit.
6 Titrate frequency of visits to compliance need.

Rewards
7 Recognize patient's efforts to comply at each visit.
8 Decrease visit frequency if compliance high.

Social support
9 Involve patient's spouse or other partner.

Haynes, R. Brian (1984) A critical review of interventions to improve compliance with special reference to the role of physicians, in: *Improving Medication Compliance*. Proceedings of a Symposium, National Pharmaceutical Council, Washington DC, November.

have shown that the main reason professional advice is not taken is that professionals talk too much and listen too little; they do not enter into negotiation but simply give advice which they expect to be followed. The main responsibility for poor compliance rests clearly with the medical profession because deficiencies in communication and treatment planning are common. The steps that professionals can take are shown in Fig. 16.3. Compliance in taking medication is further discussed in Chapter 17, p. 213.

Informal care

Friends and neighbours

The behaviour of neighbours can have an influence on a person's psychological problems. Helpful neighbours can help the person cope; intolerant neighbours can accelerate the person's decline. This is particularly the case with elderly people suffering from the effects of Alzheimer's disease.

Professionals very often overlook the actual or potential support of neighbours. Friends are also very important and the person with good friends is better able to cope with crises and adverse events although, of course, some people are better able to establish good relationships than others, and it may be that this characteristic and the characteristic of being able to cope with crises are both derived from the same set of factors.

The fact that men have more opportunities of meeting friends than women, for example by dropping into the pub, or at work, is one of the factors responsible for the fact that women consult professionals more frequently with psychological disorders.

Family

The part that the family plays in either creating psychological problems or in helping individuals cope is described in numerous parts of this book but professionals still underestimate the importance of the family and too often see the patient in isolation.

Voluntary groups

A number of voluntary groups offer help to people in distress and both prevent and alleviate the effects of psychological problems.

Much of the support provided for people without family support and without homes is provided by voluntary associations such as the Church Army, Salvation Army and the Cyrenians. Voluntary groups also help people with homes and jobs and although the influence the Samaritans have on the suicide rate is a matter of dispute, there is little doubt that they help many people in distress. Marriage Guidance Councils also help individuals and families in difficulty. It is essential not to underestimate the contribution that churches and other religious organizations make which is often done by professionals in health and social services who are, as a group, inclined to overlook the spiritual dimension of life.

Fig. 16.4 Mutual aid societies

MIND

MIND merits a special mention because of its unique position and function. Nationally MIND is a focus for research and action with a particular interest in raising national policy issues and a particular skill in lobbying Westminster. There are many local branches of MIND and these work in different ways according to local problems and opportunties. In almost all cases a local branch of MIND will act on behalf of mentally ill people to press the public services for more effective and sympathetic care.

Other mutual aid societies with local branches
National Schizophrenia Fellowship
PAD – People Against Depression
Alcoholics Anonymous
Alzheimer's Disease Society
Gingerbread (one-parent families)
Families Anonymous
CRUSE

Mutual aid societies

Mutual aid societies consist of groups of people who share the same problem. There are increasing numbers of such societies (Fig. 16.4).

The societies provide useful information to individuals based on the experience of others who have had to cope with a problem and have very effective means of passing on tips on how to cope, either with the problem itself or with the unhelpful professional. Not all mutual aid societies' activities are beneficial in the eyes of the professional and there is no doubt that their activities have some drawbacks and deficiencies, but their general effect has been very helpful.

Primary care

In the UK the term 'primary care' usually means the services delivered by a primary care team consisting of a general practitioner, health visitor, district nurse, community midwife and their support staff.

The functions of the primary care team

Solving problems

Some of the problems that are brought to primary care can be solved by members of the primary care team.

The general practitioner deals with a wide range of problems, as discussed in Chapter 12; the health visitor usually concentrates on mothers with young children, dealing not only with specific entities such as puerperal depression (see p. 146) but also dealing with problems caused by bringing up children in poverty and bad housing; the district nurse works mostly with older people but some of her work is with young disabled people and she is obviously involved in helping them to cope with emotional reactions to disability.

Supporting problems

Not all problems are soluble but the primary care team can help individuals cope with long-term insoluble problems and general practitioners are involved on a long-term basis with many people with schizophrenia, personality disorders or intractable emotional disorders.

Sharing problems

Some of the problems brought to primary care workers cannot be solved by primary care teams and are therefore shared with the hospital service. The factors influencing referral are discussed in Chapter 12 (p. 150) as well as later in this chapter (p. 206).

The strengths and weaknesses of primary care teams

Primary care teams are one of the characteristic features of the National Health Service and in very few other countries do doctors and nurses work together in such an intimate or effective manner. This arrangement has both strengths and weaknesses but on balance the strengths usually outweigh the weaknesses (Fig. 16.5).

Primary contact care

The primary care team is more appropriately called a 'primary health care team' for it consists entirely of people working within the National Health Service, yet many other professionals make direct contact with people with mental health problems.

1 *Social workers* have many clients with mental health problems and are involved in certain aspects of the operation of the Mental Health Act (see p. 316).

2 *Medical social workers* supporting patients in hospital can help individuals and families cope with disability or bereavement and thus prevent mental health problems.

3 *Psychiatric social workers* work in hospital but are members of Social Services Departments.

4 *Home helps* and home help organizers provide support for many elderly people suffering from Alzheimer's disease,

sometimes visiting more than once a day, 7 days a week (see p. 158).

5 *Probation officers* try to support a number of people who have mental illness or problems with alcohol or drug abuse whose health problems bring them into contact with the court because of the associated crimes.

6 *Educational psychologists*, often working in teams with psychiatric social workers and clinical psychologists, play a part in the Child Psychiatric Service (see p. 189, Case 1).

7 *Homeless families unit* and *housing department staff* are in contact with many people with mental health problems.

A new vision of primary health care

Primary health care has developed in the last few years, in part from the work done by the World Health Organization with developing countries. Primary health care in a developing country where professionals are very few in number is not defined by where those professionals work or who first makes contact with a person with a health problem; it is defined by a set of principles and these principles are increasingly being used in the UK as a basis for service development.

There are four main planks in the primary health care platform.

1 Care should always be organized for whole populations; often health professionals devote all their energy to the individuals who make contact with them when it is well known from epidemiological studies that there are always individuals who do not make contact who are in equal, if not greater, need of professional help and support.

2 There should be effective and efficient use of resources; it is not wrong to think about finding out whether particular services are useful or if those services are being provided as cheaply as possible; in fact it can be argued that it is wrong not to ask these questions because money that is wasted on ineffective services or on the inefficient delivery of an effective service is money that cannot be used to help other people in need.

3 There should be cooperation between all the agencies involved in mental health care; too often different professional services work in isolation or even in competition.

4 People with mental health problems and their relatives should be involved at every level in the planning and delivery of care.

Fig. 16.5 Strengths and weaknesses of the primary care team

1 Patients register with a general practitioner and stay with that doctor no matter how many specialists they see until they move to another part of the country; but the drawback is that it is very hard for a mentally ill person to change general practitioner if he or his relatives have lost confidence.

2 It is relatively easy to make contact with a doctor or nurse in primary care; but because the primary care team is a filter for specialist care a person with a mental health problem may find it more difficult to reach specialist help than the individual in more competitive health systems where direct access to expert help is more common.

3 The quality of general practice is improving as more talented and able students elect to enter general practice and as vocational training becomes more widespread; but there is wide variation in the quality of care offered and some practices offer poor care to individuals with mental health problems.

4 Teamwork is one of the strengths of primary care in the UK; but some teams have problems with communication and this can create difficulties for patients and their relatives.

Hospital care

In the past, psychiatric hospitals were built far away from the communities they served, in part because these large institutions required large tracts of land, in part because the communities wanted 'the lunatics' to be incarcerated as far away as possible. The world was therefore clearly divided into 'the sane' and 'the insane' with 'the community' the land outside the hospital wall. The hospital served its community by admitting those deemed insane, and was the hub at the centre of the services.

Some of these remote institutions have been closed, with more appropriate and local facilities being opened but even

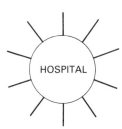

where the old buildings remain those who work within them are trying to change the relationship between the hospital and other services which help people with mental illness. The hospital is now a node in a network rather than a hub whose principal function was simply to admit or discharge patients.

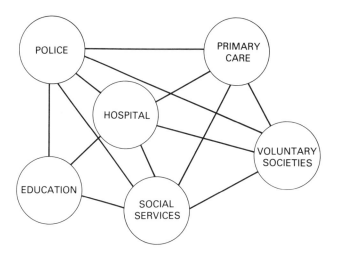

Fig. 16.6 Venn diagram showing relationship between the first three levels of care

A=Consult their doctor during year
B=Psychiatrically ill during year (level 1)
C=Identified by their doctor as psychiatrically ill (level 2)
D=Referred to a psychiatrist (level 3)
▨ Do not pass 1st filter (ill, but do not consult)
▦ Do not pass 2nd filter (illness unrecognized by doctor)
▨ Do not pass 3rd filter (not referred to a psychiatrist)

Filters between types of care

The different types of care that have been described are not, as has been emphasized, mutually exclusive but an individual is often receiving more than one type of care. The moves from self-care to informal care, and then to primary care, and then to hospital care, are in part determined by the seriousness of the symptom, but the decision to change from one type of care to another is also influenced by many other factors.

Much of the work describing the factors that influence what have been called the size of the pores of the filters between different types of care has been done by Goldberg and Huxley (Fig. 16.6).

The filter between self-care and informal care
Frequently a person is unable to gain family support because the family lives too far away, for population mobility is a feature of modern life. However, even where the family lives close by there can be barriers in seeking family support. In some families relationships are not sufficiently close to allow individuals to seek help easily whereas in others there are close relationships but family members find it difficult to

express feelings and distress to one another. Both these characteristics can prevent an individual receiving family support.

Similar factors influence the probability that an individual will receive support from friends.

Support groups have an important part to play but only a proportion of those who would benefit join such groups. Some are aware of the existence of such groups but do not wish to join a group, and others never hear about their existence and thus never make contact.

The filter between self-care and primary care
For every case known to primary care workers there is at least one other case not known to them. Sometimes the problem is simply one of access, for example if a distressed young person is not able to communicate with the general practitioner they trust on a Saturday morning they may either seek another informal source of help or take an overdose.

The probability that an individual will consult a general practitioner depends in part upon the degree of support that they are receiving from other people, in part on the beliefs and attitudes of the patient about friends and family, and the general practitioner concerned. Of course even when a person has made contact with a general practitioner there may still be a barrier to care as the general practitioner may not recognize the person as having a psychiatric problem;

conversely some people may be included as 'psychiatric cases' by a general practitioner when they have in fact a treatable physical disorder such as menopausal hormone imbalance.

The filter between primary care and specialist service

The probability that a general practitioner will refer a case to the psychiatric service depends in part on the severity of the symptoms presented but is also influenced by the following factors.

1 Access; people are more likely to be referred the nearer they live to a specialist service.

2 Other facilities available to general practitioners; if a general practitioner can refer directly to a clinical psychologist who attends the health centre regularly, he will be less likely to refer a patient to a hospital for treatment of, for example, a phobic disorder.

3 The beliefs and attitudes of the patient, their friends and family, the general practitioner, and of course the specialist referral service which can influence the culture in which it operates by increasing or damping down demand.

Future patterns of mental health care

Community care in the 1990s

In the 1980s, the NHS continued to develop community care, principally by closing large psychiatric asylums and transferring services to more locally based facilities such as day centres, smaller in-patient units and community-based teams. In parallel with this, the government introduced changes which allowed more people to claim social security for living in nursing homes or other forms of residential care. This led to a dramatic and rapid expansion in the number of private residential care places. This was most marked in the services available for elderly people with Alzheimer's disease but also applied to younger people with long-term psychiatric problems.

Because there was concern about the uncontrolled growth of long-term care, the government undertook a review and introduced legislation – the NHS Community Care Act 1990 – which transferred all responsibility for long-term care to health and social services, requring individuals to have a multidisciplinary assessment before they could be placed in long-term care and supported by the state. This was undoubtedly an advance because many people were admitted to long-term care in the 1980s without an adequate assessment of their need for long-term care and the options for looking after them in their own homes or in a hostel. This Act came into place on 1 April 1993.

Purchasing and providing

The NHS reorganization that took place at about the same time as the changes outlined above involved the division of responsibility for identifying need and allocating resources – purchasing – on the one hand from the provision of services on the other – providing. Health authorities would remain purchasers of care but GP fundholders, who will cover about half the population by 1994, were given the right to purchase some services. The GP fundholders were initially only given powers to purchase elective surgery but in 1993 were given the power to pay for certain types of psychiatric service.

Providing mental health services in the 1990s

Major changes are taking place, both in the mental health services and in the way in which they are funded. These changes will increase uncertainty and make long-term planning more difficult, but there is an increased commitment of people working in different agencies, notably health and social services, to work together rather than in parallel. More radical approaches are also being tried with home treatment for acute psychiatric disorders but, although care in the community will undoubtedly become a reality, as well as rhetoric, in the 1990s, there will continue to be a need for in-patient facilities; community care will fail unless it is adequately supported by well-resourced and well-organized in-patient facilities.

As was emphasized earlier in this chapter, in-patient facilities should not be seen as a competitor with community facilities but as a service for the community. Thus community care involves a wide range of facilities including facilities for the acutely ill person requiring urgent admission for in-patient psychiatric treatment. Without this comprehensive approach the needs of people with psychiatric disorders will not be adequately met.

Fig. 16.7 Community care

Both these words have imprecise meanings so it is not surprising that the term 'community care' should differ from one part of the country to another. The types of activity which are embraced by this term are:

1 decentralization of specialist psychiatric services from a single central hospital to locally based units;

2 closer collaboration between hospital staff and primary care workers;

3 the transfer of patients from long-stay beds in large psychiatric hospitals to group homes or hostels;

4 the provision of hospital facilities as close to the community served as possible;

5 increased recognition and support of the part played by carers and voluntary groups.

It is essential to remember that community care is not necessarily cheaper than the traditional approach to psychiatric care: on the contrary, it is often more expensive.

QUESTIONS

1 What should be the top priority for the development of mental health services?

2 What could be done to prevent mental health problems?

3 What could be done to improve the management of mental health problems in primary care?

4 What would you say the three most important characteristics of a 'good' mental health service were?

5 What would you say were the most important characteristics which would allow you to identify a 'bad' mental health service?

FURTHER READING

Goldberg D. & Huxley P. (1980) *Mental Illness in the Community.* Tavistock Publications, London. [This describes the pattern of mental illness in the whole population and the ways in which people are, or are not, referred for specialist care.]

17
The Physical Treatments

Fact sheet

Physical treatments

The most commonly used physical treatment in psychiatry is drug therapy. Anxiolytics and hypnotics are used most widely, especially in general practice. ECT is employed in a small proportion of hospital inpatients. Psychosurgery is used very rarely.

Electroconvulsive therapy

Indications

Severe depressive illness when drug treatment has failed or circumstances (suicide risk, physical deterioration) require a quick and certain response. Mania, unresponsive to drug treatment.

Side effects

Headache, some retrograde amnesia. No firm evidence for enduring memory deficit.

Antipsychotic drugs

Indications

Schizophrenia, both acute management and maintenance treatment; acute management of mania; organic psychosis.

Classes of drugs

Phenothiazenes, thioxanthenes, butyrophenones, substituted benzamides, dibenzazepines, benzisotazoles.

Side effects

Anticholinergic (dry mouth, blurred vision, constipation, micturition difficulties), anti-adrenergic (sedation, postural hypotension) and antihistaminic (drowsiness, weight gain). Therapeutic effect caused by dopamine receptor blocking properties which also cause movement disorders (acute dystonias, akathisia, Parkinsonian symptoms and tardive dyskinesia). Clozapine can cause agranulocytosis.

Antidepressant drugs

Indications

Depressive illness, anxiety disorders, obsessive compulsive disorder (5-HT uptake blockers).

Classes of drugs

Tricyclic antidepressants (TCAs), monoamine oxidase inhibitors (MAOIs), newer antidepressants, including selective 5-HT uptake inhibitors.

Side effects

TCAs: anticholinergic, anti-adrenergic, antihistaminic, cardiotoxic. MAOIs: postural hypotension, many drug and food interactions (except moclobemide). Newer antidepressants: better tolerated than TCAs or MAOIs, less anticholinergic and cardiotoxic. Effectiveness in severely ill patients and long-term safety not fully evaluated.

Mood stabilizing drugs

Indications

Prophylaxis of recurrent affective disorders, especially manic depressive illness; acute treatment of mania.

Classes of drugs

Lithium, carbamazepine

Side effects

Lithium: tremor, thirst, polyuria, impairment of renal function, hypothyroidism. Carbamazepine: nausea, dizziness, low white cell count.

Anxiolytics and hypnotics

Drugs used are almost exclusively of benzodiazepine class, but buspirone, a 5-HT receptor agonist, is a recent addition. Zopiclone, a cyclopyrrolone binds to site close to the benzodiazepine receptor.

Indications

Short-term treatment of anxiety and insomnia where counselling and reassurance are ineffective.

Side effects

Drowsiness, ataxia, psychomotor impairment, psychological and physical dependence, withdrawal reactions (probably not buspirone).

Psychosurgery

Indications

Intractable obsessional and depressive disorders.

Side effects

Apathy, disinhibition (not usually seen with modern procedures).

What are the physical treatments?

Physical treatments in psychiatry are those which are designed to alleviate psychiatric disorders by directly altering brain function. Such treatments usually take the form of administration of chemical substances, that is pharmacotherapy, but other procedures are also employed, for example the induction of seizures as in ECT, or rarely, psychosurgery. Physical treatments of various kinds have been used in psychiatry for thousands of years. In retrospect, many of these procedures seem bizarre in the extreme. However, even comparatively recently, treatments such as insulin coma therapy were once enthusiastically advocated, only to be abandoned a few years later as valueless and even harmful. The reason for this unhappy situation has been twofold. Firstly, until a few years ago there were no effective treatments for severe psychiatric illness; secondly, the aetiology of the conditions has been unknown.

We still know little about the biochemical basis of major psychiatric disorders and most of the treatments currently employed were discovered by chance, or more accurately, astute clinical observation. This is, of course, not unusual in medicine; the use of digitalis to treat dropsy far preceded knowledge of the aetiology of heart failure. In these circumstances the evaluation of therapy becomes particularly important and the advent of the controlled clinical trial has had major consequences for psychiatric treatment.

In essence, a controlled trial assesses the effect of a particular treatment by controlling for all the other variables in a therapeutic encounter. Thus in a drug trial, one group of patients will receive the drug treatment under investigation while another carefully matched group of subjects will receive identical care and assessment while being treated with an inert substance of the same appearance as the active drug ('placebo'). The study should be designed so that neither the patient nor the doctor giving the treatment or making the assessment knows which patients are receiving the active drug and which the placebo ('double-blind').

Assessment of psychiatric treatment is particularly difficult because of the powerful effect of non-specific factors such as suggestion and the tendency of some conditions to remit spontaneously. The proper application of controlled trials has allowed the satisfactory assessment of nearly all the treatments described in this chapter.

What conditions are helped by physical treatments?

The indications for particular physical treatments are described in the chapters dealing with the specific disorders. In general physical treatments are particularly useful in the management of major psychiatric illnesses such as schizophrenia and severe mood disorders. Drug therapy is often prescribed for patients with less serious conditions such as anxiety states or mild depression, but for these disorders one of the various forms of psychotherapy is usually more appropriate.

There is no reason why physical and other methods of treatment should not be combined. In fact a number of studies in depressed patients have shown that a combination

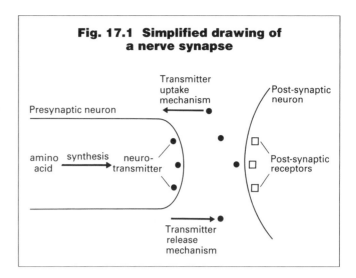

Fig. 17.1 Simplified drawing of a nerve synapse

of drug treatment and psychotherapy may be more effective than either given alone.

How do physical treatments work?

Most of our knowledge of effects of physical treatments on the brain comes from studies on laboratory animals. Whilst this information tells us much about the neuropharmacological effects of the treatments, we do not know with any certainty which, if any, of these actions is responsible for the therapeutic effect in patients.

In general psychotropic drugs and perhaps ECT appear to act by producing changes at nerve synapses (Fig. 17.1). At the synapse they either inhibit or increase the effect of one of the chemical transmitter substances that act as messengers between individual neurons. The substances particularly implicated are noradrenaline, 5-hydroxytryptamine (5-HT) and dopamine. The neurons which use these transmitters originate in the brain-stem and mid-brain, from which they fan out to innervate much of the cortex and limbic system. In animal studies, altering the function of these transmitters can affect fundamental processes such as eating, sleeping and reward. The effects of various physical treatments on these neuronal pathways will be discussed in more detail subsequently.

Electroconvulsive therapy

When should ECT be used?

The use of ECT in psychiatry has always been associated with a degree of controversy. Criticism has tended to be directed both towards a supposed lack of effectiveness and the unpleasant nature of the procedure. Such criticism has had a positive effect in stimulating clinical and basic research and as a result of carefully controlled trials there is now indisputable evidence that ECT is a highly effective treatment for severe depression. Importantly, ECT is often successful where treatment with antidepressant medication has failed, or is of limited value, for example, in patients with psychotic depression. In addition where a depressive illness is associated with life-threatening complications such as failure to eat and drink or high risk of suicide, ECT should be considered as the first line of treatment because of this rapid effectiveness (Fig. 17.2).

ECT is usually administered twice weekly and whilst there is much variation, the usual number of treatments given is between six and eight, this being decided by the clinical response of the patient. Improvement in appetite and motor retardation often precede alleviation of depressed mood; for this reason there is said to be an increased risk of suicide in the initial stages of treatment. ECT can be combined with antidepressant drugs and it is usual to continue patients on antidepressants after a course of ECT to help prevent relapse.

Is ECT safe?

The evidence suggests that ECT is a safe treatment and in certain populations, for example older people, it may be safer than antidepressant drugs. The major risk is not the application of the current or the resulting seizure but rather the accompanying anaesthetic procedure. The contraindications for ECT are therefore those of high anaesthetic risk. In addition raised intracranial pressure is regarded as a contraindication, but the presence of an epileptic disorder is not.

ECT machines now recommended for clinical use deliver low-energy electrical current in the form of brief pulses. The amount of electrical energy administered during treatment is much less than was given by older machines and side effects

such as post-ECT confusion and retrograde amnesia are correspondingly diminished. With brief-pulse machines, bilateral placement of the stimulating electrodes usually offers the right balance between therapeutic efficacy and low incidence of side effects. However, in patients experiencing troublesome side effects during treatment, unilateral application of the electrodes to the non-dominant hemisphere (usually the right side of the head) will cause less post-treatment confusion and amnesia. With older ECT machines, particularly those delivering modified sine wave current, unilateral ECT should still be preferred.

There is no evidence from either clinical studies or relevant animal investigations that ECT causes structural brain damage or is associated with the development of spontaneous seizures. Equally in general ECT does not appear to cause memory difficulties after the end of treatment.

Is ECT unpleasant?

A survey of depressed patients who had been given ECT indicated that most found the treatment helpful. When asked to compare ECT with dental treatment the majority felt the latter to be more unpleasant. Their major complaints about ECT tended to concern factors which could fairly easily be remedied such as lack of privacy and prolonged periods of waiting.

How does ECT work?

The clinical findings suggest that the crucial factor in the effectiveness of ECT is the induction of a bilateral seizure. There is historical evidence that seizures caused by the administration of drugs or photic stimulation were also effective therapeutically. However, electricity is preferred as the seizure-inducing agent because of its safety and ease of administration.

Not surprisingly a generalized seizure has major effects on many different brain pathways and neurotransmitter systems. It is therefore of great interest that, in animal investigations, ECT given in the same way as to depressed patients produces changes in certain noradrenaline receptors that are identical to those produced by antidepressant drugs (see

Fig. 17.3 Classification of clinical psychotropic drugs

Name	Examples of classes	Indications
Antipsychotic	Phenothiazines Butyrophenones Substituted benzamides	Acute treatment of schizophrenia and mania, prophylaxis of schizophrenia
Antidepressant	Tricyclic antidepressants Monoamine oxidase inhibitors Selective 5-HT uptake blockers	Major depression (acute treatment and prophylaxis), anxiety disorders, obsessive compulsive disorder (5-HT uptake blockers)
Mood stabilizer	Lithium Carbamazepine	Acute treatment of mania. Prophylaxis of recurrent affective disorder
Anxiolytic	Benzodiazepines Azapirones (buspirone)	Generalized anxiety disorder
Hypnotic	Benzodiazepines Cyclopyrrolones (zopiclone)	Insomnia

below). In addition, ECT, unlike drug treatment, increases dopamine function, perhaps explaining why it is particularly effective in patients with severe motor retardation.

Pharmacotherapy

Physical treatment in psychiatry mainly takes the form of drug therapy (Fig. 17.3). Drugs which are psychologically active tend to be lipophilic substances which penetrate well into the brain. This lipid solubility ensures that they are well absorbed from the gastrointestinal tract and widely distributed in body tissues. Because of this most psychotropic drugs are rather slowly eliminated, being metabolized by the liver to inactive, water-soluble glucuronides, before excretion by the kidney. Accordingly the presence of hepatic or renal disease necessitates caution in prescribing. Psychotropic drugs may potentiate the effect of alcohol which should be used in moderation or preferably avoided during psychotropic drug treatment.

Compliance with medication is a particular difficulty in the treatment of psychiatric disorders. Many patients with severe illnesses may not see the need for treatment or believe that it can help them. Careful explanations supplemented by written instructions are of value. Where psychotropic medication is discontinued it should usually be withdrawn gradually since sudden discontinuation of some drugs, especially anxiolytics and antidepressants can give rise to abstinence syndromes. Compliance is further discussed in Chapter 16, p. 202 (see also Fig. 17.4).

Antipsychotic drugs

How do antipsychotic drugs work?

There is little doubt that the antipsychotic effect of conventional antipsychotic drugs is attributable to blockade of dopamine receptors probably in mesolimbic or mesocortical brain regions. However, while this blockade becomes apparent during the first few hours of treatment a number of weeks may pass before a striking antipsychotic effect is apparent. This has led to proposals that the acute pharmacological effect of neuroleptics is followed by adaptive changes in the brain that produce the antipsychotic effect. It has been suggested for example that a depolarizing blockade of presynaptic dopamine neurons eventually evolves which, together with the postsynaptic receptor blockade, produces the pronounced reduction in dopamine transmission necessary for the antipsychotic effect.

Another important advance in understanding the mode of

Fig. 17.4 Compliance in taking medication

1 Administration of treatment. Simplify daily drug regime. Reduce number and frequency of drugs administered.
2 Side effects. Many drugs cause side effects often before therapeutic effect apparent. Explain and reassure patient accordingly.
3 Psychological factors. Explain need for treatment and give explanation of therapy. If necessary ask relative to supervize medication.
4 Behaviour of doctor. Education of patient improves compliance. Written notes may be useful as is enthusiastic and confident attitude!

---

action of antipsychotic drugs has been the recent description of multiple dopamine receptor subtypes in mammalian brain. For example, conventional neuroleptics bind strongly to the D_2 dopamine receptor subtype, but only weakly to D_4 receptors. In contrast, clozapine has a relatively higher affinity for D_4 receptors. This difference in binding profile may account for the efficacy of clozapine in patients unresponsive to other neuroleptics.

When are antipsychotic drugs used?

Antipsychotic drugs, also known as neuroleptics and major tranquillizers, are used to treat psychotic disorders, principally schizophrenia and mania. In the acute phase of the illness antipsychotic drugs have a useful sedative effect but in addition they ameliorate psychotic symptoms such as delusions, hallucinations and thought disorder. Especially in schizophrenia, maintenance treatment reduces the risk of acute relapse.

Pharmacology

The first discovered group of antipsychotic agents, the phenothiazines, are divided into three classes (aliphatic, piperidine and piperazine) depending on the side chain attached to the nitrogen atom in the middle ring of the tricyclic nucleus (Fig. 17.5). Thioxanthenes such as flupenthixol are based on a similar three-ring structure, but butyrophenones such as haloperidol are structurally dissimilar.

All antipsychotic drugs currently employed block dopamine receptors in the brain, a property which appears necessary for their antipsychotic activity, and is also responsible for their tendency to produce extrapyramidal movement disorders. The substituted benzamides are a class of drugs related in structure to metoclopramide. The two agents of this class in clinical use, sulpiride and remoxapride, bind selectively to dopamine receptors and are less likely than most other antipsychotic agents to produce movement disorders, or sedation. However, **remoxapride**, has recently been associated with cases of **aplastic anaemia** and its use is now restricted to patients in whom no other antipsychotic drug is deemed suitable.

Clozapine is a dibenzazepine which is relatively weak blocker of dopamine receptors but has strong antagonist effects at certain 5-HT receptors. The importance of clozapine is that it may produce significant clinical benefit in patients unresponsive to other antipsychotic drugs. It also produces less extrapyramidal movement disorders. However, these potential benefits have to be weighed against its toxicity to white blood cells (see below).

Risperidone is a recently introduced benzisoxazole derivative which produces a potent blockade of both dopamine D_2 and 5-HT_2 receptors. Controlled studies have indicated that risperidone produces fewer extrapyramidal side effects than haloperidol and may also ameliorate negative symptoms of schizophrenia to some extent. Whether risperidone, like clozapine, may offer therapeutic benefit in patients who are unresponsive to conventional antipsychotic drugs is not yet clear.

Fig. 17.5 Structure and pharmacology of neuroleptics

Chlorpromazine

Flupenthixol

Haloperidol

Class of drug	Drug	Properties
Aliphatic	Chlorpromazine Promazine	Block dopamine receptors with relatively low potency; however, antagonize α-adrenergic, H₁-histaminergic and muscarinic cholinergic receptors (especially thioridazine).
Piperdine	Thioridazine Pipothiazine	Lower incidence of extrapyramidal movement disorders but more sedation, hypotension and anticholinergic effects. More likely to cause photosensitivity reaction and lower seizure threshold.
Piperazine	Trifluperazine Fluphenazine	Potent blockers of dopamine receptors; relatively little effect on α-adrenergic and muscarinic cholinergic receptors. High incidence of extrapyramidal movement disorders. Less sedative and anticholinergic effects. Fewer skin reactions, less effect on seizure threshold.
Thioxanthene	Flupenthixol Clopenthixol	
Butyrophenone	Haloperidol	
Substituted benzamide	Sulpiride Remoxapride	Selective blockers of dopamine receptors. Little sedation. Not anticholinergic. Less liable to cause Parkinsonism and perhaps tardive dyskinensia.
Dibenzazepine	Clozapine	Weak blocker of dopamine receptors. Strong 5-HT receptor antagonist. Effective in patients refractory to other neuroleptics but risk of leucopenia (2–3%), makes weekly blood counts manadatory. Other side effects – hypersalivation, drowsiness, weight gain, seizures. Low risk of extrapyramidal disorders.

How to use antipsychotic drugs

Antipsychotic drugs are used to control psychomotor excitement, hostility and other abnormal behaviour resulting from schizophrenia, mania or organic psychosis. If the patient is very excited, and displaying abnormally aggressive behaviour, the aim should be to bring the behaviour under control as quickly and safely as possible. Chlorpromazine (orally or intramuscularly) has previously been recommended for this purpose but has the disadvantage of producing autonomic side effects such as hypotension. Current practice favours the use of low doses of drugs such as haloperidol (2–10 mg) or droperidol (2–5 mg) with diazepam (5–20 mg) or lorazepam (1–4 mg). These drugs can be given orally or parenterally (diazepam is poorly absorbed intramuscularly). The intravenous route, if it can be used, has the advantage of allowing small bolus doses to be given so that the amount of drug administered can be titrated carefully against the sought-for effect on behaviour. It is important to check for possible respiratory depression, particularly in the elderly or those with concomitant physical illness.

After a day or two it is usually possible to substitute oral medication. While patients often become more settled shortly after starting antipsychotic drugs, improvement in psychotic symptoms is usually slow, with resolution of symptoms often taking a number of weeks. Again, current trends are to maintain the dose of antipsychotic drugs at a modest steady level (for example, 5–15 mg daily of haloperidol) and not to escalate the dose in the hope of speeding up the rate of improvement. For patients in whom agitation and distress continue to cause concern it may be appropriate to add short-term intermittent treatment with a benzodiazepine rather than increase the dose of antipsychotic agent.

It is usual for antipsychotic drugs to be continued for some months after the acute episode has resolved. In addition, some patients will require long-term treatment because they will relapse without it. In these circumstances, depot preparations should be considered. These are antipsychotic agents which are esterified with fatty acids; following intramuscular injection the active drug is slowly released over a period of weeks. Thus, injections need to be given relatively infrequently, often only once or twice monthly, which can markedly improve compliance. The most commonly used depot preparations are the decanoates of clopenthixol, flupenthixol, fluphenazine and haloperidol.

Movement disorders caused by antipsychotic drugs

All antipsychotic drugs currently employed can cause extrapyramidal movement disorders. Early in treatment patients may experience **acute dystonias** which are involuntary muscle contractions, particularly of the jaw, the neck (opisthotonos) or the external ocular muscles (oculogyric crisis). Treatment with a parenterally administered anticholinergic drug, for example, benztropine 1 mg, will usually rapidly resolve the disorder.

Continued treatment with antipsychotic drugs can lead to a **Parkinsonian syndrome** with the usual clinical features of tremor, rigidity and bradykinesia. It is worthwhile trying to reduce the dose of the antipsychotic drug, but if this is inadvisable or unsuccessful, treatment with anticholinergic drugs may be beneficial. Anticholinergic drugs possess an abuse potential and for this reason should not be given routinely with antipsychotic agents. Parkinsonian symptoms frequently wax and wane during antipsychotic drug therapy and it is therefore worthwhile attempting to withdraw anticholinergic drugs from time to time. Another not uncommon movement disorder is **akathisia**, which is a sense of unpleasant subjective motor restlessness, often leading the patient to pace restlessly. An attempt should be made to reduce the dose of antipsychotic drug. Anticholinergic drugs are not usually helpful, but benzodiazepines and β-adrenoceptor blocking agents have been reported to be of benefit.

Tardive dyskinesia is a movement disorder of later onset which usually only arises after at least 3 months' antipsychotic drug treatment. It is distinguished by choreoathetoid movements which most commonly involve the tongue and lips causing characteristic chewing movements. In some patients the trunk and limbs are affected. There is disagreement about the prevalence of tardive dyskinesia but an average estimate would be about 15% of patients receiving long-term antipsychotic drug treatment. In addition some workers believe that the condition is in fact associated with schizophrenia and thus not directly related to antipsychotic drug treatment. However, the fact that patients with no family or personal history of schizophrenia can also develop tardive dyskinesia when treated with dopamine receptor antagonists suggest that the drugs do play a contributory role.

The major importance of tardive dyskinesia is that it is frequently irreversible and there is at present no satisfactory treatment. Anticholinergic drugs tend to make the movements worse. Withdrawal of the antipsychotic agent medication, if this is possible, may be followed by a remission of the disorder. Other treatments that have been advocated include the dopamine depleting agent, tetrabenazine, the antipsychotic drug, sulpiride and calcium channel blockers.

Other side effects of antipsychotic drugs
The dopamine receptor blocking properties of antipsychotic agents can result in elevations in plasma prolactin. This in turn can lead to gynaecomastia and, in female patients, amenorrhoea and galactorrhoea. Certain antipsychotic drugs, particularly aliphatic and piperidine phenothiazines, produce autonomic symptoms which can be attributed to their blockade of cholinergic and α-adrenoceptors. Antihistaminic effects can also be seen (Fig. 17.6). A potentially serious problem with antipsychotic agents is their tendency to lower seizure threshold, which can result in fits in predisposed individuals or the aggravation of pre-existing epilepsy.

Phenothiazine drugs can also cause photosensitivity reactions and skin rashes may occur with any of the neuroleptics. A cholestatic hepatitis is seen occasionally, chlorpromazine being the drug most often implicated. Other rare side effects include blood cell dyscrasias and lens opacities. Thioridazine in doses of more than 800 mg daily has been reported to cause retinitis pigmentosa. A further rare complication which is important because of its serious nature, is the **neuroleptic malignant syndrome** which is characterized by hyperpyrexia, fever, muscle rigidity and lowered conscious level. The mortality rate is about 20% and supportive care in an intensive care unit is advisable. Treatment with the dopamine agonist, bromocriptine, may be helpful.

Treatment with **clozapine** is associated with a significant incidence (about 2–3% of patients treated annually) of low white cell count (leucopenia). This adverse effect can progress to **agranulocytosis** (virtual absence of white cells) which is potentially very hazardous, and fatalities have occurred during clozapine treatment. At present, patients receiving clozapine must undergo weekly white cell counts. If this practice is followed and clozapine treatment suspended immediately leucopenia appears, the white cell count will almost invariably return to normal. However, in the UK, clozapine use has been associated with fatality due to agranulocytosis despite this monitoring system. Clearly, the potential benefits and risks of clozapine require very careful weighing by doctor and patient before treatment is instituted.

Clozapine rarely causes extrapyramidal movement disorders but its use is associated with hypersalivation, weight gain, sweating and seizures at higher doses. Myocarditis has also been reported.

As noted above, **remoxapride** has been associated with the development of aplastic anaemia.

Drug interactions
Antipsychotic drugs will potentiate the actions of other centrally acting sedatives, particularly those with anticholinergic properties. In addition since they are metabolized by the liver they may increase the plasma levels of other drugs sharing a similar metabolic pathway. If for example a patient is treated with both an antipsychotic drug and a tricyclic antidepressant the plasma level of each drug will be higher than if either had been given alone.

How do antidepressants work?
It seems likely that the therapeutic effect of antidepressant drugs is attributable to adaptive changes in the brain which follow repeated administration of the compounds. Recent studies in animals have demonstrated that chronic administration of a number of different antidepressant drugs including tricyclics, MAOIs and mianserin appear to desensitize post-synaptic β-adrenoceptors or the associated adenylate cyclase. In addition most antidepressants facilitate some aspects of brain 5-HT neurotransmission. Recently, it has been shown that an acute dietary manipulation which lowers brain 5-HT function can reverse the antidepressant effects

---

Fig. 17.6 Side effects caused by blockade of muscarinic cholinergic, α-adrenergic and histamine H₁-receptors

Anticholinergic	Confusion, dry mouth, blurred vision, precipitation of glaucoma, tachycardia, constipation, ileus, urine retention, impaired sexual function.
Anti-adrenergic	Drowsiness, psychomotor impairment, postural hypotension, impaired sexual function.
Anti-histaminic	Drowsiness, weight gain.

of some antidepressant drugs. This suggests that the antidepressant activity of some drugs is dependent on intact brain 5-HT pathways.

When are antidepressants prescribed?

Antidepressant drugs are prescribed for patients suffering from depressive disorders. In general, patients with biological symptoms respond well, although patients with severe symptoms, especially those who are psychotically depressed may not be helped as much. When prescribing for depressed patients the risk of deliberate overdose must always be considered. Usually medication should be dispensed in small amounts or entrusted to a relative.

Recently several newer antidepressants have been introduced which are safer in overdose than tricyclics and, in general, better tolerated (see below). There is debate as to whether these newer antidepressants should now be prescribed in preference to tricyclics. At present it is probably best to try to decide what is the most suitable drug for a particular patient. The antidepressant efficacy of the newer drugs is not as well established as the tricyclics for more severely depressed patients. Accordingly it may be appropriate at present to prefer tricyclics in seriously depressed patients, particularly in-patients, unless there are specific contraindications to their use or if the risk of overdose cannot be minimized.

Antidepressants

There is growing evidence that various classes of antidepressant drugs are effective in the management of anxiety disorders. In the treatment of generalized anxiety disorder, for example, tricyclic antidepressants appear as effective as benzodiazepines and may be preferred when significant depressive symptomatology is also present. In addition, in patients with panic disorder, tricyclics, selective 5-HT uptake inhibitors (SSRIs) and MAOIs have all be shown to produce significant clinical benefit. Drug treatment should therefore be considered for patients in whom cognitive therapy is ineffective or unavailable. Finally, recent studies have shown that SSRIs and clomipramine (a tricyclic antidepressant that potently inhibits 5-HT uptake) are effective in ameliorating the symptoms of obsessive compulsive disorder.

Tricyclic antidepressants

Pharmacology

Tricyclic antidepressants are structurally similar to the phenothiazines but their pharmacological properties have important differences (Fig. 17.7). Thus whilst tricyclics have minimal acute effects on dopamine pathways they inhibit the uptake of noradrenaline and 5-HT into presynaptic nerve endings. Therefore the action of these transmitters is enhanced. Like some phenothiazines tricyclics also block muscarinic cholinergic, α-adrenergic and H_1 histamine receptors thereby giving rise to similar autonomic symptoms (see Fig. 17.6).

How to use tricyclic antidepressants

Most depressed patients present with co-existing anxiety and sleep disturbance, and treatment with a sedative tricyclic such as amitriptyline is appropriate. For patients who exhibit a significant degree of psychomotor retardation, treatment with a more stimulating preparation such as desmethylimipramine can be considered. It is customary to begin treatment with a low dose of amitriptyline, for example, 50 mg at bed time, and to build up the dose over 1–2 weeks so that tolerance to side effects can develop. Since tricyclics have long half-lives the entire daily dose can be given at night which will usually help sleep and may obviate the need for a hypnotic. The usual dose at which an antidepressant effect is apparent is between 75 and 150 mg, although some in-

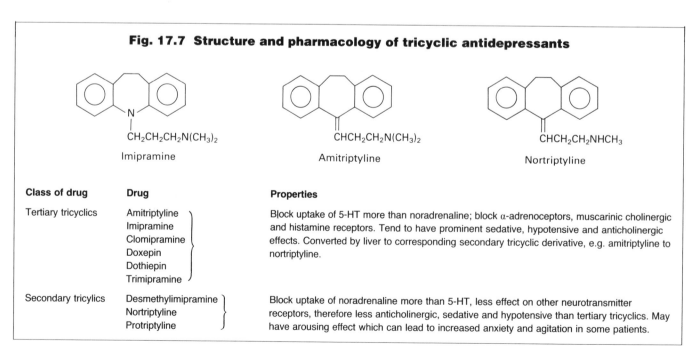

Fig. 17.7 Structure and pharmacology of tricyclic antidepressants

Imipramine

Amitriptyline

Nortriptyline

Class of drug	Drug	Properties
Tertiary tricyclics	Amitriptyline Imipramine Clomipramine Doxepin Dothiepin Trimipramine	Block uptake of 5-HT more than noradrenaline; block α-adrenoceptors, muscarinic cholinergic and histamine receptors. Tend to have prominent sedative, hypotensive and anticholinergic effects. Converted by liver to corresponding secondary tricyclic derivative, e.g. amitriptyline to nortriptyline.
Secondary tricyclics	Desmethylimipramine Nortriptyline Protriptyline	Block uptake of noradrenaline more than 5-HT, less effect on other neurotransmitter receptors, therefore less anticholinergic, sedative and hypotensive than tertiary tricyclics. May have arousing effect which can lead to increased anxiety and agitation in some patients.

patients are treated with higher doses, up to 300 mg daily, which may result in an antidepressant response where a lower dose did not.

The antidepressant effect of drug therapy is not usually apparent until 2 or 3 weeks after the start of treatment. In part, this reflects the practice of building up drug dosage slowly but in addition it appears that there is an inbuilt delay in clinical response, perhaps because the response is associated with adaptive changes in the brain rather than the acute pharmacological effects of the antidepressant. The practical importance is that patients should be warned about the delay in improvement in mood and encouraged to maintain treatment through the temporary period when unpleasant side effects are present but a therapeutic effect is not.

If treatment is successful it is usual to continue the antidepressant for about 6 months. Recent studies suggest that it is probably wise to maintain the full dose of the antidepressant during this period if tolerance allows. Some patients with frequent relapses are maintained on long-term antidepressant treatment but if a bipolar affective disorder is present then lithium is preferable.

Side effects
The major side effects of tricyclic antidepressants are the autonomic symptoms consequent on cholinergic and α-adrenoceptor blockade, which were described earlier. Antihistaminic effects may be prominent with tertiary tricyclics. Like neuroleptics, tricyclics also lower the seizure threshold.

A major problem with the use of tricyclics is their effect on the heart. The most serious difficulties occur in cases of overdose where fatal arrhythmias may result. However, even normal clinical doses can cause problems in patients with pre-existing cardiac disease, and a recent myocardial infarction is a contraindication for the use of tricyclics. In these circumstances one of the newer antidepressants should be preferred.

The effects of tricyclics on the heart are caused partly by their anticholinergic activity and partly by a direct effect on cardiac muscle. Changes in the electrocardiogram are common; QT prolongation and T wave inversion or flattening are generally regarded as benign and reversible, whereas broadened PR and QRS intervals, ST segment depression, intraventricular conduction defects and frequent premature ventricular contractions are regarded as signs of toxicity. Rare side effects of tricyclic antidepressants include blood cell dyscrasias, skin rashes and an allergic hepatitis.

Drug interactions
Tricyclic antidepressants antagonize the hypotensive effects of clonidine; they can, however, be safely combined with thiazide diuretics and β-adrenoceptor blockers. Because of their blockade of noradrenaline uptake, tricyclics can potentiate the effect of parenterally administered adrenaline and noradrenaline. This is most likely to cause difficulties with the administration of certain local anaesthetic preparations, particularly those used by dentists.

Tricyclics are metabolized in the liver and therefore like neuroleptics can increase plasma concentrations of other drugs metabolized by a similar pathway. An important clinical example is the elevation of plasma phenytoin levels which is sometimes associated with simultaneous administration of tricyclics.

Newer antidepressants
The use of tricyclic antidepressants has a number of disadvantages, in particular their slow onset of action and high incidence of adverse effects. In an attempt to improve the drug treatment of depression a number of new drugs have been introduced over the last few years (Fig. 17.8). Unfortunately there is no evidence that any of the newer drugs are therapeutically superior to the tricyclics; however, in the broad range of depressed patients their activity appears equivalent. Another point to be borne in mind is that the long-term toxicity of the newer compounds has not been fully evaluated and problems with unexpected side effects have led to the withdrawal of two agents, zimelidine and nomifensine.

Newer antidepressants should be used in patients where the use of tricyclic antidepressants is contraindicated because of their anticholinergic and cardiotoxic effects. In addition some patients unable to tolerate a clinically effective dose of tricyclic may find one of the newer drugs causes fewer side effects. The lack of sedation associated with some

Fig. 17.8 Pharmacological actions and adverse effects of some newer antidepressants

		Anticholinergic activity	Cardiovascular toxicity	Dose (daily) (mg)	Adverse effects
5-HT uptake inhibitors	Fluoxetine	0	0	20–60	Nausea, vomiting, anxiety, insomnia, headache,
	Fluvoxamine	0	0	100–300	reduced appetite, sweating, skin rash, generalized
	Sertraline	0	0	50–200	allergic reaction (rare), seizures (rare),
	Paroxetine	0	0	20–50	extrapyramidal movement disorders (rare).
Modified tricyclics	Lofepramine	+	0	140–210	Anxiety, insomnia, seizures (rare).
Sedating antidepressants	Trazodone	0	+/0	150–300	Cognitive impairment, postural hypotension, priapism (rare), cardiac arrhythmias (rare).
	Mianserin	0	0	30–120	Cognitive impairment, postural hypotension, weight gain, bone marrow depression (rare), seizures (rare).

of the newer antidepressants can be beneficial in outpatients striving to carry out their usual activities. Finally, in patients where the risk of overdose cannot be minimized, the newer drugs may be preferred because of their lower acute toxicity.

Selective 5-HT uptake inhibitors (SSRIs)
Four SSRIs, fluoxetine, fluvoxamine, paroxetine, and sertraline are presently available for use in the UK. These compounds are a structurally diverse group but have in common the ability to inhibit the uptake of 5-HT with high potency and selectivity. None of these agents has an appreciable affinity for the NA uptake site and present data suggest very low affinity for neurotransmitter receptors.

The adverse effects of SSRIs differ from the tricyclics (Fig. 17.8), with the most common adverse effect being nausea. SSRIs are not sedating but may be experienced by the patient as somewhat activating which can result in increased anxiety and insomnia early in treatment. Rarely the use of SSRIs is associated with severe restlessness and an akathisia-like syndrome can develop. This adverse effect is important to recognize because it may result in worsening dysphoria, which can in turn lead to an exacerbation of suicidal thinking and behaviour. Unlike tricyclics, SSRIs do not cause weight gain; in fact some patients may lose weight.

Systematic comparisons between different SSRIs have not yet been carried out. At present a distinction can be drawn on the basis of pharmacokinetic profile in that whilst fluvoxamine, paroxetine and sertraline have half-lives of about 24 hours with little or no significant metabolism to active compounds, fluoxetine posses an active metabolite, nofluoxetine, which has a half-life of 7–15 days. Accordingly after fluoxetine is stopped detectable effects on 5-HT neurotransmission may be present for several weeks.

The SSRIs delay the hepatic metabolism and thereby increase the activity of several other drugs including anticonvulsants, antipsychotic drugs and tricyclic antidepressants. The anticoagulant activity of warfarin can also be prolonged. Severe interactions have been reported between SSRIs and monoamine oxidase inhibitors with the development of a fatal 5-HT toxicity syndrome. Lithium and SSRIs should be co-administered with caution because neurotoxicity with myoclonus and seizures has occasionally been reported in patients receiving this combination.

Modified tricyclics
Lofepramine is a modified tricyclic antidepressant that is notable for lack of cardiotoxicity in overdose. Otherwise its clinical profile resembles that of a tricyclic antidepressant but it is less anticholinergic and not sedating (see Fig. 17.8). The drug interactions of lofepramine are similar to those of other tricyclic antidepressants.

Sedating antidepressants
Under this heading can be listed two antidepressants, mianserin and trazodone. These drugs do not inhibit the uptake of noradrenaline or 5-HT to any extent but instead block certain postsynaptic noradrenaline and 5-HT receptors. Trazodone and mianserin are not anticholinergic but both possess strong sedative properties (see Fig. 17.8). Whilst this may benefit sleep it can also lead to daytime drowsiness.

Mianserin has been associated with leucopenia and it is recommended that the white count be monitored at monthly intervals during the first 3 months of treatment. Trazodone has occasionally been reported to worsen cardiac arrhythmias in patients with pre-existing cardiac disease and rarely causes priapism. It may, however, lower seizure threshold somewhat less than tricyclic antidepressants.

Monoamine oxidase inhibitors (MAOIs)
MAOIs were the first specific antidepressant drugs to be introduced but in later years their popularity declined because of supposed inefficacy and evidence of dangerous drug interactions. Recently MAOIs have been used more frequently and with a proper appreciation for their risks they can be useful drugs.

Conventional MAOIs irreversibly deactivate both major forms of monoamine oxidase (type A and type B). The function of these enzymes is to metabolize intraneuronal noradrenaline, dopamine and 5-HT, and its inactivation is followed by increases in brain concentration of these neurotransmitters. Irreversible MAOIs are divided into two main structural classes, the hydrazines such as phenelzine and isocarboxazid, and the non-hydrazines such as tranylcypromine. Tranylcypromine is a more stimulant drug with alerting and euphoriant properties. This makes it useful in some patients but dependence has occasionally been described.

Recently some new MAOIs have been described, one of which moclobemide, is available in the UK. Moclobemide has two major differences from the conventional MAOIs described above. First, it is a reversible inhibitor of monoamine oxidase which means it can be displaced from the enzyme which will then function normally. Second, it selectively inhibits type A monoamine oxidase. This leads to an increase in brain 5-HT and noradrenaline, but other amines, for example dopamine and tyramine (that are normally metabolized by type B monoamine oxidase), are much less affected. This makes moclobemide far less likely than conventional MAOIs to cause adverse reactions with foods and other drugs (see below). However, current clinical experience of moclobemide is still somewhat limited and accordingly the discussion below will focus on the conventional irreversible MAOIs.

Indications and use
Conventional MAOIs are rarely prescribed as a first choice of antidepressant treatment unless a patient is known to have shown a response previously. Their main use, therefore, is in patients with major depression who have failed to respond to tricyclic antidepressants or ECT, and not infrequently in such subjects a useful antidepressant effect will be obtained. MAOIs are also somewhat more effective than tricyclics in patients with atypical depression symptoms (mood reactivity, hypersomnia, hyperphagia and extreme sensitivity to real or imagined rejection), and in certain forms of depression seen in patients with bipolar affective disorder.

As with tricyclics, the therapeutic effect of MAOIs is often delayed until at least 2 or 3 weeks after the start of treatment. It is important to prescribe MAOIs in a sufficient dose; this can be up to 90 mg a day of phenelzine or 50 mg of tranylcypromine. However, side effects such as postural hypotension often limit the amount that can be tolerated.

Side effects
MAOIs cause a high incidence of cardiovascular side effects, the most common of which is postural hypotension. Hypertension may also occur, usually as a result of a drug or food interaction (see below). MAOIs also cause anticholinergic effects which are similar in nature to those seen with tricyclics but less severe. Central side effects such as drowsiness, dizziness and confusion have been reported; some MAOIs, particularly tranylcypromine, can cause sleeplessness. Unlike tricyclics MAOIs do not lower seizure threshold. Rare side effects include hepatocellular damage and blood cell dyscrasias.

Drug interactions
A major reason for the relative lack of use of MAOIs is their liability to interact with other drugs and certain foodstuffs (Fig. 17.9). Such interactions most commonly involve the indirect sympathomimetic, tyramine, which is present in such items as cheese and meat extracts. Normally, tyramine taken in the diet is metabolized by the monoamine oxidase present in the gut wall. However, in patients taking MAOIs large amounts of ingested tyramine enter the systemic circulation causing a marked hypertensive reaction with severe headache and occasionally cerebrovascular accident.

MAOIs also interact with other drugs especially indirect sympathomimetics, which are commonly present in commercially available 'cold cures'. A hypotensive collapse may occur following parenteral administration of opiates to patients taking MAOIs; if such drugs are required preliminary administration of a small test dose is recommended but pethidine should be avoided. The combination of tricyclic antidepressants and MAOIs whilst perhaps not as dangerous as once thought is probably best left to specialists. Clomipramine and SSRIs should not be prescribed with

MAOIs because a 5-HT toxicity syndrome with fatal hyperpyrexia may ocur.

It will be clear from the foregoing account that MAOIs should only be prescribed to patients who will adhere to the necessary dietary restrictions. In addition no new medication either medically prescribed or commercially obtained should be taken in combination with an MAOI until the possibility of an interaction has been considered and, as far as possible, excluded. If a hypertensive reaction occurs with an MAOI the best treatment is to administer an α-adrenoceptor blocking drug such as phentolamine. If this is not available, chlorpromazine 50–100 mg intramuscularly, may be given instead. When treatment with MAOIs is stopped, the dietary and pharmacological precautions outlined above should be continued for 2 weeks which is the approximate time for new monoamine oxidase to be synthesized.

Moclobemide
Clinical studies have shown that the reversible type A MAOI, moclobemide, is an effective antidepressant in the treatment of major depression and is very unlikely to cause reactions with tyramine or other sympathomimetics. This gives moclobemide an important safety advantage over the conventional MAOIs described above. Whether the antidepressant profile of moclobemide will be equivalent to that of phenelzine and tranylcypromine, particularly in the treatment of patients unresponsive to first-line treatment with tricyclic antidepressants, is not clear. Similarly it is not yet known whether the efficacy of moclobemide in atypical depression and depression in bipolar patients will match that of the conventional MAOIs.

Mood-stabilizing drugs

Lithium
Lithium is used mainly in the prophylaxis of recurrent mood disorders, especially bipolar affective disorder. Lithium is also used in the acute management of mania but is less immediately effective than neuroleptics. Recent studies have shown that the addition of lithium to antidepressant medication can produce a useful antidepressant effect in patients who have not responded to the antidepressant given on its own.

Pharmacology
Lithium is administered as a salt, usually lithium carbonate or lithium citrate. It is rapidly absorbed and widely distributed, being handled in the body like sodium. The mode of action of lithium is not clear, but recent attention has focused on its ability to alter the function of various neurotransmitter second messengers. These are biochemical pathways that link activation of a neurotransmitter receptor with the subsequent intracellular response. In addition in both animals and humans lithium produces a marked enhancement of some aspects of brain 5-HT function.

How lithium is used
Lithium is the only psychotropic drug where the monitoring of plasma concentration is of established clinical value. This is somewhat fortunate because the therapeutic range (0.5–

0.8 mmol/litre) is close to the level where toxic effects may occur (>1.5 mmol/litre). Lithium is not metabolized and its elimination from the body is dependent on the kidney. Accordingly its administration should be preceded by a clinical and laboratory assessment of renal function. If there is any evidence of renal impairment a creatinine clearance test should be performed. Lithium also affects the thyroid (see below) and initial medical screening should include evaluation of thyroid function.

There is little to choose between the different preparations of lithium; whilst slow release formulations are available their pharmacokinetic characteristics do not differ greatly from those of the standard preparation of lithium carbonate. Lithium may be given once or twice daily, the usual dose varying from 400 to 1600 mg. Estimations of plasma concentration should be made approximately 12 hours after the last dose. Once a patient is stabilized on lithium the dosage requirement is very stable and it is usually sufficient to check plasma levels every 1 or 2 months unless there is evidence to suspect impending toxicity. Thyroid function should be checked every 6 months or earlier if clinically indicated.

Side effects

Most patients taking lithium suffer from a fine tremor and especially in the early stages of treatment, nausea and diarrhoea may occur. Patients may also experience a sensation of mental slowness and poor memory. Frequent side effects are thirst and polyuria which are a consequence of the antagonism by lithium of the action of antidiuretic hormone (ADH) on the renal tubule. Thus most patients taking lithium have an impairment in urine concentrating ability but this rarely leads to serious complications. However, a few patients develop diabetes insipidus. In most patients the effect of lithium on tubular function remits when treatment is discontinued or the dose of lithium lowered. Whilst lithium toxicity has been associated with structural renal damage it is not thought that patients maintained on long-term lithium within therapeutic plasma concentrations are at risk of irreversible renal impairment.

Lithium also depresses production of thyroid hormone by a direct effect on the thyroid gland. This results in an increase in circulating levels of thyroid stimulating hormone from the pituitary which usually maintains normal thyroid function. However, some patients, probably those who have pre-existing thyroid impairment, develop hypothyroidism. If continuation of lithium therapy is indicated on clinical grounds, thyroxine replacement therapy may be added. Very rarely lithium may produce hyperparathyroidism with raised plasma calcium concentrations.

Fig. 17.10 Signs of lithium toxicity

Decreased appetite	Dysarthria	Lowered conscious level
Nausea	Coarse tremor	Convulsions
Vomiting	Myoclonus	Renal failure
Diarrhoea	Hyperreflexia	Cardiovascular collapse
Ataxia		

Lithium sometimes produces changes in the ECG, notably T wave flattening or inversion, and rarely cardiac conduction defects may arise. Lithium should not be given to patients in cardiac failure. Other relatively infrequent side effects include leucocytosis and skin rashes. Side effects of lithium should be distinguished from signs of lithium toxicity, which are summarized in Fig. 17.10.

Drug interactions

The major interaction of lithium is with diuretic drugs, especially the thiazides. These drugs reduce the reabsorption of sodium from the proximal renal tubule and since lithium competes with sodium for transport at this site, more lithium is reabsorbed and plasma levels rise. Other factors which lead to sodium depletion, for example excessive sweating and diarrhoea, can also result in elevated plasma lithium concentration. Non-steroidal anti-inflammatory drugs may increase lithium levels. Increased lithium levels have also been reported in association with erythromycin and metronidazole treatment. There is a strong clinical impression that patients receiving lithium and neuroleptics together are more likely to experience severe extrapyramidal movement disorders.

Carbamazepine

Carbamazepine is widely used in the treatment of epilepsy, but recent studies have shown that it is also effective in the acute treatment of mania and in the prophylaxis of bipolar affective disorder. It may be used in patients who have difficulty tolerating or who do not respond to lithium therapy. It is possible in the latter patients for carbamazepine to be combined with lithium if there has been a partial response to lithium treatment.

Pharmacology

Carbamazepine has a tricyclic structure but does not inhibit the uptake of monoamines. There is, however, some evidence that it can facilitate 5-HT release. Its anticonvulsant effects have been attributed to blockade of neuronal sodium channels but whether this action is involved in its mood stabilizing effects is uncertain.

How carbamazepine is used

The dose of carbamazepine employed to treat affective disorders is similar to that used in the treatment of seizure disorder, although it is advisable to titrate the dose according to clinical response. Plasma level monitoring may be used to help avoid toxicity. Initial treatment should be with 100 mg of carbamazepine twice daily and the dose increased according to tolerance over the next 2–4 weeks. The effective dose range in the treatment of bipolar disorder is generally between 600 and 1200 mg daily although some patients may require higher doses.

Side effects

Dizziness, drowsiness and nausea are common early in treatment, particularly with rapid dose titration, but tolerance to these effects usually occurs. Persistent ataxia and diplopia may represent toxic plasma levels. A moderate degree of leucopenia is often seen during carbamazepine treatment and rarely agranulocytosis may develop. For this reason it is prudent to monitor white cell counts as well as carbamazepine levels during treatment. Skin rashes are also quite common.

Other rarer adverse effects include low plasma sodium levels and liver cell damage. Circulating thyroid levels may be lowered by carbamazepine but TSH levels generally remain in the normal range and clinical hypothyroidism is unusual. Carbamazepine can impair cardiac conduction and should be used with caution in patients with cardiovascular disease. Carbamazepine increases the hepatic metabolism of a number of other drugs including tricyclic antidepressants, haloperidol, oral contraceptives and warfarin. Carbamazepine may also induce its own metabolism which can lead to a lowering of plasma levels during continued treatment. Carbamazepine levels can be increased by erythromycin, and some calcium channel blockers such as diltiazem and verapamil. Neurotoxicity has been reported when carbamazepine has been combined with lithium.

Anxiolytics and hypnotics

There has been a growing opinion in recent years that anxiolytics and hypnotics are prescribed too frequently, often where non-pharmacological treatments would be equally effective. The argument against the use of such drugs is that firstly they may prevent the patient acquiring adequate coping skills, and secondly they may lead to the development of drug dependence. Whatever the merits of the first contention there is no doubt that many anxiolytics and hypnotics can cause dependence and withdrawal reactions. It is therefore generally recommended that these drugs should be prescribed on a short-term basis to help people in acute difficulties, where anxiety or insomnia are significantly impairing ability to cope.

Benzodiazepines and related compounds

Barbiturates have now fallen into disuse because of their high risk of dependence and serious toxicity in overdose. Benzodiazepine drugs replaced the barbiturates and are still widely prescribed, though they have been shown to produce dependence, albeit of a less severe nature than that seen with barbiturates. Benzodiazepines with a suitable pharmacokinetic profile are also used as hypnotics. Other drugs, such as chloral hydrate and chlormethiazole are available as hypnotics, but in general these compounds do not offer any advantages over the benzodiazepines. A new hypnotic agent, zopiclone, is said to cause less risk of tolerance and dependence than benzodiazepines, but these claims have not yet been fully tested.

Pharmacology

Benzodiazepines, barbiturates, chlormethiazole and zopiclone have in common the ability to enhance the activity of the amino acid neurotransmitter, γ-aminobutyric acid (GABA). GABA is the major inhibitory neurotransmitter in the mammalian central nervous system and increasing its function results in anticonvulsant and anxiolytic effects in animal models. In the brain, benzodiazepines bind to a specific receptor site closely associated with the postsynaptic GABA receptor, and thereby enhance GABA transmission. It would seem likely that if there are specific benzodiazepine receptors then there is likely to be an endogenous compound which usually occupies them. Despite much research, the nature of this compound remains obscure. Barbiturates, chlormethiazole and zopiclone bind to other sites close to the GABA receptor and also increase GABA activity.

The common effect of different anxiolytics and hypnotics on GABA transmission may explain why sudden withdrawal of these drugs can cause abstinence syndromes which qualitatively resemble each other although varying in severity. Thus it might be expected that sudden withdrawal of drugs which enhance GABA transmission would lead to a period of reduced GABA activity. Such a change would explain many of the features of withdrawal from sedative or hypnotic drugs, particularly the occurrence of anxiety and seizures. Interestingly, seizures are also seen in alcohol withdrawal and alcohol too is known to increase GABA function.

Use of benzodiazepines

There are a large number of benzodiazepines available, all of which have similar pharmacological properties. The main distinction of clinical value is based on pharmacokinetic properties (Fig. 17.11). Thus 3-hydroxy derivatives, such as temazepam, have short half-lives and no active metabolites. Such compounds are best used as hypnotics as their short duration of action should ensure minimal 'hangover' effect on the following day.

Fig. 17.11 Benzodiazepines: duration of action

Short-acting (half-life less than 11 hours)	Medium-acting (half-life 12–24 hours)	Long-acting (more than 24 hours)
Temazepate	Lorazepam	Diazepam
Triazolam	Flunitrazepam	Nitrazepam
Oxazepam		Flurazepam
Lormetazepam		Chlorazepate

Fig. 17.12 Withdrawal from benzodiazepines

Incidence of withdrawal symptoms
About 25% of subjects taking regular benzodiazepine medication for more than 6 months will experience some symptoms on withdrawal. Severe symptoms most common after sudden discontinuation of short-acting drugs.

Withdrawal symptoms
Anxiety, agitation, sleeplessness, tremor, dizziness, headache, blurred vision, perceptual abnormalities, muscular twitching, psychosis, seizures.

Management
1 Taper dose slowly over 4–8 weeks.
2 Change to long-acting preparation before withdrawal.
3 Teach anxiety management techniques.
4 For patients with great difficulty withdrawing, consider use of β-blockers.

In contrast, drugs such as diazepam have long half-lives and are themselves broken down to active compounds. These drugs can be used to treat anxiety on a continuous basis either in single dose at night or in the more usual regime of thrice daily. Probably the best practice is for patients to take the drugs on an 'as required' basis, with an agreed daily limit. Whilst short-acting drugs might have some theoretical advantages in applying this regime, in practice diazepam often seems satisfactory perhaps because its rapid absorption leads to a quick onset of action (Fig. 17.11).

Side effects
Benzodiazepines are safe and well-tolerated drugs. Common side effects include sedation and ataxia, though tolerance rapidly develops to the sedative effects. It seems likely that benzodiazepines can impair some aspects of learning but the clinical importance of this is disputed. Case reports of paradoxical aggression have appeared but the incidence of this potentially serious complication is believed to be low. It seems likely that additional factors such as alcohol consumption and personality characteristics are involved. Alcohol can enhance the sedation and impairment of psychomotor function produced by benzodiazepines; some patients abuse both (Fig. 17.12) (see also p. 124).

Buspirone
Buspirone is a 5-HT receptor agonist which has recently been introduced for the treatment of generalized anxiety disorder. Buspirone is quite pharmacologically distinct from the benzodiazepines and cannot be used to manage benzodiazepine withdrawal. In fact, there is evidence that buspirone is somewhat less effective in patients who have previously been treated with benzodiazepines. In addition, buspirone does not seem to be effective in the treatment of patients with panic disorder.

Buspirone has a slow onset of action (1–3 weeks). Unlike benzodiazepines it does not cause sedation or cognitive impairment at usual clinical doses and from present data seems unlikely to cause dependence. Buspirone does not have hypnotic properties.

Psychosurgery
Psychosurgery is little used at present because it has been almost entirely superseded by drug and behaviour therapy. Its use is reserved for the management of patients with chronic obsessional and depressive disorders that have failed to respond to prolonged and vigorous treatment with the usual therapies. There has been no controlled evaluation of psychosurgery, mainly because the nature of the treatment renders such an investigation very difficult. The general consensus is that such operations can produce benefit in selected subjects, but should only be carried out after the most careful consideration and prolonged trials of other treatment.

Techniques
Psychosurgery is performed using stereotactic techniques which allow a precise localization of the intended lesion, usually produced by the implantation of radioactive yttrium seeds. In a tractotomy the lesion is directed to the posterior part of the medial third of the orbital cortex. A further procedure, limbic leucotomy, involves disrupting some of the connections between the frontal lobe and the limbic system by placing lesions in lower medial quadrant of the frontal lobe. The cingulum is also lesioned.

The usual result of the operation is a reduction of anxiety and tension. As a result treatments such as behaviour therapy that have previously been unsuccessful may not produce a remission in symptoms. Side effects of the stereotactic procedures are said to be infrequent and mild; apathy and disinhibition have been reported.

Prescribing for special groups

Older people and the physically ill
Older patients may have impaired renal and hepatic function which can reduce ability to metabolize drugs. In addition they may be more susceptible to central and cardiovascular side effects of psychotropic drugs. It is usually advisable to start drug treatment with small doses which are gradually increased under careful supervision. It is quite common for physical and psychiatric illness to co-exist. Special consideration must be given to potential side effects of psychotropic drugs which could worsen physical illness. For example, in a depressed patient with prostatic hypertrophy a newer antidepressant would be preferable to a tricyclic drug whose anticholinergic properties could lead to urinary retention (see also Prescribing for the terminally ill, p. 280).

Pregnancy and breast-feeding
Psychotropic drugs, like all medication, must be avoided if possible during pregnancy, especially in the first trimester. If a patient has a serious psychotic illness which is known to relapse without continuing treatment then a difficult clinical decision must be made, weighing the teratogenic risk of drug treatment with that of uncontrolled psychotic illness. In general there is little positive evidence that treatment with chlorpromazine is associated with congenital malformation, and the same is true of tricyclic antidepressants. On the other hand, lithium has been associated with birth defects, mainly cardiovascular.

Most psychotropic drugs will pass from the mother's circulation to her breast milk, but generally at concentrations that are regarded as too low to harm the neonate. Lithium and MAOIs, however, should not be administered to mothers who are breast-feeding. A baby who is being breast-fed by a mother receiving psychotropic medication should be carefully observed for undue sedation, reduced muscle tone or feeding difficulties; breast-feeding should be discontinued if these occur. It should be emphasized that although small concentrations of psychotropic drugs do not appear clinically to cause adverse effects to the baby, the possibility of subtle changes in future development and behaviour cannot be excluded.

QUESTIONS

1 What are the major indications for ECT and what would you tell a patient to whom you proposed to administer the treatment?

2 What steps would you take to improve the compliance of a patient with a long-standing psychotic disorder who relapses when neuroleptic treatment is discontinued?

3 What movement disorders are associated with the use of neuroleptics and what measures may be taken to ameliorate these?

4 In the treatment of depressive illness what would incline you to use a newer antidepressant compound rather than a tricyclic antidepressant?

5 What are the indications for long-term lithium prophylaxis and what investigations would you carry out before starting a patient on lithium? Describe the possible side effects of long-term lithium administration.

FURTHER READING

Kiloh L.G., Smith J.S. & Johnson G.F. (1988) *Physical Treatments in Psychiatry*. Blackwell Scientific Publications, Oxford. [A well-referenced overview of current physical treatments of psychiatric disorder.]

Lader M. & Hetherington R. (1990) *Biological Treatments in Psychiatry*. Oxford Medical Publications, Oxford University Press, Oxford. [An account of biological treatments, including ECT, in psychiatric practice in the UK.]

Schatzberg A.F. & Cole J.O. (1991) *Manual of Clinical Psychopharmacology*. American Psychiatric Press, Washington DC. [An up-to-date account of the pharmacotherapy of psychiatric disorders as practised in the USA.]

Webster R.A. & Jordan C.C. (1989) *Neurotransmitters, Drugs and Disease*. Blackwell Scientific Publications, Oxford. [A thorough but comprehensible account of the neuropharmacology and biochemistry of the central nervous system and the relevance of these disciplines to the study of psychiatric illness.]

18
The Psychological Treatments

Fact sheet

Psychological treatments are those in which the therapist draws on psychological theories and employs psychological methods to ameliorate distress and disordered psychological processes in the patient.

The term *psychotherapy* referred originally to psychoanalytic treatments, but is now often applied to a wide range of psychological treatments.

Classification of psychological treatments

A bewildering number of terms are used to name, describe and categorize the psychological treatments. The following categorical dimensions, when used in combination, permit comprehensive classification.

Model of therapy

The model of therapy is defined by the theoretical paradigm on which it is based. The major models are the following.
1 *Psychoanalytic/psychodynamic therapies.* Psychoanalysis is both a comprehensive psychological theory and an intensive method of treatment which gives prominence to the role of unconscious processes in normal and abnormal mental functioning. As treatments, both psychoanalysis and the less intensive analytic or psychodynamic therapies derived from it, involve examination of the psychological processes (including unconscious processes) that cause and maintain the patient's disorder through analysis of the ways in which these processes are manifest in the therapist–patient relationship.
2 *Systemic therapies.* Systems theory conceptualizes the individual as a component part of his family and social system. Systemic therapies address the individual's psychological problems in the context of the family or social network, aiming to modify the structural, communication or other disturbances which generate them.
3 *Behavioural therapies* are derived from learning theory, and tackle specific disruptive symptoms or behaviours by a strategy of active measures designed to modify the processes which generate and maintain them.
4 *Cognitive therapies.* Derived from modern theories of cognition, cognitive therapy engages the patient in a critical evaluation and restructuring of the irrational thoughts and assumptions which undermine personal effectiveness and contribute to specific psychological disorders.

Mode of therapy

The mode of treatment is defined by those who participate in it.
1 *Individual therapy.* One patient is treated by one therapist.
2 *Couple therapy.* The partners in a dyadic relationship (often a marriage) are treated by one or two therapists.
3 *Family therapy.* A group of relatives, comprising one or more generations in a family (or sub-groups thereof) are treated by one or more therapists.
4 *Group therapy.* A group of patients, generally unknown to each other prior to therapy, are treated by one or more therapists.

Aim of therapy

1 *Maintenance.* Treatments which aim to maintain optimal psychological functioning in patients who are incapacitated by chronic neurotic, personality or other psychiatric disorder and who otherwise would suffer more frequent relapses in reaction to day-to-day stresses. Example: supportive psychotherapy.
2 *Restoration.* Treatments which aim to restore effective psychological functioning in patients disabled by acute psychiatric illness, adverse reactions to life crisis, or symptomatic behaviours. Examples: in-patient group psychotherapy, crisis therapy, behavioural therapy.
3 *Reconstruction.* Treatments which aim to examine and reconstruct the ways in which a person feels, thinks about himself and his world, acts, or relates to others. Examples: cognitive therapy, systemic therapy, analytic psychotherapy.

Indications for psychological treatments

The indications for psychological treatments can be identified by **diagnosis** or **presenting complaint**. In addition certain **good outcome attributes** have been identified which predict a favourable outcome. Psychological treatments are **contraindicated** in a few serious psychiatric disorders.

Indications by diagnosis

Psychological treatments are indicated primarily for: (a) acute and chronic neuroses; (b) personality disorders; (c) reactions to life crises; (d) psychological trauma; (e) psychosexual problems; (f) addictive behaviours, including substance abuse, eating disorders and repeated self-harm; (g) emotional, conduct and developmental disorders in children.

Psychological treatment methods contribute also in the general management of: (a) psychosomatic disorders; (b) psychological reactions to physical illness; (c) non-organic psychoses during remission; (d) mental handicap.

Indications by presenting complaint

1 Subjective symptoms, e.g. anxiety, depression, obsessional thoughts and compulsive actions, somatization.
2 Emotional functioning, e.g. inability to experience or express feelings, excessive or inadequate emotional control.
3 Self-concept, e.g. deficiency or distortion of self-identity, lack of purpose or achievement, low self-esteem.
4 Interpersonal functioning, e.g. inability to make and maintain relationships, lack of trust, avoidance of intimacy, over-dependency.

Good outcome attributes

- Motivation for psychological change.
- Capacity to express and to verbalize feelings.
- Capacity to tolerate anxiety and frustration.
- Willingness to examine experience in psychological terms.
- Evidence of achievement in areas of study, employment and/or relationships.

Contraindications for psychological treatment

- Active psychosis.
- Severe biological depression.
- Hypomania.
- Organic brain disease.
- Severe antisocial personality disorder.

Introduction

Psychological treatments are those in which the therapist draws on psychological theories and employs psychological methods to ameliorate psychological problems in the patient. Psychological treatments can be contrasted with **physical treatments**, in which physical agents are used to alter mood states and other psychological processes (see Chapter 17), and **social methods** of treatment which draw on the normalizing influence of social groupings to encourage change in interpersonal attitudes and behaviours.

Psychological treatments exert their effect through altering one or more of the following psychological functions—emotional processes, behaviour or thought patterns, interpersonal relationships, self-awareness and self-esteem, or other personality factors. Some treatments are designed for the limited aim of reducing or eradicating troublesome symptoms, such as compulsive checking; while others have more extensive aims, such as the promotion of greater psychological maturity.

This chapter will examine the historical development, application and techniques of a number of psychological treatments. The list of treatments to be described is not exhaustive, but covers those which are practised widely in the UK in National Health Service and related settings.

The descriptions will tend to illustrate the **differences** between treatments, in terms both of theoretical underpinning and technique. It should be emphasized, however, that these treatments also have certain characteristics **in common**.

Elements common to all psychological treatments

Therapeutic relationship

The most significant common element is the **therapeutic relationship**. This is of central importance in all treatment settings, of course, whether in psychiatry or other medical practice. Similarly the relationship between the client and the professional person is fundamental in other helping contexts, such as social work and counselling. The progress of treatment will be promoted or retarded according to its quality. For example the patient who trusts his doctor, nurse, dentist or other therapist is likely to feel safe and to comply with treatment. The patient's cooperation may be less forthcoming if he feels that the person treating him does not respect, listen to or understand him (see also pp. 38–40).

A good therapeutic relationship is a prerequisite for the success of all psychological treatments, and its ingredients are summarized in Fig. 18.1.

Assumption of a psychological explanation

Another element common to all psychological treatments is the **primary assumption** that psychological factors contribute in the causation or perpetuation of the disorder that is being treated. This assumption has given rise to a number of

---

Fig. 18.1 The therapeutic relationship

Essential ingredients

In the therapist
- Respect for the patient.
- Genuine interest in the patient as a person.
- Emotional warmth.
- Tolerance, and non-judgemental acceptance of the patient.
- Receptivity, especially the capacity to listen attentively.
- Empathy—the capacity to feel one's way into what the patient is experiencing.
- Realistic confidence in one's skills and resources.
- Awareness of one's limitations.
- Adherence to an appropriate ethical code.

In the patient
- Trust in the therapist.
- Cooperation in the task of therapy.
- Some understanding of the purpose and method of the treatment.
- Motivation to bring about change.

In the relationship
- Boundaries—the attention of both therapist and patient to the relationship's boundaries in **time** (the frequency and duration of sessions; punctuality) and **space** (where treatment takes place—and where it does not).
- Contract—the explicit or implicit agreement between therapist and patient about the purpose of the treatment, the means by which its goals will be realized, and the expectations each may have realistically of the other.

---

explanatory models of psychological functioning. All suggest that the individual is influenced by experience, and that he recreates certain aspects of formative experiences over and over again even though these may be counterproductive and distressing.

The leading theoretical models offer different explanations of this latter fact, however.

Learning theory suggests that behaviours are fashioned and maintained by actual experiences, and that troublesome symptoms are the result of learned maladaptive behaviours. The potential benefits and difficulties derived from **modelling** oneself on other important figures, for example parents, are emphasized.

Cognitive theory goes a step further to suggest that our views of ourselves and our world, and our personal assumptions are fashioned and maintained by experience, and that these may give rise to maladaptive patterns of thinking which generate anxiety, mood or interpersonal disturbance.

Classical psychoanalytic theory pointed to the formative influence of early experience, but suggested that harmful results derive more from unconscious tensions generated by unacknowledged wishes and fears in relation to the actual experience. For example, the intolerable anxiety suffered by a young man might derive from his unconscious wish to retaliate against his punitive and restrictive father. **Later analytic theories** place more weight on actual experience, especially the damaging effects of early separation, loss, psychological trauma, and deficiencies in the emotional aspect of the parent–child relationship, but still emphasize the power of unconscious forces in perpetuating difficulties into adulthood.

Fig. 18.2 History of psychological treatments

Psychoanalysis

Psychological methods of treatment gained prominence in medical settings through the work of Sigmund Freud (1856–1939). Freud, who started his career in Vienna as a neurologist, experimented at first with **hypnosis** in the treatment of patients suffering hysterical neuroses, florid forms of which were then common in neurological practice. He found that such patients were relieved of symptoms when, in the hypnotic state, they could recall upsetting experiences from earlier in their lives and could express emotions appropriate to those memories (the 'cathartic method'). Freud recognized thereby the pathogenic potential of memories which, because distressing, had been rendered **unconscious.**

Later he abandoned hypnosis when he discovered that catharsis was promoted as effectively by encouraging the patient to talk openly and freely (**free association**) in a way which revived hitherto-unconscious memories spontaneously (the 'talking cure'). He recognized that the patient's **dreams** offered another valuable source of unconscious material, but also that a variety of strategies were employed unconsciously by the mind (**defence mechanisms**, of which repression and projection are examples) to resist the emergence into conscious awareness of disturbing memories and thoughts. Obviously, the patient's **resistance** obstructs catharsis and the recovery of unconscious material.

From these discoveries Freud developed a conceptual model of mental processes, one component of which was his functional subdivision of the psyche into:
1 the **id**, basic biological drives, such as appetites for food and sexual activity, aggression, and the need for comfort and intimacy;
2 the **super ego**, those critical and prohibitive forces within oneself which oppose free expression of the basic drives (the conscience);
3 the **ego**, that rational and responsible aspect of the self which mediates to ensure appropriate fulfilment of the basic biological needs without guilty conscience or society's condemnation.

Freud recognized that patients tended to relate in ways which were influenced by earlier experience, transferring onto him certain attributes (attitudes, emotions, reactions) which told him much about the patient's formative relationships, especially with parents. The analysis of this **transference** and the material derived from the patient's free associations, and resistances to such association, remains the basis of **psychoanalysis**, the treatment model developed by Freud. Psychoanalysis was found to be effective as a psychological treatment for a wide variety of neuroses.

Freud suggested that **anxiety** was a product of tension between basic drives and either internal prohibitive forces or social constraints of the outside world. **Neurosis** results when mental defence mechanisms (see above) are employed excessively to control this internal conflict and thereby to limit awareness of the anxiety generated. The manifestations of neurosis are determined by the nature of the underlying mental conflict, the constellation of defence mechanisms utilized, and the degree of residual anxiety.

Since Freud's death psychoanalytic theory and method have been developed and modified both by Freud's colleagues and students (e.g. Carl Jung (1875–1961) and Melanie Klein (1882–1960)) and their later followers. In the UK, through the work of Bowlby, Guntrip, Winnicott and others, more emphasis has been placed on the **need for human relationship** than on the gratification of basic biological drives. The experiences of successive formative relationships with others (objects, in psychoanalytic terminology) are internalized (**internal object relationships**), acting subsequently as unconscious templates for future patterns of relating. Such templates may influence the choice of relationships, how they develop, and how the subject experiences himself in relation to the other person.

Destructive, as well as beneficial, patterns of relating may be recreated unconsciously, perhaps again and again. The same unconscious patterns emerge in therapy as transferences, and thereby may be identified, explored and modified (i.e. analysed) in the therapeutic relationship itself. All **analytic psychotherapies** retain the emphasis on the therapeutic relationship and the analysis of unconscious processes, including transference and resistance.

Group psychotherapies

Group psychotherapy was developed in the UK during the Second World War. Large numbers of soldiers were returned home as psychiatric casualties, and in the military hospitals they were organized in groups for remedial and social activities. A number of army psychiatrists recognized the psychotherapeutic potential of the groups themselves. The morale generated by collective group activity was seen to boost the self-esteem of the group's members, public expression of their self-doubt and anxiety reduced neurotic symptomatology, and the group offered a normalizing influence which diminished antisocial behaviour. These experiments established the basic principles from which modern group therapy has developed. In the out-patient setting, **small group psychotherapy** has drawn on analytic methods to enhance the natural therapeutic function of the group. In hospital psychiatric wards and other residential settings, the socializing influence of the group has been emphasized in the large group activities which characterize the **therapeutic community**.

Family therapies

Family therapies have evolved since the Second World War, initially instigated by two different trends in North American psychiatry. The first was a reaction to the emphasis on the individual in both biological psychiatry and psychoanalysis, certain psychoanalysts (e.g. Ackerman) reasserting that the individual could be understood only in the context of his/her family and social network. The second impetus came from research into the communication patterns of families of schizophrenics, which was undertaken by Bateson, Lidz and others, and which contributed to the development of **systems theory**. According to this theory (which underpins much family therapy today), the family can be viewed as a system which comprises a number of sub-systems (groupings within the family, e.g. the sibling group or the parental couple) which are in dynamic relationship to each other. A change in one sub-system will provoke compensatory changes in all other sub-systems within the family. Accordingly psychopathology cannot be regarded as residing in any one individual but in the family system as a whole. A number of models of family therapy have developed in North America and Europe, drawing variously on the psychology of communication, systems theory, psychoanalysis, and behavioural methods of treatment.

Behavioural therapy and cognitive therapy

Behavioural therapy was developed first in the 1950s, initially by the application of **learning theory** to the treatment of a variety of neurotic symptoms. Studies of learning in animals had indicated that behaviours could be conditioned and maintained by particular patterns of stimulus and reward. For example, in Pavlov's early experiments, dogs had been conditioned to salivate in response to a bell which originally had been sounded at the same moment as the appearance of food ('**classical conditioning**'). B.F. Skinner showed that animals repeated behaviours which were rewarded in some way, as by the presentation of food ('**operant conditioning**'). Behaviour therapists regarded neurotic symptoms as learned maladaptive behaviours, and drew on theories of classical and operant learning to devise strategies for modifying and eradicating these behaviours. For example, Wolpe treated phobic patients by exposing them progressively to the feared situation after inducing a state of relaxation, his rationale being that their fearful response would be inhibited if the formerly feared situation were associated with pleasurable feelings ('reciprocal inhibition').

The interest of behavioural therapists focused on observable behaviours. Covert psychological processes are also disturbed in neurotic disorders, especially cognitions – that is, patterns of thinking. Cognitive psychology suggests that faulty patterns of thinking are learned, and that cognitive faults underlie much mood disturbance and maladaptive behaviour. **Cognitive therapy** which has been developed over the past decade by Beck and others involves the examination and correction of thinking patterns which lead to inappropriate degrees of self-criticism, of pessimism, and of those other negative thoughts which are characteristic of neurotic states.

Hopefully, these issues will become clearer in the pages which follow.

The major psychological treatments

BEHAVIOURAL THERAPY

Theoretical basis

The rationale for behavioural treatments derives from the belief that symptoms, whether uncomfortable feelings, unwanted thoughts or maladaptive behaviours, are **learned** responses to particular experiences. It follows that symptoms can be modified, either by reversal of the original learned process or by the encouragement of an alternative, more constructive feeling, thought or behaviour.

Historically two major components of learning theory have been applied in the modification of troublesome symptoms. Methods derived from **classical conditioning** have been used to encourage new responses to events or experiences which previously gave rise to undesired symptoms, either by extinguishing the symptom or by reinforcing a more desirable response. **Operant conditioning** has been employed to shape healthier, more effective responses and behaviours (see p. 26).

Behavioural therapy is essentially a pragmatic and empirical treatment approach, however, and its techniques are drawn as much from the therapist's practical experience of what proves effective as from established theory.

Indications

Behavioural methods are applied in the treatment of some neuroses, particularly phobic-anxiety states and obsessive–compulsive disorders; habit disorders, including tics, smoking and eating disorders; conduct disorders in children, the mentally handicapped, and chronic schizophrenic patients; and in some marital and family disorders. Treatments are designed to reduce symptoms and behaviours which are distressing and disruptive, or to promote desirable and adaptive behaviours.

In many psychiatric disorders, symptomatic behaviours trouble both the patient and those around him. For example the rituals of the obsessive–compulsive, the avoidance behaviour of the agoraphobic, and the bed-wetting of the enuretic child cause distress both to the sufferer and to his family. The impoverished behaviour of some chronic schizophrenics, on the other hand, appears to cause more frustration to those who care for the patient than to the patient himself. Many of these behaviours are amenable to modification or eradication by behavioural therapy.

Essential features of behavioural therapy

Behavioural treatments incorporate a number of diverse techniques, but have several essential features in common.
1 Behavioural treatments are aimed primarily at the modification of **current, observable behaviours**.
2 Behavioural treatments begin with a detailed **behavioural**

analysis, in which the therapist identifies the **antecedents** of a symptom (that is, the factors which provoke it), the problem **behaviour** itself (the behavioural manifestations of the symptom), and its **consequences** for the patient and those around him (the ABC of behavioural therapy). This permits the therapist to decide on the most appropriate technical intervention to apply.
3 Treatment programmes are **designed cooperatively** by therapist and patient in order to recognize and tackle the idiosyncrasies of each individual's symptoms.
4 The patient is **recruited actively** into the treatment process by being encouraged to participate in the identification of appropriate **goals** for treatment.
5 The patient **monitors** the frequency and severity of the target symptom as therapy progresses, often by keeping a **diary** of its occurrence.
6 The therapist **measures** the target behaviour before, during and after treatment in order both to ensure selection of the most effective therapeutic techniques and to evaluate the progress and outcome of treatment.
7 The patient carries out **homework tasks** between treatment sessions.
8 The patient's relatives or friends are **recruited as cotherapists** in the treatment, accompanying and encouraging the patient in the agreed homework assignments.

Examples of behavioural treatments

Reduction of undesired symptoms and behaviours

Many techniques have been used in the treatment of phobic anxiety. Initially the process of **flooding** was used extensively. The patient was exposed to the feared object or situation (e.g. spider or enclosed space), and escape from it was prevented until his anxiety level had eventually diminished. The patient could then enter the situation again without such intense fear developing. Flooding is used less now, and recently it has been recognized that such techniques may exacerbate the target symptomatology, especially in patients suffering post-traumatic stress disorder (see Chapter 20). The aim in **systematic desensitization** or **graded exposure** is similar, but here the phobic patient is exposed gradually to the feared situation or to a series of feared situations in ascending order of difficulty. The therapist may help the patient to relax deeply before asking him firstly to imagine the situation, then to enter it in reality, and later to tackle similarly a more difficult situation.

Response prevention is a term applied to methods employed in the treatment of obsessional rituals, ruminations and other compulsive behaviours such as overeating. The patient is taught to delay or prevent his habitual responses by identifying the stimuli which provoke them and by rehearsing alternative actions. For example the patient who washes compulsively after contact with dirt (real or imagined) is encouraged to find something else to occupy himself for a period of time, following which his washing rituals will be less urgent and shorter.

Enhancement of desired behaviours

A variety of methods are used to overcome problematic symptoms by the encouragement of more desirable behaviours and skills. For example, the **bell and pad** method is used to treat nocturnal enuresis. The child learns gradually to respond to cues from his full bladder by being woken by a bell which rings when the first leak of urine establishes an electrical circuit in the pad upon which he is sleeping.

Token economy programmes have been devised to tackle some of the symptoms evident in the deficit states resulting from chronic schizophrenia. Using the principles of operant conditioning, desired behaviours (such as getting out of bed when woken, washing, or undertaking simple domestic tasks) are reinforced by the award of tokens which can be exchanged later for desirable items from the hospital shop or, perhaps more constructively, for some interpersonal reward (e.g. a game of cards with a member of staff).

Operant principles have been applied also in the treatment of social anxiety and shyness. **Social skills training** is a treatment which promotes confidence and effectiveness by teaching the shy or unskilled patient to behave appropriately in a variety of social situations. Appropriate behaviours are **modelled** by the therapist and then practised by the patients, generally in a group. Direct feedback and video-replay shows the patient where he is going wrong, and desirable behaviours are **reinforced** by praise and encouragement.

Group methods in behavioural therapy
Some behavioural treatments are carried out in a group context, as when a number of agoraphobic patients are taken on a bus together by their therapist. The group is not necessarily encouraged as a therapeutic experience in itself, though the mutual support and understanding between patients may be a valued side-product.

Practicalities
Behavioural therapies have been developed by clinical psychologists and a few psychiatrists, but are practised increasingly also by nurses and other professionals in a variety of settings. Traditionally the relationship between the patient and therapist is promoted in behavioural therapy only in order to ensure the patient's trust and cooperation. No attention is paid to the unconscious features of the relationship, such as the patient's transference to the therapist.

Case 1: behavioural therapy

Celia, a 34-year-old housewife without children, had been incapacitated by *agoraphobia* for years. She *could not leave the flat without her husband*, and had been *unable to enter trains or crowded shops* even in his company. She was treated by *graded exposure*, and *her husband was recruited as a cotherapist*. The psychologist drew up, with Celia and her husband, *a hierarchy of goals* which began with walking to the front gate while her husband watched from the door, and progressed through walking alone to the corner of the street to making shopping trips alone. At each session Celia's *achievements were reviewed and praised*, and the *next homework tasks were set*. After 10 sessions she was able to walk alone to the local shops, to enter all but the busiest supermarket and, with her husband, to travel by train into the city.

COGNITIVE AND COGNITIVE– BEHAVIOURAL THERAPY

Cognitive therapy was developed originally as a treatment for depression; but subsequently it has been applied, in conjunction with behavioural methods, in the treatment of anxiety (generalized, panic and phobic anxiety), obsessional, eating and somatization disorders.

The cognitive approach derives from the recognition that depressed mood, anxiety states and certain disordered behaviours are associated with **negative patterns of thinking** which themselves exacerbate and perpetuate the problem. Negative and irrational thinking is seen to derive from the person's faulty **attitudes** and **assumptions** about himself, which often were generated early in life by experiences which left him with a negative view of himself and his capabilities. Such negative and potentially pathogenic perceptions are perpetuated by internal representations or **schemas** of the destructive early experience. The concept of cognitive schemas is akin to the earlier psychoanalytic concept of internal object relations (see above), and is fundamental to the recent cognitive conceptualization of personality disorders.

The first step in a cognitive therapy involves helping the patient to recognize patterns of negative thinking and dysfunctional behaviour. The precipitants and consequences of irrational thoughts are analysed, especially those which are self-critical and self-defeating. As therapy progresses attention is drawn to the dysfunctional personal assumptions which underlie the negative thoughts; and these similarly are evaluated critically. The **origins** of distorted patterns of thinking and assumption are not usually examined systematically in cognitive therapy, however.

Eventually the patient is helped to **think** more positively about himself, and thereby to **feel** better about and in himself. Positive experiences and achievements are emphasized to reinforce the cognitive change. Cognitive therapies are often relatively short.

There is an element of cognitive appraisal in a number of other treatment strategies, often applied in conjunction with behavioural methods.

Problem-solving therapy is a short, pragmatic psychological treatment which draws on cognitive methods to address the patient's particular emotional problem or crisis. The patient is encouraged to identify his problem and to tackle its component parts in small, manageable steps, formulating adaptive methods of coping and reviewing their effectiveness at each stage. This is a common sense approach which can be taught easily, and which maximizes the patient's sense of achievement and control. Problem-solving promotes creative and positive thinking, which may be generalized successfully to subsequent challenges.

Specific **cognitive–behavioural treatment** programmes have been developed for the treatment of patients with eating disorders, or the problems deriving from childhood sexual abuse. Cognitive therapy is applied now also in a group context.

Cognitive therapy has been practised in the UK particularly by clinical psychologists, though some of its modifications are applied increasingly by other health workers in primary care and other settings.

Case 2: cognitive therapy

Peter, 24, had become *depressed* following his failure to achieve promotion at work. His mood was depressed, he had *withdrawn* from his friends and former social activities, and he had a very *negative view of himself and his future.* Having assessed Peter's pattern of thinking about himself, the *psychologist drew attention to his frequent self-critical remarks* (e.g. 'I'm no good at anything really', 'People don't like me') *and asked if they were really justified.* At first Peter insisted that he really was ineffectual and unattractive but, encouraged by the therapist to provide evidence of this, he could point to nothing more than his promotion failure. *The psychologist drew attention to his previous successes,* both socially and in his work, with the result that Peter began to think more positively about himself again. Then *they explored together some of Peter's assumptions about himself,* such as that he was likeable only if he was successful, and he agreed that this was inaccurate and irrational. As he began to think better of himself, his mood lifted and he recovered his former optimism and sociability. The therapist anticipated that *Peter's rejection of his false assumptions would make it less likely that he would become depressed again in the future if he failed at something.*

SUPPORTIVE PSYCHOTHERAPY

Many people who are disabled by personality deficits, chronic neurosis or psychotic illness can cope from day to day only with consistent support, especially in times of adversity. Often this support is available from family or friends, but **supportive psychotherapy** will be necessary if the vulnerable individual is isolated socially or if he tends to exhaust (or reject unintentionally) the help of those around him.

The term psychotherapy is employed here because, although it is the **maintenance** of emotional stability that is aimed for rather than psychological change, this is achieved by the creation of a supportive relationship with the therapist. Change is not aimed for with these vulnerable patients because of their persistent psychological fragility and because they lack generally the capacity for understanding their difficulties in psychological terms, an attribute which is a necessary prerequisite for most other psychological treatments.

In supportive psychotherapy, a psychoanalytic understanding of the patient is helpful for the therapist in order to maintain the therapeutic relationship, especially when the patient arouses feelings of frustration, helplessness or even hostility in those around him including the therapist. The therapist is unlikely to be exhausted by the patient, or provoked to retaliate, if he understands psychologically the reasons for the patient's behaviour and his own emotional reaction. In supportive psychotherapy, unlike analytic psychotherapy, the therapist's psychological understanding would not be communicated to the patient.

Support is an important component of most psychological treatments. In behaviour therapy and analytic psychotherapy, for example, the therapist supports the patient whilst employing other techniques to promote change. In supportive psychotherapy support is the central technique, and is used to prevent the potentially harmful effects of change. There are a number of practical components of support in this context.

1 Empathy, the therapist's capacity to feel his way into the patient's experience, allows the patient to feel understood and accepted and, when communicated sensitively, is the most supportive component of the therapeutic relationship.

2 Encouragement of the patient's strengths and capabilities promotes self-esteem and combats demoralization.

3 Explanation can be helpful when the patient misunderstands important issues relating to his circumstances or health.

4 Guidance, which may take the form of open advice or covert suggestion, is appropriate when obstacles are faced or decisions are necessary.

5 Practical support can be effective both by modifying disruptive factors in the patient's life and by modelling to the patient how this can be done.

Supportive psychotherapy is practised in a variety of settings, often without formal recognition. Psychiatrists may support individuals over long periods with regular, but not necessarily frequent, appointments in the out-patient clinic. Social workers and community nurses develop supportive relationships with vulnerable clients who may be seen at intervals in their own homes. General practitioners support many vulnerable patients indefinitely with regular or occasional surgery attendances or home visits. It should be emphasized that, although practised widely, supportive psychotherapy requires skill and considerable patience.

Case 3: supportive psychotherapy

Len, a 56-year-old former clerk, had been clinically *depressed at intervals since his wife left him* 3 years earlier. A diffident man, he had been *prone to depression for many years.* His active and outgoing wife had supported him emotionally until, after being made redundant, he had become morose and bad-tempered. Eventually, undermined by his criticism and demands, she had left him; and their two grown-up children had avoided him. *His tendency to depression was explained by his childhood experience,* his mother having died when he was 9 from a long, incapacitating illness and his father having been ineffectual and remote emotionally.

Len's *depression had been treated with tricyclic antidepressive medication,* and the biological features were reduced; but *he remained vulnerable and incapable.* Recognizing this, the psychiatrist had decided to see him monthly in the out-patient clinic for *supportive psychotherapy.* During the 30-minute apppointments, Len was *encouraged to discuss his difficulties* with the doctor, who offered explanations and advice when necessary. On occasion *practical intervention* had been appropriate, as when the psychiatrist negotiated with the Housing Department for Len's transfer to a block of flats occupied by a number of single, middle-aged people. With the *psychiatrist's emotional support and encouragement,* he had been able to look after himself and to join a local social club, and the frequency of his depressive relapses had diminished. He was a bitter and ungrateful man, and the psychiatrist required all of his understanding and skill to maintain the therapeutic relationship.

The professional worker's preparedness to see the vulnerable person, and to accept him the way he is, permits the patient to become **dependent**. Many professionals regard the patient's dependency as a problem to be avoided but, in fact, it is inevitable and unavoidable in the population for whom supportive psychotherapy is indicated, particularly in those patients suffering personality and chronic neurotic difficulties. Psychoanalytically, they can be viewed as individuals whose emotional needs were not satisfied in early life and who consequently remain vulnerable and dependent in adulthood. When, for practical reasons, it is inappropriate to allow the patient to become dependent on an individual (perhaps because the doctor will be working in the clinic for a short period only; or because the patient might regress to a state of intense, dysfunctional dependency), the patient might be encouraged to depend on the **institution** by attending a day hospital or centre or a supportive social club.

COUNSELLING

The term **counselling** is used very broadly and, in some contexts, is synonymous with psychotherapy. Psychodynamic counselling, for example, is almost indistinguishable from analytic psychotherapy (see below). More basic counselling, however, is a process whereby a person who faces a specific challenge is helped to clarify and find solutions to the problem. The solution often involves making an important life decision or coming to terms with a significant life-event. The prinicples and basic techniques of counselling have a place in all helping relationships.

Indications

Counselling is indicated when a person is faced by the need either to make a major decision or to adapt to a major event (generally a loss) in his life.

In the medical context, such decisions may centre on whether or not to have a pregnancy terminated, whether to have children if there is a risk of genetic disorder, or whether to undergo cosmetic surgery. Counselling may be indicated also for patients who have undergone mastectomy, amputation of a limb, or other mutilating surgery; who have developed chronic incapacitating illness or disability; who have been traumatized emotionally by an accident or assault; who have lost a close relative through illness or accident; or who are trying to overcome dependence on alcohol or drugs.

In non-medical contexts counselling may be available to assist a person with choice of career, tackling relationship problems, preparation for retirement, or adaptation to a new culture. Much bereavement counselling is practised outside of medical settings by non-medical personnel.

Process of counselling

In practice, whether in a medical or non-medical context, counselling involves enabling the patient or client to make his own decision or adaptation to the challenge which he faces. The counsellor helps the client to **clarify** and examine the issues faced, and this may involve the **release of emotions** appropriate to the situation (for example, grief in bereavement). Having examined the problem the client is helped to make a **decision**, where necessary, or to **come to terms with** the event experienced. This process may closely resemble the problem-solving therapy described above.

However, counselling is **non-directive** in that the counsellor does not instruct the client, advise him or offer answers. The counsellor's skills are deployed in encouraging the client to think and talk about his circumstances. The **therapeutic relationship** (see p. 227) is fundamental to this process and particularly the counsellor's preparedness to **listen to, empathize with** and **accept** the client. Specific **facilitating** techniques are employed by the counsellor to enable the client to disclose and discuss painful issues which otherwise might be avoided. In a way, the counsellor acts as a **sounding board** for the client's ideas, feelings and tentative solutions.

Practice of counselling

Counselling is practised in educational, industrial and commercial establishments, as well as in medical settings and social work departments. In the UK, there has been a considerable expansion of counselling in the primary care setting in the last few years. In some institutions, trained counsellors are employed for this specific task; but, in other settings, counselling may be practised at varying levels of formality by doctors, social workers, nurses and others.

In recent years, counselling services and centres have been developed in the community to assist people facing specific difficulties. These are staffed generally by non-professional or voluntary counsellors, who often may have faced and coped with the specific problem themselves. For example, sophisticated bereavement counselling is now available in

---

Cases 4 & 5: counselling

A trained counsellor was employed by a large and busy general medical practice. Part of her task was to support the doctors, nurses and health visitors in the management of their patients' emotional needs. She was available also to see patients when more specific counselling was indicated; and, on occasion, initiated referral of more disturbed patients to the local mental health services with which she had regular contact.

The counsellor was asked to see Jo, a young woman with systemic lupus erythematosus (SLE) who had consulted her doctor because she was pregnant. Her boyfriend had left her when he discovered she was pregnant, and she was very upset and confused about her predicament. Not surprisingly, Jo's SLE had flared up. In discussion with the counsellor, she was able to *express her anger* towards the young man who had abandoned her *and her unhappiness* about the prospect of ending the pregnancy. Initially Jo had wanted to continue the pregnancy, but she was able to recognize that her physical health was already compromised and that she could not raise a child alone. She decided to ask her doctor for a termination of pregnancy, after which the counsellor saw her again to *assist her adjustment to her losses.*

A second case presented the counsellor with a *difficult ethical dilemma.* She was asked to see Ron, a 36-year-old man, who had consulted his doctor repeatedly with his 5-year-old daughter. The father was anxious because his daughter, who had started school 6 months earlier, had suffered a series of minor infections; and he had become convinced that she had a serious underlying illness. The doctor found nothing wrong with the child, but recognized that Ron was over-anxious and possessive of his daughter. By contrast the mother, when eventually persuaded to attend the surgery, was detached and irritable towards both husband and child.

At his first appointment with the counsellor, the patient admitted there were serious problems in his marriage but was reluctant to ask his wife to participate with him in marital therapy. Instead he dwelled ruminatively on his daughter's health, eventually expressing his *fear that he would 'lose her'.* The counsellor,

Continued

concerned by Ron's unjustified preoccupation and apparently over-close relationship with his daughter, asked him directly at the next appointment about his physical contact with her. He broke down in tears, and confessed that over the past year he had touched her sexually and, when on his own, had masturbated to sexual fantasies about her. He volunteered that this was wrong and potentially destructive to his daughter, and asked for help in curtailing this *sexual abuse* of her.

The counsellor *felt obliged ethically to inform the statutory authorities* of Ron's sexual abuse of his daughter, and told him so; but because he had asked for help, wanted very much to avoid intrusive medical and legal interventions which might prove even more destructive to the child and family. She discussed the situation openly with Ron, who acknowledged eventually that he had wanted someone to intervene in order to protect his daughter. This was why he had consulted the doctor repeatedly. With his agreement, the counsellor invited his wife to the next appointment. She was upset and angry, but admitted that she had been aware of what was going on. It emerged that *both she and Ron had been abused sexually* by their fathers in childhood.

With the couple's agreement, the counsellor informed social services of Ron's abuse of his daughter. The doctor and social worker examined the child, but found no evidence of penetrative abuse or injury. Ron was interviewed by the police, but no legal action was taken against him. Instead, the family was referred to a child psychiatrist for therapeutic intervention which involved couple therapy and, later, individual analytic psychotherapy for Ron. The counsellor maintained intermittent contact with the family.

the community from voluntary, self-help organizations such as CRUSE (see also Chapter 22).

CRISIS THERAPY

In psychological terms **crisis** refers to the reaction of an individual to events which he does not have the resources, either personally or in his social network, to cope with.

Causes of crises

Crisis may be precipitated by any event which demands adaptation, whether adverse (e.g. bereavement) or positive (e.g. childbirth). Such experiences are classified as **developmental** if they are encountered naturally and inevitably during the human lifecycle (e.g. adolescence, menopause, retirement), or **accidental** when untimely or not universal (e.g. redundancy, premature death of a spouse or child, loss of a limb). The coincidence of developmental and accidental experiences, as when an adolescent's parent dies or when a child is born prematurely, is a particularly potent cause of crisis.

We all experience crises in our lives, so the state of crisis cannot be regarded as abnormal. Indeed the successful re-solution of crisis involves the development of new coping resources and promotes psychological growth. Psychological health depends on the encounter and resolution of crises. People in crises only come to the attention of psychiatric ser-vices when they resort to certain maladaptive ways of coping (e.g. taking an overdose of tablets) or suffer a **breakdown**.

Characteristic course of crises

Faced by a threatening experience, the individual feels anxious. If his usual ways of coping do not equip him to deal with the situation, he may be able to devise new strat-egies which are effective or call on the effective help of family or friends. Failure to find a solution will lead to the escalation of anxiety, sleep disturbance and impairment of concentration, all of which undermine further his morale and effectiveness. In this state of turmoil, maladaptive beha-viours may emerge – alcohol abuse, self-injurious actions, violence to others. Further escalation of anxiety provokes eventually the breakdown of normal psychological function-ing, the manifestations of which depend on the particular vulnerabilities of the person concerned. One might suffer an acute neurotic breakdown whilst another experiences the relapse of a chronic psychotic illness.

Treatment of crises

If serious breakdown occurs, hospitalization and appropriate physical treatment may be necessary. **Crisis therapy** aims to enable the individual to overcome the crisis before break-down or maladaptive solutions occur. This requires early and effective intervention, which psychiatric and social work teams are gearing themselves increasingly to provide.

Crisis therapy involves the following ingredients.

1 Clarification: the patient is encouraged to discuss his situation in order to **clarify** the problems which require solution. This process modifies the patient's perception of his problems and encourages his own coping resources.

2 Expression of emotions: discussion of the crisis also encourages the patient to express feelings which are appro-priate to the situation (e.g. grief in bereavement).

3 Support: emotional and practical support from family and friends is mobilized, thereby overcoming the sense of iso-lation which often accompanies crisis.

4 Examination of coping resources: existing coping methods are encouraged when adaptive and applicable.

5 Maladaptive assumptions and behaviours are discour-aged by the judicious employment of cognitive techniques, where possible, but by direct discouragement if necessary.

6 Alternative coping strategies for tackling the problems are identified in discussion, tried out, and then reinforced until the crisis resolves and the patient's confidence is restored.

7 Ending: therapy is ended before dependence on the therapist is established, issues relating to separation and loss being examined in discussion where these are pertinent to the crisis.

It can be seen that crisis therapy involves application of the techniques of counselling and problem-solving therapy (see above). Crisis therapy does not involve tackling long-standing personality or neurotic problems though these might be helped coincidentally by the psychological growth which occurs when crises are resolved successfully.

Crisis therapy is practised in a variety of settings including hospital emergency departments, GP surgeries and the pa-tient's own home, often by multidisciplinary teams. The emphasis is on brief, intensive intervention; so the patient may be seen, with members of his family, six times in 3 weeks before treatment is terminated. Crisis therapy is un-likely to be effective more than 6 or 8 weeks after the onset

Tina, a 19-year-old secretary, was admitted to hospital after taking an *overdose* of 20 aspirin tablets when she *discovered that her boyfriend was seeing another woman*. When interviewed later by a nurse from the psychiatric service, she acknowledged that she *had not really wanted to kill herself*. She had felt desperate and had taken the tablets on impulse. In discussion with the nurse, Tina got in touch with the *feelings of sadness and anger* which were so appropriate, and decided to return to her family home. There she was able to *talk about her situation with her parents and, later, an old friend*. When she returned to the hospital to see the nurse 3 days later, she had *decided to break off her relationship* with the boyfriend and to move out of the flat which they had shared. She had chosen to move in with her old friend, and returned to work shortly after. When interviewed again a week later she was sad about the breakdown of her relationship, ashamed of her overdose, and determined to resume some of the former friendships and activities which she had given up when she met her boyfriend. She was discharged from the crisis clinic.

of crisis, at which point other treatment strategies may be considered.

ANALYTIC PSYCHOTHERAPY

Indications

Many patients with neurotic or personality disorders present to psychiatric services with problems which are long-standing and pervasive in all their relationships and actions. Their symptoms are multiple and often diffuse, and defy amelioration by medication or by behavioural and cognitive treatments. Some patients display even an apparent reluctance to overcome their difficulties, failing to cooperate with directive treatment strategies. In these cases, analytic psychotherapy may be indicated; though some paranoid or anti-social personalities are unable to establish the therapeutic relationship in which to accomplish the work of analysis.

The process of analytic psychotherapy

The essential basis of analytic psychotherapy is the **therapeutic relationship**. In the first stage of treatment the therapist works actively to develop a trusting relationship, in which the patient can feel accepted and understood even when he is expressing or talking about his less pleasant characteristics. The patient is helped thereby to disclose intimate and painful aspects of himself and his experience. Inevitably this process of self-disclosure is accompanied by the expression of associated feelings, this combination often proving therapeutic in itself.

Analytic psychotherapy emphasizes examination of the meaning of symptoms, and aims to help the patient to make sense of his experience. The expression of hitherto-hidden facets of the patient enables him to explore, with the therapist, the ways in which his characteristic assumptions and manner may interfere with his relationships and personal achievements – as, for example, at work or in other creative or physical pursuits. This exploration often enables the patient to make spontaneous connections between his current feelings, thoughts or behaviour and significant experiences in his recent or distant past. These connections lead to increased self-understanding or **insight**. The combination of self-disclosure, emotional expression and enhanced self-understanding in the context of an accepting relationship forms the basis of the therapeutic effect in analytic psychotherapy. The patient comes to know himself better.

The patient's self-understanding is promoted primarily by analysis of the unconscious aspects of his relationships and actions. Particular attention is paid to analysis of his unconscious **transference** onto the therapist of attributes which derive from other significant relationships, especially the patient's relationships with his parents and other important figures in his early life. The patient is encouraged by the therapist to identify his thoughts and feelings for the therapist, to explore their origins, and to assess how similar patterns might complicate and interfere with other current relationships. The analysis of unconscious processes can be unsettling and painful, with the result that patients develop unconscious **resistances** to the therapeutic task. The therapist's aim always is to help the patient to develop awareness spontaneously; but, when resistances impede this process, the therapist may offer explanations (**interpretations**) to the patient about the unconscious processes which are operating. The purpose of an analytic interpretation is to overcome the patient's natural reluctance to see something uncomfortable about himself.

Long-term analytic psychotherapy

The development of greater self-understanding allows the patient to view himself and others differently and leads, in most cases, to changes in his behaviour and relationships. Greater personal effectiveness, and more satisfying relationships, reinforce positive changes in the patient's personality and self-esteem. Inevitably this process takes time, so analytic psychotherapies have tended to be prolonged. Typically patient and therapist meet for one hour each week, for periods of 1–3 years.

Short-term analytic psychotherapy

For pragmatic and financial reasons, great interest has been generated over recent years by modifications of analytic technique which allow benefits to be achieved more rapidly. **Short-term analytic psychotherapy** is sometimes called **focal psychotherapy** because attention is focused selectively on one area of the patient's experience, to the apparent exclusion of other issues. Fortunately insights and changes in one area of the patient's functioning often generalize to other areas (see clinical illustration below). Nevertheless, for this shorter treatment to be effective, the patient needs to be well motivated and able to focus on a circumscribed area of difficulty. To achieve more rapid therapeutic response, the therapist adopts a more active and interpretive stance than has been conventional in analytic psychotherapy. Particular emphasis is placed on analysis of the patient's transference to the therapist, and of the way in which he deals with the imminent ending of treatment. This method requires the patient to withstand considerable anxiety, so cannot be applied in the treatment of more fragile or disturbed patients. Typically short-term analytic psychotherapy involves 10 to 20 hour-long sessions at weekly intervals.

Case 7: short-term analytic psychotherapy

Raymond, a 34-year-old architect, was referred for psychotherapy with a history of *recent depression* and of *long-standing difficulties in relationships*. He tended to be deferential to men, particularly to older men such as his employers, and *self-consciously awkward with women. At work* he had *failed to achieve promotion or reward.* He had one long-standing male friend with whom he enjoyed outdoor pursuits, but his attempts to establish heterosexual relationships had been frustrated by his own anxiety. He was the *only child of a harshly critical father and a timid, ineffectual mother.* The psychotherapist, a man rather older than the patient, recommended a short-term analytic treatment and *identified the patient's relationships with men as a focus for work.* The patient developed rapidly an *intense transference to the therapist, behaving in a deferential and compliant manner.* Encouraged by the therapist the *patient explored his expectation of criticism and ridicule,* and recognized spontaneously its *origins in his relationship with his father.* This insight brought about no change in the patient's manner or behaviour until the therapist, prompted by a feeling of irritation in himself, suggested to the patient that his *deferential manner was also a way of covering up the intense anger with his father* which resulted from being undermined repeatedly. At first the patient was angry with the therapist for making such a suggestion but, as the penny dropped, he became able to feel his enormous resentment towards his father. This proved to be a turning point in therapy, which was concluded 4 weeks later after the fifteenth session. Raymond was no longer depressed, felt more confident, and applied himself more effectively at work. At a follow-up appointment 6 months later, he reported *greatly improved relationships with his boss and with his father,* and *greater confidence in his relationships with women.* Indeed he had established a satisfying sexual relationship with a former woman colleague.

Some degree of specialized training is necessary to practise analytic psychotherapy, and many practitioners undergo analytic psychotherapy themselves as part of this training. In the NHS, it is practised by psychotherapy-trained psychiatrists, psychologists, social workers and others in a variety of settings.

GROUP PSYCHOTHERAPY

In group psychotherapy a number of patients are brought together with one or more therapists for the purposes of mutual support, exploration, and learning through social interaction. The relationships between the patients in the group have as much therapeutic potential as those between each patient and the therapist.

Humans are born into a social network, the family, and most grow up, live and work in a social context. Satisfying personal relationships are necessary for mental health. Relationship difficulties contribute commonly to mental disorder and, conversely, mental disorder commonly causes difficulties in the patient's relationships. Group psychotherapy offers an opportunity to explore and to remedy interpersonal problems as they come alive in the social context of the group.

Group psychotherapy may be classified by its aim as maintaining (supportive), restorative or reconstructive.

Supportive group psychotherapy

Supportive group psychotherapy is useful in the management of chronically vulnerable patients, and is a common feature of the treatment programme in day hospitals and day centres. Its aims are the same as outlined above for individual supportive psychotherapy; but a group offers additional advantage in that the patients support each other to some extent, and their mutual support can continue between formal meetings of the group.

Case 8: supportive group psychotherapy

Len had been *prone to depression throughout his life*, but had suffered a *major depressive illness since being made redundant at work and then abandoned by his long-suffering wife.* A psychiatrist had treated him with *antidepressive medication*, and had maintained a *supportive relationship* with him at monthly out-patient appointments. Len had been helped to establish limited social contact with other single people in the block of flats in which he lived and, with considerable effort, began to attend a *social club* which met weekly in a *local day centre.* In this context, Len *obtained support and encouragement* both from the staff and from the other members, all of whom met together as a group during the club session.

Len discovered that other group members had experienced redundancy and marital separation, and derived comfort both from being able to talk in the *group meetings about his own difficulties and from hearing how others had coped with theirs.* These discussions continued outside of the group meetings, and Len became progressively more open and less bitter as the weeks passed. In due course he was discharged from the psychiatric out-patient clinic, but continued satisfactorily with his attendance at the supportive psychotherapy group.

Restorative group psychotherapy

The aim of restorative group psychotherapy is the restoration of interpersonal functioning, which tends to be damaged in acute psychiatric illness. Group therapy is conducted in many psychiatric admissions units in conjunction with physical treatments for this reason, and tackles the social withdrawal and other major disturbances in relating to others which are apparent in the in-patient population. However, it is often necessary to provide more than one 'level' of group therapy because of the extremes of interpersonal disability encountered in the acute ward. The most severely ill patients (e.g. the stuporose, aggressive or floridly psychotic) do not benefit from any form of psychological treatment, but other seriously depressed and psychotic patients do benefit from the educative and resocializing function of an activity-oriented group. Such groups are often conducted on acute

Case 9: restorative group psychotherapy

Joan, aged 38, *had always been rather sensitive and prickly* but became frankly *mistrustful and suspicious of others when she developed a paranoid psychosis some months after the sudden death of her mother.* She was admitted to a psychiatric unit for urgent treatment when, after successive angry confrontations with her husband and neighbours, she *tried to hang herself.*

Antipsychotic medication brought about a rapid abatement of Joan's paranoid delusions, but she *remained over-sensitive* and was

Continued on p. 236

also very upset about the destructive effect of her illness on her marital and social relationships. As her psychotic symptoms diminished, she was asked to join a *small psychotherapy group which met on the ward* each day of the week for 1 hour. *Initially Joan was mistrustful* of the other members and remained virtually silent, insisting that a group could be of no help to her. Gradually, however, other members of the group succeeded in showing her that this attitude was a product of the same process which had alienated her from her husband and friends. At this point, she began to soften and tried to engage more in the group discussion. *She derived hope from seeing other patients get better and leave the ward*, and *started to talk about her fears of returning home*. Some patients offered advice about how she might rebuild her relationships and resume her job but, when eventually the therapist pointed out her progress, Joan recognized that she had *already learned how to relate satisfactorily to others again through her experience in the group.*

---

wards by occupational therapists, using a creative task, game, music or dance to stimulate personal expression and interaction in the patients.

Patients who are recovering from psychotic or affective illnesses, or who were admitted to hospital in a crisis or with an acute exacerbation of a neurotic or personality disorder, may be selected for a 'talking group'. Its aims are more advanced, and may involve exploration both of the circumstances which precipitated the patient's problems and the patient's experience of hospitalization itself. The encouragement of the group, and the opportunity to discuss anxieties about returning home, can be invaluable to the patient as he approaches discharge from the ward; and sometimes patients are encouraged to continue attending the group for a limited period after discharge. Inevitably, however, the rapid turnover of patients in an admissions ward means that the composition of therapy groups is constantly changing. The therapist needs to take account of this, working hard to foster trust and openness in the group whilst guarding against over-ambitious attempts at reconstructive therapy.

Reconstructive group psychotherapy

Neuroses and personality disorders are caused by deficiencies and conflicts in early relationships, and such patients invariably experience difficulties in their adult relationships. It is for these conditions that reconstructive or analytic group psychotherapy is primarily indicated, the rationale of treatment being that the interpersonal foundation and manifestation of the disorder can be tackled directly because there is opportunity for a range of relationships in the treatment context itself. As in other forms of group therapy, great benefit derives for each patient from being able to talk about his feelings and worries, from the experience of being accepted and encouraged by the group, from the discovery that his problem may not be unique, and from being able to do something to help other group members. Each patient learns something from the experience and behaviour of the other patients, and from their observations about him. In reconstructive group psychotherapy, in addition, the patient learns about himself by analysing the relationships he develops with the other members of the group, including the therapist. These will betray the same unconsciously motivated

assumptions, feelings and behaviours which mar his relationships with family, friends and colleagues outside of the group. In the relative safety of the group, these transferences can be examined and understood in a way which equips the patient to discard old patterns of relating in favour of new, healthier relationships. The group therapist's task is to promote an atmosphere in the group in which interaction and examination proceed spontaneously, the therapeutic function of the group then being carried out largely by the patients themselves. The therapist contributes interpretations, as in individual analytic psychotherapy, only when the group as a whole is unable to overcome a particular obstacle to understanding.

Case 10: reconstructive group psychotherapy

Colin had a severely *obsessional personality*. His perfectionism served him well in his work as a clerk but, because he was so *rigid and critical of others*, it brought him into *conflict with his colleagues and undermined potential friendships*. He was selected for an *out-patient psychotherapy group* conducted on reconstructive lines. In early sessions he was quiet and resisted efforts to involve him in discussion. Later he became openly hostile towards the other male patients in the group, while remaining deferential towards the female therapist and indifferent towards the female patients. Eventually one of the women patients told him gently that she resented his dismissive manner, and suggested that *he should examine the way he related to members of the group if he wanted to obtain benefit from therapy*. Colin was taken aback by this challenge, but reflected on his feelings and behaviour with the encouragement of the group. *He recognized quickly that his relationships in the group were very much like those at work, and agreed that his critical and dismissive manner contributed to his social isolation and unhappiness*. Discussion in the group focused on Colin's plight several times during the next few sessions, and he became more friendly towards his female peers in the group and at work. His wariness of the male patients persisted, however, until, after several weeks, the therapist suggested that this pattern of relationships might be the product of *Colin's persisting jealousy of the other male patients'* apparently easy and friendly relationships with herself, the therapist. Colin recognized the accuracy of this interpretation immediately and *made a link spontaneously with his tremendous jealousy of his father* who had been so openly affectionate with his mother but so indifferent towards his son. This *insight enabled Colin to understand his own behaviour much more clearly*, and fuelled his determination to behave differently. In the group he started to relate more openly with the other men, expressing his feelings with increasing confidence. Having cleared up some of his angry and competitive feelings, he found that his positive feelings for the other groups members were reciprocated.

Practicalities

The duration and frequency of group meetings differs according to type. Out-patient supportive and reconstructive groups generally meet weekly, the latter for a longer period ($1\frac{1}{4}$–$1\frac{1}{2}$ hours) than the former. In-patient groups may meet several times each week, for 45–60-minute sessions. Therapy groups are conducted by staff of all disciplines, though nurses and occupational therapists play a prominent role in in-patient and day-patient settings. Reconstructive groups are conducted in hospital out-patient clinics, and in those residential units which are organized as **therapeutic communities**, where the psychological attributes of the residents and the duration of their admission (perhaps 6–12 months) make this approach viable.

FAMILY THERAPY, INCLUDING COUPLE THERAPY

The previous psychological treatments described, with the exception of crisis therapy, involve the patient as an individual being – albeit one who unconsciously carries aspects of his family life inside himself. In group psychotherapy a social context is created for treatment; but in certain circumstances it is more appropriate to treat the patient in his natural social context, the family, or to regard the family itself as the 'patient'. Family therapy involves treatment of two or more related members, who may represent one or more generations of a family. Couple or marital therapy is a form of family therapy applied to married couples, or partners in equivalent relationships.

As with individual and group psychotherapies, the aims of family therapy may be maintenance, restoration or reconstruction of the functional system.

Family support

Because the family unit has a natural capacity for psychological growth and coping, **supportive family therapy** is necessary to maintain effective functioning only in the less resourceful family or one that is faced by a prolonged major challenge. Long-term support by professional workers may be necessary, for example, for a family in which one or more members are mentally impaired, mentally ill, or physically disabled. Here the task is to assist the family in coping with the demands generated at any particular moment by illness or disability in its members. These change over time with the family's lifecycle. The problems presented to a young family by the birth of a mentally impaired child are very different to those faced years later when that child is grown up and the parents ageing.

Case 11: supportive family therapy

The parents and sister of a young schizophrenic man, who had suffered numerous psychotic episodes, were helped considerably by the *community psychiatric nurse* who visited fortnightly to administer his depot medication. The *nurse discussed how best to manage his unpredictable and sometimes frightening behaviour*. Her support, encouragement and advice to the family proved invaluable both in enabling the family to live with him without rejection or retaliation and, thereby, in reducing the frequency of his relapses.

Restorative family therapy

A family or couple is sometimes so undermined by a crisis that therapeutic intervention is required to **restore** healthy functioning. Illness and death are common causes of family crisis, but other destructive life-events such as redundancy or imprisonment of a family member may cause major problems too. A family may require help in adjusting even to essentially positive events such as childbirth or marriage. The principles of restorative family therapy are, essentially, those of crisis therapy.

Case 12: restorative family therapy

Three months after the birth of her first child, Maria was referred for psychiatric assessment by her health visitor who found her *crying and unable to cope with her baby*. It was clear immediately that Maria was *not clinically depressed*, and that this was not simply a case of 'maternity blues'. She told the psychiatrist that Simon, *her husband, had been irritable and distant for months*, that he had refused to be with her at the birth, and that he did nothing with the baby or to support her. Simon was asked to attend the next appointment with Maria, when it emerged that the *pregnancy had not been intended and that he had not wanted a baby at this time*. He was *encouraged to express his resentment openly*, and went on to describe how *he felt displaced from Maria's affections by the baby and unsure of himself as a father*. Reciprocally Maria *voiced her sadness at his lack of support and understanding*, and *described some ways in which he could help her to look after their daughter*. Soon Maria and Simon felt much closer to each other again, had resumed their sexual relationship, and were cooperating in care for the baby. Simon found that he could enjoy doing things with his daughter, even when changing her nappy, and that positive feelings for both Maria and the baby were increasing. They had been helped to negotiate the difficult transitional step to parenthood.

Reconstructive family therapy

Reconstructive family or couple therapy is indicated when a persisting fault in the basic psychological structure or functioning of the family causes psychiatric disorder in one or more members, or prevents the family from adjusting to a life crisis or challenge. There is a basic assumption underlying this approach, derived from the principles of systems theory, that members of a family unit function inter-dependently such that the behaviour and experience (including illness) of the individual cannot be understood in isolation from that of the other family members.

Therapy of this kind has been practised widely with families in which a child or adolescent member presents with illness or a conduct disorder. For this reason, much family therapy is done in child guidance clinics and in hospital departments of child and family psychiatry.

Family therapy is now being used also in the treatment of psychiatric disorders in adults. Psychological processes in the disturbed family are often so complex and involved that treatment is conducted generally by a multidisciplinary team. The therapists working face-to-face with the family are backed up by colleagues who observe the treatment sessions and offer observations and therapeutic recommendations from a more neutral standpoint.

A number of therapeutic strategies have been adopted in reconstructive family therapy. The simplest tackles faulty or inadequate **communication** patterns in the family, for much suffering and disturbance in relationships results from family members not being able to talk to each other or to relate emotionally. **Structural** family therapy tackles basic faults in the psychological and hierarchical structure of the family, as when the differences between generations are distorted (see Case 13). **Strategic** methods of family therapy involve the development of strategies to dismantle disturbed patterns of assumptions, communications and relationships within the family which are resistant to the more straightforward treatment approaches described above.

Behavioural methods are commonly used in family therapy, both alone and with the other approaches described. They are particularly valuable in couple therapy, when each partner may be asked to identify desired behaviours in the other and to find ways of reinforcing these.

Lastly the **psychoanalytic** approach is applied in work with families, and paticularly with couples. This involves the family members in mutual exploration of their problems and the pattern of their relationships, with analysis of the unconscious conflicts and assumptions which underpin them.

Couple therapy is conducted by a variety of practitioners in a variety of settings, including psychiatric clinics, social work and probation offices, and voluntary counselling agencies such as RELATE.

Case 13: reconstructive family therapy

Tracy, a 13-year-old school student, was referred to a child guidance clinic because her *behaviour at school was disruptive and abusive.* She was unruly in class and had threatened violence to her teachers. Tracy was interviewed with her parents and *two younger brothers, who were also showing early signs of disturbance.* At the assessment interview, Tracy's *mother seemed to be depressed and ineffectual.* She was shouted down repeatedly by Tracy, who swore at her contemptuously. Tracy's *father not only failed to discipline his daughter, but he also disagreed vociferously with his wife's suggestions* for managing Tracy. The therapists took the line that *Tracy was unhappy deep down,* and *unready to assume the adult responsibility that was being forced upon her by inadequacies in her parents' relationship.* They insisted that her *parents should resume the responsibilities of parenthood* for Tracy's sake, and encouraged them to *agree a way of dealing with her disrupive behaviour.* It was necessary to point out to her mother that she backed down in confrontations with Tracy, and to her father that his criticism of his wife merely fuelled Tracy's confusion. In effect the father was siding with his daughter rather than with his wife. Both parents understood this point and returned to the next session having discussed appropriate disciplinary measures for when Tracy misbehaved. Tracy fought against her parents at first, accusing her father of betraying her; but their *united stand eventually led to the cessation of her disturbed behaviour at home and at school.* At the fifth and final session, both Tracy and her parents reported that they were happier at home. Tracy's mother was no longer depressed, and Tracy was even affectionate towards her.

The practice of psychotherapy

Psychological assessment

The psychological formulation of a patient's problems, and the selection of an appropriate treatment, depend on an accurate clinical assessment. As a minimum, the interviewer aims to elucidate the patient's presenting problems, the antecedents of the problems (both precipitating and predisposing factors), the personal and interpersonal context in which the patient's problems developed; and to appraise the patient's strengths, achievements, coping style and personality. The selection procedure for an analytic psychotherapy would involve exploration of the historical and current internal origins of the patient's disorder, as well as assessment of his style of relating to the interviewer and his capacity to examine the possible contribution of unconscious processes to his problems.

The assessment procedure leads to a formulation of the patient's problems, which should be understood and agreed by the patient, and to the selection of an appropriate and feasible treatment plan.

Prognostic or good outcome attributes

An important additional component of the assessment procedure, emphasized particularly for the selection of analytic psychotherapies, is the appraisal of attributes of the patient which have been shown to influence the likely outcome of therapy. Positive prognostic features include the patient's motivation for the work of therapy and for desired change; his capacity to express feelings, including in words; his capacity to tolerate anxiety and frustration (both of which are inevitable during the course of a therapy) without destructive action; and his willingness and ability to conceptualize his experience in psychological terms, rather than somatizing or attributing his problems externally. Achievements in study, work, relationships and other pursuits serve as evidence of personal effectiveness, commitment and maturity.

On the other side of the balance, there are features which serve as absolute current contraindications for psychological treatment. These include serious psychiatric illness, such as active psychosis, severe biological depression, hypomania, and organic brain disease, and severe antisocial personality disorder.

Matching treatment to patient

From the accounts above, it might seem that each of the psychological treatments described is a discrete therapeutic entity, to be prescribed selectively for specific psychiatric disorders. Such specificity is possible often, but this simple picture omits the need to match the treatment to the patient rather than to the illness. For example many depressed patients can be treated successfully by cognitive therapy; but there are some, particularly those with underlying personality problems, who might be treated more effectively by a psychoanalytic psychotherapy.

Combined and integrated treatment approaches

The different treatments described in this chapter are not necessarily mutually exclusive. In clinical practice, there is often scope for some combination or cross-fertilization of technique. For example, a patient in the closing stages of an analytic psychotherapy may be encouraged by the therapist to rehearse modified behaviours between sessions, as in a behavioural therapy.

On an empirical basis, different modes of therapy may be combined in a comprehensive treatment programme. For example, concurrent individual and group analytic psychotherapies have been used successfully in the treatments of women who had been abused sexually in childhood and of women with eating disorders. Combined individual and couple cognitive behavioural therapies have been employed also, with benefit, for sexually abused women.

Integrated models of psychotherapy have been developed at a theoretical level, and applied effectively as treatments. Cognitive behavioural therapy has been described above. Another recent development in the UK is cognitive analytic therapy which integrates principles and methods of cognitive, behavioural and analytic therapies in a short, active and relatively structured treatment which has broad clinical application.

Factors common to all psychological treatments

The relationship between patient and therapist is an important therapeutic ingredient in all psychological treatments. Equally attention to psychological influences, including the unconscious forces which mould the patient, can be essential in any treatment. Failure to **listen** to the patient, to understand his predicament, and failure to appreciate the power of unconscious forces such as transferences can undermine treatment in psychiatry and in other medical settings.

Ethical code

Increasingly it has been recognized that the practitioners of psychological treatments must adhere to an explicit code of ethics. In part, this is because the opportunities for exploitation or abuse of the patient are so prominent when he or she enters a therapeutic relationship in which trust, dependency and self-disclosure may be intense. The risks are particularly great for patients who were sexually abused in childhood, because therapists may be provoked unconsciously to re-enact elements of the original abusive experience. It is essential that therapists, regardless of the model of therapy practised, should understand the unconscious processes at play in the therapeutic relationship.

The ethical code of conduct for psychological treatment practitioners includes:
- explanation to the patient of what he can expect of the therapy and the therapist;
- maintenance of confidentiality;
- a commitment to the safety and integrity of the patient and (in certain circumstances) others;
- appropriate professional limits on personal, social and physical contact with the patient.

Psychological and physical treatments

Psychological treatments are practised sometimes in conjunction with physical treatments. Indeed some disorders, particularly anxiety and depression, cannot be treated wholly by physical methods alone. Attention to psychological factors is imperative, particularly if the likelihood of relapse is to be minimized. There is no essential contradiction in the concurrent prescription of medication and psychological treatment, and the combination may be necessary when biological symptoms are prominent and impair the patient's capacity to think about and to construe his predicament psychologically. For example a depressed patient who has been exhausted by sleep disturbance may require sedative antidepressive medication before cognitive or psycho-analytic treatments could be effective.

Problems occur, however, if the side effects of medication impair the patient's capacity to think and act responsibly. The drowsiness generated by excessive dosage of benzodia-zepines or by sedative tricyclic antidepressants can hinder the patient's active participation in psychological treatment. Even small doses of sedative medications can reduce the patient's motivation to help himself, and the dependent patient's reliance on pills may preclude the development of the self-reliance which is a goal of most psychological treatment.

'Formal' and 'informal' treatment

As has been indicated in the text, psychological treatments are practised in a variety of settings by a variety of health workers. It should be added here that these practitioners vary in their levels of expertise, but also that psychological treatments are practised expertly at various levels of formality. **Formal** treatment is likely to be conducted in hospital or clinic settings at fixed, regular appointment times for a finite duration, by staff who are trained or are training in the use of a particular treatment model. **Informal** therapy is done successfully outside of these boundaries, often by staff who have no formal training in psychological treatments but whose psychological work may be 'supervized' by someone who has. Effective analytic psychotherapy can be accomplished by general practitioners, for example, in successive brief interviews at irregular intervals. Alternatively, community psychiatric nurses might effect valuable change in a chronically disabled patient by the judicious application of techniques derived from behavioural treatment or family psychotherapy. The adjective 'informal' does not imply therefore that treatment is simple or that it is unsophisticated.

Conclusion

Whether practised formally or informally, all psychological treatments rely for their effectiveness on the skill and enthusiasm of the therapist, on the accurate selection of the treatment appropriate for that patient, and on the patient's receptivity to psychological intervention. Any psychological treatment can be hindered by a lack of motivation in the patient to change his experience, or by his failure to comprehend the purpose or method of the treatment. Even when these conditions are optimal, however, a successful outcome cannot be guaranteed.

The human mind is a complex entity and its function is not yet entirely predictable, even by expert practitioners who have worked for years in the field of mental health.

QUESTIONS

1 List some indications for behavioural therapy. How might behavioural therapy be applied in the treatment of a young woman who presented with a phobia of pigeons?
2 What is meant by the psychological term 'crisis', and in what circumstances might crisis therapy be indicated?
3 Explain how a patient's transference to his general practitioner might impede the therapeutic process.
4 Outline the potential benefits of group psychotherapy for an emotionally reserved woman whose ambitions for marriage and motherhood had been unfulfilled.

5 How might you treat a hitherto successful student who had taken a minor overdose after failing her first-year examinations?

FURTHER READING

Barker P. (1992) *Basic Family Therapy.* 3rd Edition. Blackwell Scientific Publications, Oxford. [A comprehensive and impartial account of family psychology and the main methods of family and couple therapy. Includes a useful chapter on ethics.]

Bloch S. (ed.) (1986) *An Introduction to the Psychotherapies.* 2nd Edition. Oxford University Press, Oxford. [Clearly written introductory chapters on each of the psychological treatments, except counselling, outlined here; and with one or two more in addition.]

Brown D. & Pedder J. (1991) *Introduction to Psychotherapy: An Outline of Psychodynamic Principles and Practice.* 2nd Edition. Tavistock Publications, London. [A concise but comprehensive account of psychodynamic psychotherapy in both individual and group contexts.]

Hawton K., Salkovskis P.M., Kirk J. & Clark D.M. (1989) *Cognitive Behaviour Therapy for Psychiatric Problems: A Practical Guide.* Oxford University Press, Oxford. [An authoritative text which offers practical instruction on the clinical practice of CBT. Chapters include assessment, and treatment of anxiety, depression, eating disorders and marital problems.]

Holmes J. (ed.) (1991) *Textbook of Psychotherapy in Psychiatric Practice.* Churchill Livingstone, Edinburgh. [Comprehensive coverage of the major psychological treatments.]

Storr A. (1990) *The Art of Psychotherapy.* 2nd Edition. Heinemann, Oxford. [A very readable account of individual psychoanalytic psychotherapy, its application, methods and potential pitfalls.]

Wright H. (1989) *Groupwork: Perspectives and Practice.* Scutari Press, Harrow. [Basic but lucid introduction to theory and practice of group therapy.]

V
SPECIAL PROBLEMS

19
Suicide and Attempted Suicide

Fact sheet

Definitions
- *Suicide* describes any fatal deliberate act of self-harm, although official suicide verdicts require substantial evidence that death was intended and the act was deliberate.
- *Attempted suicide* describes any non-fatal deliberate act of self-harm. Most cases involve self-poisoning.

Incidence
- *Suicide* became less common after 1962. In recent years rates of suicide have risen in males and declined in females. The main increase has been in young men. Approximately 4500 official suicides per year in the United Kingdom. However, official statistics considerably underestimate the true suicide rate.
- *Attempted suicide* became very common in the late 1960s and early 1970s. Some decrease in early 1980s, but rates stable or possibly increasing since then. Accounts for at least 100 000 general hospital admissions per year.

Distribution
- Suicide is more common in males than females, persons of older age (although rates in young males have increased lately and those in older men and women have decreased), the single, widowed, divorced and the unemployed.
- Attempted suicide is more common in females than males, people under the age of 35 years, lower social classes, the single and divorced, people living in areas of social deprivation, and the unemployed.

Factors associated with suicide
- Psychiatric disorder, especially depression, alcohol and drug abuse, schizophrenia and personality disorders.
- Physical illness, especially chronic disabling disease, AIDS.
- Unemployment.
- Previous suicide attempts.

Factors associated with attempted suicide
- Relationship difficulties.
- Psychiatric disorder, as for suicide.
- Physical illness.
- Unemployment.
- Social deprivation.
- Financial problems.

Management of attempted suicide
Careful assessment, especially of current problems, psychiatric disorders, risk of repetition, risk of suicide, coping resources and supportive relationships, willingness to accept help. Should involve interviews with relatives, friends and general practitioner.

Aftercare
- Psychiatric hospital in-patient admission for those with severe psychiatric disorder and/or major suicide risk.
- Out-patient or community-based counselling for those with social and interpersonal difficulties.

Prevention of suicidal behaviour
- Detection and appropriate treatment of those at risk, especially people with depression and substance abuse.
- Continuing care of patients with chronic mental illness.
- Availability of emergency psychiatric or voluntary agencies.
- Reduced availability of means for suicidal behaviour.
- Responsible media reporting of suicides.

Prognosis in attempted suicide
- Social and psychiatric problems improve in the majority of cases shortly after attempts.
- Further attempts by approximately 15% in subsequent year.
- Suicide in at least 1% in first year and 3% in 5 years after attempts.

The nature of suicide and attempted suicide

The term **suicide** is used to describe any deliberate act of self-harm which results in death. By contrast, **attempted suicide** includes any deliberate act of self-harm which does not result in death. While the term attempted suicide is often a misnomer, because many acts in this category do not involve serious suicidal intent, other terms which have been suggested (e.g. 'parasuicide', 'deliberate self-harm') can also be misleading. The traditional term, attempted suicide, is therefore used in this chapter.

Attempted suicide includes two categories of act: **deliberate self-poisoning** (or 'overdose') and **deliberate self-injury**. Deliberate self-poisoning describes the intentional ingestion of more than the prescribed amount of medical substances, or ingestion of substances never intended for human consumption, irrespective of the intended outcome of the act. Deliberate self-injury describes any intentional self-inflicted injury, again irrespective of the intended outcome.

It is important to recognize that both suicide and attempted suicide are forms of behaviour; they are not in themselves illnesses, nor do they necessarily reflect illness.

Stengel first emphasized the importance of distinguishing suicide from attempted suicide. This is partly because of the obvious difference in outcome between the two types of act, but also because there are important differences, described below, in terms of the characteristics of people who engage in these behaviours. However, there is also a considerable overlap between suicide and attempted suicide, death sometimes occurring unintentionally, and attempts sometimes being 'failed suicides'. Moreover, there is a significant risk of suicide after attempted suicide.

Suicide

Ascertainment of suicide statistics

Official methods of identifying suicides for statistical purposes vary greatly between different countries. In England and Wales, suicide verdicts are decided by coroners who require:

1 Clear evidence that the act was self-inflicted.
2 Evidence that death was intended (e.g. a suicide note).
There is good reason to believe that a considerable number of probable suicides are not recorded in official suicide statistics, but allocated to the categories of 'accidental' (this applies especially to poisoning and drowning) or 'undetermined cause'. Evidence for this assertion comes from studies of individuals whose deaths have been assigned to these categories, which have shown characteristics similar to official suicides. Whilst official suicide statistics clearly underestimate the true suicide rate, possibly by as much as 50 to 100%, there is also evidence that they may nonetheless be useful for examining epidemiological patterns and trends over time and between different countries.

Trends in suicide rates

Suicide rates for England and Wales have shown much variation during this century, decreasing markedly during the two World Wars and increasing during the Depression of the 1930s. Recent trends are of particular interest. Between 1962 and 1975 there was a substantial decrease in annual suicide rates. The most likely explanation for this were the introduction of non-toxic domestic gas and the reduced prescribing of barbiturates, both common methods of suicide prior to this period. Since 1975 there has been a gradual increase in suicide rates in men and a decrease in rates in women (Fig. 19.1). The reasons for this are unclear, although increasing rates of unemployment, alcohol and drug abuse, mental disorders and AIDS together with social changes have been suggested as possible factors. In 1991 there were 3893 official suicides in England and Wales. In addition there were 2054 deaths from undetermined causes.

Demographic characteristics

At all times throughout this century suicide has been more common among males than females. Suicide is rare under the age of 15 years, steadily rising with increasing age, and reaching a peak in women in their late 50s and in men in their late 60s. During the past 20 years, suicide rates in young men have increased very markedly, whilst those in older people of both sexes have decreased. Thus increasing age is less of a risk factor for suicide than it used to be, particularly in young men.

There are no very marked variations in suicide rates between different social class categories. However, suicide rates

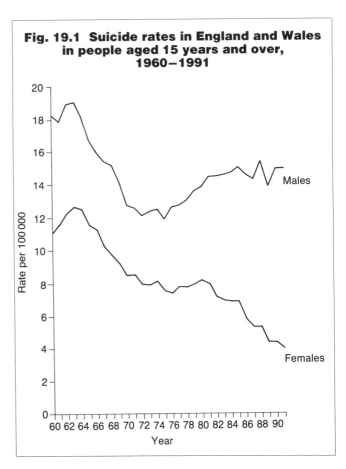

Fig. 19.1 Suicide rates in England and Wales in people aged 15 years and over, 1960–1991

vary considerably with marital status, being highest amongst the single, divorced and widowed.

Seasonal variations

There are seasonal variations in suicide rates. The highest rates occur in the late spring and early summer, probably reflecting the increased prevalence of affective disorders at this time. In females there also appears to be a smaller peak in the number of suicides in the autumn.

Methods used for suicide

Availability is a major determinant of methods of suicide. Thus, until detoxification of domestic gas during the 1960s, domestic gas poisoning was the most common method used for suicide in this country. Now the most common methods used for suicide in males are car exhaust poisoning and hanging, whereas in females they are self-poisoning (especially with psychotropics and analgesics) and hanging. Violent methods of suicide (e.g. hanging and shooting) are more commonly used by men. The influence of availability of method is demonstrated by much greater use of firearms for suicide in the USA (where guns are easily obtained) compared with their use in this country.

What causes suicide?

Suicide rarely results from a single factor, most suicides following a gradual accumulation of problems, with sometimes a final event immediately preceding the fatal act. Because a complex interaction of problems and events often leads up to suicide, it is usually difficult to point to definite causes. The principal factors which have been suggested can be subdivided into those of a psychiatric, social, and physical nature (Fig. 19.2).

Psychiatric disorders

All studies of completed suicides have found that a large proportion of individuals (at least half) were suffering from **depression** at the time of their death. Averaging the findings from follow-up studies of individuals with major affective disorders reveals a risk of suicide of approximately 15%, which is thirty times the general population risk. Suicide risk appears to be greatest relatively early in the course of the illness. Specific risk factors in individuals with depression are social isolation, a history of suicide attempts, insomnia, self-neglect and a profound sense of hopelessness.

The suicide risk in **alcoholism** has also been estimated at 15%, the risk increasing the longer the disorder persists. Most alcoholics who kill themselves are also depressed. Specific risk factors in alcoholism include poor physical health, unemployment, previous suicide attempts and the recent loss of a close relationship through separation or death. **Drug addicts** also have a high mortality from suicide.

Approximately 10–15% of people with **schizophrenia** die by suicide. The risk is greatest in young males, particularly those who are unemployed. Although the risk is highest in people with chronic disorder, suicide tends to occur relatively early in the course of the illness. Young able people who have achieved academic success prior to the onset of their disorder, but who are severely distressed by intellectual handicaps caused by the condition, are particularly at risk. Suicide rarely occurs during acute episodes, but usually during a relatively non-psychotic phase of illness, especially when there is depression, feelings of hopelessness and of isolation. The risk is greatly increased if there is a history of previous attempts.

Studies of suicides reveal a substantial number of people with **abnormal personalities**, especially of a sociopathic kind. Aggressiveness, impulsivity, lability of mood and alienation from peers may characterize those most at risk, especially in the presence of alcohol or drug abuse.

Social factors

Loss of social ties and supports has long been recognized as a major cause of suicide, although it was Durkheim at the end of the last century who laid special emphasis on this in his well-known but ill-defined concept of 'anomie'. Social isolation, whilst rarely defined operationally, is frequently highlighted as a major factor in suicide. Such isolation often results from loss through bereavement or separation, especially if social or family support is lacking.

Unemployment and suicide are statistically associated, but the nature of this association is unclear. It is likely that in some individuals unemployment does indirectly lead to suicide because of domestic and financial consequences, which may result in depression, alcohol abuse and a sense of hopelessness, whilst in others the association may be the result of psychiatric disorder rendering a person unfit for employment, the psychiatric condition rather than the lack of work being the link factor.

Physical factors

Poor physical health is common amongst suicides, especially the elderly, with suicide risk being particularly increased in people suffering from malignant disease or neurological disorder (e.g. the risk is increased fourfold in epilepsy). Peptic ulcer is also relatively common in suicides, but this probably reflects the increased risk in alcoholism. People with AIDS have a greatly increased risk of suicide.

Recently there has been interest in evidence from CSF and post-mortem brain studies that suicide may be associated with reduced cerebral serotonin (5-HT) activity. The evidence for this has largely been indirect, and it is unclear

Fig. 19.2 Causes of suicide

Psychiatric disorders	Social	Physical
Depression	Isolation	Physical illnesses—malignancies, neurological disorders, AIDS
Alcoholism	Loss—bereavement, separation	Reduced cerebral serotonin (5-HT) activity
Drug addiction		
Schizophrenia	Unemployment	
Personality disorder		

whether it might be related more to aggressiveness and impulsivity rather than having a direct link with suicide.

Can suicide be prevented?

In order to prevent suicide, either the social and other factors which increase risk have to be altered, or individuals who are already on the pathway to suicide must be identified and helped in ways which ameliorate their difficulties. The first approach probably concerns social changes which might result from major political initiatives, and is beyond the scope of this text. The second approach requires consideration of the important risk factors for suicide, the extent to which people who kill themselves contact professionals and other agencies beforehand, the effectiveness of suicide prevention agencies, the avoidability of means for suicide, the role of the media, and the role of psychiatry.

Risk factors for suicide

The well-established risk factors for suicide, most of which have already been mentioned, are listed in Fig. 19.3. An important point to note is that the common belief that people who threaten suicide never do it is entirely false. Perhaps as many as three-quarters of suicides have previously intimated or overtly expressed their intention to others beforehand.

Although we are now well aware of the important risk factors, this does little to ease the problem of identifying those individuals who are most likely to kill themselves because the occurrence of suicide is, fortunately, relatively rare, while the factors shown in Fig. 19.3 are all relatively common. In other words, in identifying a probable high-risk group, this will only include a tiny minority who are at definite risk.

Contacts with helping agencies prior to suicide

Several studies have shown that most people who kill themselves have recently been in contact with a medical agency, usually their family doctor. In one study, 40% had seen their family doctor within a week, and nearly 60% within a month of killing themselves. Almost one in five had seen a psychiatrist in the month beforehand, and 69% had seen either their family doctor and/or a psychiatrist in this period. This indicates that suicide prevention at such times might be feasible, but begs the questions of how these individuals could have been identified accurately and whether effective preventive measures were available. Suicide very often occurred whilst active treatment of psychiatric disorder was being undertaken, although whether the treatment was always the most appropriate is less clear.

Undoubtedly it is very important that general practitioners and other primary care and community workers be well-trained in the detection, assessment and management of suicide risk. General practitioners must also be skilled in the recognition and treatment of depression. An intensive educational programme on the management of depression provided for general practitioners on the Swedish Island of Gotland was associated with a significant although temporary decline in the island's suicide rate.

The effectiveness of suicide prevention agencies

In Britain the most well-known voluntary agency advertising itself as being available to provide help for distressed and suicidal people is the Samaritans, which has branches in most major cities. Whilst probably providing a useful befriending service, research so far has not demonstrated that this organization has a significant preventive effect on suicide. Nevertheless, common sense and the known social isolation of many suicides suggest that the increasing availability of helping agencies for people in distress is likely to prevent at least some suicides, as well as serving other useful functions.

Availability of means for suicide

It is well recognized that suicide risk is influenced by availability of means for suicide. Thus when toxic domestic gas was gradually replaced by non-toxic North Sea gas in the 1960s the suicide rate showed a steady decline, gas having been a very common method for suicide. Current suicide rates might be affected by reducing availability of some of the common substances used in suicide and by making favourite places for suicide (e.g. certain bridges) less accessible.

Role of the media

There is empirical support for the notion that dramatic publicity about suicides might facilitate further suicides, especially in young people. A responsible media policy for reporting of suicides might therefore help prevent suicides.

The role of psychiatry

Identifying and helping people at risk of suicide is one of the psychiatrist's most important and difficult tasks. Enquiry about suicidal ideas is necessary when assessing most patients with psychiatric disorders, especially if the clinician has the slightest suspicion that such ideas may be present. This enquiry should be made of **all** patients with depression. There is no evidence that asking about suicide ever causes someone who has not previously thought about it to begin doing so. Furthermore, many depressed patients feel suicidal to some extent and are often relieved by being able to discuss these ideas with an understanding clinician. The most important thing to assess is whether the patient is entertaining suicidal ideas at the present time. There are various ways of going about such an enquiry, but useful opening questions are: 'How do you feel about the future? Can you see your situation improving?' The clinician should be alert to any indication that the patient feels pessimistic or hopeless about the situation or chances of recovery. These questions can be followed by another, such as: 'Have you ever thought

---

Fig. 19.3 Risk factors for suicide

Male sex	Previous suicide attempt(s), suicide threats
Older age (less of a risk factor than it used to be, especially in males)	Chronic or life-threatening physical illness
Single, widowed, divorced	Social isolation
Psychiatric illness (especially depression, alcoholism, schizophrenia)	Unemployment

life is not worth living?' If the patient answers positively to his question it should be followed by detailed enquiry concerning whether the patient had contemplated harming himself/herself, whether a specific method has been thought of, and what has stopped the patient doing such a thing. Other factors which should be taken into account include the risk factors which have already been discussed, a family history of suicide, wishes for reunion with a dead parent or spouse, and the availability of suppportive relationships.

When suicide risk is severe, the Mental Health Act (1983) enables psychiatrists, if necessary, to admit people with psychiatric disorders to hospital compulsorily. The effectiveness of ECT and antidepressant medication usually allows the alleviation of major depressive disorders with reasonable rapidity. Nevertheless, virtually all psychiatrists who have for even just a few years been involved in the care of patients with major psychiatric conditions will have experienced the suicide of at least one patient whilst in treatment. Suicides occur from time to time in psychiatric hospitals, the first week after admission being a time of particular risk, as is the period immediately following discharge. The introduction of prophylactic medication, especially lithium carbonate and depot phenothiazines, has probably increased the ability of psychiatrists to prevent suicides in patients with recurrent affective disorders and schizophrenia. Continuing community support of patients with chronic mental illness, particularly by community psychiatric nurses, should also contribute to suicide prevention.

It must be acknowledged that however efficient psychiatric services are in their efforts to alleviate illness and prevent suicide, some suicides will always occur in psychiatric patients.

What effect does suicide have on other people?
Suicidal deaths cause greater difficulties for relatives and friends than most other forms of death. All the well-recognized features of grief occur following suicide, but may be compounded by their severity and by the reactions of other people. Coming to terms with the death by suicide of a young person is particularly difficult, especially for parents. Reactions of people who experience a suicide in someone close to them typically include the features listed in Fig. 19.4. Many people who have had this experience comment how they were shunned or blamed for the death by other people. The effects of a suicide on a family are often devastating, leading to marital disharmony, and neglect of, or restrictive attitudes towards, children.

Fig. 19.4 Reactions to suicide

- **Denial** – including inability to accept the death, or that it was due to suicide.
- **Anger** – towards the deceased, friends of the deceased, medical agencies, and the coroner.
- **Shame** – because of the considerable stigma associated with suicide.
- **Guilt** – about whether the individual contributed to the suicide, or could have prevented it.
- **Fear** – about the individual's own self-destructive impulses.
- **Suicidal thoughts** – including the idea of joining the deceased.

Only recently have efforts been made to establish counselling for people affected by a suicide. Helpful strategies include encouraging communication between family members, assistance with accepting feelings of guilt without these becoming unduly distorted, encouraging ventilation of anger, and exploring how adjustment to the death might be made in the long term. Unfortunately, professional health workers often have considerable difficulty in providing this counselling, probably because they themselves find suicide such a distressing topic. Support groups are available for relatives of people who have died by suicide (e.g. Survivors of Suicide).

Attempted suicide

How common is attempted suicide?
Identification of cases of attempted suicide is usually based upon referrals to general hospitals. There is evidence, however, that this method of identification considerably underestimates the full extent of the problem. Cases managed by general practitioners or within institutions, such as psychiatric hospitals and prisons, will be missed. Nevertheless, whilst statistics based on hospital referrals will underestimate the extent of attempted suicice, they are useful in examining trends over time. Unfortunately, national statistics for attempted suicide are not available; reliance has to be placed on information from centres which maintain special monitoring services.

During the 1960s and most of the 1970s there was a vast increase in the numbers of people referred to hospitals each year following suicide attempts. Most of the increase was due to a rise in the numbers of attempts involving self-poisoning. Subsequently there was a modest decline in rates of attempted suicide although recently the members of cases appear to have increased again. There are at least 100 000 general hospital referrals in the UK each year because of self-poisoning, which is now the most common reason for acute medical admission of women to hospital and second only to ischaemic heart disease as the most common reason for admission of men. This phenomenon appears to have occurred in many parts of the Western world.

What methods are used in attempted suicide?
Approximately 90% of cases of attempted suicide that are seen in general hospitals involve **self-poisoning**, usually by medicinal drugs. The most common drugs used to be minor tranquillizers, but are now analgesics, particularly paracetamol and aspirin. These drugs have either been prescribed for the individual, or bought from shops, or are readily available in the home. Paracetamol, antidepressant and aspirin overdoses can be particularly dangerous, sometimes causing unintended death.

Self-injuries may be of three types. First, and most commonly, superficial self-cutting, usually of the wrist or forearm. Secondly, violent methods (e.g. hanging, jumping in front of moving vehicles, shooting) or deep lacerations, especially of the throat or chest, which are usually associated with serious suicidal intent. Thirdly, and least commonly, bizarre self-mutilation (e.g. of the eyes or genitals), which

Fig. 19.5 Characteristics of attempted suicide patients, and common problems and precipitants preceding attempts

Characteristics	Problems	Precipitants
Females > males	Marital/relationship difficulties	Major row
Mostly young people especially teenage females and males in their 20s	Unemployment	Separation
	Financial problems	
Social classes IV and V have highest rates	Alcohol abuse	
Single and divorced have high rates	Psychiatric disorder, especially depression, anxiety, alcoholism, drug addiction and schizophrenia	
Most common in areas of social deprivation	Physical ill-health	

usually indicates major psychiatric disturbance, often schizophrenia.

In many cases, whether overdoses or self-injuries, the act is preceded by heavy drinking, which may have increased impulsivity and hence facilitated the behaviour. Alcohol is also often consumed as part of the act and adds to its dangers.

Who is most at risk for attempted suicide?

Age and sex
The characteristics of people most commonly involved in attempted suicide are summarized in Fig. 19.5. In contrast to completed suicide, attempted suicide occur more often amongst females, who outnumber male attempters by approximately 1.5:1. A further contrast with suicide is that the behaviour is most frequent in younger people, approximately two-thirds being under the age of 35. It is extremely rare in children under the age of 12 years, but becomes increasingly common during the teenage years, especially in girls. The sex ratio for adolescent attempters is even more skewed towards females than amongst adult attempters. The reason for this is unclear, but may reflect the greater range of alternative means of dealing with distress amongst boys (including alcohol abuse and aggressive behaviour), some kind of 'popularity' of this means of coping amongst girls, and, possibly, greater social and psychological pressures on adolescent girls. The peak incidence is amongst 15−24-year-old females, and 20−35-year-old males.

Social factors
Another contrast with completed suicide is that the incidence of attempted suicide is very much greater amongst people of lower socio-economic status than among those in other socio-economic groups. High-rate geographical areas include urban districts characterized by social deprivation

and overcrowding. The marital status groups most at risk are the single and divorced.

Family background
People who attempt suicide have very often experienced a disrupted parental relationship, usually because of separation. In addition, the family background may have been chaotic. A history of child abuse or neglect is not uncommon. Psychiatric disorder, suicidal behaviour and alcohol abuse also often occur in other family members.

Problems and precipitants preceding attempts
The usual pattern is for an attempt to occur following a specific precipitant in the context of longer term difficulties (Fig. 19.5), although sometimes a suicidal act occurs after an acute crisis. The most common constellation of events and difficulties, especially in females, is the disruption of a close relationship, usually with the partner, following persistent difficulties in the relationship. In young adolescents the relationship with the parents is very often disturbed and there may be a history of sexual abuse. A very high proportion of attempters are unemployed, the risk being especially high amongst the long-term unemployed, although, as for suicide, it is difficult to tease out the specific nature of the contribution of unemployment to attempted suicide. However, attempters often have severe financial difficulties. Psychiatric symptoms, especially those of depression and anxiety, are very common in attempters when seen shortly after their attempts, and amount to clinical psychiatric disorder in about one-third of patients. Alcoholism and alcohol abuse are particularly frequent amongst attempters, especially males. Physical illness is also remarkably common. A specific association has been demonstrated between epilepsy and attempted suicide.

What are the motives for attempted suicide?
The intentions behind a non-fatal suicidal act are often unclear or complex. Some cases, perhaps a minority, involve definite suicidal intent (wish to die). Other common motives include communication of distress and despair, attempts to alter the behaviour of others, revenge, and escape either from intolerable stress or from a difficult situation.

The extent of premeditation before attempts varies greatly, from a few minutes to several days or weeks. However, apparently impulsive acts, with very brief premeditation, are

---

Fig. 19.6 Topics to cover during the assessment of an attempted suicide patient

1 Events that preceded the act.
2 Reasons for the act, including suicidal intent.
3 Problems faced by the patient.
4 Does the patient have a psychiatric disorder?
5 Family and personal history.
6 Psychiatric history, including previous suicide attempts.
7 The risk of a further attempt.
8 The risk of suicide.
9 Coping resources and supports.
10 What kind of help might be appropriate, and is the patient willing to accept it?

Case 1: failed suicide

Mr B., aged 59 years, was admitted to a general hospital after being discovered in the garage by his wife when she returned early from work. He was sitting with the engine running and a tube from the exhaust pipe running in through the driver's window. Mr B. made an uneventful physical recovery. However, he reported symptoms of depression, including early morning waking, loss of appetite and weight, and a profound sense of hopelessness about the future. He still felt suicidal and wished he had succeeded in killing himself. Mr B. had recently retired early from his work as a bank manager because of his chronic ulcerative colitis. Since retirement he had become increasingly dejected

This type of case represents a 'failed suicide' in that only chance intervention probably prevented Mr B.'s death.

Major depression is common among suicides and those who make serious suicide attempts.

Hopelessness is a major factor associated with suicide risk.

Suicide is more common among people who are retired or unemployed and those with chronic physical illness.

Case 2: the forgotten wedding anniversary

Mrs W., a 32-year-old housewife, was admitted to a general hospital having taken an overdose of hypnotic tablets together with some whisky.
The overdose followed a row with her husband. They had been married for 12 years, but during the 2 years since Mr W. became landlord of a public house they had frequently argued about the time he was spending in the pub.
Mrs W. had been drinking more than usual, often on her own, and had been sleeping poorly.
Ten days before her overdose Mrs W. had gone to her general practitioner and told him how she was feeling. He had then prescribed the hypnotic. When seen in hospital by a psychiatrist Mrs W. admitted that she

Overdoses often occur following a row in the setting of marital difficulties.

Alcohol abuse is often associated with self-poisoning.

Two-thirds of self-poisoners visit their GPs during the month preceding their overdoses.

Case 3: the distressed art student

Miss E. was a 20-year-old art student. She was seen in a casualty department with multiple cuts to her wrist and forearm. This was the fourth time she had been seen in casualty following wrist-cutting, and she admitted having cut herself on other occasions.
Miss E.'s upbringing had been very chequered, her parents having separated when she was aged four following which she was fostered because of suspicions of physical abuse by her mother.
She had been sexually promiscuous since the age of 15, but had never been able to establish a close relationship with a boy. Her periods were irregular and she was prone to episodes of binge eating when feeling depressed.

Wrist cutting often involves multiple cuts and is commonly repeated.

A history of a broken home is frequent among suicide attempters as is a history of child abuse.

Sexual problems, difficulties in establishing close relationships, menstrual abnormalities and eating disorders are common in female wristcutters.

and had lost all enthusiasm for his usual interests. His wife had tried all she could to help him. On two or more occasions recently he had said that he felt a burden on his wife and that she would be better off without him.

Suicide communications precede most suicides.

Mr B. was diagnosed as suffering from major depression and admitted to a psychiatric unit. After treatment with ECT and antidepressants his depression lifted.

ECT would often be the treatment of choice in someone with severe depression and serious suicidal risk.

He and his wife were seen by a psychiatrist on several occasions during which they discussed how they might change things at home so that they could have more time together but also allow Mr B. to have a useful role. Eventually they decided that Mrs B. would also retire from her job and that they would use their retirement lump sum payments to purchase a small guest house which they would run jointly.

Treatment following suicidal attempts should not just be concerned with psychiatric disorder but with other factors which may have precipitated it.

had taken the overdose partly to block out her feelings and partly to show her husband how bad she felt. The psychiatrist noted that the overdose was impulsive, Mrs W.'s husband had been in another room at the time, and a few minutes after taking the tablets she told him what she had done.

Many overdoses appear to be communications with other people.

These features suggest low suicidal intent.

The psychiatrist did not think Mrs W. had a formal psychiatric disorder but judged her to be distressed because of her marital difficulties, the situation being complicated by her alcohol abuse. The psychiatrist arranged to see Mrs W. and her husband for six counselling sessions during which he helped them to discuss their difficulties. Mr W. eventually arranged to take on further help in the pub in order to allow he and his wife more time together.

Many self-poisoners do not have formal psychiatric disorders but are responding to chronic or acute stress.

Brief counselling of a problem-solving kind is often the treatment of choice following overdoses.

Miss E. had first cut herself when aged 17 after row with a casual boyfriend. Subsequent episodes of cutting occurred at times when she was feeling tense, usually because of difficulty in a relationship. The cuts, made with a razor blade, were mostly superficial, painless, and had a calming effect on her. However, she also felt disgusted by her behaviour.

Self-cutting often seems to function as a tension-relieving behaviour. It is often painless and is not usually life-threatening.

Following psychiatric referral she was engaged in a psychotherapeutic relationship. This took a stormy course, Miss E. cutting herself twice when she felt the therapist was rejecting her. However, she eventually was able to come to trust her therapist. Her cutting ceased but she still tended to binge eat.

In a girl with such a disturbed background the formation of a relationship with someone she can begin to trust may offer the best hope for the development of the ability to form other stable relationships. The psychotherapist will often find that the therapeutic relationship is tested by the patient.

extremely common, particularly in adolescents. Alcohol is often an important factor in such behaviour.

Sometimes the motivation underlying an attempt can be judged from its impact on people close to the individual. Commonly evoked emotions include guilt, sympathy and anger.

What help should suicide attempters receive?

Assessment

Before any plans can be made for aftercare a careful assessment should always be carried out. Most suicide attempters are referred to the general hospital and here there should be available rapid assessment, once the physical effects of an attempt have worn off. Current official guidelines support policies whereby the initial assessment is carried out either by physicians, or by specially trained psychiatric nurses or social workers, provided that psychiatric expertise is also readily available.

During the assessment the points listed in Fig. 19.6 should be addressed. The assessment interview should, wherever possible, be carried out in privacy, away from the busy medical ward. Suicide attempters are often initially hostile and defensive, and therefore the asessor needs to try to establish rapport with the patient before proceeding to ask detailed questions. Information should always be sought, if possible, from relatives and friends, the patient's general practitioner, and any other professionals involved.

In order to begin understanding why the attempt occurred it is useful to ask the patient for a sequential account of the events during the 48 hours or so preceding the attempt, including the circumstances leading up to hospital admission.

Factors which suggest **suicidal intent** are listed in Fig. 19.7. A common and serious mistake is to assume that the degree of suicidal intent can be gauged from the physical danger of the act. This assumption can be very misleading, especially with overdoses, because many people have little idea of what effects particular tablets or substances might have. Thus a person with serious suicidal intent might take a small overdose of sleeping tablets, whilst another, with no thoughts of actual suicide, might impulsively consume all the tablets in a large bottle of aspirin. Only when a person has reasonable knowledge of the danger involved is the size and nature of an overdose a useful guide to suicidal intent.

Information about most of the **patient's problems** will be gained from the detailed enquiry about events leading up to the attempt. However, it is also useful to check through a list of potential problem areas, including:
• relationship with partner, spouse, or other family members (including children);
• employment or studies;
• finances;
• housing;
• legal problems;
• social isolation and relationships with friends;
• alcohol and drugs;
• psychiatric disorder;
• physical illness;
• sexual difficulties;
• bereavement or impending loss.

In assessing **psychiatric disorder** attention should be paid to symptoms of depression and anxiety (pp. 75, 89) as well as to assessment of the patient's current mental state (p. 34). All patients should be asked about their drinking habits and use of drugs (see Chapter 10).

Factors known to increase the **risk of a further attempt** are listed in Fig. 19.8. The more factors shown by an individual the greater the risk. It is also important to assess the extent to which a patient's problem appears likely to change as a result of the act. The risk of suicide following an attempt is significant (see below). Factors associated with increased **risk of suicide** are listed in Fig. 19.9.

The patient's **coping resources and supports** can be assessed by asking about:
1 How the patient has coped with stressful events in the past.
2 What the patient thinks he or she can do to overcome the current difficulties.
3 Who the patient can turn to for help (including friends and relatives as well as professional sources of help).

Aftercare

Having completed a careful assessment the assessor is then in a position to plan what can be done to help the patient after discharge from hospital. A small proportion of patients will require in-patient psychiatric hospital care. These include those with severe psychiatric disorders and those judged to be at considerable risk of suicide. When admission is definitely indicated but the patient refuses this then a section of the Mental Health Act (1983) may have to be used (p. 316). Some patients who are in a state of extreme crisis may benefit from a brief period of hospital admission.

Out-patient care will be appropriate for a substantial proportion of patients. These include patients who are facing social, interpersonal and practical difficulties and who appear prepared to tackle these. Counselling (see p. 232) using a problem-solving approach, is often indicated. Other family members should be included whenever possible. Occasionally, psychotropic medication, especially antidepressants, may be necessary (p. 215), but the risks of the medication being used in an overdose must always be assessed.

Some patients will already be in the care of helping agencies (e.g. another psychiatric team, social services, probation) at the time of their attempts and, unless there are specific contraindications (e.g. in-patient care required), it will be usual to return the patient to this care.

Specific intervention is not required for all patients. Some, for example, will refuse any aftercare. In other cases, particularly when an attempt has occurred in response to an acute crisis which appears to be resolving as a result of the act, the assessment procedure, especially if family members or friends are actively involved, may be sufficient and the patient can be returned to the care of the general practitioner, following discussion of the assessment. Sometimes general practitioners will in any case wish to provide aftercare themselves.

Whilst in-patient care of patients with severe psychiatric disorders usually appears to be effective, the results of other forms of care, especially out-patient treatment, are less clear. Few studies of psychological and social management have demonstrated effects on rates of repetition of attempts, although the time to repetition may be delayed by intensive treatment. However, benefits have been found in terms of social problems and psychiatric symptoms, particularly for women.

What is the long-term outcome following attempted suicide?
Repetition of attempts is fairly common, occurring in approximately 15% of individuals during the year following an attempt, the risk being highest during the first 3 months. The characteristics of those most likely to repeat are indicated in Fig. 19.8. In spite of the relatively high repetition rate, many patients experience considerable improvement in their social and psychological difficulties soon after their attempts, although it is often unclear whether this is the result of treatment, natural resolution of a crisis, or the effect of the attempt itself (e.g. on the behaviour of other people).

As noted earlier, people who make attempts are at considerable risk of eventual suicide. At least 1% will kill themselves during the first year (a risk that is 100 times that of the general population) and 3% or more during the 5 years following an attempt. The risk factors for eventual suicide are listed in Fig. 19.9.

Can attempted suicide be prevented?
Major preventive measures probably depend on widespread social and economic changes, although modifying the attitudes of people to the use of mood-altering substances in general and to suicidal behaviour in particular are also likely to be relevant. It is noteworthy that the reduction in the

incidence of self-poisoning which occurred during the early 1980s was when minor tranquillizer prescribing was on the decline, although it is difficult to demonstrate a causal association.

Several other measures may be relevant to prevention. These include making emergency access to help readily available for people in crisis, better control of substances commonly used in self-poisoning, and improved identification and management by health and social agencies of those at risk. General practitioners may be in an important position with regard to prevention because almost two-thirds of patients will have consulted their general practitioners during the month before an attempt, and a third within 1 week. Whilst much is known about the characteristics of those at risk, it is often difficult for general practitioners to distinguish those patients most at risk from the large number of other patients with social and interpersonal difficulties. However, it is wise for general practitioners always to consider and assess the risk of suicidal behaviour in any patient who presents with symptoms of depression or anxiety, especially when prescription of a psychotropic drug is contemplated.

QUESTIONS

1 What are the main differences between people who kill themselves and people who make attempts?
2 What are the reasons for alcoholics being at special risk of suicidal behaviour?
3 What might you do if you were a medical house officer and one of your patients threatened to leave hospital immediately after recovering consciousness following an overdose of hypnotics?
4 You are working in general practice and one of your female patients presents saying that she is feeling depressed and hopeless, and thinking of killing herself, because things are going very badly in her marriage. What might be your response and subsequent actions?
5 When prescribing an antidepressant to a depressed patient who has expressed suicidal ideas, how might you reduce the risk of the patient taking an overdose of the medication?

FURTHER READING

Blumenthal J. & Kupfer D.J. (eds) (1990) *Suicide over the Life Cycle: Risk Factors, Assessment and Treatment of Suicidal Patients.* American Psychiatric Press, Washington. [A comprehensive overview of suicidal behaviour and its treatment during various life stages.]

Hawton K. (1987) Assessment of suicide risk. *Br. J. Psychiatr.* **150**, 145−53. [A brief review of suicide risk factors and their assessment.]

Hawton K. & Catalan J. (1987) *Attempted Suicide: A Practical Guide to Its Nature and Management.* 2nd Edition, Oxford University Press, Oxford. [Following an account of the problem of attempted suicide this book provides a description of practical approaches to assessment, treatment and prevention.]

Maltsberger J.T. (1986) *Suicide Risk: The Formulation of Clinical Judgement*, New York University Press, New York. [A sensitive detailed account of factors to consider in assessing suicide risk.]

Roy A. (ed.) (1986) *Suicide*. Williams & Wilkins, Baltimore. [An excellent source book for those wishing for detailed reviews of many aspects of suicide.]

20
Post-traumatic Disorders

Fact sheet

Traumatic stress

Trauma may be physical or psychological. Psychological trauma refers to the deep emotional wounds resulting from intensely stressful events. Psychological and physical injury may be inflicted by the same traumatic event, but the severity of psychological trauma is not related directly to the occurrence or severity of physical injury. Traumatic stress may lead to prolonged psychiatric disorder.

Causes

The causes of traumatic stress include: (a) traumatic bereavement; (b) physical and sexual assault; (c) childhood sexual abuse; (d) accidents and fire; (e) disaster; (f) terrorist activities; (g) war.

The **process of traumatization** involves the interaction between features of the *traumatic event* itself, the *characteristics of the person* who experiences it, and qualities of that person's *context and experience* in the aftermath of the traumatic event.

Reaction

Reactions to traumatic stress may be categorized as: (a) normal emotional reactions; (b) acute stress reaction ('shock'); (c) post-traumatic stress disorder; (d) post-traumatic personality disorder.

Post-traumatic stress disorders are a range of neurotic syndromes, the core symptomatic features of which cluster as (1) *re-experiencing phenomena*, such as intrusive recollections or dreams of the event; (2) *avoidance phenomena*, including emotional numbness, avoidance of reminders of the event, and emotional or social withdrawal; and (3) persistent *physiological arousal*, as evidenced by anxiety, insomnia and impaired concentration.

Post-traumatic personality disorder develops insidiously over the months and years following prolonged or repeated traumatic events, and is characterized by personality deterioration, marked irritability, dysfunction of relationships and substance abuse.

Epidemiology

Following very traumatic events such as serious accidents or disasters, at least 30–50% of survivors and others affected by the incident manifest symptoms of traumatic stress, and 10–30% develop post-traumatic stress disorder.

Conservative figures show that 10–25% of women and 5–15% of men report having been abused sexually in childhood; and up to 20% of abused women and 10% of abused men report serious lasting damage as a result of the abuse.

Examples of specific traumas

Traumatic bereavement

Traumatic bereavement is the product of the sudden, unexpected and perhaps violent death of a loved one. The traumatic effect of the death is exacerbated by: (a) death of a child; (b) horrific or painful death; (c) mutilation of the body; (d) no body being recovered; (e) multiple losses.

Compared with other bereavements, traumatic bereavement is associated with a greater incidence of: (a) disbelief, delayed or inhibited grief; (b) chronic, unresolved grief; (c) physical or psychiatric illness.

Disaster

A disaster is a destructive event on a massive scale, challenging the coping resources of all affected by it. The psychological impact of disasters affects: (a) the survivors, injured and uninjured; (b) witnesses of the impact; (c) relatives, including the bereaved; (d) emergency services; (e) frontline medical and hospital personnel; (f) carers and counsellors.

Accidents sometimes involve tragedy on a smaller scale, but may have a powerful traumatic impact on those affected.

Childhood sexual abuse (CSA)

Childhood sexual abuse is the exploitation of children and adolescents for the sexual gratification of the abuser. *Incest* refers to sexual abuse by a close relative.

Risk factors. Features of CSA which are associated with enhanced risk of later psychopathology include: (a) young age at onset; (b) repeated abuse; (c) prolonged duration of abuse; (d) incestuous abuse; (e) multiple abusers; (f) contact, especially penetrative, abuse; (g) violent or degrading abuse; (h) betrayal by other adults.

Lasting effects of CSA. Women who have been abused sexually in childhood manifest an enhanced incidence of: (a) anxiety and depression; (b) low self-esteem, shame and guilt; (c) dissociative disorders; (d) self-injury; (e) bulimia nervosa; (f) substance misuse; (g) sexual promiscuity and psychosexual disorders; (h) interpersonal problems; (i) physical problems; (j) re-victimization; (k) personality disorder.

The management of post-traumatic disorders

Prevention

- Primary prevention.
- Secondary prevention: defusing, debriefing, advice and information, self-help groups.

Treatment

- Medication.
- Psychological treatment: cognitive-behavioural and psychodynamic psychotherapies; short-term psychotherapy for uncomplicated disorders; long-term psychotherapy for disorders following complex trauma; group therapy where traumatic experience is shared; couple or family therapy when others involved in or affected by trauma.

Introduction

In the past few years, increasing attention has been paid by psychiatrists to the psychological effects of traumatic experiences. This has followed in particular from growing awareness of the short- and long-term effects of sexual abuse in childhood, war and large-scale 'disasters'. Clinical experience has led to the recognition and nosological description of post-traumatic stress disorders (PTSD).

The psychological reactions of individuals to traumatic stress are of concern also to medical and non-medical staff in primary care and general hospital services. This is both because the traumatic event may have caused physical injury as well as psychological problems; and because PTSDs, not unusually, have physical concomitants or presentations.

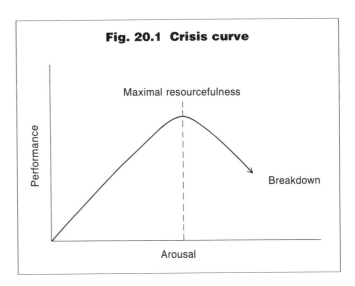

Fig. 20.1 Crisis curve

Theory of traumatic stress

Stress

Stress, the psychophysiological response to challenge, is natural and inevitable in human life. We all face adversity at intervals. Indeed, progressive exposures throughout life to manageable challenges are necessary for the development and maintenance of healthy, effective styles of *coping*. Adversity mobilizes, tests and promotes the individual's coping resources. The most resourceful people are those who have struggled with and mastered successive challenges.

Problems develop when people face adversities with which they cannot cope. The psychological state of *crisis* is generated by experiences which threaten or overwhelm personal resources, and may lead to cognitive disorganization, maladaptive patterns of behaviour (e.g. substance misuse, violence), or frank psychiatric *breakdown*.

The natural history of crisis may be represented graphically by the relationship between increasing arousal and performance – the crisis curve (Fig. 20.1). The individual facing a challenge is aroused, and arousal promotes enhanced performance. The problem may be analysed cognitively in a way which generates effective action. If the adversity cannot be overcome, arousal increases beyond a level of maximal resourcefulness, precipitating disorganization, distress and dysfunction, i.e. breakdown.

We all experience emotional crises at intervals in our lives. Developmental crises are those associated with the demands of life transitions, e.g. adolescence, marriage, retirement and other expected losses. Accidental crises are those generated by *critical incidents* which are premature and phase-inappropriate in the lifecycle (e.g. for parents when a child dies), or the product of accidents.

Some individuals, particularly those with chronic neurotic disorders or vulnerable personalities (many of whom were exposed to unmanageable experiences early in life such as emotional, physical and sexual abuse), possess limited coping resources and break down in the face of relatively minor demands. On the other hand, certain experiences are so stressful that they will sorely challenge even the most resourceful person.

Trauma

Derived from the Greek for 'penetrate' or 'wound', the term trauma is familiar to all health professionals. *Traumatic events* are those critical incidents which do not just challenge but actually cut through the individual's usual repetoire of coping skills. *Psychological trauma* refers to the effect of those experiences which penetrate the individual's psychological *defences* (see Chapter 18), wounding the very core of the self.

Psychological models of traumatization

The psychological process of traumatization can be conceptualized in a number of ways. Different psychological models perhaps represent the different aspects of the process.

Traumatic events involve violence to or violation of the person, the experience penetrating the individual's psychological defences (Freud's 'stimulus barrier') and generating sudden and intense fear, even terror. Of itself, this fearful intrusion may disrupt or disintegrate existing mental organization and function. For a time, the individual's very being is threatened. Years of adaptation and psychological development can be stripped away in a moment, leaving the individual exposed emotionally, terrified. Usual coping resources, including the capacities to think about, process and communicate experience, are overwhelmed.

Traumatic experience generates a 'fear structure'. The experience disrupts internal cognitive representations, the patterns of beliefs and assumptions, derived from earlier experience, which form the basis for the individual's perceptions of himself and of events in his world. For most people, these include assumptions that the world is a relatively predictable, orderly and safe place. Such expectations of personal security may be shattered by the traumatic experience.

At the same time, cognitive and emotional functions are disrupted, thereby preventing the processing and assimilation of experience. Memories of the event, and their associated affects, remain raw; and the original fear is 'regenerated' again and again. The traumatized person generally attempts to avoid thinking of the experience, or dissociates unconsciously from the memory of it. Inevitably, however,

Fig. 20.3 Typology of traumatic experiences (Terr)

Type	Nature of incident(s)	Typical reactions
1	Single, intense, unanticipated (e.g. accident, assault).	Full detailed memory; preoccupation; flashbacks and other intrusive phenomena.
2	Prolonged ± repeated ± anticipated (e.g. childhood sexual abuse, torture, war combat).	Intense dread; massive avoidance: repression/ denial/dissociation; rage/ passivity; unremitting sadness.
Crossover	Single event resulting in prolonged or repeated adversity (e.g. accidental injury followed by severe disfigurement).	Mixed picture of intrusive and avoidant phenomena.

recollections of the event flood back into consciousness in various forms (thoughts, visual images, sounds, even smells), associated with intense arousal or fear. So, a cycle of *avoidance*, *intrusion* and *arousal* is established – the basis of the post-traumatic stress reaction.

The disruption to processing of the traumatic experience is often compounded by reactivation of the *residues* of earlier unresolved traumatic experiences, including overwhelming early losses, abuse in childhood or bereavements.

Traumatic experience also disrupts the individual's affectional bonds (Bowlby: 'attachments'). The traumatized person experiences himself as alone, separate, dislocated – even when his family and friends remain loyal and close. His detachment, loss of loving feelings, preoccupation and irritability may eventually estrange others, even those hitherto closest to him.

Simultaneously, the victim of trauma may experience intense, irrational *guilt* and *shame* for his actions or omissions during the traumatic event. 'Survivor guilt' refers to the disaster-victim's sense of guilt for even having survived when others perished.

Causes of traumatic stress

Psychological trauma results from experiences which derive from *outside* ourselves and which pose an overwhelming threat to our physical and psychological integrity (Fig. 20.2). It has been said that 'traumatic stress is the normal reaction of normal people to abnormal events'.

Traumatic bereavements are those which are *sudden*, *unexpected* and *violent* – from accident, suicide or murder. Sudden deaths from illness, especially if unanticipated, can be very distressing but traumatize the bereaved less often unless associated with particular pain or horror. Grief may be particularly complicated, following traumatic bereavements, if the violent death was witnessed, or if the body is severely mutilated or missing.

'Man-made' disasters and accidents are recognized to have greater traumatic potential than 'natural' incidents. Amongst trauma specialists, there is a move away from use of the term 'accident', because many such incidents are the result of avoidable actions or omissions.

Typology of traumatic stressors

The individual's experience of traumatic incidents, and his psychological reaction and potential adjustment to them, will depend significantly on the duration of the ordeal and whether it is single or repeated. Terr has distinguished two types of trauma, which can be seen perhaps as two poles of a continuum, with differing typical effects (Fig. 20.3). As will be addressed later, this typology has implications for treatment. Type 1 reactions tend to be uncomplicated and are more readily responsive to treatment; whereas type 2 reactions are often complex, and sometimes intractable.

Interactive nature of traumatization

Psychological traumatization is not the product simply of a critical incident or traumatic event, though some incidents are so disturbing that anyone would be traumatized potentially by them. These are universal stressors or critical incidents. Instead we conceptualize traumatization as an *interactive* psychological process, the subjective outcome of dynamic interaction between the traumatic event itself and specific aspects of the internal (psychological) and external (social) worlds of the person experiencing it (Fig. 20.4).

The individual's experience of the traumatic event is influenced powerfully by pre-existing personal attributes, both positive (coping resources, strengths) and negative (specific vulnerabilities), and by the social or interpersonal context in which he recovers from the ordeal – the 'recovery

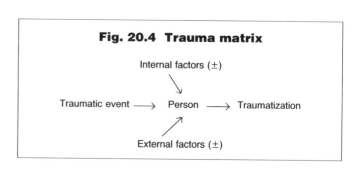

Fig. 20.4 Trauma matrix

environment'. Some features of this interactive process are outlined in Fig. 20.5.

Traumatic stress reactions

As has been emphasized already, a person's experience of and reaction to a traumatic event is influenced by a number of factors. Consequently, different people will respond differently following exposure to the same traumatic incident.

It is important clinically to differentiate normal from abnormal psychological reactions to traumatic stress. Some level of distress and symptomatology is normal in the early weeks after a trauma, though certain symptomatic features may suggest later psychological problems.

It is important to remember, however, that post-traumatic reactions are not simply a collection of symptoms. 'These symptoms are the outward indicators of an internal process' (Hodgkinson & Stewart).

A proportion of those exposed to traumatic events will develop post-traumatic psychopathology. Studies of disasters and other traumatic events have shown that one-quarter to one-half of victims develop lasting post-traumatic stress reactions, another one-third experience transient but limited psychological symptomatology, whilst the remainder have little or no discernible psychological reaction to the experience.

It is important also to note that, whilst some individuals are disabled lastingly by traumatic experience, others report later that they are stronger, wiser, more resourceful because of the experience. These individuals may be described justifiably as *survivors*.

The psychological reactions to traumatic events can be categorized as early or late. (1) Early: normal emotional reactions; acute stress reaction ('shock'). (2) Late: PTSD, chronic or delayed; post-traumatic personality disorder (PTPD).

Early normal emotional reactions to traumatic stress

The immediate reaction to a terrifying experience is often emotional numbness and disbelief, followed by euphoric relief at having survived. This gives way generally to distress and renewed fear as the victim reflects on his experience and its consequences for him, which may include bereavement or disability.

In the first few weeks, repeated recollections of the ordeal are common, as are intense, intrusive visual and other sensory images of the incident. The most powerful intrusive re-experiencing of the event generates a 'flashback', during which the victim has the terrifying illusion of going through the ordeal again. Sleep is often disturbed by nightmares, and increasing fatigue may further impair psychological adjustment to the trauma.

During this phase of disorganization, people are distracted and vulnerable to accidents. With appropriate psychosocial support, including the opportunity to talk and think about the traumatic experience, the level of distress and physical arousal diminishes over the weeks after the event. By 3–6 months, many victims will be coming to terms with the experience.

Acute stress reaction

A number of victims of traumatic incidents, including those who receive news of a traumatic bereavement, experience intense emotional and cognitive disorganization within the first hours. This acute stress reaction, commonly called 'shock', may be manifest by:
- disorientation;
- severe numbing or dissociation;
- marked emotional and social withdrawal;
- intense distress;
- panic;
- tics and other movement disorders;
- psychotic symptoms (delusions, hallucinations).

Such individuals may require hospitalization and sedation, though it is important to avoid over-sedation which obstructs realization of the traumatic event.

Post-traumatic stress disorder

Some psychological symptoms, although they might be regarded as normal concomitants of adjustment in the weeks after a traumatic event, are indicative of psychopathology when experienced months or years later.

Post-traumatic stress reactions are characterized by three clusters of symptoms: (1) re-experiencing phenomena; (2) persistent symptoms of increased arousal; and (3) persisting numbing or avoidance (Fig. 20.6). *PTSD* (PTSD: DSM-III, ICD-10) is diagnosed formally when all three symptom clusters are manifest; but post-traumatic stress reactions may be severe and disabling even if they do not fulfil the diagnostic criteria for PTSD. For example, phobic avoidance of travel after a road accident may be disabling even when not accompanied by intrusive images of the accident.

Clinically PTSD is diagnosed only if the symptom pattern persists or emerges more than 3 months after the traumatic labelled PTPD, the typical features of which are listed in Fig. 20.7.

PTPD develops gradually, perhaps insidiously, over the months or years following (type 2) trauma, particularly when this is complex, prolonged and occurs early in life, in childhood or early adulthood. Intrusive re-experiencing of the trauma (particularly flashbacks) and hyperarousal are fundamental to PTPD, the latter giving rise to irritability and explosiveness which undermines relationships. Avoidance phenomena are prominent, manifest particularly by emotional dissociation, loss of intimacy in relationships, and avoidance of interpersonal contact. Substance misuse is common, and can be seen as an attempt at affect regulation.

PTPD is associated with significant rates of revictimization and mortality from accidents, suicide and homicide.

Examples of specific traumas

Traumatic bereavement
The death of a loved relative or friend is almost invariably distressing. The bereaved person must grieve the loss, and adjust to life without the deceased (see Chapter 22).

Bereavement represents a crisis, therefore, an intense emotional and adaptational challenge. The challenge is particularly great and sometimes overwhelming when the death is sudden, unexpected and violent. Sudden deaths from illness, accident, suicide or homicide may traumatize the bereaved.

Certain features of the death are associated with a traumatic effect on the bereaved:
- sudden and unexpected death;
- death involving intense pain and/or horror;
- mutilation of the body;
- no body recovered;
- death caused by the actions, or omissions of others;
- 'untimely and premature' death, that is the death of a child or young person;
- multiple losses or bereavements in the same incident.
The tasks of grieving are made more difficult if the death was characterized by one or more of these features. Particular problems may ensue when the body cannot be viewed by bereaved relatives, as when the body is severely mutilated or not recovered. In such circumstances, the bereaved may be

experience. The onset of the disorder may be *delayed*, in some individuals emerging years after the traumatic event. Reactivation of the traumatic stress disorder may be precipitated by subsequent stresses, including the involutional stresses associated with ageing (many veterans of the world wars have become symptomatic in late age) and other experiences which simulate the original trauma in some way, however little the actual threat posed.

The diagnosis and management of post-traumatic stress reactions is often complicated by *co-morbidity* with other psychiatric disorders, especially depressive, phobic and substance misuse disorders. Whether, nosologically, these can be regarded as associated or concurrent disorders is immaterial to management, for they may require adjunctive treatment in their own right.

Post-traumatic personality disorder
In some individuals, personality disorder may have been evident before a traumatic experience. The disordered personality may contribute, therefore, to the genesis and manifestations of post-traumatic stress reactions.

In recent years, however, it has been recognized (particularly from the study of Vietnam War veterans) that severe and prolonged PTSD may be associated with disturbance and disorders of personality functioning. This has been unable to believe that the deceased is really dead. Evidence suggests that most bereaved persons benefit from viewing the recovered body before burial or cremation, even if it is mutilated; though this should never be forced.

Traumatic bereavement is associated with a greater incidence of:
- delayed or inhibited grief, characterized by disbelief;
- chronic, unresolved grief, characterized often by anger or guilt;
- physical illness;
- psychiatric illness;
- (probably) suicide.

Accidents and disasters

In terms of psychological impact on those involved, small- and large-scale accidents have much in common, the result of the suddenness, horror and destruction involved.

A disaster is a destructive event or occurrence on a large or massive scale. The scale of destruction, deaths, injuries and disruption poses a threat to the coping resources of the individuals and communities affected by it; and disaster has a significant emotional impact on the whole society in which it occurs.

Disasters have been categorized as follows:
- natural (e.g. earthquake, flood, hurricane)/man-made (e.g. technological disaster, war);
- accidental (e.g. rail or air crash)/intentional (e.g. terrorist explosion);
- sudden onset (e.g. transportation accident, fire)/gradual onset (e.g. hurricane, famine);
- medium scale, affecting dozens of people/large scale, affecting 100 or so people/massive, affecting hundreds or thousands.

A road or domestic accident may involve one or a few people; but obviously many people will be affected emotionally, and potentially traumatized, by a disaster. The destructive psychological impact is not confined to those who are injured, or even to those present and directly involved in the incident. Traumatic experiences spread like a *ripple effect*, over space and time, to affect people progressively further away from the point and moment of the destructive incident. Psychologically, trauma is contagious.

Fig. 20.8 Psychological victims of disaster

- Primary victims, the survivors – injured and uninjured.
- Witnesses, bystanders.
- Relatives and close friends of the survivors.
- The bereaved (some of whom may have survived the ordeal themselves).
- 'Victims by proxy', those who might have been there.
Those who feel responsible for the incident, justifiably or not.
- Emergency services personnel.
- Emergency medical teams.
- Other workers at the disaster site, including media personnel.
- Front line hospital staff.
- Intensive treatment unit (ITU) or trauma ward staff.
- Body handlers and mortuary staff.
- Carers and counsellors.

The survivor of an accident or disaster, in which others die, and who may have been close to death himself, is left with an 'imprint of death' (Lifton). This burden is transmitted unconsciously to all with whom he was contact.

Following a disaster, many groups of people will be affected in addition to those who experienced the disaster at first hand (Fig. 20.8).

Risk factors

Certain features of the victim's experience in an accident or disaster may constitute particular obstacles to eventual psychological adjustment:
- prolonged exposure to personal danger or threat to life;
- witnessing the injury, pain, death and mutilation of others, especially relatives or friends: intrusive recollections may be vivid and problematic later;
- injuries requiring prolonged treatment, repeated surgery, or resulting in permanent disability or disfigurement;
- the perception (whether justified or not) that one's own actions or omissions contributed to the disaster or other people's suffering or death: shame and guilt may be prominent later;
- identification of others (individuals, agencies or organizations) who are perceived to have caused the incident, particularly when ensuing legal action and compensation claims are prolonged: anger is often intense.

Epidemiology

Research evidence confirms that more than 50% of people sustaining serious injury in road traffic accidents (RTA) develop psychological problems as a result, including the symptoms of post-traumatic stress and phobic avoidance of driving or road travel. One study showed that 10% of patients displayed the full diagnostic picture of PTSD during the year after the accident. Psychological morbidity was not related to the severity of physical injury, but did correlate with horrific memories of the accident.

Scientific study of the survivors of several, disparate disasters suggests that 30–45% will develop significant psychological problems, particularly PTSD and depression.

Childhood sexual abuse

Childhood sexual abuse (CSA) has been defined as the involvement of dependent, developmentally immature children or adolescents in sexual activities which they do not truly comprehend, to which they are unable to give informed consent, and which violate established social taboos.

The essential features of CSA are that a young person is exploited sexually by, and primarily for the sexual gratification of, an older person. Most sexual abuse of children is perpetrated by men, though there is growing recognition of the abuse of sons by mothers. Children are also abused sexually by adolescent boys, many of whom were or are themselves currently the victims of sexual abuse by an adult. Most sexually abusive adults have sexual contact also with other adults, either heterosexual or homosexual (or occasionally both); but *paedophiles* have a perverse and sometimes exclusive sexual preference for sex with children.

Attention has been drawn in recent years to the serious

but less prevalent problem of *ritual satanic abuse*, which involves ceremonialized, quasi-religious physical violence and sexual abuse.

Epidemiology

Girls are abused more than boys. Community surveys of adults show that 10–25% of women and 5–15% of men report the experience of having been abused sexually in childhood. The range in prevalence figures reflects differences in the definition of CSA and methodology.

More is known about the epidemiology and effects of sexual abuse of girls than of boys. A history of CSA is more prevalent in certain clinical populations, including women with eating disorders, psychogenic pelvic pain and severe sexual dysfunction; and those who display repeated self-harm or multiple personality disorders.

Of those abused, 13–20% of women and 4–10% of men report serious, lasting psychological damage. Features associated with lasting damage are summarized in Fig. 20.9. A conservative estimate suggests that between 300 000 and 500 000 women in the UK suffer lasting distress, difficulty and psychopathology as a result of sexual abuse during childhood.

Sexual abuse is sometimes categorized in the following ways.

Familial (incest) versus non-familial abuse. Incestuous sexual abuse is perpetrated by fathers and step-fathers more than mothers, siblings and other relatives. Abuse by non-relatives which involves physical contact is perpetrated more often by adults known to the victim than by strangers.

Contact versus non-contact abuse. Contact abuse implies genital or other physical contact, including touching, fondl-ing, masturbation, or *penetration* by the abuser (with finger, penis or inanimate object) of the victim's vagina, anus or mouth.

Non-contact abuse may involve, for example, provocative suggestion, exhibitionistic exposure, or voyeuristic demands by the abuser, or the involvement of the victim in pornographic activities.

Single or repeated abusive episodes.

Disclosure of abuse

Some victims disclose their experience of sexual abuse to another person. Children may disclose current abuse because it is frightening or painful; or because they realize, at some level, that it is wrong and want it to stop. Sometimes adults recognize clinical signs in children suggestive of CSA (Fig. 20.10). Adults may disclose past experience of abuse because they want help with its lasting destructive effects. Disclosure has been made easier by growing public awareness and discussion of CSA.

However, many victims are not able to tell anyone of their ordeal, either whilst the abuse is happening or later. Sometimes they come later to professional attention only because of suggestive physical and psychiatric signs which are recognized as features of a 'disguised presentation' (Fig. 20.11).

The victims of sexual abuse have often maintained the *secrecy* demanded by the abuser because they fear both the *threats* of the abuser (threats of violence, loss of favour, destruction of the family, being taken into care) and the possible or actual *betrayal* by the person to whom they might turn, whether parent, teacher or other. All too many children and adults have met with disbelief, blame or outright rejection when they have tried to talk of their experience.

There have been many reports of sexually abused children or adults being further abused by those to whom they turn for help, including doctors, social workers and other professionals. Disbelief, rejection or accusation of complicity in the abuse will confirm the victim's sense of betrayal. At worst, the victim may find herself being exploited, seduced or assaulted sexually by her therapist, thereby compounding the original traumatization. Some victims of sexual abuse may relate in a sexualized manner, and some are flirtatious or provocative; but the doctor or therapist is required to understand enough about the effects of sexual abuse (and the unconscious processes associated with them) to avoid un-

---

Fig. 20.9 Risk factors

Lasting destructive psychological effects are associated with the following features of child sexual abuse:

- young age at onset;
- repeated episodes of abuse;
- prolonged duration of abusive experience;
- incestuous abuse, especially by father;
- multiple abusers;
- physical contact, especially penetrative abuse;
- associated violence, degradation;
- 'betrayal' by other adults to whom victim turns.

Fig. 20.10 Clinical signs in children

Signs in children and adolescents which are suggestive of recent or current sexual abuse:

- anxiety states;
- conduct disorders;
- deterioration in learning ability and educational performance;
- inappropriate sexual display;
- 'frozen watchfulness';
- promiscuity;
- early pregnancy.

Fig. 20.11 Disguised presentation of lasting effects of child sexual abuse

- Intractable, 'characterological' depression.
- Low self-esteem.
- Mistrust and fear in relationships.
- Psychosexual problems.
- Dissociative tendency.
- Repeated self-destructive behaviours.
- History of 'parentification', i.e. inappropriate, early responsibility for domestic chores, care of siblings and emotional support of parents.
- psychogenic abdominal or pelvic pain, menstrual disorders, irritable bowel syndrome.

The management of post-traumatic stress reactions

Women who were sexually abused in childhood have been shown to have an enhanced risk of:

- anxiety;
- depression;
- low self-esteem;
- negative self-concept, including shame and guilt;
- dissociative disorders, ranging from emotional numbness through hysterical disorders to multiple personality disorder;
- self-injury;
- eating disorders, especially bulimia nervosa;
- substance misuse;
- promiscuity, associated infection, early pregnancy;
- psychosexual disorders, e.g. impaired interest, vaginismus and orgasmic dysfunction;
- interpersonal problems;
- revictimization – assault, rape; abuse of own children by self or partner;
- physical problems, e.g. psychogenic, gynaecological and gastro-enterological disorders;
- personality disorder.

Prevention

The *primary prevention* of post-traumatic stress reactions would require prevention of the traumatic incidents which generate them. Although this may appear to be beyond the remit of psychiatry, the study of human attitudes and reactions to specific dangers and traumas has generated knowledge upon which programmes of prevention may be based.

For example, understanding of the transgenerational repetition of CSA indicates the importance, when treating adult victims of CSA, of examining the unconscious self-destructive processes which lead potentially to the abuse of the patient's own children. Appreciation of the psychological processes whereby people repress awareness of the dangers of road accidents may contribute to safer standards of driving. The exposure of drivers to video-recordings of the aftermath of road accidents, followed by discussion of factors contributing to careless driving, may diminish such repression. The growing challenge to use of the term 'accident' demonstrates a new awareness that many such traumatic incidents are not truly accidental, and that much can be done to prevent them.

Secondary prevention of post-traumatic stress reactions is more widely possible. Scientific evidence is emerging to confirm the clinical impression that early psychological intervention can assist people's adjustment to traumatic experiences.

Ideally, the psychological needs of the victim should be addressed in the immediate post-impact phase. The provision of a safe, quiet and supportive environment may be enough to facilitate a reduction in the victim's fear and distress. This process if often facilitated by enabling the person to talk about what happened to them, the aim being to *defuse* emotional tension. In some settings, this process occurs spontaneously as a group event. Firefighters or accident department staff, for example, often talk through a particularly distressing incident afterwards. For workers in high-stress settings, this opportunity should be actively encouraged.

The process of adjustment to traumatic experiences is further facilitated by a *debriefing* intervention after 24–72 hours. At this stage, talking through the incident may dislodge early obstructive defences such as denial and dissociation, enabling the reality of the experience to be faced and appropriate affects mobilized. Information about the incident can be reviewed. By these means, emotional and cognitive processing can be promoted. When a number of people have experienced a traumatic event together, debriefing is undertaken most effectively in a group.

Certain *practical interventions* may promote the first stages of adjustment for the victims of particular traumas. For example, those who have suffered a traumatic bereavement may grieve more readily if they have seen the body of the deceased. When the corpse is mutilated, specific emotional

professional, unethical and anti-therapeutic behaviour towards the patient.

The child's helplessness and perceived isolation in the face of abuse and betrayal, leads to her '*accommodation*' to it. She cannot disclose her experience or escape from it, so she acquiesces to the abuse and protects herself from the fear, pain and trauma by means of powerful psychological *defences*, particularly repression, denial and dissociation. These defences may become part of the child's character structure or personality, and persist into adulthood. The internal residues of trauma and protective defences manifest in adulthood in a number of ways (Fig. 20.12), most seriously as severe borderline personality disorder or multiple personality.

As with any trauma, the repressed memories or dissociated affects may be reactivated by specific later experience. This may be the case if the victim is raped or assaulted in adulthood, or if she or he hears about the sexual abuse of others. Memories of the abuse may flood into a woman's consciousness when she is being examined internally by a doctor, or when having intercourse with her partner. Sometimes a delayed PTSD may emerge; and, in serious cases, the intrusive memories of the earlier ordeal may lead to the victim's suicide, perhaps years after the abuse ended.

In some victims, the repressed memories of abuse are re-enacted unconsciously rather than remembered. When compared with non-abused persons, the victims of CSA are more likely to:

- experience further sexual assault and rape;
- abuse physically or sexually their own children;
- establish relationships with partners who abuse the victim and her children.

The main lasting effects of CSA are summarized in Fig. 20.12.

preparation of the bereaved will be necessary before the body is viewed.

Following disasters, it has been found that some survivors are helped considerably by membership of a *self-help group*. Such groups or networks can disseminate helpful information, promote exchanges of experience, and offer valuable peer support. This helps to reduce each survivor's sense of isolation and resultant interpersonal problems, as well again as promoting adjustment to the traumatic experience.

Treatment

Fundamental principles

The effective management of people presenting with post-traumatic states depends on a number of principles, specific and general. A specific requirement is for accurate *diagnosis* of the pathological reaction, and *formulation* of the patient's traumatic experience. Of significance here is to establish the following.

1 The *type* of trauma experienced. Relatively uncomplicated PTSD following type 1 trauma can be treated successfully with short-term psychodynamic or cognitive-behavioural therapies. Complex PTSD and PTPD following type 2 traumas may require more prolonged psychodynamic psychotherapy in which the patient is supported psychologically whilst re-examining gradually the traumatic experience and its various sequelae.

2 The *stage* of the reaction. Management of an acute stress reaction within hours of the traumatic experience is very different from that of an entrenched PTSD, months or years after the traumatic event.

3 The symptomatological *nature* of the stress reaction. Specific behavioural or other techniques may be necessary for the treatment of certain symptomatic components of the disorder, such as phobic avoidance.

4 The personal and social *resources* available to the patient; for, early or long after the trauma, the aim is to assist the person's own adjustment to and integration of the experience.

Second are the *general principles* which underlie the treatment of any traumatized person, but which may need to be emphasized to differing degrees according to the characteristics of the person, trauma and context.

1 *Protection* from further danger. This is particularly important for victims of sexual abuse, who may be abused currently by the original or a contemporary abuser. Similarly victims of trauma are at greater risk from accidents and self-harm, and appropriate protective interventions may be necessary.

2 *Respect* and *belief* for the victim's story, however unpalatable or unlikely it may seem. Few people make up stories of traumatic experience; and, although some may unconsciously elaborate the story, it is essential for the development of a trusting therapeutic relationship that the therapist should accept what is told unless there is compelling evidence to the contrary. Distortions often resolve during the course of therapeutic exploration.

3 Central to the psychological treatment of post-traumatic stress reactions is to enable the victim to *recount* or narrate the traumatic experience. It is this process, repeated successively in various forms, that facilitates necessary emotional expression, cognitive appraisal and gradual integration of the experience.

4 Appropriate *pacing*. The patient should not be forced to disclose and described the traumatic experience until, with gentle encouragement, ready to do so. Forced disclosure and flooding techniques risk retraumatization of the patient.

5 *Active* strategy. It is sometimes not enough to listen as a patient recounts a traumatic experience, for he or she may feel left helplessly with the reliving of it in a way that is retraumatizing. For this reason, reflective counselling may be anti-therapeutic. The therapist may need to enquire actively, but non-intrusively, about the patient's experience; and to propose active techniques to address specific symptoms.

6 *De-sexualization* of sexual abuse. Many victims of sexual abuse find it helpful to reframe the traumatic experience as the perpetrator's abuse of power over the child victim, rather than as a sexual experience for the victim.

7 *Therapist 'supervision'*. No clinicians can work with the victims of traumatic experiences without, sooner or later, being touched by their distress. In order to maintain therapeutic effectiveness, the clinician requires his or her own emotional outlets and an opportunity to talk with colleagues about the work.

Aspects of treatment

Setting

Patients who present with acute stress reactions ('shock') require measures to reduce their level of arousal. The provision of a quiet, safe and supportive environment is essential, by admission to hospital if necessary. The treatment of later post-traumatic states also progresses more satisfactorily if undertaken in quiet surroundings, free from intrusive interruption.

Medication

Sedative medication may be necessary in the immediate management of patients with acute stress reactions, and in the treatment of patients with PTSD for whom insomnia and fatigue compounds the problems and obstructs recovery. The advantages of sedation must always be weighed against the disadvantages of reducing the patient's capacity to think and process feelings, and the dosage titrated accordingly.

Tricyclic and newer antidepressants have been shown to be effective in treating intrusive images, including nightmares, as well as concomitant depression.

Psychological treatments

1 *Short-term psychotherapy* is effective for patients with uncomplicated PTSD. Cognitive-behavioural techniques may be useful for tackling specific symptomatic components of the disorder, particularly phobic avoidance and panics. Psychodynamic exploration, linking present to past and 'external' to 'internal' experience, may be necessary especially when unresolved earlier traumatic experiences are rekindled.

2 *Short-term group psychotherapy*, again drawing flexibly on psychodynamic and cognitive-behavioural techniques, may be very effective in helping patients overcome a sense of isolation. Groups are composed of individuals who have

something in common, either the traumatic experience itself (a particular disaster or CSA) or some particular result of it (e.g. interpersonal problems, disfigurement).

3 *Long-term psychotherapy* is necessary for patients with complex PTSD or PTPD. For such individuals, it may take time to develop a trusting therapeutic relationship, to establish the links between present difficulties and the original traumatic experience(s), to integrate the trauma, and to tackle its sequelae.

4 *Couple* or *family* therapies are appropriate when more than one member of a family is exposed to a traumatic event, or when an individual's reaction to a trauma threatens relationships within the family.

Qualities of the therapist

Although the treatment of severely traumatized patients will require the skills of a therapist who has expertise in trauma work, many preventive and primary therapeutic interventions can be undertaken effectively by GPs, nurses, counsellors and others, if they have a basic knowledge of trauma psychology.

To be effective, whether working at a primary or specialized level of expertise, the therapist working with the victim of trauma requires:

- a knowledge of trauma psychology;
- a capacity to listen empathically to descriptions of horrific and sometimes degrading experiences without over-identification with or distancing oneself from the patient;
- the skill to monitor one's own emotional responses as a source of information about the patient's experience;
- resolution of one's own traumatic experiences;
- access to supportive colleagues with whom to discuss the work;
- close emotional relationships with family or friends.

Case 1

A middle-aged lorry driver was referred for psychiatric opinion 6 months after an accident in which a motor-cyclist was killed. In the accident, he had taken evasive action when the motor-cycle careered towards him, out of control. He was *haunted day and night by images* of the motor-cyclist's terrified face, moments before the impact, and of his crushed body afterwards at the rear of the vehicle.

The patient, hitherto an emotionally-contained man, was deeply ashamed because he had broken down and cried after the accident. He was encouraged to resume driving, but *could not bear to get into the cab* of his articulated lorry. He *avoided* the site of the accident, and swerved involuntarily whenever approached by a motor-cycle. After the accident he lost all interest in his former leisure pursuits, became withdrawn, morose and increasingly irritable. He sought help after a violent outburst towards his wife.

The psychiatrist learned that the patient had been *involved previously in an accident* in which a motor-cyclist died 20 years before, and then had manifest *no emotional reaction*. It also emerged that the patient had recently argued with his motor-cyclist son, culminating in a threat to 'knock his block off'.

As a boy, the patient had been called 'cry baby' and punished violently by his father for crying after his mother's sudden and unexpected death. He had *learned to keep his distress well hidden* thereafter, and had come to feel proud of his emotional control.

The psychiatrist recognized that the accident had been deeply traumatic to the patient, and diagnosed PTSD. He identified the

Continued

Case 1 (*Continued*)

contribution of the patient's traumatic bereavement in childhood, his subsequent characterological repression of feeling, the significance of the confrontation with his son, and the source of his shame for crying. These factors were explored and related to the recent traumatic experience in the course of a short-term dynamic psychotherapy. The patient made rapid progress.

Case 2

A 23-year-old woman was admitted to hospital having taken a massive overdose 2 days after her husband attempted forcibly to consummate their year-old marriage. His attempted penetration of her led to immediate *flashbacks to her step-father's repeated violent rapes* of her during childhood, during which she would dissociate from the pain and terror by imagining herself floating at the ceiling. Her mother had seemed not to notice the step-father's sexual abuse of the patient until he began to involve a younger daughter.

Following the step-father's imprisonment, no mention was made again of the abuse; and the patient 'forgot' all about it. However, she was moody throughout her adolescence, was prone to cutting herself, and abused alcohol in her late teens. She had few friends, and surprised everyone by marrying suddenly. She enjoyed her husband's physical embrace, but could not achieve sexual arousal and experienced severe vaginismus.

In hospital, she disclosed her history of sexual abuse to her primary nurse; but then withdrew and behaved as if the nurse had let her down. This was understood by the staff to be a transference recreation of her sense of betrayal by her mother, and the nurse was able to suggest this connection to the patient with benefit. *Slowly the patient developed trust in her nurse*, who always listened attentively but never pushed for information.

Having eventually talked in detail about her childhood abuse, the patient then agreed to *couple therapy with her husband*. He was open and supportive, and acknowledged with regret his own sexual impatience. Although the patient became hostile towards her husband at intervals during the therapy, she was helped to see that her anger and fear were related more to her step-father. She was able to develop a satisfactory sexual relationship with her husband in the months that followed.

QUESTIONS

1 What is meant by the psychological use of the terms 'stress', 'crisis' and 'traumatization', and how do they interrelate?

2 What features of a bereavement may render it traumatic?

3 How would you manage clinically a middle-aged woman who had just survived with minor injuries a road accident in which others died, and who was highly agitated, unable to think straight, and unresponsive to reassurance?

4 What are the diagnostic features of post-traumatic stress disorder?

5 How would you manage a young woman who, while recovering from general anaesthetic for dilatation and curettage, is heard to cry 'Don't hurt me, daddy' repeatedly?

6 Why are group interventions and treatments of potential value for the survivors of a disaster?

FURTHER READING

Garland C. (1991) External disasters and the internal world: an approach to psychotherapeutic understanding of survivors. In:

Holmes J (ed.) *Textbook of Psychotherapy in Psychiatric Practice*. Churchill-Livingstone, Edinburgh. [Detailed outline of psychodynamic theory and treatment of post-traumatic stress following disaster.]

Grant S. (1991) Psychotherapy with people who have been sexually abused. In: Holmes J. (ed.) *Textbook of Psychotherapy in Psychiatric Practice*. Churchill-Livingstone, Edinburgh. [Chapter outlining some principles of psychodynamic treatment of CSA victims.]

Hobbs M. (1990) Childhood sexual abuse: how can women be helped to overcome its long-term effects? In: Hawton K. & Cowen P. (eds) *Dilemmas and Difficulties in the Management of Psychiatric Patients*. Oxford University Press, Oxford. [Chapter summarizing epidemiology, psychiatric effects and treatment of women survivors of CSA.]

Hodgkinson P.E. & Stewart M. (1991) *Coping with Catastrophe: a Handbook of Disaster Management*. Routledge, London. [Useful outline of trauma psychology and guide to basic psychological and organizational principles of disaster management.]

Scott M.J. & Stradling S.G. (1992) *Counselling for Post-Traumatic Stress Disorder*. SAGE, London. [Readable text, with plenty of clinical examples, but account of treatment limited restrictively to cognitive-behavioural methods.]

Terr L.C. (1991) Childhood traumas: an outline and overview. *Am J Psychiatry* 148:10−20.

Wright B. (1991) *Sudden death: Intervention Skills for the Caring Professions*. Churchill-Livingstone, Edinburgh. [Slim book containing a wealth of clinical experience and wise advice.]

21
Terminal Illness

Fact sheet

Anxiety about suffering, death, and separation from attachment figures, and anticipatory **grief** are seen in almost all dying patients. There is no sharp division between their symptoms and those of psychiatric patients.

Medical intervention is sought when:
- symptoms are severe and disabling to the patient or distressing to others;
- it is believed that such suffering can or should be relieved.

How much dying patients suffer depend on:
- the nature of the illness and the adequacy of symptom control;
- previous personality, coping mechanisms, etc.;
- previous history of suffering and loss;
- adequacy of support from family and friends.

Psychological problems in dying patients present as:
- anxiety;
- depression;
- disturbance of behaviour (e.g. mental confusion, paranoia);
- physical symptoms not responding to usual treatments.

Symptoms

May be stress-related (non-organic), organic or a mixture of both.

Causes of stress-related symptoms
- Difficulty in coming to terms with death.
- Poor communication about the illness.
- Difficulty in adjustment to role change.
- Pre-existing problems.

Causes of organic symptoms
- Side effects of treatment, e.g. drugs, hormones.
- Biochemical disturbances, e.g. hypercalcaemia.
- Direct effect of disease, e.g. cerebral secondary.

Diagnosis

Based on problem-orientated history.

Onset related to:
- recognition that the illness could be terminal;
- exacerbation of the disease;
- initiation of new treatment, or appearance of side effects.

Investigations should be done where:
- a reversible organic condition is suspected and results might lead to modification of treatment.

Management

Depends on accurate diagnosis. Possible interventions include:
- changes of treatment;
- individual and/or family psychotherapy aimed at improving communication and facilitating adjustment;
- provision of practical assistance with social problems;
- psychotropic drugs.

It is worth attempting treatment even when life expectancy is short. Mistakes in prognosis are often made and unnecessary suffering should always be relieved.

Outcome

Psychological symptoms may improve markedly even when the physical condition continues to deteriorate. Where they were the main reason for admission to hospital, a return home is often possible.

Bereavement reactions are less severe if there is no 'unfinished business' between the patient and family, and when the death has been peaceful.

What kind of terminal illness is complicated by psychological problems?

'Terminal illness' in this chapter refers to illness which confronts the patient with the probability that the condition from which he is now suffering will lead to his death in the foreseeable future. In practice it mainly involves those conditions that run a chronic or intermittent course ending in death, i.e. the malignancies and progressive neurological diseases. An historical perspective on the care of the dying is given in Fig. 21.1.

In those illnesses which present as crises where the issue of life or death is resolved in one way or the other in a relatively short time (e.g. myocardial infarction), resuscitative measures are usually continued almost to the moment of death. The patient, if he is conscious, has little opportunity to recognize that he may be dying and even less to contemplate this and speak about it to others. Potentially fatal diseases which may remit (e.g. the leukaemias) fall somewhere in between. The clinician and/or the patient may choose to continue efforts to bring about a remission right up to the end, thus avoiding the distress of facing death, and also depriving the patient of the opportunity to come to terms with it.

People who have been through a crisis and recognize that they might have died are 'survivors'. Some accept their situation with gratitude and even discover that they are less afraid of death than before. Others may emerge disabled by anxiety and hypochrondriasis, even when there is good physical recovery.

Patients who have AIDS are especially prone to psychological problems. As well as facing the probability of death, some also have to cope for the first time with their family discovering that they are gay or bisexual. They may become intensely angry with the person who they believe infected them, and feel guilty that they have passed on the virus to a partner or child. The recognition that such tragedies could have been avoided may add to their despair and guilt and lead to suicidal feelings or attempts. The possibility of AIDS-related dementia is so distressing that some would prefer to die before that complication occurred. The social implications of the disease and the ensuing isolation adds to the stress. Group methods of providing support, and good facilities for care at home are essential if these patients are to have a reasonable quality of life for as long as possible.

How do psychological problems present?

Because patients and families have no way of knowing how much emotional distress is 'normal' in terminal illness, they seldom complain about this in the way they do about physical symptoms. Too often professional carers fail to recognize anxiety or depression, or they assume they are an inevitable

---

Fig. 21.1 Historical perspectives

The care of the dying began to develop as a medical specialty when Dr Cicely Saunders started to work with the nuns at St Joseph's Hospice in the East End of London, and then went on to open St Christopher's Hospice in 1967. In previous centuries terminal care was regarded as part of general medicine, a continuation of the effort by doctors to 'Cure sometimes, relieve often, and comfort always'. Treatments available for cure or relief were simple and the importance of the quality of the doctor–patient relationship was well recognized.

As more scientific medicine developed, more diseases became curable and the art of providing relief and comfort was to some extent neglected. It had been the province of the religious leaders in the community for many centuries and to them individuals have turned when the doctors have said that 'nothing more can be done'. With the current decline in religious beliefs and practices, such people are now looking more often to the medical profession for relief of suffering of many kinds.

The hospice movement first fostered the development of expertise in the control of symptoms, especially pain, and we have now reached a point where the greater part of the physical distress usually associated with terminal illness can be relieved, provided that the available methods are fully used. This is a magnificent achievement, but a new problem is beginning to emerge. No longer overwhelmed by pain, vomiting, breathlessness, etc., the patient has been set free to contemplate what is happening to him and has time to look death in the face. The psychological suffering of which some have always been acutely aware is now being unmasked for others, and the insights and techniques of psychiatry and psychotherapy can be a great help to them, enabling them and their families to adjust successfully as the illness progresses.

Fig. 21.2 Psychological symptoms in dying patients

These present as

Anxiety
- with clinging, demanding behaviour;
- fear of being left alone or going to sleep;
- panic attacks.

Depression
- apathy and inability to enjoy activities that still remain possible to the patient;
- feeling a burden and 'not worth bothering with' even when they are much loved.

Disturbed behaviour
- persistent anger, aggression;
- refusal of medication that is essential to relieve pain;
- paranoia, confusional states.

Physical symptoms unresponsive to treatment
- pain;
- vomiting;
- breathlessness.

Most of these conditions should be regarded initially as symptoms of underlying psychosocial problems and not as evidence that a psychiatric illness is present.

part of dying. Research using the HAD scale shows that about a quarter of cancer patients in a hospital or hospice are depressed, a quarter anxious, and about half in each group score significantly in the other parameter also. All the symptoms listed in Fig. 21.2 should be investigated if they cause persistent concern to the patient or family. Some will be found to be completely reversible and much can be done to relieve others. Where there is little possibility of change within the patient, helping the family and other care givers to understand the problem and to manage it in the best way, eases much of the stress on them.

Assessment of psychological problems in the terminally ill

Assessment begins with history taking, and technique may have to be modified to take account of the weakness and poor concentration seen in a very ill patient. The interviewer should be familiar with the common problems facing the dying and make sure that he covers these areas (Fig. 21.3). If the patient welcomes the interview and uses it as an opportunity to unburden, this should be encouraged and formal questioning be kept to the minimum necessary to clarify the problems and ensure that nothing vital is missed. If he has little to say, it is useful to take a new history of the illness with the emphasis on the patient's experience and on communication. Questions such as 'When you found the lump, what did you think it was? What did the doctor say? Did you tell your husband about it?' give an opportunity to establish good rapport and at the same time reveal communication problems and the attitude of the patient to the illness. Further questions guide the patient to cover other

---

Fig. 21.3 Common problems facing dying patients

- Coming to terms with death.
- Communication between patient, staff and family.
- Problems related to the disease and to treatment.
- Problems related to role adjustment.
- Pre-existing family and social problems.

Fig. 21.4 Adjustment reactions
(see also Chapter 20, p. 259)

Definition
A disorder ocurring in response to an identifiable psychosocial stressor, with onset within 3 months of exposure to stressor, persisting not longer than 6 months.

A maladaptive reaction resulting in impairment in occupational functioning, social activities or relationships, or in symptoms worse than would be expected for the magnitude of the stressor.

Main types: adjustment disorder with anxious mood, depressed mood, disturbed conduct, physical complaints, or a mixture of these.

---

areas as the story unfolds. To assess the mental state the interviewer notes verbal and non-verbal cues which prompt him to ask questions which will exclude or reveal depression, paranoia, hallucinations, dementia, etc. with the minimum distress to the patient. When the medical part of the history suggests that psychological problems may be due to drugs, biochemical changes, or other complications of the underlying disease, discussion with colleagues is essential to clarify this and plan necessary investigations.

Diagnosis

By far the most frequent psychiatric diagnosis applicable to dying patients is adjustment disorder. Also common are drug psychosis, and transient organic psychotic conditions (confusional states). The non-organic psychoses (attributable to recent life experiences) include depressive and excitative types, acute paranoid reaction, and reactive confusion. Almost any psychiatric syndrome can be seen in the dying, either stress-related or organic, and quite often a mixture of the two. For instance a patient with features of mania who has breast cancer may be responding to stress, but the symptoms are just as likely in this instance to be caused by a cerebral secondary tumour or by the dexamethasone being used to control it.

Coming to terms with death

Although everyone knows that death is inescapable, most people assume that they will live to be old and plan their lives accordingly. They are **shocked** when they realize that their life may end soon, and some feel emotionally numb for a short time. They just **cannot believe** what is happening to them and may deny that they are seriously ill or that they have been told what is wrong with them. This **denial** protects them from suffering the full impact of the crisis at once. It defends them against some of the anxiety and usually disappears gradually with the passage of time. It becomes a problem if it leads to refusal of essential treatment or persistence in making unrealistic plans for the future. Sometimes denial co-exists with signs of distressing anxiety. These patients usually benefit from gentle confrontation with the truth. Their inability to acknowledge the diagnosis openly makes it impossible for them to ask questions like 'Will dying be very painful?' which have been at the back of their mind, and which can often be answered in a reassuring way.

The presence of physical symptoms that do not respond to adequate treatment is related to denial. They provide an alternative and less threatening focus of anxiety. The patient says in effect, 'There is nothing the matter with me except my pain', but he cannot begin to lose that pain until he has the courage to face its meaning. If psychotherapy can help him do this, the symptom becomes controllable or disappears.

Many patients become distressed that something is happening to them which they cannot control, and which will deprive them of everything in life which they hold most dear. They ask 'Why?' as if they need to make sense of their predicament and work out who, if anyone, is to blame. Some conclude that it is mainly the fault of others and in them **anger** is a prominent response. Others, rightly or wrongly, blame themselves and feel **guilty**.

If anger becomes displaced on to family or other care givers, relationships become strained and the patient may lose the support he needs and become isolated. Occasionally it takes a regressive stubborn form which hinders the patient from living to the full. For example, someone who becomes paraplegic from spinal secondaries may refuse to accept a wheelchair, declaring vehemently 'If I can't go home on my own two feet, I don't want to go home at all!' Psychotherapy may help such a patient through this detrimental phase.

As the anger wanes, **grief** usually takes over. This is a necessary part of coming to terms with mortality and many patients come through it to a stage of quiet **resignation**, whilst a few achieve a positive **acceptance**. This is characterized by a determination to fight the illness as effectively as they can, and to make the most of the life that is left. Grief may persist or progress to frank depression. Suicidal thoughts may be prompted by the wish to escape suffering, or to retain control, and are not always a sign of depressive illness in the dying.

These responses to the knowledge of mortality do not often progress in the orderly fashion described here, nor are they gone through once and for all. They tend to recur with greater or less severity each time the patient is confronted with clear evidence that the disease is progressing, forcing him to give up yet another of his accustomed activities.

Anxiety is present to some degree throughout the process of coming to terms with death. Some is characteristic separation anxiety; a response to the threatened loss of close relationships. Other components include anxiety about the progress of the illness and worries over how the rest of the family will cope when the patient deteriorates and dies. Psychotherapy and anxiolytic drugs may help those whose anxiety is the direct result of the illness, but patients who have been anxious for much of their lives seldom improve and a few get worse, requiring quite heavy sedation to make the last lap of their life tolerable.

Communication

When physical symptoms are controlled, communication problems are the commonest remediable cause of anxiety and depression in the dying. Many patients complain that it has been difficult or impossible to obtain sufficient infor-

mation about their illness from their doctor. A few who say this will have been told their diagnosis and are now denying it, but more often they have asked direct questions which have been met with vague or euphemistic answers. The patient usually knows from his symptoms and from the anxious or over-cheerful behaviour of those around him, that something serious is wrong, but he may refrain from asking more for fear of the emotional upset that may ensue. But it is common for patients to express relief when the truth is openly acknowledged. Then they can ask questions about the prognosis and the likely history of the disease, and plan accordingly. Decisions can be made and support from the extended family and community can be more easily mobilized.

Patients are often anxious about communication with close relatives. They wish to confide and to prepare them for what is to come, but they also wish to protect everyone from the impact of painful news for as long as possible. People tend to confide in those whom they see as strong and protect those whom they perceive as weak or dependent on them. They may underestimate the capacity of others to bear pain and cope with the crisis. Many patients value the opportunity to discuss with their doctor how to talk about the future with their children or elderly parents, and some ask for help in doing this. Conjoint family sessions can be most effective and rewarding, breaking through the isolation which each person has been feeling as he has been worrying alone.

Ethical issues related to confidentiality often have to be considered during terminal illness. When investigations are complete and a diagnosis has been made, the doctor knows more than the patient about the state of his body and his future prospects. In any other situation, most people would not want anyone else to know more than they do about themselves and what is likely to happen to them. Here the doctor (and often other members of the clinical team) possess information that family members and others may also wish to know. Usually the patient wants to remain in control of the spread of such news, deciding for himself how much shall be told, to whom and when. Respecting the rights and needs of everyone concerned and balancing them appropriately requires considerable tact and skill. Saying too much can be as harmful as saying too little.

To give an accurate **prognosis** is almost impossible, and the consequences of getting it wrong can be deleterious, causing people to prepare for death prematurely or to be unduly shocked when it comes unexpectedly soon. The doctor should not yield to pressure to be specific. Instead it is better to provide regular opportunities to talk over the progress of the disease and support the patient in bearing the uncertainty.

Problems related to the disease and its treatment

Many patients have already been helped by the surgical team to adjust to the effects of operations like mastectomy and colostomy, and others have been supported through the vicissitudes of radiotherapy and chemotherapy, but some

Case 1: the woman who refused treatment

Mrs H., aged 38, married with a teenage son and daughter, had a *3-year history of breast cancer*. She was attending out-patients regularly for chemotherapy and seemed to be doing well until she suddenly surprised her consultant by *refusing further treatment*. He thought she seemed depressed and referred her for psychiatric assessment. The following problems emerged. The patient was indeed *depressed*, weepy, and wishing she were dead. Her husband had not understood the doctor's explanation to him about his wife's illness and prognosis (*communication problem*). He thought she would die soon and that he might prolong her life if he allowed her to rest completely. He got up early to do the housework and to get the children off to school and he said she must leave preparation of the evening meal to him. Lonely and idle all day, she felt miserable, useless, and guilty that he was getting so tired (*role adjustment, family problem*).

He said that he was now so busy that there was no time to take her to see her elderly parents any more. Previously she had cleaned and shopped for them and enjoyed their company. Now she was cut off from them and felt guilty that she was letting them down (*role adjustment*).

Her husband and son quarrelled continuously (*pre-existing problem exacerbated by mother's illness*) and she was grieving over the prospect of her daughter growing up motherless (*facing own mortality*).

She felt ugly since her mastectomy. She had been very sick for several days

Case 2: the old soldier who hit out

Mr R., aged 82, had *multiple bony secondaries* from carcinoma of the prostate. He was a cheerful patient who said he had seen death in the First World War and was not afraid of it. However, the psychiatrist was urgently called when he *used his walking stick to attack visitors to the patient opposite*. He looked *frightened, vigilant*, and *suspicious*. Eventually he confided that he knew they were plotting to kill him. He became angry when this belief was gently challenged so he was reassured that the problem would be looked into and that he would be protected from such danger.

Diagnosis

The patient was denying his own fear of death and was also unable to acknowledge that the threat to his life was within his own body. Instead he attributed it to other people (projection) and felt that his survival depended on attacking them. The use of this psychological mechanism resulted in a *paranoid reaction*.

Management

At first he refused medication, but eventually accepted 3 mg of haloperidol to please the psychiatrist, who told him he deserved 'something to calm his nerves if such distressing things were happening'. The next day he was calmer and became able to face, talk about, and weep over the fact that he was dying and afraid. As he became able to accept the reality of his situation his suspicions ceased and he withdrew his accusations.

Case 3: the man who was only worried about his wife

Mr J. was 70 and had carcinoma of the colon. He looked *anxious*, was *restless and slept badly*. He was being treated with diazepam, which made him sleepy. He *denied any worries except those about his wife*, who was alone while he was in hospital. *Each time she came he questioned her aggressively about all her activities and became very angry if she was only a few minutes late*. She found him so difficult that she curtailed her visits and then he began to complain that she had ceased to care. The nurses noted the distress of them both and involved the psychiatrist. On questioning, Mr J. said he knew he was going to die but he was not worried about it. He had not spoken to his wife about it 'Because it might upset her'. Later he changed this to 'Because I might cry, and I have always been the strong one'.

Diagnosis

Anxiety state. This patient recognized that he was anxious but attributed the whole of it to his concern about his wife. The unrecognized anxiety about himself was directed towards her (displacement) and allowed him to avoid facing his own fear of death. In addition, the couple had problems in communication and role adjustment.

Management

Psychotherapy helped him to accept that he was anxious about himself as well as his wife and to withdraw the displacement. He refused a conjoint session but agreed to tell her he knew he was dying, so that they could plan together how she would cope

Case 4: the doctor who was too busy

A doctor in an oncology ward noticed that he had become unusually reluctant to go to work. He particularly avoided spending time with a man in his forties who had lung cancer and who was married with young children. After this patient died, the *doctor felt guilty* that he had always been too busy to talk to the patient's wife, although she had several times asked to see him. This preyed on his mind and once he dreamed of the couple and then found it quite difficult to get back to sleep. He began to wonder if he was unsuited to this kind of work, and *he felt a failure*.

Fortunately, he sought out a friend who had known him for a long time. Together they recognized that the *case had reminded him of his own father's death* when he was 6. He had been frightened by his mother's tears, and his avoidance of the patient's wife protected him from the resurgence of this memory. He realized that he and his mother had never talked about the painful weeks following his father's death, and resolved to do so on his next visit home. She was not as upset as he expected, and told him she had always wondered if there was anything wrong with the way he had been 'such a brave boy'. Suddenly he felt it was alright to grieve for his father, and this he also shared with his friend. Soon he lost his doubts about his choice of oncology as a specialty, and continued in it with increasing satisfaction.

following her last two chemotherapy treatments and had not reported this to the doctor, assuming that it was inevitable (*effects of treatment and poor communication*).

She decided it was time to give up the struggle. In other circumstances she might have contemplated suicide; just letting the illness have its way seemed an easy and blameless way out.

Diagnosis
Adjustment disorder (depressive).

Management
Discussion of treatment programme with oncologist. Interviews with patient and husband, separately and together (family session would have been ideal but husband refused). Antidepressants were not used.

Outcome
The oncologist agreed to delay next course of chemotherapy. He offered to modify it slightly and admit the patient to monitor and treat immediate side effects if and when she decided to resume.

Her husband understood the prognosis better, and her need to retain a role. She asserted herself more and he learned to leave her to do things, even if it made her tired. Visits to parents were reinstated, though less often. Her husband made more effort to understand his son.

In 1 month she was less depressed and accepted further treatment. She returned to work part-time, did more for her family, and achieved her goal of being able to talk with her daughter at the time of her menarche. She lived reasonably well for a further 2 years.

Outcome
He still became frightened from time to time in the evenings but knew that he was afraid of dying and could accept comfort. 1.5 mg of haloperidol was given at 6.0 p.m. for a week and then discontinued. He died peacefully a few days later.

alone in the future. He risked crying in front of his wife for the first time in his life.

Outcome
When they talked, both wept and comforted each other. The next day he said triumphantly to the psychiatrist 'you were right, it was OK'. Undue anxiety about his wife's visits ceased and she began to stay most of the day, sitting beside him knitting or reading. His anxiety diminished, diazepam was reduced, and he was less drowsy.

reach the terminal stage still struggling with, and disabled by these problems. Even then, psychotherapeutic help may be effective. Toward the end of a long illness, decisions may have to be made about whether to stop or modify chemotherapy which has distressing side effects, giving the patient a more comfortable last few weeks, or whether to continue the fight to prolong life right up to the end. Every patient who wants to share in this decision process should be allowed to do so. Some persist in therapy to please an enthusiastic oncologist, or because they are terrified of death. They are relieved when they realize it is acceptable to give up the struggle. Others refuse treatment while it is still likely to be effective, because other problems have made their life seem unbearable. Someone who is not directly concerned with treatment may be able to help to clarify the issues involved, helping both groups to become more certain about what they really want.

Adjustment to role change

Good adjustment in this context can be defined as the capacity to go on living as well as possible within the limitations of the illness. Some patients become aggressively independent, refusing to accept help when they need it, and suffering unnecessarily as a result. Others take up the sick role too soon, becoming bored or depressed. The relatives of both groups find these behaviours difficult and everyone benefits when psychotherapy helps the person to get the level of dependency right. Guidance is often needed with decisions about when to stop work or the provision of care for children. Anger about what is being lost may interfere with enjoyment of what is still possible, and envy of others who have to take over the roles which the patient relinquishes may strain relationships. Here also individual or family psychotherapy may be effective.

Toward the end of a person's life, relatives who cannot bear the thought of losing the patient may pressurize him to eat, talk, or make efforts to recover when he is ready to withdraw and rest. They need: a reminder that it is more loving to leave him in peace, encouragement to let him go, and support in their grief.

Management

Whether the patient is at home or in hospital, good management depends on accurate identification of any problems and their causes. It will usually involve **liaison** with other members of the caring team, to improve communication or to discuss changes in treatment. Occasionally the most important work will be with the caring relatives or the staff whose own anxiety interferes with their appraisal of the patient's needs. They may be unfamiliar with psychological explanations for angry and aggressive behaviour and for intractable symptoms, and may prefer sedation to long conversations as a means of producing a more peaceful patient. Particularly difficult for them may be intervention which enables the patient to mourn, so that the initial outcome is more obvious distress. Quite often staff are just too busy to be able to give the psychological care that they fully recognize is needed. Establishing a good rapport with them is an essential component of liaison psychiatry, of which the care of the dying should be a part.

Psychological treatment
Many of the treatments described in Chapter 18 are useful in terminal illness. Particularly at the time of diagnosis, crisis therapy can facilitate adaptation to the threat of loss, illness, change and death. When patient and therapist agree that there are problems in communication or role adjustment, these may be effectively resolved by meeting with a partner or the family. Patients who are struggling to find meaning in their predicament often appreciate being put in touch with a priest or other person who is competent to listen and help.

Most psychotherapy with the terminally ill will of necessity be brief and supportive. Techniques must be adapted to take account of physical weakness, poor concentration, and the need to focus on whatever is the most urgent concern of the patient at that moment. Familiarity with psychoanalytic ideas about the unconscious and defence mechanisms is very helpful in understanding and treating patients in whom denial or anger is causing suffering, and those whose physical symptoms are being exacerbated by emotional factors. Dying patients often have vivid dreams and are grateful for an opportunity to talk about their meaning as they come to terms with death.

Some of the depression associated with terminal illness is amenable to a cognitive approach. This can help the patient to realize that, even though he may be going to die in the near future, he need not remain overwhelmed by this threat. He may discover that he can retain more control over his life than he first thought, and that there are still good things that he can do and enjoy in the present.

Anxiety management and relaxation techniques can often help those whose lives are being spoiled by fear or panic. They are especially useful to assist in the control of breathlessness, some kinds of pain and insomnia, and in such cases they may reduce the need for medication.

Psychotropic drugs
Care has to be taken in prescribing these drugs as most terminally ill patients will be receiving medication already and many will also have impaired hepatic or renal function. Most of the biological indicators of depression are likely to be obscured by the illness or treatment, but early morning waking is often a feature. The presence of low self-esteem, inappropriate guilt, or symptoms of psychotic depression all suggest that a good response to medication is likely. Amitriptyline is still the first choice where it is tolerated; it is usually given at night and may replace some or all night sedation. One of the newer antidepressants may be needed where drowsiness, dry mouth, constipation, etc., are already a problem. (Even in very ill patients, ECT can be safe and effective, and its speed of action may be a great advantage, giving a few good days or weeks before death.)

Haloperidol is the drug of choice in confusional states and psychoses, especially when the patient is agitated or hallucinating. If the patient is on an anti-emetic already it may also be a satisfactory replacement for that. A few very anxious patients do not respond satisfactorily even to high doses of benzodiazepines, but show a distressing combination of drowsiness and agitation. They may do better on a major tranquillizer such as thioridazine. When the patient is near death, hyoscine is used because it has anti-emetic and tranquillizing properties and also dries secretions. Together with morphine or diamorphine it is usually the drug of choice for the near moribund patient. The presence of a familiar person who can hold his hand and perhaps talk quietly to him from time to time contributes greatly to a peaceful state, and this personal aspect of care of the dying should never be forgotten.

If a patient or relative raises the question of euthanasia, the reasons behind this should be carefully explored. Sometimes patients reveal much more about their suffering to the relatives than to professionals, and assume nothing more can be done to bring relief when in fact more adequate symptom control is quite possible. The patient who is depressed or feels that he has become too much of a burden to his family may also ask that death be hastened. When such problems are addressed patients may regain their wish to go on living. If suffering does become intractable, the ethical question of how it should be relieved must be considered carefully (see Chapter 4).

Outcome

It is never possible, nor would it be desirable, to relieve all the emotional suffering in patients and families coping with terminal illness. To do so would be to deny the humanity of the situation; the reality of what is being lost. The aim of intervention is to relieve all unnecessary and disabling symptoms so that the work of anticipatory grieving can be accomplished leaving everyone concerned able to function as well as possible.

When time is short, some people change considerably. Crisis intervention techniques may resolve old problems and occasionally reconcile divided families. Where the patient himself cannot change, helping those around him to understand and give support can still make a painful situation more bearable.

Psychological symptoms and emotional distress may improve markedly even when the physical condition continues to deteriorate. Where they were the main reason for admission to a hospital or hospice, a return home is often possible and some patients die there.

Bereavement is easier to bear and complicated grief is less likely if the memories of the last illness are not traumatic, the necessary things have been said or done, and the death has been peaceful.

Professional responses to dying patients

Most of us cannot work closely with patients who are dying and remain unaffected by their suffering. Often without our realizing it, they awaken our own fear of death. This fear is an essential part of human nature, an expression of the instinct for survival which prompts people to take appropriate care of themselves and avoid undue risks. Because dying patients remind us of our mortality, they tend to make us anxious and we are likely to respond with one of the two basic reactions to threat: fight or flight.

The 'flight' responses include all the ways we have of avoiding facing the suffering of the dying: being too busy to talk and listen, telling ourselves that patients do not really want to know anyway, delegating to others the breaking of bad news, and concentrating on the physical aspects of diagnosis and symptom control. Thus we satisfy our consciences without becoming very involved in our patients.

The 'fight' response can make us try to prove to ourselves through what we do for our patients, that the suffering associated with dying can be overcome. This motivates good care and is advantageous unless we have such intense investment in it that it leads to overinvolvement or identification. Then personal anxiety and distress increases, boundaries become blurred, and judgement distorted, so that the care giver becomes less effective.

An awareness that these problems exist and a willingness to recognize their manifestations in ourselves can lead to a more appropriate attitude, based on acceptance of this fear and the effects it has on us. Talking through these issues with a friend or colleague can help, as can support groups for staff whose work often brings them face to face with death. Adjusting to the knowledge that we ourselves will one day die is part of our own maturation. It is important that we learn to cope with this in such a way that our patients and our families do not suffer unduly from our adjustment reactions!

QUESTIONS

1 A woman of 62 with a 3-year history of breast cancer now has lung and bone metastases. She says she is not at all worried about herself, but she always looks anxious and sometimes has horrific nightmares of being buried. How can you help her?

2 A man of 60 is found at operation to have inoperable carcinoma of the colon with liver secondaries. Before he regains consciousness, his wife asks to see the doctor. She has guessed that he is seriously ill and asks the house surgeon to promise not to tell her husband his diagnosis. How would you handle your interview with her?

3 A woman of 27 has carcinoma of the ovary. She is married with children of 8 and 6. Her symptoms are well controlled and she could go home, but she is reluctant to get up and does not seem interested in anything. What problems is she likely to have and how could you help her?

FURTHER READING

Doyle D., *et al.* (Eds) (1993) *Oxford Textbook of Palliative Medicine* Oxford University Press, Oxford. [Includes descriptions of emotional and psychiatric problems associated with all kinds of cancer (including paediatric) and their management.]

Holland J. & Rowland J. (Eds) (1990) *Handbook of Psychooncology* Oxford University Press, Oxford. [Thorough coverage of the psychological care of the patient with cancer. Includes large section on oncology staff: psychological and ethical issues.]

Stedeford A. (1984) *Facing Death. Patients, Families and Profes-sionals.* 2nd Edition. Sobell Publications, Oxford. [A detailed coverage of psychological problems in terminal illness, with extensive use of cases. Chapters on bereavement and professional responses to death are also included.]

USEFUL ADDRESSES

British Association of Cancer United Patients (BACUP), 3 Bath Place, Rivington Street, London EC2A 3JR (tel: 071-696 9003).

22
Bereavement

Fact sheet

Facts about bereavement

Bereavement is associated with increased psychological and physical morbidity. Normal grief is disabling but symptoms resolve in due course provided the bereaved person has adequate support. In abnormal grief the symptoms may be altered in timing and intensity and the processes of mourning may fail to begin or to progress. Bereavement can precipitate or exacerbate almost all psychiatric syndromes.

Indicators that grief is abnormal

Delayed onset:
- by more than a week or two;
- behaving as if the deceased has not died.

Persistent:
- agitation, anxiety, clinging behaviour;
- anger which alienates carers;
- despair leading to self-neglect and suicidal threats;
- hypochondriasis.

Inability to:
- return to work (after weeks);
- resume usual social activities or interests (after months or years, depending on nature of relationship lost).

Antisocial behaviour, promiscuity
(Usually adolescents).

Alcoholism

Psychiatric illness:
- anxiety state, with panic attacks or phobic features;
- mania (rare);
- depression;
- paranoid reaction.

The transition between normal grief and depression is not clearly marked. Important indicators of depression are low self-esteem, inappropriate guilt, early morning waking and suicidal ideas/plans where the patient does have other potentially rewarding relationships, etc. Antidepressants are usually effective in such cases.

Factors associated with poor outcome in the bereaved

Personal
- Children, adolescents, young adults with dependent parents and children.

- Parents bereaved of adolescent or young adult child.
- Especial vulnerability to separation and loss.
- History of psychiatric illness.
- Other recent or concurrent losses or crises.
- Excessive use of drugs and alcohol.

Circumstances
- Low socio-economic status.
- Presence of young children at home.
- Lack of confiding relationship or other perceived support.

Observed during the terminal illness
- Unusually clinging or dependent behaviour.
- Unusual anger, guilt, or self-reproach.
- General impression on the part of the carers that bereavement will go badly.

Characteristics of the loss
- Sudden unexpected death.
- Death following a very long or distressing illness.
- Circumstances which preclude seeing the body, attending the funeral, etc.
- Suicide.

Characteristics of the relationship
- Ambivalence.
- Unduly controlling, dependent or clinging.

Management

- *Bereavement counselling* given to those who are vulnerable reduces the morbidity of abnormal grief.
- *Individual and family therapy* are useful, the latter particularly so when a family is unable to share grief.
- *Techniques which facilitate the expression of feelings* in a safe setting are especially helpful.
- *Psychotropic medication* is not indicated in normal grief except perhaps as a sedative for a caring relative who is exhausted and wishes to recover sufficiently to face the funeral. Medication may be used when psychiatric illness supervenes, to restore normal grieving and facilitate resolution.
- *Bereavement can play a significant part in precipitating or exacerbating almost all psychiatric syndromes.* Its significance is often unrecognized by the patient and it is often missed in the history, especially if it occurred several years previously. Failure on the part of professionals to recognize this leads to inaccurate diagnosis and inadequate or ineffective treatment.

Introduction

The verb 'to bereave' means to rob or to leave desolate, and bereavement usually refers to the experiences through which people pass when they have lost, through death, someone who is important to them. These experiences are normal in the sense that they happen to almost everyone in the course of a lifetime. Nevertheless, it is appropriate to consider them in a textbook of psychiatry because bereavement causes disabling psychological symptoms and occasionally precipitates or complicates almost all of the psychiatric syndromes described in this book.

A major bereavement is a distressing and disruptive experience, especially frightening to anyone who is going through it for the first time. Such a person often needs to be told that what it happening to him is normal, if it is. He may need help bearing it and making sense of it, and reassurance that he will eventually recover. This kind of support is often provided by family and friends. The professional person who is involved should be able to assess whether the grief is proceeding as expected and whether the bereaved person is receiving the help which he needs from others. In addition, he should be able to recognize complications, know how and when to intervene, and when to seek more expert help in management. In order to do these things he must be familiar with normal grief.

Normal grief

Normal grief is best described from two points of view: the psychological, emotional, and spiritual **symptoms** experienced by the bereaved person, and the psychological **tasks** which he must accomplish as he adjusts to his new

---

Fig. 22.1 Normal grief

Before onset
- Shock, numbness and disbelief.

Acute phase
- Waves or 'pangs' of grief.
- Physical symptoms, mainly of anxiety.
- Searching for the deceased, crying.
- Anger.
- Going over the past, guilt.
- Pre-occupation with the memory of the deceased.
- Hallucinations and/or a sense of the presence of the deceased.

Intermediate phase
- Pining.
- Physical symptoms, mainly of depression.
- Loss of purpose, hopelessness.
- Withdrawal.

Resolution
- Physical symptoms diminish.
- Mood improves.
- Customary activities resumed and/or new ones begun.
- Symptoms may recur at anniversaries for years.

Case 1: the grief of Mrs W.

Mrs W. was 50 when her husband, John, died. He had been ill for 6 months and she thought she was prepared for his death, but when it actually happened, it came as a **shock**. For a few hours she **could not believe** he was really dead, although she began to inform her relatives and to make the necessary arrangements. Soon she began to weep, and she felt as if her tears would never stop. Eventually they did, leaving her exhausted and feeling dead inside. As the days passed she was to become familiar with these pangs of grief. They came like an illness or a pain, except that she could not put a finger on the part of her that was hurting. They lasted for minutes or even up to an hour, and then subsided but returned when someone offered sympathy or something reminded her of John. They were at their worst in the days after the funeral when all the helpful people had gone away, and of the first time she realized how very alone she was.

At night she slept badly. Sometimes she thought she heard John calling her or she dreamed he was in bed beside her and woke bitterly disappointed to find the empty space. She was restless, sometimes deriving comfort from looking at his things, but seeing them often intensified her grief as she realized he would never need them again.

In the days after the funeral she felt tired and ached all over. She wasn't hungry and when she did eat she had indigestion. She began to wonder if she was becoming ill. Sometimes she almost wished she was. If she could die too, the terrible loneliness would be over. Then she remembered that the rest of her family still loved her. Usually that led her to reproach herself for wanting to die but sometimes she felt angry with them, feeling that they were forcing her to keep going.

When she went out, she would catch herself scanning the people in the street, searching for her husband. Sometimes she thought she saw him and would set off to greet him, only to realize it was a stranger. At home she often began to set the table for two, or peeled too many potatoes. Over and over again she would be reminded of his absence and would be temporarily overcome by grief and longing.

She was surprised at how **angry** she was with him for dying. How could he go and leave her like this? Didn't he know how much she still needed him? And then she felt **guilty** for she realized that he had not chosen to die. She would go over the events of the past, especially his last illness, wondering if there was anything more she could have done to help him. She recalled times when she was critical and impatient, and deeply regretted them. Sometimes her anger was directed at God. If he existed and was good, why did he let this happen to her? When she prayed there seemed to be no one there to listen anymore, and this emptiness added to her pain. She felt envious of friends who still had husbands, and awkward in their company. She did not want to go out.

Quite slowly these turbulent painful feelings became less frequent and less intense, but they returned with unexpected force when someone offered sympathy or something reminded her of her loss. Mostly she felt flat and miserable. Her husband had been the main focus of her life after her children had left home, and now there seemed no purpose in living. She got up late, neglected her appearance, and could not be bothered to clean her house. Friends asked her out and she sometimes went to please them, but did not enjoy their company. She began to wonder if she was doomed to feel like this forever. This was the experience of **grief**.

After many months there came a sunny day when she realized she was enjoying the brightness. She decided to clean up her house so that it looked better next time her family came. Suddenly she noticed that there was time now to take up a hobby which she had neglected ever since her children had been born. More and more often she felt her normal self again and friends began to say 'She has got over it now'. She did not agree with them, for she still thought of

Continued on p. 280

her husband often and missed him very much, but now gratitude was mixed with the sadness. Bad memories of his illness and death were fading, to be replaced by good ones of their marriage and family life. She discovered, to her surprise, that there were some advantages in being independent, which partly compensated for her loneliness.

The first anniversary of his death was very distressing, almost as if it was all happening again. She felt ill and went to her doctor, who was not surprised to see her at that time. For years she had a resurgence of grief around John's birthday, and occasionally something reminded her most painfully of his death and her sadness was intensely but briefly renewed. Mainly she had become content. She had **accepted** her new identity, and felt that there was a place for her amongst her family and friends, even though she had been forced to change so much as she made the transition from being a wife to being a widow.

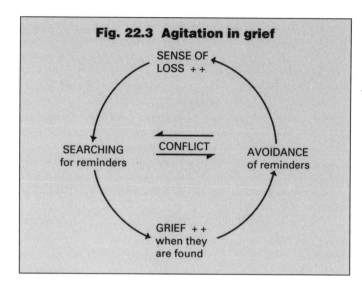

Fig. 22.3 Agitation in grief

identity. The symptoms of normal grief are summarized in Fig. 22.1 and most of them are described in the case of Mrs W. She went through many of the phases or responses referred to in Chapter 21; i.e. shock and numbness, disbelief, anger, grief and acceptance. Denial in its fully developed form is not seen for long in normal grief, though many bereaved people feel for weeks or months that the deceased has only gone away and will eventually return and restore 'normality' to their lives. The anger and irritability often seen in grief may be the most difficult part for the family and friends to cope with, and here the understanding and support of the professional outsider may be especially helpful. Figure 22.2 shows the outcomes of the various responses to anger on the part of the bereaved and those around him.

Many stable, competent people, finding themselves rendered temporarily disorganized by acute grief, become afraid that they are about to break down. An explanation of their predicament in terms of the disabling effects of an approach/ avoidance conflict (shown in Fig. 22.3) helps them to understand why they feel as they do. They can be reassured that their response is a normal one in the circumstances and that

it will pass in time. Similarly Fig. 22.4 depicting the nature of grief work helps to explain why the changes which the bereaved person has to undergo seem so radical and exhausting.

The **tasks of mourning** (Fig. 22.5) begin with the acceptance of the reality of the loss. Being present at the death, seeing the body after death, and the rituals of a funeral all help to bring this home to the bereaved.

All intrapsychic change is stressful and most people at some stage try to avoid the pain of grief. They may search for a substitute for the relationship that is lost, e.g. they may remarry quickly or adopt a 'replacement' child. Figure 22.4 illustrates why this is usually unsatisfactory for both parties, because the bereaved person tries to impose on the other the shape of the missing person. It is much wiser, though initially more lonely and painful, to wait until grieving is complete before attempting to form a new relationship.

Adjusting to a world in which the dead person is missing entails changing many of the rituals of daily life and may include taking on some of the functions previously assumed by the deceased. For instance, young parents sometimes relate to their children differently. A father may be more often the disciplinarian and a mother more often a comforter. If father dies, mother finds that she has to play some of father's roles too, and in doing so she becomes a more whole and balanced person. This should often be the outcome when mourning is successfully completed, as depicted in Fig. 22.4.

In the early stages of mourning the bereaved person is preoccupied with the memory of the one who has died. It is as if the psyche has to re-evaluate all aspects of the relationship and get it into perspective, accepting and forgiving the bad, and appreciating the good, before letting go. Only after this has happened does the emotional energy tied up in that relationship become free. Then it can be re-invested either in a new relationship or in a series of activities, friendships, etc., through which the person develops a new independence. The deceased is not forgotten, but the bereaved person comes to realize that there is no disloyalty in beginning to live well and to love again.

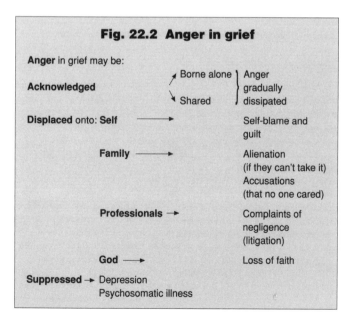

Fig. 22.2 Anger in grief

Anger in grief may be:

Acknowledged — Borne alone / Shared } Anger gradually dissipated

Displaced onto: Self — Self-blame and guilt

Family — Alienation (if they can't take it) Accusations (that no one cared)

Professionals — Complaints of negligence (litigation)

God — Loss of faith

Suppressed — Depression Psychosomatic illness

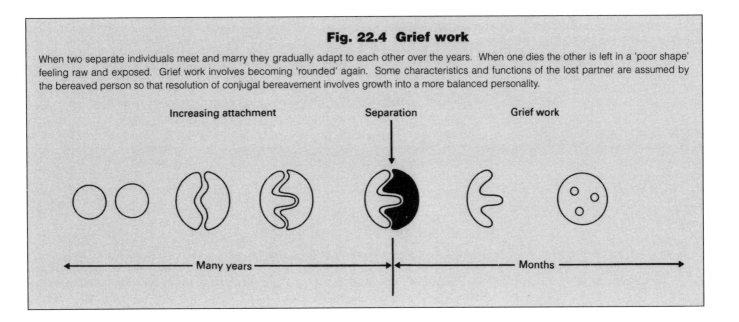

Fig. 22.4 Grief work

When two separate individuals meet and marry they gradually adapt to each other over the years. When one dies the other is left in a 'poor shape' feeling raw and exposed. Grief work involves becoming 'rounded' again. Some characteristics and functions of the lost partner are assumed by the bereaved person so that resolution of conjugal bereavement involves growth into a more balanced personality.

Increasing attachment   Separation   Grief work

←————— Many years —————→   ←————— Months —————→

Abnormal grief

The transition from normal to abnormal grief is a gradual one and in assessing each case the appropriate question is not 'Is this normal?' but 'What might be expected for this person with this loss?' The same symptoms occur in normal and abnormal grief but are modified in timing and intensity. The processes of mourning may get stuck at any stage so that symptoms and behaviour that would be appropriate in early bereavement may be abnormal if still present a year later.

Characteristics which determine an individual's response to bereavement include age, personality, and previous experiences of loss. Children grieve differently from adults. The child who seems to behave in a very 'grown up' way after the death of a parent may be responding to pressure to support the surviving parent, with a resulting inhibition of his own grief. Bereaved children suffer multiple losses if the death of a parent brings with it changes in social circumstances such as moving to a new house or school. In addition, the surviving parent may withdraw into his own grief leaving the child doubly bereft. Grief in the elderly often remains unresolved, the surviving spouse continuing to live as if the separation is temporary, for the elderly have less motivation to detach themselves from a lifetime partner and make a new beginning.

The coping mechanisms that a person usually uses at times of stress will come into play again in bereavement and a range of responses may be seen. Regressive collapse into helplessness, a refusal to accept that the death has occurred or denial that it has affected the person's life, stoicism, or frantic overactivity may all prevent progress towards resolution.

The process of grieving may also be interfered with by the pressure of society or the family on the bereaved. They may be encouraged to be brave and controlled, and to return to their usual routine as quickly as possible, as if nothing very important has happened. To counteract this, some people need permission to grieve and reassurance that it is alright to be distressed and unable to function at their usual level for a time. The acceptance of vulnerability and need, and the ability to use the support of others during bereavement are marks of maturity. When they are regarded as weakness, unneccessary guilt is engendered.

The history of previous losses influences the response to a new one. A man or woman who first comes into close contact with death in middle-age will find it more frightening and disruptive than will the person who has become familiar with it gradually during childhood and adolescence. The deaths of pets, elderly neighbours, grandparents, etc., provide opportunities for the reality of death to be faced when personal security is not seriously threatened, so that learning about grief and recovery can take place and coping skills can develop. But however prepared a person may be, the experience of several losses in quick succession is likely to produce a state of numbness, as if the individual cannot tolerate any more, or a catastrophic response of overwhelming grief from which recovery is much delayed.

The grief response also varies according to the circumstances of the loss and the nature of the relationship lost. Sudden unexpected death, whether it be cot death, the death of an adolescent on a motorcycle, or the collapse of a woman at work, almost always produces a severe reaction. Numbness and disbelief may delay the onset of grieving, and when it does begin it is intense and prolonged, the features of anger and anxiety being especially prominent. A short illness provides time for anticipatory grief, for reparation

Fig. 22.5 Tasks of mourning (modified from Worden)

1 Accept reality of loss.
2 Experience (and bear) the pain of grief.
3 Adjust to a world in which the dead person is missing.
4 Emotionally relocate the deceased and move on with life.

and reconciliation, for saying goodbye, and for making plans for the future. A very long illness may provoke premature detachment on the part of the family. Alternatively, those who are bereaved in these circumstances may be exhausted by years of caring, lack of holidays, and multiple false alarms which lead to an inappropriate but defensive sense of security so that death, when it does come, shocks them as if it was unexpected. When a disabling terminal illness extends over years, the patient may become the central focus for those around who give up outside interests and activities in order to devote themselves to him. Such relatives, when bereaved, may feel they no longer have anything to live for and need much encouragement to make new beginnings.

Where there has been long-standing ambivalence in a relationship, death may first bring a feeling of relief. Only later, when grieving begins, does the bereaved person recognize how intense the bonds of attachment were, and how much the partner is missed. Then guilt over the negative parts of the relationship emerges and may take a self-punitive form, the survivor continuing to grieve for a long time as if this could make reparation for the past. On the other hand, relief at the ending of an ambivalent relationship which has been recognized as such during life, may be genuine and uncomplicated. The survivor is able to take advantage of new freedom and develop in new ways.

A clinging, dependent relationship usually bodes ill for either partner. If the dominant partner dies, the spouse is left helpless; if the less dominant partner is the survivor, he or she no longer has anyone to care for. In either case the outcome is often chronic grief. Occasionally the label 'chronic grief' provides a convenient refuge for the bereaved person who feels unable to face the changes required of him by a new identity, or who has other less acceptable problems which he is shielded from acknowledging whilst he remains disabled by his grief.

Certain losses almost always carry with them an increase in morbidity. Where there is reason for blame or guilt, and where the support of the family or society may be withheld, e.g. in cot death, suicide or the death of a homosexual partner, there will be much suffering. Parents who lose a child on the brink of maturity often fail to recover for years, and the young parent left to cope alone with bringing up children seems to suffer more than the childless person who has recently married. Elderly parents whose adult son or daughter dies are often especially distraught, wishing they could have gone instead. Their grief is eased when family relations are good and they can help, e.g. with the care of grandchildren.

Case 2

Mr O., aged 30, became very *distressed after his dog died* in the kitchen one night during a fit. Two weeks later he was still preoccupied with thoughts of her, was *anxious and unable to concentrate* at work, and *woke several times most nights* thinking that he had heard her crying downstairs. He had been very fond of her and felt guilty that she had died alone, but he recognized that his grief was quite out of proportion to his loss.

A year previously, his brother-in-law had been killed in an accident. Mr O. immediately went to support his sister and her children, took over all the funeral arrangements, and was a 'tower of strength' to the whole family as they experienced the grief of this tragedy. His *wife noticed at the time that he showed little feeling.* In the following months he made numerous trips to help his sister, but he himself seemed unaffected by his brother-in-law's death.

Diagnosis
This case illustrates the appropriateness of asking 'What would be expected for this person with this loss?' and shows how grieving can be abnormal in timing and intensity. The onset of grief for the brother-in-law had been delayed and was eventually precipitated by the death of the dog on to whom feelings about the relative were displaced.

Management
Offering this diagnosis as a possible explanation for his symptoms proved enough in itself to initiate grief for his brother-in-law. He then allowed himself to begin to go over for the first time the events following that death. Soon he found himself facing his own mortality as he recognized that something similar could happen to him, and he considered what that would be like for his own wife and children. His family, who had been glad of his composure and strength at the time of the tragedy, were sympathetic when his own grief began, so he was able to share it with them and be supported himself.

Outcome
The recurrent dreams/hallucinations of the dog in the kitchen ceased from the time of the initial consultation and a normal grief reaction ensued.

Other conditions precipitated or exacerbated by grief

So far in this chapter attention has been focused on the psychological changes in grief, noting in passing that many of the physical symptoms seen in anxiety or depression are also present. Bereavement is a stressful event and as such some of its effects are likely to be mediated through interference with the endocrine and immune systems. It is not surprising therefore that people are more prone to illness of various kinds during bereavement. Consultation rates at the GP's surgery and hospital admissions are known to rise at this time. Widowers over 54 years of age have a 40% increase in mortality from cardiovascular disease in the 6 months after bereavement, compared with married men of the same age. Other studies suggest an increase in psychosomatic illness. Bereaved people use tranquillizers and sedatives more, and are liable to increase their smoking and drinking. Alcohol provides temporary solace from grief but drinking is often followed by depression, and the alcoholic seems unable to progress through his grief while he is drinking. The risk of suicide is increased following the death of a parent or spouse, but this is not paralleled by a similar rise in attempted suicide.

Unresolved grief is an important factor in marital breakdown. Failure of one partner to understand and support the other when one of their parents dies is often interpreted by the bereaved spouse as a lack of love. The problem may not lie in the marriage, but in the personality of the other spouse who, because of his own background or upbringing, either cannot face death himself or cannot express openly the deep feelings he or she has. Marital problems sometimes begin with a miscarriage or stillbirth, especially when the husband feels the loss less acutely than his wife or denies his own grief. Following the death of a child, especially a cot death or an accident, the anger of grief may be displaced onto one or other parent, provoking an atmosphere of blame and guilt and preventing them from supporting each other and grieving together.

The bereaved patient who complains of physical illness presents a diagnostic dilemma. For instance, a change in bowel habit in a middle-aged widow may be the result of anxiety or depression. If the spouse died of carcinoma of the colon, the symptom may be produced by identification with the deceased. (Temporarily taking on mannerisms of the person who has died is part of normal grief, but experiencing their symptoms for any length of time is not.) Hypochondriasis sometimes occurs in grief. This may be morbid but, particularly in the case of a young single parent, it may be understandable in terms of their increased anxiety about remaining well in order to care for children and maintain the family income. The need to exclude physical illness must be balanced against the need to avoid over-investigation which can increase anxiety still further.

Phobic anxiety increases in bereavement, especially fears of illness, infection, and cancer. Avoidance of going out may be agoraphobic, but may also be related to fear of meeting people in case they respond by avoidance or in other ways upsetting to the newly bereaved. Both manic and depressive psychoses may be precipitated by the death of someone close, as may a paranoid reaction, the latter being more common in the elderly.

Assessment

There is no sharp dividing line between normal and abnormal grief; the suffering experienced ranges from the mild and transient to severe and disabling. Many people progress through bereavement satisfactorily, sustained by their own inner resources and supported by family and friends. For them outside intervention is unnecessary and could even undermine their confidence in their own ability to cope. At the other end of the scale are those whose suffering is intense and lasting and whose lives become so disorganized that it is clear that professional help of some kind is needed. In the middle is a large number of people who are at risk of a pathological reaction which could be modified or prevented by the right intervention.

The fact sheet at the beginning of this chapter lists features associated with poor outcome, which can be noted before the death occurs, alerting a carer to special vulnerability. Under the heading 'Indicators that grief is abnormal' are others which can be observed during the terminal illness and in the early days or weeks of bereavement. Whenever several features in either list are applicable to a newly bereaved person, he or she is at risk. Regular visits or consultations to monitor the progress of grief and intervene if necessary may make all the difference between a good

readjustment and outcome, and continuing morbidity for many months or even years.

Management

Bereavement counsellors include general practitioners, health visitors, social workers, priests, and lay people with a special training. The counsellor aims to support a bereaved person through his grief by listening, reducing his sense of isolation, helping him to make sense of what is happening, maintaining his hope, and encouraging resolution in due course. He is also alert for signs of abnormal grief and either provides therapy himself or refers the individual on. All forms of psychological treatment referred to in Chapter 18 have a place in the management of abnormal grief. The aim is to overcome defences which block the normal processes of mourning, and to provide support as they emerge. Physical treatments may be required when clearly defined complications such as paranoia, psychotic depression, or mania

---

Case 3: the woman who was forbidden to grieve

Mrs J., aged 64, was referred to a psychiatrist *a year after her bereavement*. She complained of *insomnia*, *restlessness* and *lack of interest* in any of her previous activities. She said she had got over the effects of her husband's death, but she looked very unhappy. Her GP had tried an antidepressant but it had no effect. At the initial interview she told the psychiatrist that her husband had said 'I don't want you to grieve for me' and she had tried to behave as her husband wished. *She never spoke of him* to her son (on whom she had become very dependent) or to her friends, and *she did not cry*. She thought she might feel better if she did, but her husband had been 'so good' that she felt she owed it to him to be brave. During the consultation she described their relationship in such idyllic terms that the psychiatrist suspected that it was rather ambivalent.

Diagnosis
Delayed grief in an ambivalent relationship.

Management
During the initial consultation the psychiatrist explained to Mrs J. why it was necessary for her to grieve, drawing for her the diagram of Fig. 22.4. He used the techniques of guided mourning; asking her to let herself realize how much she missed her husband, to look at and bring with her photographs and mementoes of him, and to talk about him with her son. He warned her that she would be more upset than before, and arranged to see her regularly. When he gained her confidence he reduced and then discontinued the antidepressant.

She began to grieve and as sessions progressed it became clear that her husband's 'goodness' had entailed doing so much for her that she felt helpless and unduly dependent. Idealization turned to anger, which in turn led to guilt. She transferred her dependence to the psychiatrist who supported her as she worked through her grief, encouraging her to say goodbye to her husband, and then to himself as the sessions ended.

Outcome
Initial increase in distress followed by improvement over a period of 6 months. She began to take an active part in the life of her village, and depended less on her son who then felt able to leave home permanently for the first time.

are precipitated by bereavement. Phobic anxiety states, hypochondriasis, and psychosomatic illnesses require treatment in their own right, but usual measures may be unsuccessful unless the bereavement factor which precipitated or exacerbated the problem is given due weight. The bereaved alcoholic poses special difficulties as he is liable to make many demands on the caring services but be unable to progress through his grief until his drinking comes under control. Patients of this kind need an experienced therapist who can combine an understanding and supportive attitude with the capacity to set limits and avoid over-involvement.

Outcome

The outcome of normal grief is, by definition, resolution. How long this takes is difficult to state since there is no clear end to grief. Early writers tended to think in terms of months or a year, but it is now recognized that the bereaved may have symptoms from time to time for much longer. Most of them do not expect to get over bereavement in the way one recovers from an illness or an accident, but rather to adjust to it, achieving a new life-style which may be different from the one before bereavement, but is also satisfactory and rewarding.

QUESTIONS

1 A man of 60, whose wife suddenly died of coronary heart disease 3 months previously, complains of breathlessness, palpitations, and vague chest pain. What are the possible causes of his symptoms? What questions would you ask to assess the quality of his grief, and what investigations and care might he need?

2 Two months after her 8-year-old son was killed in a road accident, a woman of 30 complains that she feels very restless but is unable to sleep. Her husband, who only drank occasionally before, now spends most evenings in the pub, and she sees him as callous and unsympathetic to her grief. Their 6-year-old daughter clings to her mother and is unwilling to go to school. How might you interpret these changes in her husband and child to her? What sort of help is likely to benefit this family?

3 A woman of 69 has been a widow for a year, but she seems as upset as she was in the first month after her husband's death. Her daughter says 'Mum should be getting over it by now.' What are the probable causes of this syndrome, and how might you help this widow and her daughter?

FURTHER READING

Worden W. (1991) *Grief Counselling and Grief Therapy*. Tavistock Publications, London. [A practical and comprehensive book covering the diagnosis and management of normal and abnormal grief, including short sections on special types of loss such as stillbirth, suicide, etc.]

Murray-Parkes C. (1986) *Bereavement: Studies of Grief in Adult Life*. Tavistock Publications, London. [A description of the phenomenology, determinants, and outcomes of bereavement, mainly in widows, with less emphasis on management.]

Stroebe M.S., Stroebe W. & Hansson R.O. (eds) (1993) *Handbook of Bereavement: Theory, Research and Intervention*. Cambridge University Press, Cambridge. [Comprehensive coverage of all aspects of the subject.]

USEFUL ADDRESSES

CRUSE – The National Organisation for the Bereaved, Cruse House, 126 Sheen Road, Richmond, Surrey TW6 1UR (tel: 081-940 4818/9047). [Provides counselling and advisory service and opportunities for social contact.]

National Association of Bereavement Services, 20 Norton Folgate, London E1 6DB (tel: 071-247 1080/0617). [Produce a National Directory of Bereavement and Loss Services which is being continually updated. It lists local services and also services for particular groups, e.g. widows and widowers, parents, gays, those bereaved by cot death, sudden infant death, suicide, etc.]

23
Sexual Problems

Fact sheet

Sexual dysfunctions

Females
- Low sexual desire.
- Impaired sexual arousal.
- Orgasmic dysfunction.
- Vaginismus.
- Dyspareunia.

Males
- Low sexual desire.
- Erectile dysfunction.
- Premature ejaculation.
- Retarded ejaculation.

Prevalence
- *Females*: perhaps 10% of women consider themselves to have a problem, but only a small proportion of these wish help. Most frequent problem is low sexual desire. Sexual problems common in gynaecology and menopause clinics.
- *Males*: Most common dysfunction is probably premature ejaculation, but erectile dysfunction is most common problem among those seeking help. In the general population, erectile dysfunction in less than 1% of men age 30; over 25% at age 70. Erectile difficulties frequent among attenders at diabetic and genito-urinary clinics.

Causes
- Usually multiple.
- *Predisposing factors* include early environmental influences and events.
- *Precipitants* include times of life change, stress, conflict, physical and psychiatric illness, surgery and medication.
- *Maintaining factors* include anxiety, dysfunctional thoughts (e.g. performance concerns) and beliefs, conflict, poor communication and lack of information.

Assessment
Personal, sexual and psychiatric history of each partner. Physical examination and further tests when necessary.

Treatment
- *Sex therapy*: combination of homework assignments, counselling and education. Up to two-thirds of couples derive benefits.
- *Brief counselling* and *education*.
- *Marital therapy*.
- *Physical treatments*.

Sexual deviations

Variations in sexual behaviour include
- Exhibitionism.
- Voyeurism.
- Sadism.
- Masochism.

Disorders of sexual object include
- Fetishism.
- Transvestism.
- Paedophilia.

Disturbance of gender role
- Transsexualism.

Prevalence
- Rare in women, except sadism, masochism and transsexualism.
- Exhibitionism is most common offence due to sexual deviance in England and Wales.
- Prevalence of most deviations uncertain as rarely come to medical attention.

Causes
Many factors have been suggested, including genetic, early environmental influences, conditioning, social anxiety and inadequacy, and personality disorders. Causes in most cases remain obscure.

Reasons for coming to medical attention
Guilt, shame, fear of conviction, depression, being charged with an offence, partner requests help.

Assessment
Personal, sexual and psychiatric history. Need to assess role of the deviant behaviour in the individual's life. Motivation.

Treatment
Possible aims:
- reduction in deviant interest (behaviour therapy or libido-reducing medication);
- increasing heterosexual adjustment;
- adjustment to deviant behaviour.

Homosexuality
Sexual attraction to members of one's own sex. Considerable variations between individuals in extent of homosexual and heterosexual interest.

Prevalence
Approximately 7% of males age 30; 2–4% of females.

Legal
Age of consent for male homosexual behaviour is 18 years.

Causes
Many genetic, early environmental and learning theory explanations have been put forward. None has been substantiated.

Reasons for medical attention
Now rarely for concerns about sexual orientation. Increasingly because of AIDS, including fears of disease, advice on prevention, and help with the physical and psychological consequences of carrying the AIDS virus or having contracted the disease.

What are sexual problems?

Sexual problems are of two types – **sexual dysfunctions** and **sexual deviations**. Both are difficult to define.

Sexual dysfunctions include any persistent impairment of the normal patterns of sexual interest or response. However, this definition can be criticized on two counts. First, it is virtually impossible to indicate precise limits of normality in sexual functioning because, as Kinsey and colleagues' studies in the USA a few decades ago demonstrated, the variations in sexual behaviour in the general population are vast. Secondly, the extent to which an individual's sexuality seems dysfunctional will depend on many factors, including whether the person thinks there is a problem, his or her expectations and needs, current social values and the responses of professionals to requests for help.

Sexual deviance is a term applied to any sexual interest or activity that is preferred to, or displaces, adult heterosexual interest or behaviour, or that is considered unusual or bizarre, and that violates laws or prevailing social codes. It is possible for a form of sexuality considered deviant at one point in time largely to cease to be so in another era. Homosexuality provides the best example, although for completeness and because of its importance it is included in this chapter.

Sexual dysfunctions

How are sexual dysfunctions classified?

Many sexual dysfunctions can be categorized according to the phase of sexual response which is affected. As a result of their pioneering studies of sexuality during the 1950s and 1960s, Masters and Johnson identified three phases of sexual response – **excitement**, **orgasm** and **resolution**. During the **excitement** (or **arousal**) phase various physiological changes occur, but especially erection in the male and genital engorgement and lubrication in the female. **Orgasm** in both sexes includes subjective sensations and physiological events, particularly seminal emission and ejaculation in the male and pelvic muscle contractions in the female. During **resolution** the physiological changes of arousal are gradually reversed. In males this phase includes a refractory period of variable length, from minutes to hours or more according to age, before sexual arousal and orgasm can occur again. The refractory period may not occur in females, some experiencing further orgasms in close succession. Sexual dysfunctions cannot be classified in terms of sexual response alone, because another very important aspect of sexuality is **sexual interest** or desire. This refers to a person's sexual drive or willingness to engage in sexual behaviour with the partner.

The types of sexual dysfunction usually recognized are listed in Fig. 23.1 (note: different terms may be used to describe the same dysfunction, e.g. 'low libido' instead of 'low sexual desire'). Each sexual dysfunction can also be categorized according to whether it has been present from the onset of sexual activity (**primary**) or began after a period

Fig. 23.1 Sexual dysfunctions

Aspects of sexuality affected	Females	Males
Sexual interest	Low sexual desire	Low sexual desire
Sexual arousal	Impaired sexual arousal	Erectile dysfunction
Orgasm	Orgasmic dysfunction	Premature ejaculation Retarded ejaculation
Other types of dysfunction	Vaginismus Dyspareunia	

of normal sexual functioning (**secondary**), and whether it occurs in all settings (**total**) or in some settings (e.g. with a partner) but not others (e.g. masturbation) (**situational**).

The female sexual dysfunctions

Low sexual desire

As with most types of sexual dysfunction this category includes a wide range of difficulties, ranging from a lack of spontaneous interest in sex but an ability to respond to the partner's approaches with pleasurable arousal, to a lack of interest in initiating sexual activity and being averse to the sexual approaches of the partner. Levels of sexual desire vary greatly from one woman to another (the same is true of men), and it is impossible to draw a clear distinction between normal and abnormal. Sexual interest is not only manifested in behaviour with a partner, but also in sexual thoughts and fantasies, attraction to other people, and masturbation. (Note: the term 'frigidity' should not be used as it is non-specific and has perjorative connotations.)

Impaired sexual arousal

Problems concerning sexual arousal are characterized by failure of the physiological responses and sensations which normally occur during sexual activity. They are relatively uncommon in women who have unimpaired sexual interest, except soon after childbirth and following the menopause. However, some women, due to sexual inhibitions, are unable to respond to sexual stimulation in spite of being interested in sex.

Orgasmic dysfunction

A substantial proportion of women do not experience orgasm on all or many occasions of sexual activity, but nevertheless enjoy their sexual relationships and should not be regarded as having a sexual problem. The extent to which a woman views herself as having a problem concerning orgasm will depend on her and her partner's expectations. Primary total orgasmic dysfunction is, however, regarded by most individuals as a problem. When a woman has previously been able to experience orgasm but now no longer can, this also is likely to be a problem.

Vaginismus

In this condition, sexual intercourse is impossible or extremely painful because, whenever vaginal penetration is attempted, spasm occurs in the muscles surrounding the entrance to the vagina. This is nearly always the result of a specific phobia concerning vaginal penetration. The response of the vaginal muscles is automatic, the woman having little or no control over it. Vaginismus is usually a primary problem, although it can occasionally occur as a secondary problem following a sexual trauma (e.g. rape) or vaginal infection. Most women with this problem can enjoy other aspects of sexual activity.

Dyspareunia

This means that pain is experienced during sexual intercourse. Sometimes the pain is located at the entrance to the vagina in which case it may be due to mild vaginismus or a physical disorder (e.g. vaginal infection or a Bartholin's cyst). When dyspareunia is experienced on deep penetration a physical cause (e.g. endometriosis or salpingitis) should be suspected. However, it can also occur because of lack of sexual arousal, the inner part of the vagina normally expanding and the cervix elevating during arousal.

The male sexual dysfunctions

Low sexual desire

Men far less often seek help for this problem than do women, probably because men with severe loss of interest are likely to have erectile dysfunction and will ask for help with this instead.

Erectile dysfunction

The erectile response is very vulnerable to a wide range of physical disorders, medication and drugs, and also to psychological influences, especially anxiety and distracting thoughts. Erectile dysfunction can range from a total problem (in which case it is usually due to a physical cause) to one only occurring when sexual intercourse is attempted. Sometimes, especially in men with physical disorders, only partial erections can be obtained.

Case 1: fear of failure

Mr J. was a 55-year-old businessman. After *drinking heavily* at a party one evening he tried to make love to his wife but became concerned when he found that he could not get an erection. A few days later he once more tried making love, but was so *anxious*, fearing that the same thing would happen, that again he could not get an erection. Subsequent episodes of failure followed. *Unable to discuss the problem* with his wife he eventually avoided sex altogether. Three months later his wife persuaded him to go to his doctor.
In discussion with the doctor

Alcohol often diminishes sexual performance.

Erectile difficulties often follow an initial failure experience which leads to performance anxiety.

Communication difficulties may confound the problem.

Continued

Case 1 (*Continued*)

Mr J. was initially very embarrassed, saying he felt humiliated by the problem. He found it difficult to understand as, until recently, he had always kept himself physically fit. However, he did say that his alcohol consumption had risen substantially in the past 2 years, ever since he had been under increasing stress at work. No abnormality was found on *physical examination* except slight obesity and a moderately enlarged liver. Blood tests for *fasting blood glucose* and sex hormone levels were normal but liver function tests were mildly abnormal. Mrs J. was a shy attractive woman, 10 years younger than her husband. She was keen to help with the problem but found her husband difficult to talk to about sex. The doctor first offered Mr J. *advice on gaining control over his drinking*. When Mr J. had reduced his consumption to a social level the doctor referred he and his wife to a specialist who offered them sex therapy. During treatment it became apparent that Mr J. was obsessed with his *sexual performance*. In addition he expressed the fear that his wife might look for another partner. Therapy focused *on helping the couple discuss their sexual relationship* and on encouraging Mr J. to engage in sexual activity without constant self-monitoring.
After 4 months' treatment the problem was largely resolved, although Mr J. had two setbacks when he tried to make love when feeling very tired after stressful days at work. A further catastrophic response to these was prevented because Mr and Mrs J. were now able to discuss what had happened and reassure each other.

Physical investigations are often indicated in cases of erectile dysfunction. This problem can occasionally be the presenting symptom of diabetes mellitus.

Before attempting any specific treatment for a sexual problem alcohol consumption should be under control.

Performance anxieties, especially fear of failure, commonly become apparent during treatment of erectile dysfunction. Encouraging communication between partners is a major ingredient in sex therapy.

Premature ejaculation

There is no entirely satisfactory definition of premature ejaculation. While a man who always or usually ejaculates before sexual intercourse begins would clearly be regarded as having a problem, it is not appropriate to say how long a man should be able to prolong sexual intercourse before ejaculation occurs. Most clinicians rely on the extent to which a man and his partner think he has reasonable control over his speed of ejaculation. Rapid ejaculation is extremely

Case 2: the unconsummated marriage

Mrs P. was a 26-year-old shop assistant who presented to her general practitioner because she had *not been able to conceive* following 3 years of marriage. Upon further enquiry it became apparent that she and her husband had *never had full sexual intercourse*. Despite being able to enjoy foreplay, during which she became aroused, whenever sexual intercourse was attempted Mrs P. became tense and vaginal penetration was impossible. Sexual activity between Mr and Mrs P. had gradually become less and less frequent, although they remained very fond of each other. Both partners were extremely distressed by the problem. Mrs P. regarded herself as a freak and *assumed that her husband might seek out another partner.* Mr P. thought the problem might have something to do with his having had a circumcision at the age of 16 because of a tight foreskin. When her doctor obtained a sexual history from Mrs P. it became apparent that she had been brought up in a *family where sex was never discussed.* She had *not been prepared for menstruation* and when her first menstrual period began she thought she was dying. She had found it impossible to use tampons, attempts at inserting them having been painful. At the age of 15 *an uncle had twice attempted to engage her in sexual activity*, including trying sexual intercourse, which had frightened and disgusted her. Mrs P. had never told her husband about this. She had two boyfriends before she met her husband but always refused sexual contact except mild petting. Mr P. was also sexually inexperienced when he met his wife. When they first attempted sexual intercourse on their honeymoon this was a disaster, both of them feeling awkward and embarrassed. *Mr P. tried to have sexual intercourse when his wife was unaroused, but this was unsuccessful and very painful for Mrs P.* Gradually they became able to enjoy foreplay, but intercourse was never possible. Eventually they abandoned trying to have intercourse and sexual contact became less and less frequent. They were both keen to have children, although *Mrs P. was terrified by the idea of childbirth.* She thought that her vagina was far too small to accomodate her husband's penis let alone a baby.

When her general practitioner attempted a vaginal examination Mrs P. became very tense and the examination could only be completed with difficulty. However, apart from obvious spasm of the vaginal muscles the doctor could detect no other abnormalities. It was clear that Mrs P. had vaginismus. During subsequent discussion it became obvious that Mrs P. was largely ignorant about her sexual anatomy. After taking a full history from both partners the doctor gained the impression that, apart from this sexual problem, Mr and Mrs P. had a satisfactory relationship and were both keen to overcome the sexual difficulty. She therefore began a course of sex therapy.

She decided first to concentrate on helping Mrs P. become more comfortable with her sexual anatomy, using pictures from a book to increase her understanding. Subsequently she encouraged Mrs P. to examine her genitals with a mirror and later to explore her vagina with her fingers. She also taught her to gain more control over her vaginal muscles by learning to contract and relax them. After several weeks of practice Mrs P. became more confident, accepting that her genitals were normal and that sexual intercourse should be possible.

At this stage *the doctor explained the sensate focus exercises to both partners* and encouraged them to practise these in order to start rebuilding their sexual relationship. Later Mr P. was able to explore his wife's vagina with a finger under her guidance. Once this stage was established the couple were instructed to try vaginal containment, using the female

Non-consummation sometimes first comes to medical attention when a couple complain of infertility.

Fear of losing the partner is often a reason for seeking help for sexual difficulties.

Sexual problems are often associated with an inhibited upbringing.

A history of incest or child sexual abuse is common among women with sexual difficulties.

A sexual problem of this kind can be precipitated by a traumatic first attempt at sexual intercourse.

Extreme fear concerning childbirth and distorted ideas about vaginal anatomy may contribute to such a sexual problem.

The diagnosis of vaginismus, suggested by the history, can be confirmed by vaginal examination. This can also exclude other causes of the problem (e.g. unruptured hymen, congenital abnormality).

Education is often an important component in treating people with sexual difficulties.

Sensate focus is a useful way for couples to begin to re-establish their sexual relationship.

Continued on p. 290

superior position.
This proved difficult and Mrs P.
became very distressed.
When she next saw the doctor
she broke down weeping in the
surgery, and it took careful
explanation and encouragement
by the doctor to help her admit
to her husband the fact of her
uncle's attempted sexual

Blocks to progress are often
encountered during sex therapy
and careful counselling is then
necessary to help establish and
overcome the reasons for these.

intercourse and the fear this
had caused her. Mr P. was very
understanding and the couple
left the surgery more confident
of success. Vaginal containment
was soon successful and after a
further couple of weeks *they*
were able to have sexual
intercourse.

Sex therapy is nearly always
successful in the treatment of
vaginismus.

---

common in young men having their first sexual experiences with a partner and should not be regarded at that stage as constituting a dysfunction.

Retarded ejaculation

This problem affects ejaculation and the experience of orgasm, with both either not occurring at all during sexual activity or only with great difficulty. Most men with this problem experience nocturnal emissions but do not ejaculate either in masturbation or during sexual activity with a partner, whilst in some the problem is confined to activity with a partner. There are other types of ejaculatory problems not commonly seen in psychiatric practice. These include **retrograde ejaculation**, when orgasm occurs but the ejaculate passes into the bladder instead of along the urethra (this is usually the result of either surgery, especially prostatectomy, or medication), and **painful ejaculation**, which is usually the result of an infection (e.g. non-specific urethritis).

In addition to the sexual dysfunctions of males and females considered above, some people experience a general lack of enjoyment or satisfaction from their sexual relationships and may seek help for this.

How common are sexual dysfunctions?

Little attention has been paid to the extent of sexual difficulties in the general population. From the research which has been conducted it appears that they are common, especially in females. Thus in one study a third of women had some sort of sexual dysfunction. However, only 10% of the whole sample regarded themselves as having an actual problem and only a third of these wished to have help for it. Low sexual desire and orgasmic dysfunction are the most frequent problems found in such surveys. Not surprisingly, sexual dysfunctions are likely to be more common in certain clinical populations, especially women attending gynaecology clinics, notably menopause clinics. Very little is known about the extent of sexual dysfunctions amongst men in the general population. Whilst premature ejaculation is probably the most common problem, Kinsey and his colleagues found that the prevalence of erectile dysfunction increases markedly with age, from less than 1% at age 30 to over 25% at age 70. Clinical settings in which erectile dysfunction is especially frequent include urology and diabetic clinics.

In clinics specializing in the treatment of sexual difficulties the most common reasons for referral are low sexual desire in women and erectile dysfunction in men.

What are the causes of sexual dysfunction?

Sexual dysfunctions can result from a wide variety of psychological and physical causes. Even when a dysfunction has a physical basis, psychological factors may also be relevant, and vice versa. In each case it is helpful to consider physical, psychological and interpersonal dimensions of the problem, rather than a dichotomous view (i.e. 'Is it physical *or* is it psychological?'). A chronological subdivision of causes into **predisposing factors**, **precipitants** and **maintaining factors** is a useful way of viewing aetiology (Fig. 23.2).

Many people with sexual difficulties have been brought up in a family environment in which sexuality is a taboo subject, or where very negative attitudes have been apparent. Sexual traumas, such as childhood sexual abuse, incest and sexual assault, can undoubtedly lead to sexual difficulties but we do not know in what proportion of cases this is so. Primary sexual dysfunctions may have lacked an obvious precipitant. However, for many secondary dysfunctions it is usually possible to identify a fairly clear precipitant. Common precipitants include times of life change (e.g. marriage, childbirth, menopause), conflict in a relationship, physical illness, and psychiatric disorders, especially depression. There are clear associations between sexuality and mood. Thus sexual interest often covaries with a person's sense of well-being, low sexual desire is a common symptom of depression, and persistent low sexual desire often follows an episode of depression, particularly post-natal depression.

Fig. 23.2 Examples of causes of sexual dysfunction

Predisposing factors
Inhibited upbringing
Inadequate sex education
Sexual trauma

Precipitants

Childbirth	Depression	Physical illness
Infidelity	Menopause	Surgery
Conflict	Sexual trauma	Medication
		Alcohol abuse

Maintaining factors

Expectation of failure	Physical illness
Distracting performance-orientated thoughts	Medication
Anxiety	Depression
Discord in general relationship	Lack of information
Poor communication	

Fig. 23.3 Examples of physical disorders and treatments which may cause sexual dysfunctions

Physical disorders

System	Disorder	Possible sexual dysfunction
Cardiovascular	Arteriosclerosis	Erectile dysfunction
	Hypertension	Erectile dysfunction
	Myocardial infarction	Loss of interest
Endocrine	Diabetes	Erectile dysfunction; impaired interest and arousal in women
	Hypogonadism	Impaired sexual interest and arousal
	Hyperprolactinaemia	Erectile dysfunction
Genito-urinary	Peyronie's disease	Erectile dysfunction
	Priapism	Erectile dysfunction
	Pelvic or genital infection	Dyspareunia
Musculoskeletal	Arthritis	Mechanical difficulties
Neurological	Epilepsy	Impaired sexual interest
	Spinal cord injury	Impaired sexual arousal and orgasm
	Multiple sclerosis	(as above)
Renal	Renal failure	Loss of interest

Surgery

	Procedure	Possible effects
	Rectal resection	Erectile dysfunction
	Prostatectomy	Retrograde ejaculation (radical prostatectomy often causes erectile dysfunction)
	Mastectomy	Loss of interest
	Oophorectomy	(see hypogonadism)
	Vaginal operations for malignancy	Dyspareunia
	Episiotomy	Dyspareunia
	Amputations	Mechanical difficulties

Medication

Class	Example	Possible effects
Antihypertensives	Most	Erectile dysfunction
	Propranolol	Erectile dysfunction and loss of interest
Diuretics	Bendrofluazide	Erectile dysfunction
Hypnotics and minor tranquillizers	Diazepam Nitrazepam	Loss of interest
Major tranquillizers	Chlorpromazine	Loss of interest, impaired arousal, erectile dysfunction and retrograde ejaculation
Tricylic antidepressants	Amitriptyline	Erectile dysfunction
Serotonergic antidepressants	Fluoxetine	Retarded ejaculation, orgasmic dysfunction

Once established, a sexual dysfunction may persist in spite of resolution of the cause – this may be because of lack of confidence, anxiety and persisting dysfunctional thoughts. However, continuing discord and poor communication are often very important. Sexual problems in men commonly reflect concerns with sexual performance, whereas those of women are more often due to concerns about the overall relationship, especially lack of emotional intimacy.

Many physical disorders and their treaments can interfere with sexual function, some of the more important examples being listed in Fig. 23.3. Diabetes mellitus is a particularly important cause of sexual dysfunction in men, erectile dysfunction occurring in approximately a quarter of 30-year-old men with this condition, and thereafter becoming increasingly common. Some physical illnesses or surgical procedures may cause sexual problems because of consequent anxiety (e.g. myocardial infarction), embarrassment (e.g. ileostomy or colostomy), or disturbance of body image (e.g. mastectomy). Antihypertensives are the most important group of drugs which interfere with sexual function. Propranolol, for example, may cause loss of interest or erectile dysfunction in as many as 17% of users. Neuroleptics, especially when used long term, frequently cause sexual problems; this can be an important factor leading to non-compliance.

Alcohol and drug abuse are further important causes of sexual difficulties. Alcohol may affect sexual function by many means, including peripheral neuropathy, liver and testicular damage, and the catastrophic effects that alcohol abuse can have on relationships.

How do people with sexual dysfunctions present to doctors?
As attitudes to sexuality have changed and it has become more widely known that people with sexual dysfunction can often be helped, direct requests for help have become more common. However, often the presentation is more covert and whether or not a problem is detected may depend on the skills of the doctor and his or her willingness to discuss sexuality with a patient. Sometimes a patient draws attention to a sexual problem by a physical complaint, such as a vaginal discharge. In other cases a problem will only be detected if the doctor asks specifically about sexual function, such as when assessing the effects of an illness, operation or medication. Specific enquiry in family planning, infertility or menopause clinics will often uncover sexual difficulties.

Doctors differ greatly in their attitudes regarding the importance of sexual dysfunctions. Yet for many patient these problems are devastating and may lead to severe emotional problems and/or breakdown of relationships. It is imperative that doctors appreciate these facts. Sometimes doctors themselves find it difficult to discuss sexual matters with patients, thus making it difficult or impossible for patients with problems to receive help. Guidance and help with this aspect of medical care should be part of every doctor's training.

Assessment of people with sexual dysfunctions
Before one can plan treatment a careful **assessment** must be carried out. When assessing a couple the partners should be interviewed separately, at least initially, because most people are more frank in their answers when seen alone. The

Fig. 23.4 Topics to be covered during the assessment of sexual dysfunction

- Nature and development of the sexual problem.
- Family background and early childhood – especially parental relationship, and family attitudes to sexuality.
- Early sexual development and experiences, including homosexuality and any sexual traumas (e.g. sexual abuse).
- Sexual information – source and extent.
- Masturbation – occurrence and whether dysfunction experienced (especially orgasmic dysfunction, erectile dysfunction or retarded ejaculation).
- Previous sexual relationships – especially whether current problem occurred.
- Relationship with partner – its development, sexual relationship, general relationship, children and contraception, infidelity, commitment.
- Schooling, occupation, interests, religious beliefs.
- Medical and psychiatric history.
- Use of alcohol, drugs and medication.
- Mental state (although formal mental state examination usually unnecessary).
- Goals (what changes are desired) and motivation (willingness to engage in treatment).
- Physical examination and investigations (if necessary).

important areas to cover are listed in Fig. 23.4. Many people will naturally be embarrassed when discussing their sexual difficulties and experiences. This should not cause the interviewer to avoid topics but does mean that the interview should be conducted in a relaxed and reassuring manner. It is often helpful to acknowledge the patient's embarrassment and explain how this is understandable. When a particular topic proves exceedingly difficult, this can be put aside and broached again later. With tact and understanding on the part of the interviewer most people are able to discuss their difficulties openly and are often very relieved by having done so.

A physical examination is by no means always necessary, but is indicated in men with erectile dysfunction, and in some cases of low sexual desire when the history suggests a possible physical cause. Physical examination of men with erectile problems should particularly include testing of peripheral sensation, reflexes, circulation and blood pressure, and examination of the genitals, together with a careful search for any general signs of illness. The diagnosis of vaginismus can be confirmed to physical examination because spasm of the vaginal muscles will usually occur when vaginal examination is attempted. When dyspareunia is the presenting complaint a gynaecological or genito-urinary assessment may be necessary.

In the USA and elswhere, but only in a few centres in the UK, specialized investigations for erectile dysfunction (e.g. nocturnal penile tumescence recordings, corpus cavernosgraphy, and arteriography of the genital blood supply) may be used to assist in the differential diagnosis of cases with a likely organic cause. When indicated, blood tests should be ordered for sex hormones (especially testosterone and luteinizing hormone), prolactin, and fasting blood glucose (or a glucose tolerance test arranged).

Treatment approaches for people with sexual dysfunctions

Psychological methods

Psychological treatment of sexual dysfunctions is now carried out by a wide variety of professionals, including some marriage guidance counsellors, family planning doctors, general practitioners, psychiatrists, clinical psychologists and gynaecologists.

Sex therapy

Until a couple of decades ago sexual dysfunctions were regarded as symptoms of disturbances of personality originating in early childhood experiences. Thus Freud postulated that failure of normal maturation in one of the phases of childhood sexuality, which interfered with the development of an individual's relationship with one or both parents, was the root of most sexual problems. Such problems were therefore regarded as difficult to treat, requiring lengthy psychoanalysis or insight-orientated psychotherapy. During the late 1950s and 1960s, behavioural approaches such as systematic desensitization were tried with some success, but it was not until 1970 when Masters and Johnson published their treatment approach that a real breakthrough occurred. This approach, now known as sex therapy, incorporates three elements – homework assignments, education and counselling – and is focused on couples rather than individual partners.

The homework assignments in sex therapy are summarized in Fig. 23.5. These behavioural components in the programme enable a couple to tackle their sexual difficulties step-by-step. Education is an important element in treatment and involves providing basic information about sexual anatomy and response, and correcting misinformation. Counselling is the crucial factor in most cases, and involves helping a couple communicate more openly, examination of attitudes which are preventing enjoyment of sex, including, when necessary, investigating the origins of such attitudes, and helping the couple resolve general relationship conflicts which may be contributing to the problem.

Sex therapy normally lasts between six and 18 sessions over 2 to 6 months. Up to two-thirds of couples derive substantial benefits from treatment, often with consequent improvement in their general relationship. The results of treatment are excellent for vaginismus (with a 90% success rate), and very satisfactory for psychogenic erectile dysfunc-

Fig. 23.5 Homework assignments in sex therapy

- Ban on sexual intercourse and intimate sexual activity.
- Sensate focus – partners take turns at exploring each others' bodies non-sexually.
- Genital sensate focus – genitals and breasts included in exploration.
- Specific techniques for particular problems – e.g. squeeze or stop-start techniques for premature ejaculation, waxing and waning for erectile dysfunction, graded vaginal penetration using fingers or dilators for vaginismus.
- Gradual return to sexual intercourse – via an intermediate stage of 'vaginal containment'.

tion (although this approach can also be of assistance where the cause is partly physical), premature ejaculation and orgasmic dysfunction. Low sexual desire has a varied outcome, reflecting the fact that this problem may be related to general relationship issues, severe psychological conflicts or constitutional factors.

Whilst sex therapy was originally developed for couples, its principles can be applied in the treatment of individuals without partners although the results of such treatment are difficult to ascertain.

Brief counselling and education

A full sex therapy programme is unnecessary for many people with sexual dysfunctions. Instead, brief counselling, including advice, recommending self-help books and simple educational measures may suffice. This should be within the scope of many doctors, especially general practitioners.

Marital therapy

When assessing couples with sexual difficulties it is essential to distinguish between those whose sexual problem is the main difficulty (and for whom one of the approaches mentioned above will be appropriate) and those where the principal problem lies in their general relationship – marital therapy will be the treatment of choice in these latter cases (see p. 236). If necessary, sex therapy can be offered later when the relationship has improved.

Physical methods

Several advances have recently occurred in the physical treatment of sexual dysfunctions. Some of these are listed in Fig. 23.6. Penile prostheses have been in vogue in the USA. However, the long-term outcome with these is uncertain. Use of injectable pharmacological agents in the treatment of erectile dysfunction is a new approach which requires further evaluation. Vacuum devices are gaining in

popularity, being safe, non-invasive and relatively effective. Hormonal treatments should only be used where there is evidence of hormonal abnormality.

Can sexual dysfunctions be prevented?
The contributions of inadequate information about sexuality and inhibited attitudes to the development of sexual dysfunctions have already been noted. Appropriate sex education might therefore have a major role in preventing some sexual problems in adulthood. Whilst ideally this would be provided by parents, many themselves lack the necessary knowledge and are not comfortable with sexuality. Therefore this needs to be provided in schools. Such education would probably be most effective if it was incorporated in a broad educational programme concerning human relationships, including attention to personal responsibility, and moral and religious aspects of sexuality. The media have considerable potential for prevention of sexual difficulties. For example, responsible use of television, magazines and newspapers for increasing awareness about sexuality could help promote healthy and informed attitudes.

Sexual deviations

What is the nature and prevalence of sexual deviations?
There are many types of sexual deviation, some of which very rarely come to medical attention. Here only the more common deviations will be considered. In addition, a separate section is devoted to homosexuality. A striking fact is that most sexual deviations are entirely or almost entirely confined to males. The only exceptions are transsexualism, sadism and masochism.

Sexual deviation can be grouped into three categories (Fig. 23.7), the most frequent examples of which are considered below.

Exhibitionism
This is exposure of the genitals to unprepared members of the opposite sex, usually strangers, for the purpose of sexual gratification. Rarely does the exhibitionist attempt to engage the 'victim' in further sexual behaviour. Exhibitionism is

---

Fig. 23.6 Some physical methods used in treating sexual dysfunctions

Erectile dysfunction
- Penile prostheses – flexible or inflatable prosthesis implanted in corpora cavernosa. Usual indication: irreversible organic erectile dysfunction, especially in younger men.
- Intra-cavernosal injections of smooth muscle relaxants (e.g. papaverine) – produce erections of sufficient duration for sexual intercourse. Usual indications as above.
- Vacuum devices – usually produce a full erection, which is then sustained with a constriction ring. Helpful for men with severe or moderate erectile problems related to physical factors, and may be helpful for some with psychogenic problems.
- Penile ring – helpful for some men with poor genital circulation but who can obtain partial erections.

Impaired sexual interest and arousal
- Hormone replacement (testosterone, oestrogens) where evidence of hypogonadism.
- Bromocriptine in cases of hyperprolactinaemia.

Orgasmic dysfunction or retarded ejaculation
- Vibrator.

Fig. 23.7 Classification of sexual deviations and the more common examples in each group

Variations in sexual behaviour
Exhibitionism
Voyeurism
Sadism
Masochism

Disorders of sexual object
Fetishism
Transvestism
Paedophilia

Disturbance of gender role
Transsexualism

Fig. 23.8 Two types of exhibitionist

1	2
Inhibited young man	Sociopathic personality
Relatively normal personality	Exposes in aroused state, with erect penis and usually masturbating
Struggles against impulse to expose	
Exposes with flaccid penis	Sadistic element to behaviour
Does not masturbate during exposure	Derives pleasure from the act and experiences little shame or guilt
Derives little pleasure from act and feels guilty and humiliated by his behaviour	

almost entirely confined to males, although there have been occasional reports of female exhibitionists who expose their breasts or, very rarely, their genitalia. Most exhibitionists frequently repeat the behaviour. Indecent exposure describes the legal offence, which is the most common offence due to deviant sexual behaviour in England and Wales, making up about a quarter of sexual offences dealt with by the courts.

Two broad types of exhibitionist have been described (Fig. 23.8). Most acts of exhibitionism are preceded by a mounting feeling of tension. During the act the individual usually seeks to evoke a strong emotional reaction in the victim, such as surprise or shock. Some exhibitionists take considerable risks of being caught. There appears to be an association between exhibitionism and making obscene telephone calls.

Voyeurism

The voyeur ('peeping Tom') derives sexual pleasure from observing the sexual behaviour of other people or from observing women undressing, taking care not to be noticed by those he is watching. The act is usually accompanied or followed by masturbation. Voyeurism is confined to men, although the prevalence of this condition is not known. Most voyeurs are young, shy men who have difficulty in establishing relationships with women.

Sadism and masochism

Sadism means deriving sexual arousal and pleasure from inflicting pain on, or causing fear to, another person. Common sadistic practices include beating, whipping and bondage (tying up the other individual). Severe sadism may lead to sadistic murder, with mutilation of the victim's body, especially the genitals.

Masochism describes the association of sexual pleasure with suffering, such as through being beaten, bound or chained, or humiliated. In its extreme form masochism may be extremely dangerous, especially when practised alone, such as in males who seek sexual arousal from anoxia by strangulation or covering the head with a plastic bag.

Mild sadistic and masochistic practices are probably quite common in the sexual repertoires of some couples. It is unclear how often sadism or masochism are the predominant

Case 3: the washing line thief

Mr M. was a 25-year-old factory worker. He was referred for a psychiatric opinion after being charged with stealing women's underwear from a washing line. At interview he presented as a shy individual. He explained that during his teens he had experienced *great difficulty in forming relationships with girls*, mostly because of *feelings of inadequacy*. He first became excited by female underwear when he *masturbated using a pair of his elder sister's knickers*. During his later teens he had occasionally obtained female underwear from shops or from washing lines. His fetishistic interest diminished when he met his wife Pauline at the age of 21.

However, their *sexual relationship was unsatisfactory*, mostly because Pauline was very inhibited. Mr M. became frustrated and soon his fetishistic interest and behaviour returned, this leading to the current offence. Treatment was offered to the couple, *focusing on the difficulties in their sexual relationship*. After 3 months of sex therapy Pauline had become more relaxed about sex and hence began to enjoy it. Her husband's fetishistic interest had disappeared.

Three years later, however, Mr M. was *again caught stealing* a woman's underwear from a washing line. This offence occurred when his relationship with his wife was again in difficulties because she had become depressed after the birth of their first child.

Fetishists and exhibitionists often suffer from social inadequacy which make it difficult for them to form relationships with females.

Fetishistic interest may follow a chance association of sexual arousal with an article of clothing.

Deviant sexual interest may be fuelled by sexual dysfunction. In such cases the latter might be the initial focus of treatment.

Recidivism of deviant sexual behaviour is common. Sometimes the behaviour appears to serve a comforting function at times of stress.

sexual behaviours. Both forms of behaviour, but especially masochism, are found in women as well as men.

Fetishism

The fetishist prefers inanimate objects or individuals not usually regarded as attractive in order to become sexually aroused. Whilst many men become aroused by particular items of clothing or parts of the female body not normally associated with sexual arousal, fetishism is used to describe an extreme form of such interest where the fetishistic object displaces other means of sexual arousal. Often the sexual stimuli that arouse the individual fetishist are of a narrow variety, such as rubber clothing, women's underclothes, shoes or a particular attribute of a person, such as lameness or other deformity, or obesity.

The fetishistic interest may be acted out alone, usually through masturbation in the presence of the desired object. Sometimes the individual will wear a particular item of clothing that is arousing. The fetishist may resort to stealing in order to obtain the object (e.g. female clothing may be stolen from washing lines). A fetishist who has a sexual partner may try to get the partner to collaborate in the deviant behaviour, such as by wearing clothing that is arousing. This may also be achieved by the collaboration of a prostitute.

Fetishism is almost entirely confined to men, but the prevalence is not known, especially since this type of deviation rarely comes to medical attention except through the complaints of a partner.

Transvestism

Transvestism, or cross-dressing, is closely related to fetishism. The transvestite repeatedly dresses in the clothes of the opposite sex. Often this is done for sexual pleasure alone (fetishistic transvestism). Many transvestites are married, but may keep their cross-dressing behaviour secret from their partners. Discovery of the cross-dressing by the partner usually causes disgust and requests for professional help, but some partners will collude with the behaviour, perhaps allowing the clothing to be worn during sexual activity. Some men who cross-dress are transsexuals (see below), or effeminate homosexuals. Many women who cross-dress are lesbians or transsexuals.

Heterosexual transvestites are usually men. The prevalence is unknown, but it is not uncommon for psychiatric help to be requested for this problem, especially when it is disrupting a couple's relationship.

Paedophilia

This describes adult sexual interest in, or sexual activity with, prepubertal children. It is largely confined to men. While the prevalence is unclear, the extent of popularity of pornography involving children suggests that it is not rare. In many cases the behaviour is confined to fondling or masturbation, but in some sexual intercourse is practised or attempted and may, especially in very young children, cause injury. The paedophile may be attracted to children of the same or opposite sex, or occasionally both. Often the paedophile is an acquaintance or relative of the child. The behaviour is commonly repeated, and in many cases the child appears to cooperate with it, whether through interest or fear. Paedophilia overlaps with child sexual abuse by parents. In the latter, which mostly but not always involves sexual activity between fathers and daughters, there often appears to be some collusion on the part of the mother, who may appear to ignore the behaviour.

Paedophilia should be distinguished from opportunistic and 'secondary preferred' sexual contact with children where the perpetrator is learning disabled or mentally ill (unless coincidentally known to be a 'primary' paedophile). For example, the learning disabled adult who offends may, through his general handicap, be unconfident in approaching adult sexual partners. Similarly, acts with an adolescent girl

or boy on the part of a normal adult whose usual preference is for adults of that sex does not strictly amount diagnostically to 'primary' paedophilia. There is also a major distinction between personality disordered paedophiles (sexual psychopaths) and those who have an enjoyment of children (often played out in their profession) and who are unable otherwise to relate sexually to others. The former are unconcerned for, and often aggressive towards their victim, whilst the latter are 'kind' towards the children they abuse, albeit they often fail to see that their behaviour is wrong and, in fact, harmful. Paedophilic acts secondary to brain damage or to severe mental illness are also to be distinguished from primary paedophilia.

Transsexualism

A transsexual believes that he or she is of the opposite sex, usually has an overwhelming desire to live as a member of the opposite sex, and will often seek hormones, surgery and other procedures to achieve a 'sex change'. Estimates of the prevalence of transsexualism have been of the order of 1 in 30 000 to 1 in 100 000. Transsexualism is not confined to men, there being perhaps one female transsexual for every three or four male transsexuals.

Whilst the prevalence is relatively low, many transsexuals come to medical attention, usually requesting help with sex reassignment. Although transsexualism occasionally appears to evolve from transvestite interest, more often transsexuals report having felt unhappy with their assigned gender from a very early age. Some transsexuals, especially females, are homosexual. Clinicians often find transsexuals difficult patients, largely because of the many demands they make and moral dilemmas they may pose. However, transsexuals are usually very distressed by their predicament and depression and suicide attempts are not uncommon.

What are the causes of sexual deviations?

Whilst many aetiological theories have been put forward to explain sexual deviations, in most cases the causes are not clear. The aetiology of transsexualism is particularly puzzling.

Genetic factors appear to play little role in the direct aetiology of sexual deviation, although genetically determined aspects of personality may have some relevance. **Psychoanalytic** explanations usually focus upon disturbances during the development of childhood sexuality, which lead to fears concerning adult sexuality. **Learning theory** suggests that the deviant interest may first develop because of positive conditioning between the object of the deviant behaviour and early sexual arousal, in some cases because of a chance association. Inhibitions upon normal sexual development, possibly because of social and sexual anxiety, and reinforcement of the deviant interest through masturbation with deviant fantasies, may then strengthen and maintain the drive in the deviant direction. There is little doubt that **social anxiety** and **inadequacy** and **personality factors** may be important, at least in maintenance of deviant interest. Occasionally, **organic factors** may be relevant. For example, exhibitionism may first occur in older age because of early dementia or uraemia.

How do individuals with deviant sexual interest come to medical attention?

Deviant sexuality may come to medical attention in a variety of ways. Occasionally, a person makes a direct request for help, either because he feels ashamed or guilty about his sexual interest, or because the behaviour is against the law and he fears being caught. Such a request is more likely when a person becomes depressed. However, the desire to be rid of the deviant interest may fade once the person's mood improves. More commonly, medical assessment is requested because a person has been charged with an offence. A request for help often comes from a spouse who has just discovered her partner's deviant sexual behaviour, or has tolerated it for some time but no longer feels she can cope. A common concern is the possibility that children will become aware of the problem. Finally, deviant sexuality may come to light during assessment for sexual dysfunction.

Some doctors have very pejorative attitudes towards people with sexual deviations and these may influence their responses both to their sexual behaviour and to other health problems such people might have. It might be unreasonable to expect all doctors to share very liberal attitudes to variant sexual interest and behaviour. It is important, however, that doctors recognize any pejorative attitudes they might have and be prepared to distance themselves from these in their clinical management of their patients. Alternatively they might ask a colleague who is more comfortable with such problems to see these patients.

Management

Assessment

A careful initial assessment should cover the points listed in Fig. 23.9. In assessing the nature of the problem a behavioural analysis of the person's current sexual behaviour and attitudes should be carried out. This will include enquiring about:

1 the level of sexual drive: frequency of sexual acts (deviant and otherwise), masturbation, and sexual thoughts.

2 Stimuli that are found arousing, potentially erotic stimuli which are aversive, and the nature of sexual fantasies.

3 The antecedents, nature and consequences of a typical incident involving the deviant sexual behaviour. It is often helpful to ask the person to keep a diary record for a few weeks in order to complete this analysis.

It is especially important to establish why the person is seeking help and what he really wants. The role of the deviation in the individual's life is likely to be important in assessing whether treatment is justified. Thus to attempt to help a person rid himself of a deviation which is a central part of his life and which is a major source of comfort is unlikely to succeed or may cause considerable distress.

Whenever appropriate and possible the person's regular sexual partner should be included in the assessment. Sometimes a sexual deviation is maintained by difficulties in the sexual relationship with the partner, in which case such difficulties can be a major focus of treatment (see Case 3).

Assessment of sexual deviancy in relation to dangerousness requires painstaking detailed history taking of sexual development, experience, fantasies and behaviour. A crucial aspect is the degree of acceptance by the offender that what he does is wrong and that he wishes to change his behaviour. Where someone faces a current alleged offence history taking is generally complicated by a reluctance of the offender to be frank and, even after treatment, by (often) telling the assessor what he thinks (s)he 'wants' to hear. In relation to serious offenders penile plethysmography (PPG) is often undertaken, whereby sexual arousal is monitored against visual images of different types of sexual activities (including violence) and different sexual 'objects' (for example, children and adults of different sexes). Such tests are informative but are by no means definitive either of orientation and specific deviancy or of response to treatment. In particular, it is possible to 'fake' negative responses through 'suppression' and 'distraction'. However, PPG can be a useful adjunct to interview assessment. Initial and subsequent assessment should also take into account the fact that many offenders are vulnerable to depressive reaction during effective treatment.

Treatment

When the assessment has been completed the possible objectives and implications of treatment should then be discussed. In particular, it must be emphasized that, whatever the aim, treatment is likely to require considerable efforts on the part of the patient. Any major psychiatric disorder should be dealt with before specific treatment of a sexual deviation is attempted. Broadly speaking, treatment can have one of three aims (although they are not necessarily exclusive).

1 Facilitation of non-deviant sexual interest and behaviour.

2 A decrease in deviant sexual interest and behaviour.

3 Adjustment to the deviant behaviour. Some of the treatment approaches available to help with each of these objectives are summarized in Fig. 23.10.

Whilst a direct treatment approach to the deviant sexual interest might appear to be the obvious first step, in practice this is often not the best approach. Initially it is usually preferable to help the patient identify and improve aspects

---

Fig. 23.9 Assessment of individuals presenting because of deviant sexuality

1 The nature of the problem:
- what is the deviation?
- when did it begin?
- what is its extent, in terms of frequency, strength of drive and the results of the individual trying to control it?
- does it cause harm to others?

2 Sexual history (see Fig. 23.4), especially heterosexual adjustment.

3 Psychiatric history and current mental state (NB exclude depression, alcoholism, dementia and mania).

4 What part does the deviation play in the individual's life, e.g. source of sexual gratification, comfort from feelings of loneliness, anxiety or depression?

5 Why does the individual want to change (e.g. fear of prosecution, actual offence, pressure from spouse, depression)?

6 What does the individual want, e.g. to be rid of the deviation, help in accepting it or in partner accepting it?

7 Extent of motivation to engage in treatment programme.

Fig. 23.10 Treatment approaches for sexual deviations

Objective	Methods of treatment
Facilitation of non-deviant sexual interest and behaviour	• Advice on *increasing social contacts and reducing boredom*, e.g. joining social organizations, taking up hobbies. • *Social skills training* – if patient has major social anxieties or deficient social skills. • *Treatment of sexual dysfunction* – if dysfunction is contributing to deviant interest. • *Self-monitoring* of deviant and non-deviant sexual interest and behaviour. • *Modification of masturbation fantasies* – from deviant to non-deviant fantasies.
Decrease in deviant interest and behaviour	• *Self-control procedures* – plan and rehearse in imagination an alternative sequence of behaviour to put into action when the urge to engage in a deviant act occurs. Advice on reducing associated behaviours (e.g. heavy drinking, use of drugs). • *Modification of masturbation fantasies.* • *Aversion therapy* (largely abandoned because unpleasant and of doubtful efficacy). • *Covert sensitization* – pairing of images of deviant act with images of aversive consequences (e.g. being caught by police). • *Anti-libido medication*, e.g. cyproterone acetate – last resort when behaviour dangerous or otherwise uncontrollable.
Adjustment to the deviant behaviour	• *Advice* on minimizing danger or offence that behaviour might cause to others. • *Self-help group* – where can meet other people with similar interests.

of his current lifestyle which are fuelling the deviant interest. Several approaches are available for directly reducing deviant sexual interest, although none is highly effective. Self-control procedures are probably the best. The most realistic approach in many cases is to help the individual accept his sexual deviation. Group therapy with other individuals with similar deviant interest may also be useful.

Treatment of sex offenders is increasingly pursued through group therapy. Minor offenders often attend groups which are run by probation officers, sometimes with psychiatric pre-assessment and treatment back-up (e.g. where an offender develops a depressive illness during treatment). Treatment centres on 'confrontation' (about the extent and significance of offending), 'acceptance' (of responsibility), 'understanding' (of the methods of planning and facilitating the offence which the offender uses), 'recognition' of the risk he poses and the need to 'empathize' with victims. Otherwise, treatment methods are as defined in Fig. 23.10. As regards 'serious' sex offenders there is a decreasing tendency to offer

admission to special hospitals, rather than allowing them to go to prison. This reflects increasing pessimism about the treatability of psychopaths generally (albeit that there is little evidence of either systematic treatment *per se* or of research into treatment outcome). Indeed it is only if a (broader) 'psychopathic disorder' (in terms of the Mental Health Act) can be defined as present that detention for treatment is legally possible.

The management of transsexuals may necessitate very different measures. Introduction to a self-help group for transsexuals may be helpful. Attempts to modify the patient's conviction that he or she is of the wrong sex rarely, if ever, succeed. Most transsexuals remain persistent in their demands for help with their desired physical changes. Sex reassignment can include extensive counselling, advice on living as a member of the opposite sex, social skills training, electrolysis for male transsexuals to remove beard growth, hormone treatment (oestrogens for male transsexuals in order to produce breast enlargement, and androgens for female transsexuals to produce voice change and beard growth) and surgery (e.g. mastectomy, hysterectomy, genital surgery). This last step should only be undertaken when psychiatrist, surgeon and patient are all convinced that such a drastic step is going to be beneficial, especially as there is considerable uncertainty about the long-term outcome following sex-reassignment surgery.

Homosexuality

It is important to correct the common misunderstanding that homosexuality (sexual attraction to other individuals of one's own sex) is an all-or-none phenomenon, i.e. that a person is either heterosexual or homosexual. Thus, Kinsey and his colleagues developed a scale in which the extent of homosexuality and heterosexuality in any one individual can be scored. Some individuals are entirely homosexual in their orientation, only have sexual interest in, and sexual relationships with, members of their own sex. Others are bisexual, showing similar degrees of sexual attraction to their own and the opposite sex, whilst some individuals are predominantly homosexual (but have some heterosexual interest). The majority of people are entirely heterosexual. However, some heterosexual individuals will engage in homosexual behaviour under certain circumstances when access to the opposite sex is prevented (e.g. in prison). Distinction should be made between homosexual interest or behaviour, and homosexual identity, where erotic homosexual feelings or activity are accepted by an individual as an integral part of his or her personality.

Homosexual behaviour is extremely common in adolescence, especially in single-sex schools. The prevalence of homosexuality in adulthood is uncertain. Kinsey and colleagues found that 7% of men aged 30 were largely or entirely homosexual. It has been estimated that between 2 and 4% of females are homosexual.

Until the Sexual Offences Act of 1967 all forms of male homosexuality were illegal in this country. Under the Act the legal age of consent for male homosexuality was 21, but in 1994 was reduced to 18 years. The age of consent for heterosexual behaviour is 16 years. No laws exist specifically concerning female homosexuality, except in the armed forces.

The possible causes of homosexuality have been the subject of extensive but inconclusive debate. It has been suggested, for example, that genetic and/or, pre-natal or early post-natal hormonal influences make a person susceptible to becoming homosexual, especially if subsequently exposed to certain environmental influences. However, no reliable differences have been found between homosexuals and heterosexuals in either their hormonal make-up or physique. It has also been postulated that homosexuality may result from disturbed early relationships with parents, especially the parent of the opposite sex. Again, this theory has not been substantiated. Finally, it has been suggested that anxieties about heterosexuality ('heterophobia') and positive conditioning of homosexual fantasies through masturbation may be important. In the absence of any conclusive facts about the aetiology of homosexuality many people now simply accept homosexuality simply as being a variant of human sexual interest and behaviour, rather like left-handedness.

In the past, when homosexuality was more stigmatized than it is today, requests for psychiatric help, especially by men, were common. Now such requests are infrequent, although this may partly be the result of the establishment of special counselling agencies for homosexuals. Some people seek help to rid themselves of their homosexual interest, whilst others wish for assistance in adjusting to it. Sexual dysfunction may be another reason for requesting help. With the spreading fears concerning AIDS amongst male homosexuals there are a host of new reasons for seeking medical advice, especially concerning 'safe sex', testing for evidence of the HIV virus, and how to cope with being a carrier of the virus or having developed the full infection.

At one time, strenuous efforts were made to try to diminish homosexual interest. Aversion therapy was in vogue for a while, and other behavioural approaches, such as systematic desensitization to heterosexual situations, were also tried. These approaches, which were of doubtful effectiveness, have largely been abandoned, partly because help for sexual re-orientation is now rarely sought.

QUESTIONS

1 What are the more important causes of erectile dysfunction in a 55-year-old man?

2 Alcohol can interfere with sexual function in several ways. What are they?

3 You are working in general practice, and in the middle of a busy surgery a female patient tells you that she has a sexual difficulty which she has kept secret from her husband, to whom she is devoted. How might you proceed in assessing whether you can help her?

4 For what reasons might individuals with deviant sexual interest seek help, and how might these influence your choice of treatment?

5 Homosexual males may seek help from doctors with regard to AIDS. What are the possible reasons for their seeking such help?

FURTHER READING

Bancroft J. (1988) *Human Sexuality and Its Problems*. 2nd Edition. Churchill Livingstone, Edinburgh. [An excellent standard textbook, which thoroughly examines sexual anatomy and response, and deviant and dysfunctional sexuality.]

Hawton K. (1985) *Sex Therapy: A Practical Guide*. Oxford University Press, Oxford. [Includes a thorough description of sexual dysfunctions and their causes, followed by a step-by-step account of sex therapy.]

24
Violent and Antisocial Behaviour

Fact sheet

Mental disorder and antisocial behaviour (ASB)
- Sometimes there is a 'causal' link.
- Sometimes merely 'coincidental'.

Assessment of dangerousness
- Properly defined as 'the probability of a given (future) violent act (and harm) occurring'.
- Notoriously difficult.
- Largely based on data relating to the individual patient.
- Three simple rules: (1) the best predictor of future behaviour is past behaviour; (2) meticulous correlation of past mental state, interactional, institutional and other 'independent variables' *with* past violence assists in the prediction of future violence; and (3) developing a 'psychological understanding' of the patient's violence can be of great assistance.
- Pursue detailed 'analysis of violence' (association of violence with past mental state and other variables *in that patient*).
- Make putative links with 'functional' or organic diagnosis and psychopathology.
- Be aware of statistical studies linking (or not) diagnosis with violence.
- Assess relevant 'psychodynamic mechanisms'.
- Describe personality factors in the patient.
- Investigate ordinary criminological data in the patient.
- Identify potential victims.
- Identity risk factors for therapists.

Management of violence
- Modification of 'patient' and 'environmental' risk factors defined in 'analysis of violence'.
- Proper determination of (1) treatment setting; (2) management strategies; and (3) legal context (see Fig. 24.1).

Domestic violence and homicide
- Mainly men against women (the man often being suspicious and jealous).
- Sometimes a non-violent man kills rejecting wife in context of an 'adjustment reaction' or 'depressive illness'.
- Rarely a battered woman kills abuser in a state of 'learned helplessness'.

Arson
- Often psychologically normal.
- Sometimes for psychological gain through (1) irresistible impulse; (2) sexual excitement; (3) tension or depression relief; and (4) psychotic drive.

Shoplifting and acquisitive offences
A small minority are related to a variety of mental disorders – including neurotic depressive illness, anxiety neurosis, compulsive states, substance abuse and (rarely) medication effects.

Sexual offending
- Sexual offending and sexual abnormality are not synonomous.
- Frequent 'multiple paraphilias'.
- Serious offending more likely to be specific and 'boundaried' (see also Chapter 23, p. 293).

Non-accidental injury to children
- Of enormous importance.
- Generally not related to mental illness or disorder.
- Be aware of suspicious signs in the child and in the parents.
- Management should emphasize separation of different professional responsibilities.
- The child must be seen regularly.
- Be aware of high risk of sexual abuse.
- Be aware of 'Munchausen by proxy syndrome'.

The assessment interview
- Must be detailed and thorough.
- Can be highly instructive.
- Approached incautiously, the patient may be made apprehensive, secretive, angry or violent.
- Pay attention to simulation or dissimulation.
- Gain as much 'objective' information as possible.
- Pursue good general psychiatric practice irrespective of coincidental antisocial behaviour.

Introduction

General psychiatry is partly concerned with potential 'harm to self'. *Forensic* psychiatry is concerned also with the risk of 'harm to others' (as well as to property). In relation to harm to self there is substantial evidence of direct links with particular diagnoses and mental states. In relation to harm to others the evidence is less clear-cut. The issue is also complicated by consideration of ordinary, non-mental health related, propensities to offend and by consideration of the possible relevance for offending of personality disorder. Indeed, psychopathic personality disorder is the 'junctional case' in forensic psychiatry, since it sits at the interface between the sometimes presumed 'mad' (mentally ill) and the presumed 'bad' (normal criminal). The failure of psychiatry to resolve for itself the clinical nature and diagnostic status of personality disorder leaves room for great variation of opinion and of clinical forensic practice. Hence, the emphasis placed on aspects of 'madness', as against 'badness', varies; there is also undoubted inter-case inconsistency of diversion to hospital, as against prison, and a good deal of evidence that treatment of, and research into treatment of, personality disorder is wholly inadequate.

Since there are insufficient research data to presume levels of dangerousness based on specific diagnostic or mental state data, assessment and management of violence is largely a clinical science, aided by 'straws in the research wind'. This chapter will, therefore, address a number of types of antisocial behaviour (ASB) from a clincial point of view, aided by reference to what *is* known in research terms.

Mental disorder and antisocial behaviour

Clinical forensic psychiatry is adequately defined as concerned with the coincidence of mental disorder and ASB (not strictly 'offending' since it is the *behaviour* and not the criminal justice system consequences which define the clinical problem). Does 'coincidence' imply causality? That is, are we concerned with 'mentally disordered offending' or with 'offending in the mentally disordered'? The significance of the answer may be partly legal. Clinically, the distinction is important in terms of *modifying* violence; however, the *absence* of a causal link does not imply that a seriously mentally disordered person should be refused hospital treatment *because* of his offending.

Specific *types* of ASB can be variously linked with clinical states or diagnostic categories. Hence, arson, some acquisitive property offences, sexual offending and non-accidental injury to children (NAIC) are considered separately from violence *per se*.

Mental disorder and violence

Explanation of violence by mental disorder, as well as assessment of dangerousness, is easier in the *absence* of previous ASB or personality factors and in the *presence* of clear organic or functional psychotic illness. The less clear the picture in these terms, the less presumptive of a causal link can the clinician be, with correspondingly less confidence in the removal of risk of future violence by successful treatment of the mental disorder.

Assessment of dangerousness

Assessment of dangerousness is notoriously difficult. There are, however, three simple rules which may assist.
1 The best predictor of future behaviour is past behaviour.
2 Meticulous correlation of past mental state, 'interactional', institutional and other 'independent variables' *with* past violence assists in the prediction of future violence.
3 Developing a 'psychological understanding' of a patient's violence can be of great assistance.
Violence is definded by a person's behaviour and is assessed after it has occurred. *Dangerousness* is 'predictive'; properly defined it is 'the probability of a given violent act (and harm) occurring'. Its assessment should not be 'contaminated' by fear on the part of the clinician or by the social unacceptability of particular possible violence. Hence, hitting the doctor should not be perceived as meaning that the patient has now shown himself or herself to be more dangerous than when he or she ('only') hits a nurse (a not uncommon misperception!).

Assessment of unmodified dangerousness merges into management recommendations to minimize dangerousness.

Relevant non-psychiatric factors

Ordinary risk factors of offending in the *absence* of mental disorder must be presumed potentially also to affect the mentally disordered. Hence, *criminological* and *social* factors relating to childhood development and ASB *per se* are relevant (see Fig. 24.1 for a detailed description). Such factors can be expected to 'interact' with psychiatric factors. This emphasizes the importance of taking a very full history and of searching for objective background information which goes beyond the purely psychiatric. The role of *alcohol* and *drug use* must also be acknowledged and assessed.

Personality

Irrespective of personality disorder *per se*, the role of premorbid personality is important in assessing past violence and determining future dangerousness, particularly in view of the relative frequency of 'dual diagnosis' (usually personality disorder *and* mental illness or learning disability). Megargee's concept of 'over-controlled' and 'under-controlled' personalities in relation to violence is useful in a

Fig. 24.1 Assessment of dangerousness

Basic principles

1 Violence is behavioural, and assessed after the event.

2 Dangerousness is predictive; it is properly defined as 'the probability of a given (future) violent act (and harm) occurring'.

3 Assessment of dangerousness is notoriously difficult.

4 Three simple rules:
- the best predictor of future behaviour is past behaviour;
- meticulous correlation of past mental state, interactional, institutional and other 'independent variables' *with* past violence assists in the prediction of future violence;
- developing a 'psychological understanding' of the patient can be of great assistance.

Detailed assessment

Relevant non-psychiatric factors

Ordinary criminological factors include the following.

Childhood factors

General offending is associated (West & Farringdon, 1973) with:
- low family income;
- large family size in childhood;
- parental criminality;
- low intelligence;
- poor parental behaviour;
- alcohol and drug abuse/dependence;

Plus
- poor relationships with parents;
- physical and sexual abuse;
- alcoholism in the parents;
- dominating mothers;
- history of interparental violence (battering parents were themselves battered).

Detailed current factors

1 Age: more young people commit offences generally; in the young violent offences are uncommon and far less likely of repetition than property offences; offences decline with age.

2 Sex: far fewer women than men commit violent offences.

3 Marital status: failure to achieve or maintain a sexual partnership plus a history of at least one violent assault on a woman is ominous.

4 Alcohol and drugs: a very high proportion of ordinary offending is associated with alcohol (especially) and drug intoxication.

5 Previous forensic history: important predictor of future violence.

Hence, histories should include:
- ordinary criminological factors;
- ordinary social factors;
- previous forensic history;
- alcohol and drug history.

Personality factors

- 'Over-controlled': associated with non-deviant personal backgrounds, extremely infrequent violence, extremely severe type, against a family member.
- 'Under-controlled': associated with deviant background, substantial previous forrensic history, repetitively violent, against strangers.
- Paranoia.
- Suspiciousness.
- Jealousy (may become 'morbid').
- Deceptiveness.
- Sadism (especially with escalating sadistic sexual fantasies and behaviour).

Plus
- 'Borderline personality disorder' tension release.
- 'Psychopathic personality disorder' *per se*.
- Frequency of 'dual diagnosis' ('personality disorder' plus mental illness or mental handicap).

Analysis of violence

1 Historical correlational data *as they relate to the individual patient*.

2 The timing, frequency and type(s) of violence *correlated with*:
- the mental state;
- environmental atmosphere;
- medication record;
- ward, hostel, day care, occupational or domestic setting;
- presence/absence of disinhibiting psychoactive substances.

3 Putative links between violence *and*:
- 'functional illness': e.g. psychotic drive arising from delusions *or* abnormalities of affect;
- 'organic disorder' e.g. brain damage (especially frontal lobe); epilepsy (a very rare cause); ?some association of violence with temporal lobe abnormality; episodic dyscontrol syndrome (a controversial diagnosis).

Plus

4 Insight into illness and treatment need.

5 Motivation for change.

Mechanisms of violence

'Statistically suggested mechanisms' (from Häffner & Böker)

1 Diagnosis and phenomenology:
- *no overall association* of mental disorder and serious violence;
- all diagnostic categories much more likely to be *dangerous to themselves* than to others;
- *diagnostically*, the risk is much higher for schizophrenia than for other diagnoses;
- *learning disability*, little evidence of increased risk of violent offending;
- in schizophrenia origins of violence lie in the *personality* as much as, if not more than, in subsequent illness;
- in affective psychosis a clear association between violence and the *illness*, rather than with personality;
- *specific phenomenology*: violence associated with systematized delusions, persecution, jealousy, increased frequency of auditory and somatic hallucinations, link with a family member.

2 Illness duration:
- 84% of schizophrenics ill for more than 1 year and 55% for more than 5 years when they kill;
- 10% of affectively ill perpetrators kill in the first 4 weeks of illness and 33% in the first 6 months of illness.

3 Treatment history: 68% of psychotic offenders receive no treatment in the 6 months preceding the offence.

4 Potential victims:
- in about 50% of all psychotics the victim forms part of the delusional system;
- even higher proportion in schizophrenics than in affective psychotics.

'Psychodynamic mechanisms'

1 'Psychopath': attacks because he or she is untrammelled by normal moral constraints and fails or is unable to empathize (includes 'sadism').

2 'Paranoid': suspicious and so fears assault on him he must effect a pre-emptive strike (includes 'jealousy').

3 'Schizoid': feels he or she will be emotionally suppressed by the victim and so attacks to preserve a separate sense of 'self'.

4 'Depressive': attacks another as a sudden reversal of the violence more usually directed inwards.

---

general way. See Fig. 24.1 for a summary of other relevant personality factors.

Analysis of violence

In the absence of clear predictive research knowledge based on specific diagnoses or specific mental state abnormalities, assessment of dangerousness, with a view to its modification, requires meticulous collection of a variety of data types *as they relate to the individual patient*. It may also be possible, still using only past data, to assess the 'predictability' of past violence on the basis of data arising from even earlier violent episodes, so that a measure of the 'degree of confidence' placed in the correlations may be possible.

Identification of the patient's psychopathology *per se* may give rise to putative links between diagnosis and violence. Hence, teasing out detailed manifestations of a person's 'functional psychosis' may suggest specific factors predictive of violence. Some researchers have propounded the concept of 'psychotic drive', whereby violence is presumed to occur as a direct result of specific delusional or hallucinatory experiences. Others suggest that affective aspects of psychosis, such as fear or flattening of affect, are more important in determining violence than are particular delusions. By contrast to both these approaches, some psychotics seem to offend as a result of the less specific effect of generalized mental deterioration on social functioning. *Organic conditions*, especially frontal lobe damage or deterioration, can give rise to a reduced threshold for violence. *Epilepsy* is a very rare direct cause of violence, sometimes associated with *temporal lobe abnormality. Episodic dyscontrol syndrome* is a controversial organic diagnosis accepted by only some as 'causal' of violence.

Insight into the need for treatment and '*motivation for change*' may be significant pointers to the modifiability of future risk.

Mechanisms of violence

Two approaches can be adopted in order systematically to assess and define the relationship between mental disorder and violence: (1) statistical correlational; and (2) psychodynamic.

Statistically suggested mechanisms

Statistical studies of general offending in relation to mental disorder vary greatly in their findings. This arises from sampling and diagnostic variation or bias. Also, many studies adopt a highly 'aggregate' approach, thereby missing the subtleties of which mental state signs or symptoms are dangerous rather than which diagnoses.

Widely accepted as the best study in the field, Häfner and Böker (1982) described detailed statistical associations between both diagnoses and mental state phenomena *and* serious violence (see Fig. 24.1 for full details). Of particular importance are the following findings.

1 No overall association of mental disorder and serious violence.

2 All diagnostic categories (including schizophrenics) were much more likely to be dangerous to themselves than to others.

3 The risk of violence to others was much higher for schizophrenia than for other diagnoses, for example, depression.

4 Aggressive behaviour prior to a schizophrenic illness was an important factor predictive of future violence, whereas in affective psychosis a clear association was demonstrated between violence and the onset of illness *per se*.

5 Violent schizophrenics tended to have been ill for several years when first violent, whilst affective psychotics were violent in the first few weeks or months of illness.

6 The majority of psychotic offenders received no treatment in the 6 months preceding the offence.

By contrast with Häfner and Böker, one recent UK study by Taylor and Gunn, seemed to show a definite overall increased association between severe violence and specifically schizophrenia.

Such studies are useful only through being *potentially* predictive of violence *in the individual patient*; it is important, therefore, to consider specific illness and mental state phenomena as predictive of violence only as they can be shown to have been so in a particular patient's history.

Psychodynamic mechanisms

The psychodynamic approach is based upon presumed psychodynamic mechanisms of violence *per se*. Hence, Storr (1970) distinguishes four *mental mechanisms* differentially producing violence; these are defined in terms of particular mechanisms and not particular diagnoses, albeit that some mechanisms occur more often in some diagnoses. Given that the phenomenological approach is unlikely to be comprehensively adequate it would be unwise to fail to attempt to 'understand' patients' violence. Hence:

1 the *psychopath* attacks because he or she is untrammelled by normal moral constraints and is unable to empathize with the victim;

2 the *paranoid* patient is suspicious and so fears assault on him or herself that he or she must effect a pre-emptive strike;

3 the *schizoid* feels he or she will be emotionally overwhelmed by the other person and lose his or her psychological integrity and so attacks to preserve a sense of separate 'self';

4 the *depressive* (very rarely and usually explosively) attacks another as a sudden reversal of the violence more usually directed inwards, often via suicide.

Although such mental mechanisms can be generally predictive of violence it may still be very difficult to define the *moment* or the '*object*' of violence.

Personality disorder and violence

Aside from 'personality factors', which can operate to the level of disorder, and 'psychodynamic mechanisms', two further aspects of personality disorder are important (for factors generally see Fig. 24.1).

Sadistic fantasies

There is often clinical concern relating to the predictive significance of sadistic sexual fantasies. It is known that, in a proportion of personality disordered patients who have committed very serious sexual violence, there has very often been prior association with the need of an inadequate man to *control* another person, escalation of the *degree* of control in masturbatory fantasy and *conversion* of fantasy into reality. However, it is not known how many other men have such fantasies, perhaps offend in a minor way, and never escalate the fantasies or convert them into reality. Hence, although such fantasies *per se*, and particularly conversion, raise a strong index of suspicion of serious risk, it is based on only partial scientific knowledge. Coincidence of such fantasies with a diagnosable personality disorder would greatly increase the index of suspicion.

Borderline personality disorder

This diagnosis (DSM-III-R) *can* be particularly associated with violent offending and with arson (see below). Hence, tension relief may be achieved not only through deliberate self-harm, cutting for example, but also through violence to others and through fire setting.

Generally, it is often very useful to request 'personality psychometry' on violent and offender patients. This may confirm and better articulate clinical impressions of personality types and mental mechanisms so as to increase understanding of the origins of violent behaviour.

Identification of potential victims (Fig. 24.1)

A potential victim of the *schizophrenic*, the *paranoid psychotic* and the *depressive psychotic* may be identified by delusional phenomena and by close family association and emotion. 'Misidentification' may be particularly dangerous in schizophrenia. In relation to any paranoid psychotic, the perceived persecutor is often at risk. The young children of a depressed woman may be at particular risk, through extension of her hopeless view of the world to incorporate the prospects for her children. The partner of a rejected depressed man may be at risk if there is emotional '*provocation*' on her part.

Breach of confidentiality is justified, and may even be an ethical (and perhaps civil legal) duty, where there is an identified victim reasonably at substantial risk of major harm (see Chapter 4).

Management of dangerousness

Minimization of violence arises from *modification* of risk factors for the individual patient as defined by the analysis of violence and of identified psychodynamic mechanisms. The more 'controllable' are the factors apparently associated with past violence, and the greater the degree of confidence in the correlations identified, the more reassured can the clinician be. A painstaking approach is the only proper route to risk minimization and to avoidance of unwarranted restriction of patients' civil rights through too cautiously over-identifying dangerousness.

Management of dangerousness comprises recognition of the roles of (1) *treatment setting*; (2) *management strategies*; and (3) *legal context*.

Treatment setting

A patient may be unmanageable and dangerous on an open ward but completely safe on a locked ward, or medium or maximum secure unit, without further intervention such as medication. Violent patients are often themselves fearful and made less so by perimeter, staff and psychological *containment*. This emphasizes the importance of the availability of *all* levels of care, from community to maximum security (that is, special hospitals). Similarly, increased staffing levels or 'specialing' may reduce risk through containment.

In the community, matching the choice of hostel or domestic environment to the patient's psychopathology can be equally crucial, as can the proper choice of day-care and occupational facilities. The availability of a specifically skilled and adequately staffed community team is crucially important.

Management strategies

Risk is minimized by knowledge of risk factors and, therefore, by *shared* knowledge; maximum inter-staff and inter-agency communication must be pursued (Fig. 24.3).

Specific strategies include any approach likely to modify risk factors of any type.

1 *Medication* may reduce mental state risk factors; there is also some evidence that carbamazepine may be of use specifically in violent patients, although this is complicated by the debate over the diagnosis episodic dyscontrol syndrome in relation to minor electroencephalographic and neurological abnormalities.

2 *Cognitive therapy* may reverse dangerous links between cognition and action (for example, through use of ABC techniques, that is, 'antecedents → behaviours → consequences', so as to understand episodes of violence in detail and apply 'anger management' techniques to modify the sequence).

3 *Behavioural modification* may assist especially when there is frequently repeated violence (or other ASB).

4 *Altered staff attitudes* may 'defuse' repetitive dangerous interactions.

5 *Removal* of another patient specifically at risk may be all that is required.

6 *Avoidance* of self-administration of disinhibiting substances may both improve the mental state of the patient and reduce the risk of violence.

Individual therapists can become of great emotional importance to violent patients, with consequent risk to the therapist. There is often inherent ambivalence, where a 'positive' transference is mixed with feelings that the therapist (for example, a responsible medical officer) is 'controlling' the patient through the legal and institutional context of treatment. Apart from feelings of *persecution* the patient may feel *rejection* by the therapist towards the end of treatment. This may be particularly relevant after long-term care in the community. Hence, great care should always be taken to elicit any strong feelings or delusional beliefs about therapists.

As in relation to suicidal ideas, there should be *no diffidence* in asking patients about violent thoughts, fantasies or actions, albeit that this should be pursued with caution and in awareness of the patient's likely *mental mechanisms*.

There should be clear decisions about *leave* and *escorting*

Fig. 24.3 Management of dangerousness

Modification of risk factors through:
- modification of correlates identified in 'analysis of violence';
- modification of 'psychodynamic mechanisms'.

Plus

1 Proper treatment setting.
- Importance of 'containment' (perimeter, staff and psychological).
- Patients' behaviour is often determined by the setting.
- Importance of the availability of *all* levels of security, from community to maximum security, and *all* levels of forensic and generalist care.

2 Management strategies
- Shared knowledge is crucial.
- Pursue *maximum information communication*, inter-staff and inter-agency.
- Be aware that *institutional and nursing regimes* can determine or avoid violent atmospheres and episodes.

Specific strategies include:
- *medication* (for primary illness, also sometimes carbamazepine);
- *cognitive therapy*;
- *behavioural therapy*;
- *removal* of another patient/person at risk;
- *avoidance* of disinhibiting substances;
- *awareness* of personal risk to therapist through patient's perception of persecution and/or rejection;

- do not be *diffident* in asking questions about violence or 'sensitive' mental symptoms;
- clear decisions about '*leave*', '*escorting*' and '*domiciliary visits*';
- clear unit policies about the *management of violent incidents* in in-patient and community settings, including knowledge of 'control and restraint' techniques if on locked/secure wards.

If confronted alone with potential or actual violence:
- impulsive speech or movement may worsen an already dangerous situation;
- attempt to continue conversation;
- be non-judgemental;
- allow/encourage the patient to feel 'safe';
- flee the patient (only) when reason is overcome by fear *and/or* where the patient is deemed uncontrollably dangerous.

Procedures after a violent incident include:
- 'debriefing';
- ensure maximum knowledge of the factors leading to the violence;
- defuse distressed emotions in staff.

3 Legal context
Legal context of treatment may assist or inhibit risk minimization, e.g. Section 3, 37/41, including 'conditional discharge', Section 7 guardianship

---

in relation to any in-patient. Decisions regarding *domiciliary visits* to community patients must specifically address the possible risk to staff.

More generally, there must be clear unit policies about the *management of violent incidents*. Staff on a secure unit or ordinary locked ward should receive training in control and restraint procedures, including the important psychological aspects. These techniques comprise methods of maximal physical control of the patient with minimal risk of injury to both patient and staff. Ultimate control and restraint may involve *seclusion*; this must only be used for control and never punitively. In general psychiatric hospitals it may be appropriate to have an emergency team who are trained in such skills, perhaps attached to the hospital locked ward which has some expertise in dealing with violent patients. Policies should extend to out-patient settings.

Where an individual therapist is confronted alone with potential or actual violence the experience may be extremely frightening. However, impulsive speech or movement may worsen an already dangerous situation. By contrast, there should be attempts to continue conversation and to be non-judgemental, all aimed at allowing the patient to feel 'safe'. A good general rule is 'think about the psychological interactions in spite of your fear'. Only when reason is overcome by fear and/or where the patient is deemed uncontrollably dangerous should an attempt be made to flee the patient.

Management strategies must also take account of *procedures after a violent incident*. It is essential that there is staff debriefing after a violent episode. The purpose of this is first, to ensure maximum knowledge of the factors apparently leading up to the incident, for future reference; and second, to defuse distressed emotions in staff (for example, feelings of failure or anger) so as to ensure continued cohesion of the staff and the unit. It may also be helpful to use a community meeting, of staff *and* patients, for a similar purpose.

Hospital management, and specifically nursing management, must acknowledge that *institutional* and *nursing regimes* can tend to determine or avoid violent atmospheres and episodes on wards and, therefore, operational policies should be defined accordingly; there is a substantial literature on 'violence in hospital', for example, Fottrell (1980).

Legal context

The legal context of treatment may assist or inhibit risk minimization. Hence, a Section 3 Treatment Order (see Chapter 25) may operate either or both to make the patient feel more psychologically 'contained' and/or 'required' to accept medication, both of which may reduce risk. Proper use of Part IV of the Mental Health Act may similarly assist. Again, the addition by a Court of a Section 41 Restriction Order to a Section 37 Hospital Order (see Chapter 25) may increase the patient's sense of 'containment' and/or 'requirement' to accept help; it will also allow for eventual 'conditional discharge' into the community with a requirement of medical and social supervision and the taking of medication. This *may* result both in improved acceptance of treatment and a more cooperative patient generally, thereby improving other aspects of risk minimization. A Section 7 Guardianship Order may provide a similar if lesser effect. Knowledge by the patient that it is unit or general practice policy to allow or encourage the police to investigate and also charge patients with offences committed on clinical premises may provide valuable 'ordinary' inhibition of violence.

Domestic violence and homicide

There is insufficient space here to deal comprehensively with domestic violence. Specifically as regards homicide, in *men* where there has been no previous violence, this is often associated with an adjustment reaction or mild to moderate depressive illness, in response to rejection or spousal infidelity (or both). Other men kill on a background of a long history of battering. In *women* there is a small number of cases of battered women who kill. Such violence may be related to minor mental disorder, or to a normal psychological reaction to stressors such as chronic post-traumatic stress disorder, but it is in a different category from other mentally disordered violence and is essentially situational in character. Commonly the woman develops a state of 'learned helplessness' resulting in cognitive distortion which locks her into an abusive relationship.

Arson

Fire setting can be an 'ordinary' criminal offence aimed at financial gain, revenge, covering another crime or used as a means of attacking another person. However, for some fire setting is a source of *psychological* gain. Faulk (1988) divides this group, itself very heterogeneous, into (1) irresistible impulse; (2) sexual excitement; and (3) tension or depression reducing. A further group (4) arises when fire setting is directed by *psychotic experiences* (Fig. 24.4). *Irresistible impulse* fire setters are frequently unable to understand or explain their behaviour. They are often 'inadequate' to ordinary life demands, hence somewhat overlapping with the tension or depression reducing group. They are often caught and the behaviour may escalate. Although often referred to in the literature, *sexual excitement* from fire setting is clinically rare. The disorder involves fantasy and reality of fire setting as a stimulus to sexual excitement and satisfaction. By contrast, the *tension or depression relieving group* is common. It may occur in the context of inadequacy and borderline intelligence or mild mental handicap or in the context of a personality disorder, quite frequently borderline personality disorder (DSM-III-R). In the latter example it is usually associated with other forms of 'acting out' behaviour, such as, cutting, swallowing or other ASB.

Arson dangerousness is defined in terms of the risk of future fires and of escalation of the scale of fire setting. Faulk

---

Fig. 24.4 Arson for 'psychological gain'

1 Irresistible impulse.
2 Sexual excitement (clinically rare).
3 Tension or depression relief.
4 Psychotic drive
Also associated with:
• personality disorder;
• mild/borderline learning disability;
• psychosis.

(1988) summarizes a number of predictive studies by indicating that the best predictors are the number of previous convictions, the parole score and the time served in prison for the last offence, this being an indication of previous conviction numbers and of the severity of the last offence. He concludes that, overall, the statistical chance of a repeat arson after a sentence or period in hospital is low.

Clinical assessment, by comparison with the 'actuarial' approach just referred to, should follow the painstakingly detailed approach recommended more generally for dangerousness assessment.

Conviction of fire setting is distinguished by virtue of the intent to threaten the life of others, recklessness towards others and arson 'simpliciter'.

Acquisitive offending

The vast majority of shoplifting and other acquisitive offenders are psychologically normal. However, such offences may be associated with the following mental disorders and in the following ways.

Neurotic depressive illness

This is the commonest disease correlate of shoplifting. Depressive preoccupation or inattention may result in taking without the intention to steal (hence there may be a psychologically based defence of 'lack of intent', see also Chapter 6, p. 80). Alternatively, the wish to 'self-harm' may extend to deliberate (therefore *with* intention) theft so as to be caught and punished. The caricature of the middle-aged woman who has a chronic mild depressive illness and who shoplifts exists but is probably less common than often thought.

Anxiety-based neuroses

Suddenly leaving a shop in a panic attack, sometimes on a background of severe social phobic disorder, may 'coincidentally' result in taking without the intention to steal. Similarly, a generalized anxiety state may result in 'non-intentional' taking.

Compulsive states

Obsessive–compulsive disorder as a valid determinant of theft is rare. However, such cases do occur, often being psychologically 'understandable' either in relation to theft *per se* or the particular goods that are stolen.

Schizophrenia

Very rarely theft may be psychotically driven, by 'positive' symptoms. More commonly it arises through social deterioration resultant from chronic illness and 'negative' symptomatology.

Affective psychosis

Mania may result in spending money the person does not have, associated with elevated mood and grandiose thinking. Depressive psychosis may result in theft as described under neurotic depressive illness, as well as rarely through delusional thinking.

Organic brain states

Either confusion or reduced social constraints may result in a variety of offending behaviour by *demented* persons. Other types of *brain deterioration or damage* may result in offending through personality deterioration. *Epilepsy* could theoretically result in theft but, in practice, such a situation is extremely rare.

Substance abuse

Substance abuse is a disorder which gives rise to acquisitive offending but usually through 'ordinary' motivation, albeit to feed an addiction. There may also be theft through general social decline. Any offending, including acquisitive offending, may arise through disinhibition coincidental with intoxication.

Medication effects

Offending through impaired concentration as arising from excessive hypnotic medication, antidepressants, steroids and anti-epileptic drugs has been reported. However, it is probably a rare cause of offending.

Amnesia

An important general distinction arises between claimed amnesia based on a memory disorder and amnesia resulting from lack of attention or of concentration coincidental with the alleged offence. The former has no implication for lack of intent whereas the latter does (see Chapter 11, p. 132).

Sexual offending

Sexual offending and sexual abnormality are not synonymous (Fig. 24.5). Hence, for example, many rapists are psychologically normal. Also, it is probably the case that the more 'severe' or 'abusive' the offending the more specific the *type* of offending. Albeit that many abnormal offenders, even some serious offenders, have multiple *paraphilias*, very serious sexual deviance and offending is more likely to be 'boundaried' and specific. A rapist who attacks adult females will not tend also to commit paedophiliac offences. Specifically as regards 'abnormal' sexual offending, there is a close association with personality disorder; it may also arise *de novo* from brain damage or chronic degenerative brain disease, as well as in association with chronic psychosis. (For details of types of deviance, offending, assessment and management see Chapter 23, p. 293.)

Fig. 24.5 Patterns of sexual offending

- Sexual offending and sexual abnormality are not synonymous.
- Many rapists, for example, are 'psychologically normal'.
- Many abnormal offenders have multiple 'paraphilias'.
- Serious sexual deviance and offending tends to be more 'boundaried' and specific.
(See Chapter 23 for detailed descriptions of offender types/sexual deviance diagnoses).

Non-accidental injury to children

NAI emphasizes the fact that assessment and prediction of dangerousness is not a task reserved for psychiatrists, particularly where there is no mental disorder. It also serves to illustrate various 'ordinary' (non-mental disorder) aspects of risk assessment. Indeed, much of what follows also applies to domestic violence in all its forms. Hospital doctors, general practitioners and social workers should be constantly alert to the risk of NAI to children. Further aspects of child maltreatment are covered in Chapter 15, p. 192.

The House of Commons Select Committee reported in 1977 that about one in 10 000 children will be killed each year and 10 times as many are severely injured as a result of child abuse.

Clinical signs which should raise the index of suspicion in the practitioner include the injuries listed in Fig. 24.6, but there must also be vigilance for two further phenomena.

Firstly, *sexual abuse* of children, which is usually committed by a family member or friend (see Chapter 23, p. 295). Secondly, '*fabricated illness*' in children (that is, illness fabricated by the parents or Munchausen by proxy syndrome). Meadows has described children who have been subjected frequently to potentially painful and dangerous investigations and treatment. They are commonly presented by the parents as having some neurological disorder, especially fits, abnormal bleeding or apnoeic attacks. Warning

---

Fig. 24.6 Signs which should cause suspicion of non-accidental injury in children

Suspicious signs
- Multiple fractures, sub-periosteal haematomata, epiphyseal separation on X-ray.
- Multiple burns, bruises or laceration of various ages. Also bite marks, torn buccal mucosa.
- Rupture of abdominal viscera.
- Delay in reporting injury or in obtaining help.
- Vague or discrepant history of injury.

The parents
Mother:
- young maternal age at birth of first child;
- low intelligence;
- unmarried.

Father:
- personality disorder;
- criminal record;
- frequently absent.

Both parents:
- poor relationship;
- low social class;
- mental illness may be present;
- socially isolated;
- violent temper;
- unrealistic expectations of child;
- may have been battered in childhood.

---

signals include inexplicable illness, uncertain diagnosis, a parent who refuses to leave the child and who seems far less concerned about her child's progress than are the staff. The definitive sign is the disappearance of symptoms in the absence of the parent (Fig. 24.6). Little is known of the psychopathology of the syndrome, although it is assumed that the parent (usually mother) achieves 'psychological gain' by the attention she receives through her 'sick' child. The management of NAI is described in Fig. 24.7.

Child risk factors

Battering is statistically more likely if the child is illegitimate, or the result of a premarital pregnancy, *and* when the child is an only child or the youngest (perhaps an unwelcome start or addition to a family). Early separation of the newborn baby from the mother (e.g. admission to a special care baby unit because of neonatal difficulty) may prevent adequate attachment between mother and child, leading to a poor relationship subsequently. Anecdotal evidence suggests battering is more likely when the child wakes easily at night or utters a piercing cry.

Some children who are abused show the sign of frozen watchfulness; others contribute an unusual amount to the management of the home.

The assessment interview

The importance of the interview is that it is at once an *investigative*, *diagnostic* and *therapeutic* aid (Fig. 24.8). It should be possible to elicit a great deal of clinical information which will be of great assistance in assessment and management. Approached incautiously, however, the patient may be made apprehensive, secretive and, on occasions, angry or even violent. Few procedures in medicine have the potential for perceived intrusiveness of the degree arising in a psy-

chiatric interview, and particularly where violent or offending behaviour is involved.

The reason for the interview should always be explained. It is sensible to approach the patient through the least sensitive material being addressed at the beginning of the interview, turning to ASB and sensitive mental symptoms and abnormalities only towards the end of the interview. The importance of a 'non-judgemental' attitude in relation to the latter is crucial (particularly where a report may be used for a court report, see Chapter 4 regarding issues of confidentiality). It is important to gain corroborative and other information from 'objective informants', including relatives, friends, previous hospital notes, work records, previous convictions (where available) and (again, where available) case depositions, often a mine of useful information about the defendant's mental state during the offence and about the detailed nature of the offence. Particular attention should be paid to simulation, particularly where there are court proceedings pending, or to dissimulation. Evasiveness about symptoms, suspiciousness and inconsistency may suggest areas of great sensitivity for the patient. The patient should be offered an opportunity at the end of the interview to explain anything that he or she thinks is important.

As in all psychiatric practice, good clinical work is based on a 'therapeutic alliance'. It is not as difficult to achieve this as might be presumed in someone who is violent and/or facing court or Mental Health Review Tribunal proceedings. Hence, throughout the clinician's dealings with the patient good general psychiatric practice should be pursued, irrespective of the complicating factor of unlawful or antisocial behaviour, past, present or predicted.

REFERENCES

Faulk M. (1988) *Basic Forensic Psychiatry*. Blackwell Scientific Publications, Oxford. [A clear short text on clinical forensic psychiatry. But definitely only a 'starter' on most topics.]

Fottrell E. (1980) A study of violent behaviour among patients in psychiatric hospitals. *Br. J. Psychiatr.* **136**, 216–21. [One of a number of studies available which deal with violence in psychiatric hospitals].

Häfner H. & Böker W. (1982) *Crimes of Violence by Mentally Abnormal Offenders. The Psychiatric Epidemiological Study in the Federal German Republic*. Cambridge University Press, Cambridge. [A massive definitive epidemiological study on the relationship between mental disorder and very serious violence. Probably the best piece of work ever conducted in the field.]

Meadow R. (1985) Munchausen syndrome by proxy. *Arch Dis Child* 57:92–8.

Megargee E.I. (1970) Undercontrolled and overcontrolled personality types in extreme antisocial aggression. In: Megargee E.I. & Hokanson J.E. (eds). *The Dynamics of Aggression*. Harper & Row, New York, pp. 108–20.

Storr A. (1970) *Human Aggression*. Penguin, Harmondsworth. [A very readable introduction to relevant 'psychodynamic' ideas relating to violence.]

West D.J. & Farrington D.P. (1973) *Who Become Delinquent?* Heinemann Educational, London. [The definitive birth cohort prospective study on the family and background correlates of subsequent deliquency.]

FURTHER READING

Bluglass R. & Bowden B. (eds) (1990) *Principles and Practice of Forensic Psychiatry*. Churchill Livingstone, Edinburgh. [A massive reference text which is extremely comprehensive and offers something on every topic in forensic psychiatry, though being thin on treatment. It is multi-authored and therefore sometimes repetitive.]

Eastman N.L.G. (1993) Forensic psychiatric services in Britain: [A current review. *Int. J. Law Psychiatr.* **16**, 1–26. A recent comprehensive update on forensic psychiatric services in Britain.]

Farrington D.P. & Gunn J. (eds) (1985) *Aggression and Dangerousness*. John Wiley & Sons. [A comprehensive multiperspective review of aggression in relation to mental disorder.]

25
Legal and Ethical Psychiatry

Fact sheet

Law and ethics
- Law and ethics, although clearly distinct, are intricately interlinked.
- Distinguish clearly psychiatric issues from legal and ethical issues.
- Law arises from courts ('common law') and Parliament (statute law).
- 'Common law' governs all patients, statute law governs specific patients (e.g. the Mental Health Act 1983 (MHA) governs detained patients and a small number of specified informal patients).
- Statute law 'trumps' common law.
- Courts and tribunals administer law, sometimes assisted by psychiatric evidence.
- Legal and psychiatric constructs are clearly distinguished, even when apparently related (e.g. 'psychopathy' in psychiatry versus 'psychopathic disorder' in the MHA).
- 'Criminal legal psychiatry' involves the State against an individual (e.g. a mentally disordered defendant).
- 'Civil legal psychiatry' involves one individual against another (one or more of whom may be mentally disordered).

Consent to treatment
Consent *requires*:
- a competent patient;
- information;
- voluntariness;
- patient assent.

A consent form is merely (one piece of) evidence as to the fact of consent, other evidence may conflict with it.

Exceptions to consent requirement include:
- implied consent;
- necessity (with incapacity);
- treatment in an emergency;
- post-suicide attempt;
- detention under the Mental Health Act 1983.

Part IV Mental Health Act 1983 divides treatments (on the basis of invasiveness and risk) into 'severe' (requiring competent consent and an MHAC medical opinion), 'moderate' (competent consent or an MHAC medical opinion) and 'mild' (requiring neither). 'Moderate treatments' include ECT and drugs beyond 3 months whilst detained. 'Severe treatments' include psychosurgery and hormone implants.

Civil capacities
Civil capacities are 'action specific'; there is no 'generalized competent mental state'. Action-specific capacities are defined by legal purpose and by specific legal criteria. Hence, a patient may be competent to marry but not to make a contract *or* competent to manage his affairs but not to make a will (or vice versa).

Detention in hospital
- Criteria for detention are *mental illness, severe mental impairment, mental impairment, psychopathic disorder* and (for detention up to a maximum of 28 days) *mental disorder* (an umbrella term covering the other four categories *plus 'any other disorder or disability of mind'*).
- Grounds for detention are 'the interest of the patient's health or safety or the protection of others' (NB: danger to self or others is not a necessary ground, ill health will do).
- Admission may be for 28 day assessment (Section 2) or for treatment (Section 3). 72 hour detention (Sections 4 or 5) may proceed to either Section 2 or Section 3.

Admission from courts and prisons
- A *remand order* may be made from *court*, either under the Mental Health Act (Section 35 for assessment or 36 for treatment) or through remand on bail with a condition of hospital residence.
- The remandee *in prison* can be transferred 'urgently' direct from prison to hospital (Section 48).
- 'Unfitness to plead' or 'insanity' *may* result in a hospital order (with or without a restriction order, see below) and *must* (with a restriction order) if the charge is murder.
- Hospital orders (Section 37) are equivalent to Section 3 detention as regards their criteria and grounds (see above); if there is a 'restriction order' (Section 41) this gives power to the Home Office over the location of patient and 'parole'.

Court reports and evidence
- Expert reports to courts and Mental Health Review Tribunals must be unbiased by the source of request.
- There are major ethical problems where 'medical' information can be *legally* relevant. The lack of confidentiality must be explained to the defendant before the interview.
- Reports address the *disposal* issue (mainly) and *verdict* issues (sometimes), for example insanity, diminished responsibility, automatism and infanticide.
- Court reports should be based on sources of information beyond defendant interviews (i.e. witness statements, previous psychiatric records, prison inmate medical records, psychometric tests, etc.).
- Reports and evidence should be presented in awareness of their solely legal context and relevance.

Essential principle of legal and ethical psychiatry: beware the boundary between things medical and things legal or ethical.

Introduction

There are legal rules and ethical principles which apply to all psychiatric patients. A small minority of patients are detained under the Mental Health Act 1983 and special legal rules apply in those circumstances. However, the majority of patients must be treated in the context of 'common law' rules (that is, rules arising from courts and not from statute). Hence, this chapter considers a variety of legal and ethical aspects of treatment of psychiatric patients as well as the provision of both criminal and civil court reports. It excludes law relating to children.

Law and ethics

Distinguish law and ethics

Law is that body of rules formally sanctioned by Parliament and the courts so as to be defined as 'law' and administered by 'legal fora' (courts and tribunals).

Ethics addresses issues involving conflicts between ethical principles and between the interests of different parties; this includes *ethical codes*, not having the status of law but being administered by self-governing professional bodies, usually themselves having the power in law to register, deregister or discipline professionals.

The relationship between law and ethics includes the following.
1 Ethics must operate on a legal backcloth; hence there may be a (natural) coherence between the two but there is *no necessary* coherence.
2 Ethics operates to 'fill the gaps' in the law, often arising because the law is 'silent' on many issues (the law, so to speak, 'exists' to cover *any* situation but, in many circumstances, cannot be determined until someone takes the issue to court).
3 Ethical principles may give rise to legal constructs, for example, (ethical) *autonomy* is the basis of (legal) *battery*, as well as being an aspect of *negligence*.

Psychiatric ethics are the 'shoulds' of psychiatric practice, by comparison with technical issues. Central to all medical ethics is the conflict between the *autonomy* of the patient (for example, concerning consent) and the *duty of care* of the doctor (for example, in negligence); many ethical dilemmas can be distilled down to this conflict.

Distinguish law and psychiatry

There is a clear distinction between psychiatric diagnoses and legal/social constructs. Hence, mania is a diagnosis where arson is a piece of behaviour amounting to a crime (you cannot, therefore, have a diagnosis of 'arsonist'). Hence also, schizophrenia is a diagnosis whilst 'abnormality of mind' giving rise to 'diminished responsibility' (in the Homicide Act 1957) is a legal construct. There is no reason why apparently related psychiatric and legal constructs (for example, in the latter illustration) should necessarily relate to one another. Hence, for example, even where the *same word* is used, for example, 'psychopathy' (in psychiatry) and 'psychopathic disorder' (in Section 1 of the Mental Health Act 1983) they are differently defined and therefore distinct from one another. Clearly law may adopt a 'term of art' from psychiatry but then redefine it so that it means something different from the original psychiatric construct.

The distinction between psychiatric and legal constructs is central to 'legal psychiatry'. It emphasizes the 'boundary' between psychiatric diagnosis/formulation *and* its legal use/ implications. The distinction is of crucial importance in both civil and criminal legal psychiatry.

Legal sources

Statute law 'trumps', and sits on a bedrock of 'common law' (for example, the Mental Health Act 1983 overrides common law in specified respects but the common law still applies even to detained patients where the Act is 'silent').

The Code of Practice, the official guidelines for applying the Mental Health Act, (see p. 319) does not have the force of law but it may be used evidentially to persuade courts towards a particular legal result.

Legal fields

Civil law involves one 'individual' against another and relates to any matter defined by Parliament or the courts as 'civil'. *Criminal law* involves the State against an individual, where Parliament and/or the courts have defined an activity as a 'crime' and given the State the right to initiate proceedings on behalf of society. As an example, a defendant with a psychopathic personality disorder may be convicted of 'diminished responsibility manslaughter' (in the *criminal* law) yet be sentenced to imprisonment because he is not detainable under the Mental Health Act 1983 (in *civil* law).

Legal fora

There is a distinction between criminal and civil fora (applying the legal fields defined above). There is also a distinction between courts *per se* and quasi-judicial bodies (for example, Mental Health Review Tribunals).

Courts are defined in a hierarchy, both in the criminal and civil context. Hence, all criminal cases begin (and most end) in the Magistrates' courts, some proceed to the Crown Court (rarely the Central Criminal Court, Old Bailey), a very few go to the Appeal Court (Criminal Division) and a tiny number go, on a point of law, to the House of Lords. In the civil courts the same hierarchy applies from the County Court, through the High Court and Appeal Court and to the House of Lords. There are specialist courts for juveniles, as well as Coroner's Courts for the specific purpose of determining the cause of death of an individual.

Mental Health Review Tribunals are specifically concerned with determining the legality of detention under the Mental Health Act 1983. By analogy Discretionary Life Panels (Criminal Justice Act 1991) operate as independent tribunals in order to address the continuing detention in prison beyond the recommended tariff of any 'discretionary' life sentence (psychiatrists now commonly offer independent reports to panels regarding 'risk', especially in cases of personality disordered prisoners).

Civil and criminal legal psychiatry

Hence, issues divide into *civil legal psychiatry* and *criminal legal psychiatry*, according to which body of law is applicable and in which legal forum. There may be a crossover between the two whereby a 'patient' can also be a 'defendant' or a 'litigant'.

Consent to treatment

All psychiatric patients are treated under the terms of the common law relating to consent to treatment (Fig. 25.1). The small number who are detained under the Mental Health Act 1983 also have specific 'consent to treatment' law applicable to them through Part IV of the Act (a very small number of informal patients are also governed by the Act in relation to psycho-surgery and hormone implants).

Common law

The ethical principle of *autonomy* (that is, the patient has the right to control his or her own body and mind) translates legally into the concept of *battery* (or assault). If a patient is 'medically touched' without consent (that is, without consent to *that* touching) there is battery. Hence, only consent avoids liability for battery. However, the threshold of consent to avoid battery is low and, in most cases, absence of consent is determined instead on the basis of the law of *negligence*. Hence, a doctor can be negligent not only in his or her technical practice but also in his or her overall dealing with the patient, including the amount of information that he or she gives to the patient about prospective treatment.

Definition of consent

The following ethical and legal model of consent (Meisel *et al.*, 1977) describes 'elements' of consent:

$$Cp + I \rightarrow U$$
$$U + V \rightarrow D$$

where: Cp = competence; I = information given; U = understanding achieved; V = voluntariness; and D = decision (affirmative).

There is no valid (ethical) consent without *all* of the elements being simultaneously satisfied. English law can also be described in terms of the requirement and definition of each of these elements of consent.

Competence

In common law, competence to consent is taken to mean that the patient is 'capable of understanding in broad terms the nature and purpose of the treatment'. The Mental Health Act 1983 goes a little further and states that the patient must be 'capable of understanding the nature, purpose and likely effects of the treatment'. Additional explanation is offered in the Code of Practice of the Mental Health Act Commission. Competence to consent to treatment is an example of a particular 'civil capacity' (see further below).

Fig. 25.1 Consent to treatment

Common law

Applicable to all patients. Consent requires:

- competent patient;
- information to patient;
- 'voluntariness';
- assent.

Exceptions to need for consent:

- 'implied consent' (minor 'procedure – e.g. take pulse);
- 'reasonable patient' would consent (patient unconscious);
- interrupting suicide;
- 'necessity' – *some* impairment of capacity *and* death or grave harm will result from non-intervention;
- 'emergency' – to prevent serious harm to patient/others/property;
- Mental Health Act Part IV for detained patient.

Mental Health Act

- Section 5.57 – 'severe' treatments: competent consent *plus* MHAC medical opinion.
- Section 5.58 – 'moderate' treatments: competent consent *or* MHAC medical opinion.
- Section 5.63 – 'mild' treatments: *neither* competent consent *nor* MHAC medical opinion.

Information

There are two *possible* standards. First, a 'patient based' standard; that is, a doctor must give that level of information necessary to allow the patient to *operate* his or her autonomy. Second, a 'profession based' standard; that is, a doctor must give that level of information which is normally given by the profession *in that medical situation*, based on his or her 'duty of care'. In English law the standard is the 'profession based' standard (Bolam *v.* Frearn Hospital), with the courts reserving the right to say that professional standards in a particular context are insufficient (Sidaway *v.* Bethlem Royal and Maudsley Hospitals). Hence, if very little, or no information is given then this would amount to a battery (see earlier); if more than that was given, but not to the required standard, then there would be negligence.

Understanding

It is unclear whether English law expects that the competent patient has listened to and understood the proper information so as to understand; however, ethics and legal common sense clearly require the doctor to ensure that the patient *does* understand. Indeed 'understanding' is the only available empirical measure of 'competence'.

Voluntariness

There is a distinction between 'overt coercion' and 'covert coercion', also between 'covert coercion' and 'reality coercion' (that is, the patient unwillingly accepts the reality of his or her situation). 'Persuasion' sits between covert coercion and reality coercion. There are often fine dividing lines in this area.

Decision

There is a distinction between a decision *per se* and *evidence* as to a decision. Hence, a consent form is no more than 'evidence'; there may be other evidence (for example, from a nurse who says that the patient coincidentally declined his or her consent verbally) which conflicts with the consent form. Also, there can be either/both 'temporal' inconsistency and 'inconsistency of modality' (of behaviour) of the patient.

Exceptions to the requirement of consent

1 *Implied consent* (by the fact and nature of consultation): this cannot be used beyond what is reasonable and is, indeed, a limited legal doctrine.

2 *Implied consent* (patient's consent 'unavailable' where the 'reasonable man' would consent): this applies, for example, to the unconscious patient.

3 *Necessity*: where there is patient incompetence and, without intervention, grave harm or death would likely occur the clinician may intervene; there is a distinction between 'necessity' and mere 'convenience' (to treat).

4 *Emergency*: in order to prevent immediate serious harm to a patient or to others, or to prevent a crime, the patient may be treated in an emergency (irrespective of detention under the Mental Health Act). There is a distinction between 'emergency treatment' under common law and 'urgent treatment' under Section 62 of the Mental Health Act 1983 (which latter applies only to detained patients).

5 *Post-suicide attempt*: because attempted suicide used to be a crime (no longer) the clinician can legally reverse the effects of a suicide attempt but cannot stop a suicidal patient walking out of casualty unless he or she is detained *for mental disorder* under the Mental Health Act.

6 *Detained under the Mental Health Act 1983*: this requires satisfaction of the criteria in the Act (that is, some form of 'mental disorder' plus at least one of the 'consequences' criteria of non-detention, see further below). It only allows treatment for mental disorder (not physical disorder). Treatment is allowed only in terms of the constraints applied by Part IV of the Act (see further below). The Mental Health Act adds 'powers to doctors' and 'safeguards for patients' which override common law provisions. The Code of Practice advises in more detail about consent to treatment.

It is important to note that there is no *legal* (by comparison with ethical) basis for 'proxy consent' of an incompetent adult patient (albeit that there is in relation to children). However, it is possible for a court to rule that non-consensual treatment of a particular patient would not be unlawful, because it is 'medically indicated' and 'in the patient's best interest'. This, of course, generally applies to treatment for physical conditions.

There is for the clinician a constant potential conflict between (1) his or her *duty of care* to the patient (relating legally to negligence); and (2) the requirement of *consent* from the patient (relating legally to battery or to negligence).

Consent to treatment under the Mental Health Act 1983

Except in relation to psychosurgery and hormone implants, Part IV of the Act applies only to patients who are detained (not merely detainable). Such patients are then governed, in relation to consent to treatment, by particular legal provisions which go beyond, and 'trump', common law provisions. Hence, the requirement of consent to treatment is not played out in the same way for a detained patient as it is for an informal patient.

Part IV essentially divides treatment into three types according to the degree of 'clinical intervention'. Hence, there are 'mild' treatments, 'moderate' treatments and 'severe' treatments on the criterion of invasiveness and physical risk. Each is treated separately by the Act. Under Section 57 'severe' treatments (in the author's terminology) require 'competent consent' *and* a 'second opinion' from a Mental Health Act Commission (MHAC) appointed doctor. These treatments include psychosurgery and hormone implants. By contrast, under Section 58, treatments which are 'moderately' invasive require *either* 'competent consent' *or* a 'second opinion'. These treatments include ECT and drug treatments beyond the first 3 months whilst detained. If a patient is either refusing treatment competently *or* is incompetent to consent or refuse, then an MHAC doctor must assess the case. The latter does not certify treatment acceptability on the basis that it is what he or she would do but, rather, on the basis that it is within a range of accepted clinical practice. Treatments that are 'mildly' invasive (or not even invasive at all) are governed by Section 63, which requires *neither* 'competent consent' *nor* a 'second opinion'. This covers any treatments not specified under regulations as relating to the other Sections. Where a 'severe' or 'moderate' treatment may need to be given urgently without obtaining competent consent or a second opinion the Act allows, under Section 62, 'urgent treatment' to be given. There is a sliding scale of 'consequences of not treating' against 'degree of invasiveness' of the treatment which, taken together, validate or fail to validate any particular urgent treatment. Most commonly this Section is used to give the first ECT treatment in a severely depressed patient whose physical well being is at risk and where an MHAC doctor cannot attend quickly.

Civil capacities

Civil capacity in English law is 'action specific'. Hence, a person may be mentally capable of legal process A but not of legal process B. The law defines its own criteria for capacity in relation to a particular process and the psychiatrist is then required to determine whether the patient's mental state results in *in*capacity in relation to those specific criteria. Capacity to consent to treatment (as above) is one example of a specific civil capacity. Others include the following.

Sexual and family relationships

Article 8 of the European Convention on Human Rights secures the right of all to respect for private and family life. The United Nations' Declaration of Rights of Mentally Retarded Persons (1971) recognizes the right of (for example) mentally handicapped persons to live in their own family but says nothing regarding the right to develop sexual and family relationships for themselves. In general terms, there is a delicate balance to be struck between the need for patient protection and the right of a patient to normal sexual and family relationships.

Sexual relationships

There is a distinction between 'the capacity to consent to sexual intercourse' and 'protection of the mentally disordered'. Patients are protected by ordinary criminal law (that is, the Sexual Offences Act) in addition to particular protections arising from the fact of their mental disorder. The capacity to consent to sexual intercourse is judged at a relatively low threshold, on the basis that the activity is well known and easily understood!

Marriage

The legal capacity to marry is not equivalent to the legal capacity to have (extra-marital) sexual intercourse. The law attempts (1) to take a relaxed view of qualification for matrimony whilst (2) preserving the idea that it must be a voluntary consensual union.

There are two grounds for annulment: (1) lack of valid (competent) consent; and (2) sufferance from mental disorder within the meaning of the Mental Health Act 1983 such that the person is 'unfitted for marriage', even though competent to consent to marry. Both grounds result in a marriage being 'voidable' (not automatically 'void'); the marriage exists until successfully challenged in the courts by one of the parties.

Before marriage any person (including a doctor) may enter a 'caveat' with a superintendent registrar which he or she must investigate; the registrar will rarely refuse to marry the person on the basis of (2) 'unfitness for marriage', but more commonly refuse on the basis of (1) 'incapacity to consent to marriage'.

The capacity to consent to divorce is similar to the capacity to consent to marriage.

Property

Testamentary capacity

This is based upon the test of a person being capable of 'making a will with understanding of the *nature* of the business in which he is engaged, a recollection of the *property* he means to dispose of, of the *persons* who are the objects of his bounty and the manner in which it is to be *distributed* between them' (Banks *v.* Goodfellow 1870). Testamentary capacity is *not* identical with incompetence to manage one's affairs more generally.

General management of affairs (Court of Protection)

The grounds (under Section 94(2) Mental Health Act 1983) are the presence of one of the four categories of mental disorder in Section 1 of the Act as well as a medical certificate (one only) that the person is 'incapable, by reason of mental disorder, of managing and administering his property and affairs'. The doctor need not have any special psychiatric expertise.

Contracts

Competence to form a contract involves the ability to understand the nature of the contract involved. Contracts for 'necessities' of life (for example, food) do not require competence.

Compulsory detention in hospital

Categories of mental disorder

Under Section 1 of the Mental Health Act 1983 a patient may be defined as suffering from one of the following.

1 *Mental illness*: this is not defined in the Act.

2 *Severe mental impairment*: this is defined as a 'state of arrested or incomplete development of mind, including severe impairment of intelligence and social functioning and is associated with abnormally aggressive or seriously irresponsible conduct on the part of the person concerned'.

3 *Mental impairment*: this is defined as for severe mental impairment but the word 'severe' is replaced by 'significant' in the definition.

4 *Psychopathic disorder*: this is defined as 'a persistent disorder or disability of mind (whether or not including significant impairment of intelligence) which results in abnormally aggressive or seriously irresponsible conduct on the part of the person concerned'.

5 *Mental disorder*: this amounts to an umbrella term which covers categories 1–4 as well as including the 'catch all' phrase 'any other disorder or disability of mind' (it is applicable only to 72 hour and 28 day assessment sections).

Section 1 of the Act specifically excludes promiscuity or other immoral conduct, sexual deviancy and dependence on alcohol or drugs as the sole evidence of mental disorder for the purpose of the Act (albeit that it may be present in conjunction with a legally valid disorder).

Types of admission

Admission (see Fig. 25.2) is based upon the presence of one of the defined disorders in conjunction with a definition of certain consequences that will arise if the patient is not compulsorily admitted. Sections are defined according to the purpose and length of admission and, by and large, the 'civil rights' protection afforded to the patient is greater the longer the period that the Section can potentially run. The following is a summary of the main Sections (not including Sections arising out of the criminal courts or precipitated by the Home Secretary).

Admission for assessment: Section 2

This Section lasts for up to 28 days and can be made on the basis of 'mental disorder' alone (that is, including 'any other disorder or disability of mind'). The application must be made by the nearest relative or an approved social worker (ASW) and must be supported by two medical recommendations, including one from a doctor approved under Section 12(2) of the Act (that is, someone having special experience in the treatment of mental disorders, often coincidental nowadays with Membership of the Royal College of Psychiatrists). The recommendations must state that the patient suffers from mental disorder of a nature or degree which warrants his or her detention in hospital for assessment, and that such detention will be in the interests of the patient's own health or safety or for the protection of others. An appeal to a Mental Health Review Tribunal within 14 days of admission is available.

Admission for treatment: Section 3

This requires definition of one of the four major categories of mental disorder (not therefore 'mental disorder' as an umbrella term). Treatment may be for up to 6 months (although it can be extended). In the case of 'psychopathic disorder' or 'mental impairment' (not the other two categories) the proposed treatment must be 'likely to alleviate or prevent deterioration of his/her condition'. Otherwise the application and grounds are similar to Section 2.

Admission for assessment in cases of emergency: Section 4

Admission for assessment for up to 72 hours may be made by the nearest relative or an ASW and supported by one doctor, who will not necessarily be Section 12(2) approved but who will preferably (not necessarily) know the patient, commonly the general practitioner. The application must state that admission under Section 2 (ethically a better basis on which to admit) would involve unacceptable delay. Otherwise the criteria are as for Section 2. A second medical recommendation (from a Section 12(2) approved doctor if the first is not so) received by the hospital managers within 72 hours will allow further detention under Section 2.

Detention of patients already admitted to hospital: Section 5

Section 5(2) allows for the detention of a patient already receiving in-patient treatment by the doctor in charge of the case (or his nominated deputy). The criteria are similar to Section 2.

Under Section 5(4) there is a 'nurses holding power' which allows detention by nursing staff of an existing patient for up to 6 hours from the time the decision is recorded. A doctor must attend as rapidly as possible.

Application for guardianship: Section 7

An application can be made by the nearest relative or ASW, again supported by two medical recommendations (one approved). The reports must define one of the four categories of mental disorder and the necessity, in the interests of the welfare of the patient, for him or her to be received into guardianship of an individual or local social services authority for up to 6 months, which can be renewed.

The powers of guardians (Section 8) include requiring the patient to reside in a specified place, to attend specified places for treatment, work or training, and to be available to be assessed at his or her residence or elsewhere. The order is a somewhat weak one and has not been extensively used. It does not give a basis for compulsory treatment of physical conditions of the patient who is incapable of consenting thereto (see also above). Neither does it amount to a psychiatric 'community treatment order' or 'community supervision order'.

Persons in public places

Under Section 136 a person in a public place may be removed to a place of safety, such as a psychiatric hospital or a police cell, for up to 72 hours for further assessment. The person should appear to be in immediate need of care and control in the person's own interest or for the protection of others.

Fig. 25.2 Compulsory Admission (Civil) Provisions of Mental Health Act (1983)

Section number	Title	Duration	Authorization	Conditions
2	Assessment	28 days	One application[1] Two medical recommendations[2]	Patient is suffering from Mental Disorder (Section 1, MHA 1983) warranting detention in hospital for assessment Patient requires detention for own health or safety or for the protection of others
3	Treatment	6 months	One application Two medical recommendations	Patient must be suffering from Mental Disorder (Section 1, MHA 1983) which requires medical treatment in hospital Patient suffering from Psychopathic Disorder or Mental Impairment – treatment must be likely to alleviate or prevent deterioration Patient requires detention for own health or safety or for the protection of others
4	Assessment in emergency	72 hours	One application One medical recommendation	As for Section 2, MHA, 1983
5	Detention of patients already in hospital	72 hours	One medical recommendation	Doctor in charge of treatment reports that an application for admission under Sections 2 or 3 (MHA 1983) ought to be made
		6 hours	One application	Patient suffering from Mental Disorder requiring immediate restraint from leaving hospital for own health or safety or the protection of others Not possible to secure the immediate attendance of above-mentioned doctor

Notes
[1] One application – either by nearest relative, or approved social worker (Section 13) who must have seen the patient in previous 14 days (Section 11).
[2] Two medical recommendations. At least one doctor should be approved (Section 12.2).

Admissions from courts and prisons

Remand from court

A mentally disordered defendant (see Fig. 25.3) may be remanded to hospital for *assessment* (Section 35 in Magistrates' or Crown Court) or for *treatment* (Section 36, in a Crown Court only). A remand on bail with a condition of hospital residence can also be made. There is evidence that these provisions are little used, largely as a result of lack of inpatient resources of the right type (sometimes secure) and as a result of inadequate numbers of court diversion or liaison schemes offered by the NHS to courts (although such schemes are increasing in number).

During remand in prison

Under Section 48 the Home Secretary can transfer a patient from prison to hospital if there is a need for 'urgent treatment'. This operates entirely separately from the powers of courts to make remand orders.

Unfitness to plead and insanity

A patient may be sent to hospital where found 'unfit to plead' under the Criminal Procedure (Insanity) Act 1964, as amended by the Criminal Procedure (Insanity and Unfitness to Plead) Act 1991. This requires two medical recommendations so as to make a Section 37 order (see below). A defendant must also have been found, on a 'trial of the facts', to have done the act with which he was charged (but not convicted, since there is not a full trial so as to include the 'mental element' of the crime). A finding of 'insanity' (the McNaughton rules) gives rise to similar potential consequences of hospital admission. Insanity is a legal concept defined as 'a defect of reason resulting from a disease of the mind such that the defendant did not know the nature or quality of his/her act *or* that (s)he did not know it was (legally) wrong'. In relation to both 'unfitness to plead' and 'insanity' there is an automatic direction to hospital if the charge was murder.

Hospital orders

The commonest order made by the courts (see Fig. 25.4) is that of a Section 37 Hospital Order. This requires two medical recommendations similar to those for Section 3 (a civil treatment order) but there is no requirement of a social worker or relative's application since the court makes the application for itself (so to speak). The duration of the order is also similar to Section 3. A Crown Court may add a Restriction Order (Section 41) 'to protect the public from serious harm'. Oral evidence from a psychiatrist must be given in court. The effect of the order is to give the Home Secretary substantial powers over the patient's place of treatment and leave. However, a Mental Health Review Tribunal can, and sometimes in law must, discharge even against the advice of the Home Secretary.

After conviction but before sentence, a court can make an Interim Hospital Order (Section 38) which allows for periods of up to 6 months in hospital, during which assessment of the patient's treatability can be made. In the author's view, this should nearly always be applied where consideration is being given to a full hospital order for a patient suffering from 'psychopathic disorder', and sometimes in relation to patients with other types of mental disorder.

Sentenced prisoners

If a sentenced prisoner becomes mentally disordered during his sentence then he may be transferred under Sections 47 and 49 of the Mental Health Act if the Home Secretary agrees. If the patient was serving a determinate prison sentence then the Section 49 (giving the Home Office powers equivalent to Section 41) 'falls off' at the 'earliest date of release' (from the prison sentence). The patient is then detained as if under an ordinary Section 3.

Mental Health Act Commission

The operation of the Act is monitored by the MHAC, which is responsible directly to the Secretary of State for Health.

Fig. 25.3 Compulsory Admission of Unsentenced Defendants, Mental Health Act (1983)

Section number	Title	Duration	Authorization	Conditions
35	Remand to hospital: for report on mental condition	Initially 28 days renewable to 3 months	One medical recommendation written or verbal	Removal to hospital within 7 days No categories of mental disorder excluded
36	Remand to hospital: for treatment	Initially 28 days renewable to 3 months	Crown Court Only Two medical recommendations written or verbal	Removal to hospital within 7 days Categories of mental disorder excluded are: mental impairment and psychopathic disorder
38	Interim Hospital Order	Initially up to 12 weeks renewable to 6 months	Two medical recommendations written or verbal Crown/Magistrates' Court	Removal to hospital within 28 days No categories of mental disorder excluded
48	Removal to hospital of unsentenced prisoners	Unspecified	Two medical recommendations (both approved) written	Removal to hospital within 14 days Categories of mental disorder excluded are: mental impairment and psychopathic disorder

Fig. 25.4 Compulsory Admission (Criminal) Provisions of Menial Health Act (1983)

Section number	Title	Duration	Authorization	Conditions
37	Hospital Order	6 months (renewable)	Two medical recommendations (one approved), written or verbal Crown/Magistrates' Court	Offender suffers from mental disorder requiring him to be detained for medical treatment: must be admitted in 28 days, and hospital order must be most suitable method of treatment
37(41)	Hospital Order with restrictions ('Restriction Order')	Any specified period, or without limit of time (Section 41,3(a))	(Crown Court only) Oral evidence from at least one medical practitioner (Section 41,2)	Evidence must show that a Restriction Order is necessary 'for the protection of the public from serious harm', having regard to (a) the offence, (b) offender's antecedents, and (c) the risk of further offences (prognosis). No leave of absence, transfer or discharge without Home Secretary's consent
46	Detention during Her Majesty's Pleasure	Without limit of time	Her Majesty's Forces Acts of Parliament	Like a restriction order, but only applies to members of forces
47	Removal to hospital of sentenced prisoners	6 months	Reports from two doctors (of whom one approved)	Prisoner suffers from mental disorder requiring him to be detained for medical treatment (which in the case of psychopathic disorder/mental impairment will lead to alleviation or prevents deterioration). Transfer within 14 days
49	Restriction on discharge of prisoners		At Home Secretary's discretion	Similar to Section 41, but ceases at what would have been earliest date of release (now becoming notional Section 37)

Case 1:

A man recently discharged from detention under Section 3 of the Mental Health Act 1983 (MHA) for 'mental illness' stops taking his medication and is then arrested for murder. The Magistrates' Court places him on remand in custody. He is found in prison to be mentally ill and, on a subsequent remand to the Magistrates' Court, is made the subject of a Section 35 Assessment Order under the MHA. He goes to a regional secure unit where he is thought to be well and he therefore returns to prison, via the court. After his case has been committed to the Crown Court he is (now) obviously mentally ill and is transferred by the Home Secretary under Section 48 for urgent treatment to a special hospital. At his trial he is found fit to plead (under the Criminal Procedure (Insanity and Unfitness to Plead) Act 1991) and then successfully pleads 'manslaughter on the grounds of diminished responsibility' under Section 2 of the Homicide Act 1957. However, by the time of sentence he has been effectively treated and is entirely well again, so that he cannot be disposed of under the MHA. He therefore receives a determinate prison sentence. During his sentence he again becomes ill and is therefore transferred to a special hospital by the Home Office under Sections 47 and 49 of the MHA. At his 'earliest date of release' (EDR) the Section 49 'falls off' so that the Home Office loses its power over the case and he becomes notionally detained as if under Section 3. Six months later he is discharged by his regional medical officer to the community.

If, alternatively, he had still been mentally ill at the time of sentencing he could have been made the subject of a Section 37 Hospital Order with a Restriction Order under Section 41 added (after a psychiatrist has given evidence to the court). Subsequently he could have been 'conditionally discharged' by a Mental Health Tribunal (for example, on condition he take medication and see his RMO); eventually he could have been absolutely discharged.

The Commission includes members of all clinical disciplines, as well as lawyers and lay persons. It is responsible for recommending to the Secretary of State for Health publication of the *Code of Practice*, which applies to the Act and to practice more broadly. The *Code* does not have the force of law but is similar to the *Highway Code* in terms of its authority. The Commission is crucially important in scrutinizing the operation of hospitals who take patients under the Act. It gives access to a complaints procedure for patients whose civil rights have been withdrawn and investigates pro-actively the operation of the Act within hospitals. Clinicians should be closely acquainted with the *Code of Practice*.

Court reports and evidence

A clinician may be called to court either as an *expert* (to give an opinion) or as a *professional witness* (to give evidence of professional fact, for example, a casualty officer in relation to injuries seen in a victim). An expert may be requested to provide a report by the *court* (in which case the opinion is available to both sides) or approached by the *Crown Prosecution Service* or by the *defence*. The opinion expressed should be unbiased by the source of the request. However, the adversarial process in court tends, once the clinician *has* an opinion, to polarize differences of view between experts. This tendency emphasizes the importance of a report being overtly balanced and also explicit in considering evidence which points in both directions, albeit on balance in one particular direction. Opinions can be applied to criminal and civil courts, as well as to quasi-judicial bodies such as Mental Health Review Tribunals.

Ethics

Where a report is provided on someone who is not an existing patient it is important to emphasize that the person is not a 'patient' and that the context is very different from an ordinary doctor–patient relationship. Hence, confidentiality does not apply (since the report will be available at least to lawyers for one side, and perhaps to the other side as well, and since there is no 'privilege' for a doctor in court as regards anything that he or she has been told by a defendant). It is therefore imperative to warn a criminal defendant that *anything* he tells the doctor *may* come out in court (even if it is not included in the report). Some psychiatrists consciously restrict, or even omit discussion of the alleged offence for this reason (see also below).

Legal issues

It is similarly crucially important to distinguish between legal and psychiatric issues. Hence, a psychiatric report represents psychiatric information for an entirely non-psychiatric (that is, legal) purpose offered. This aspect also determines that the report should be structured not as a 'case formulation' but so as clearly to point towards the relevant legal issues (either disposal or verdict issues). It is important to gain clear legal instructions from the source of referral and not to accept a referral of the type 'query psychiatric problem'. For example, there may be a *verdict* issue such

as 'insanity', 'diminished responsibility' (in homicide cases only), 'automatism', 'infanticide', 'incapacity to form specific intent' or a *disposal* issue relating to an order under the Mental Health Act, a Probation Order with a condition of treatment or relating to psychological factors in mitigation. The vast majority of court reports address only disposal, a very small minority (even of Crown Court cases) address verdict issues.

Information sources

The importance of 'objective' informants is as great in forensic as it is in general psychiatric practice ('informants' often include witness statements). It is also important to see the 'inmate medical records' in any prison hospital where a defendant may be held. Psychometry may be helpful, including nowadays the possibility of 'suggestibility' and 'compliance' assessment (often occurring in conjunction with mild learning disability) where a previous confession is rebutted.

The assessment

A good report should ensure that instructions are adequate, should be based upon reading all the relevant social and evidential papers, as well as previous psychiatric records, and should be based upon in-depth interviewing of the defendant (or party to civil litigation). It is advisable not to address the legally relevant areas until towards the end of the assessment since to do otherwise may distort the process of psychiatric assessment *per se*. Some psychiatrists believe that there should be little or no discussion of the alleged offence at all (in a criminal case) on the basis that legally relevant information which the defendant would otherwise not have wished to be available may thereby be put into court. This emphasizes the importance of explaining the context to the defendant *before* the interview proper begins (see also above).

The report

The written report should be clear, avoid over-inclusiveness, pursue legal relevance as its aim, minimize the use of (or at least define and explain) technical terms, be written in awareness of the possibility of having to defend the exact form of words in cross-examination in court, be written with conscious reference of the psychiatric boundary (for example, not 'recommending' a prison sentence) and avoid value-laden statements. It should use a system of headings which makes clear the distinction between information sources, opinion and recommendations. In the opinion section it is important to separate out psychiatric diagnosis from legal implications. It is also vital to give reasons for the opinions expressed (rather like the mathematics paper which instructs 'show your workings').

Oral evidence

In giving oral evidence many of the same elements of advice apply. There must be recognition that the context is a legal one and that the rules are legal also. It is important to *prepare* evidence and also to be aware of the arguments against the conclusion to which you have come.

Fig. 25.5 Court reports and evidence

Report

Identification	• Report on whom?
Introduction	• Source of request for report. • Information sources (interviews, depositions, other informants, previous medical records).
Information	• Interviews with defendant (or litigant). • Mental state examination. • Interviews with informants. • Extracts from depositions/previous medical records.
Opinion	• Psychiatric diagnosis. • Legal implications (e.g. relating to specific psychiatric defences).
Recommendations	• Regarding disposal.
'Rules'	• Explain any technical terms. • Include only information to aid understanding. • Keep to medical boundaries (avoid view on guilt/innocence *or* on sentence, except medical disposal). • Make only 'supported' recommendations (e.g. hospital order only if you have arranged a bed). • Be cautious about risk assessment (e.g. on Section 41 issue). • Use accepted (ICD-10, DSM-IV) diagnostic categories.

Evidence
• Speak carefully.
• 'See' where questions are leading.
• 'Educate' the jury, clear simple explanations.

Summary

This brief introduction to legal and ethical psychiatry can offer only some basic information. Hopefully, it will stimulate the reader to pursue individual topics further. If there is one message to take away from the topic it is 'be vigilant about the boundary between things medical and things legal or ethical'. Legally improper or unethical acts by clinicians often have their origin in a lack of vigilance about that boundary.

REFERENCE

Meisel A., Roth L.H. & Lidz C.W. (1977) Toward a model of the legal doctrine of informed consent. *Am. J. Psychiatr.* **134**, 285–9.

FURTHER READING

Bluglass R. (1983) *Guide to the Mental Health Act 1983*. 1st Edition. Churchill Livingstone, Edinburgh. [Useful annotated summary guide solely to the Mental Health Act (not other legislation).]

Carson D., Eastman N., Gudjonsson G. & Gunn J. (1993) Psychiatric reports to courts. In: Gunn J. & Taylor P. *Textbook of Forensic Psychiatry: Clinical, Legal and Ethical Issues.* Chapter 21, pp. 826–56. Butterworth-Heinemann Ltd., Oxford. [A comprehensive description of the interface between criminal law and psychiatry, with detailed description of 'how to do it' in relation to psychiatric reports to courts and expert evidence.]

Eastman N. (1990) Consent to psychiatric treatment. In: Bradley J.J., Harten-Ash V.J. & Page M.L. (eds) *Psychiatry and the Law.* Duphar Laboratories Ltd., Dorset Press, Dorchester. [An expanded version of the description in this chapter of the law and ethics of consent to treatment.]

Eastman N. & Hope A. (1988) The ethics of enforced medical treatment: the balance model. *J. Appl. Philos.* **5**(1). [A critique of the English law of consent to medical treatment with a suggested ethical model which more properly reflects how clinicians probably think ethically.]

Grounds A. (1985) The psychiatrist in court. *Br. J. Hosp. Med.* **July**, 855–8. [An excellent practical overview of the legal, psychiatric and ethical problems of court reports and evidence.]

Hoggett B.H. (1990) *Mental Health Law.* 3rd Edition. Sweet & Maxwell, London. [The definitive work on mental health law in the UK.]

Jones R. (1991) *Mental Health Act Manual.* 3rd Edition. Sweet & Maxwell, London. [The standard comprehensive manual, for the *aficionado.*]

Mental Health Act Commission: Code of Practice (1993) HMSO, London. [Essential reading.]

Roth L.H., Meisel A. & Lidz C.W. (1977) Tests of Competency to Consent to Treatment. *American Journal of Psychiatry*, **134**:279–84.

Skegg P.D.G. (1984) *Ethics and Medicine.* Clarendon Press, Oxford. [Includes very detailed chapters on the law of 'capacity to consent to treatment'.]

Index

clozapine 213, 215
cocaine 125–6
codeine abuse 123
cognitive–behavioural therapy 230
cognitive function
    in acute and chronic organic
        states 134–5
    disturbances 10, 131–4
cognitive theory 26–7, 227
cognitive therapy 230–1
    history 228
cohort study 21
communication in terminal illness 271
community care 201, 206
    in schizophrenia 67–9
community learning disability team 175
competence 47–8, 314
compliance 202–3
compulsory detention in hospital 316–17
concentration, testing 133
concrete thinking 135
conditioned stimulus 26
conduct disorder 186, 188, 189, 194
    and learning disability 177–8
consciousness, clouding of 10, 134
consent to treatment 314–15
    in childhood 194–5
contracts, competence to form 316
conversion disorders 144, 150
coping 202, 257
counselling 232–3
    in general practice 150
        genetic 61
couple therapy in post-traumatic stress
        reactions 265
Court of Protection 156, 316
court reports 319–20
courts 313
    admissions from 318
crack 126
criminal behaviour, genetic basis 112
criminal law 313
crisis 257
crisis curve 257
crisis therapy 233–4
critical incidents 257
cross-dressing 295

dangerousness
    assessment 301–4
    management 304–5
déjà vu 10
deliberate self-harm 245
delirium 10
delirium tremens 121
delusional disorders 12
delusional perception 10, 59
delusions 9–10
    in organic states 135
dementia 10, 11–12, 132
    causes 159
    definition 158
    diagnosis 158
    management 158–61
    secondary 12
depersonalization 10
depersonalization syndrome 95
depression 8–9

agitated 79
and anxiety 89
in childhood 189–90, 194
differential diagnosis 13
in the elderly 161–2, 164–5
endogenous 73
and learning disability 178
major/psychotic 5, 12, 73, 79
minor/neurotic 5, 12, 73, 306
and obsessive–compulsive disorders 93
reactive 73
retarded 79
and suicide 246
see also affective disorders
depressive neurosis 73, 76–8, 79–80
derealization 10
developmental language disorder 191
developmental syndromes 191–2, 194
diabetes mellitus and sexual
        dysfunction 291
diagnosis 5–7, 31
    skills involved 40–2
    and symptoms 14–16
diagnostic assessment/formulation 6–7
diagnostic category 5
Diagnostic Statistical Manual 11
digit span 133
disasters, effects of 261
disease categories 6
    adult 11–14
disintegrative psychoses 191
disorders of vegetative function 14
dissociative states 14
domestic violence 306
double-blind trials 211
Down's syndrome 172
drug abuse 116, 122–7
    and anxiety 89
    and sexual dysfunction 291
    and suicide 246
drug-related disorders 12
DSM 11
dyspareunia 288
dysthymic disorder 73, 76–8, 79–80
dystonia due to antipsychotic drugs 214

eating disorders 14, 98, 100–4
    atypical 105
    in childhood 191
    diagnostic criteria 99
    distribution 99–100
    in general practice/hospital 144
ecstasy 125
ECT 82, 211–13
    in the elderly 162
educational psychologists 204
elderly 154
    demography 155
    illnesses in 158–66
    pharmacotherapy 222
    psychiatric assessment 156–8
    special considerations 155–6
electroconvulsive therapy 82, 211–13
    in the elderly 162
emotional disorders in childhood 188–91,
        194
emotional neglect 192
encopresis 192

enduring power of attorney 156
enuresis 191–2, 230
epidemic hysteria 94
epilepsy
    differential diagnosis 136
    and learning disability 177
    and violence 303
episodic dyscontrol syndrome 303
erectile dysfunction 288
ethics 42, 46–50, 313–14
    and court reports 320
    and learning disability 179–80
    and psychotherapy 239
    and substance abuse 126–7
evidence 319–20
exhibitionism 293–4

factitious disorders 144
family
    high expressed emotion 69
    studies 22–3
    supporting role 203
family therapy 25, 195, 237–8
    history 228
    in personality disorders 111
    in post-traumatic stress reactions 265
fetishism 294–5
fire-setting 188, 306
flight of ideas 9
flooding 229
fluoxetine 217–18
flupenthixol 213, 214
fluphenazine 214
fluvoxamine 217–18
focal psychotherapy 234
food fads 191
food refusal 191
forensic psychiatry 301
formal thought disorder 9, 59
fragile X syndrome 172, 177
free floating anxiety 8
friends, supporting role 203
frontal lobe syndrome 131
frozen watchfulness 192

GABA, effects of anxiolytics on
        transmission 221
galactorrhoea due to antipsychotic
        drugs 215
gamma aminobutyric acid, effects of
        anxiolytics on transmission 221
general hospital
    accident and emergency
        department 148
    in-patient care 147–8
    out-patient clinics 147
    psychiatric disorder in 142–51
general practice see primary care
genetic counselling in schizophrenia 61
glue-sniffing 125
graded exposure treatment 90, 92, 229
grief 279–81
    abnormal 281–2
    assessment 283
    chronic 282
    conditions precipitated or exacerbated
        by 282–3

management 283–4
outcome 284
group psychotherapy 235–6
history 228
in post-traumatic stress reactions 264–5
in sexual deviation 297
gynaecomastia due to antipsychotic
drugs 215

hallucinations 10
in organic states 135
hallucinogen abuse 126
haloperidol 82, 213, 214, 274, 275
heroin abuse 123–4
history taking 6, 32–3, 36–7
HIV infection
and drug abuse 122
mental health aspects 146
home helps 204
homeless families unit 204
homicide 306
homosexuality 297–8
housing departments 204
hyoscine 283
hyperkinetic disorder 192, 193, 194
hypnotics 220–2
hypochondriasis 95, 144
hypomania 9, 12, 73
in childhood 194
in the elderly 162, 163
hysteria 93, 94–5
in childhood 189
hysterical amnesia 132

ICD 11, 186
illusions 10
imipramine 216
impaired sexual arousal 187
incest 262
indecent exposure 294
informal care services 203
information 314
insight 10
intelligence tests 134
International Classification of Diseases 11,
186
interviewing 38, 39–40
involutional melancholia 73
IQ tests 134
isocarboxazid 218

jamais vu 10
jealousy, morbid 69–70

knight's move 9
Korsakoff's syndrome 132

laboratory investigations 37–8
latah 94
late paraphrenia 163
learned helplessness 80
learning disability 168–74
ethical issues 179–80
legal framework 179–80

and physical illness 176–8
provision of services for 174–9
and psychiatric disorders 178–9
learning theory 26, 227
legal issues 312–21
Lesch–Nyhan syndrome 177
leucopenia due to antipsychotic drugs 215
life-events 25
linkage studies 22–3
lithium 82, 219–20
in childhood 195
in elderly patients 162
lofepramine 217, 218
low sexual desire 287, 288
LSD 126

malingering 94
mania 12
in the elderly 162, 163
and learning disability 178
and shoplifting 306
manic depressive disorder 73
in childhood 191
manic episodes, presentation 74–5, 76–8
MAOIs 218–19
marriage, grounds for annulment 316
masochism 294
maternity blues 146
medical social workers 204
melancholia 73
memory
in chronic organic states 134
testing 132–3, 134
Mental Health Act 1959 169
Mental Health Act 1983
admission from courts and prisons
under 318, 319
compulsory detention under 316–17
consent to treatment under 315
and learning disability 170
and personality disorder 111
Mental Health Act Commission 318–19
mental health care services 200
filters between types 205–6
future patterns 206
types 201–4
Mental Health Review Tribunals 313
mental illness as a concept 7
mental retardation see learning disability
mental state examination 6, 34–6, 37,
131
in learning disability 177–8
methadone 123–4
methylphenidate 195
metonyms 9
mianserin 217, 218
MIND 203
mini-mental state examination 160
mixed affective states 9
moclobemide 218, 219
modelling 227
monoamine oxidase inhibitors 218–19
monogenic studies 23
monosymptomatic hypochondriacal
psychosis 70
mood 8–9
in organic states 135
morbid jealousy 69–70

morphine abuse 123
mourning, tasks of 270, 271
Munchausen by proxy syndrome 307–8
Munchausen syndrome 95, 144
mutual aid societies 203

NAI 192, 307–8
narcotic drug abuse 123–4
negative formal thought disorder 9, 59
neighbours, supporting role 203
neologisms 9
neuroleptic malignant syndrome 215
neuroses 12, 14, 86
aetiology 87
assessment 87
definition 87
outcome 89
presentation in general practice/
hospital 143–4
related syndromes 95
syndromes 89–95
treatment 88
undifferentiated 87
non-accidental injury 192, 307–8
nortriptyline 216

obesity 105, 144
obsessive–compulsive disorders 9, 14,
92–3
in childhood 191, 194
and shoplifting 306
occupational therapists, assessment by 38
operant conditioning 26, 175, 229
opioid abuse 123–4
opium abuse 123
organic orderliness 135
organic psychiatric states 11–12, 130–8,
144–6, 307
orgasmic dysfunction 287
orientation testing 132

paedophilia 261, 295
pain 11
panic attacks 8
paranoid state 70
in the elderly 163
parasuicide 245
Parkinsonian syndrome due to
antipsychotic drugs 214
paroxetine 217–18
patient, attitudes towards 42
PCP 126
pemaline 195
perseveration 9, 135
persistent delusional disorders 69–70
personality
and mental illness 27
and neuroses 87
and violence 301–2
vulnerable 109
personality disorder 14, 108
aetiology 110
antisocial/sociopathic 111–13
assessment 110
borderline 303–4
classification 109